D1573139

HANDBOOK OF COGNITION AND EMOTION

HANDBOOK OF
Cognition and Emotion

Edited by

Michael D. Robinson
Edward R. Watkins
Eddie Harmon-Jones

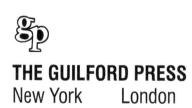

THE GUILFORD PRESS
New York   London

© 2013 The Guilford Press
A Division of Guilford Publications, Inc.
72 Spring Street, New York, NY 10012
www.guilford.com

Printed in the United States of America

This book is printed on acid-free paper.

Last digit is print number: 9 8 7 6 5 4 3 2 1

Library of Congress Cataloging-in-Publication Data

Handbook of cognition and emotion / edited by Michael D. Robinson, Edward R.
Watkins, Eddie Harmon-Jones.
    p. cm.
  Includes bibliographical references and index.
  ISBN 978-1-4625-0999-7 (hardcover)
    1. Emotions and cognition—Handbooks, manuals, etc. 2. Cognition—Handbooks,
manuals, etc. 3. Emotions—Handbooks, manuals, etc. I. Robinson, Michael D.
II. Watkins, Edward R. III. Harmon-Jones, Eddie.
  BF311.H3336 2013
  152.4—dc23

                                                 2012043610

About the Editors

Michael D. Robinson, PhD, is Professor of Psychology at North Dakota State University. He is associate editor of *Emotion*, the motivation/emotion section of *Social and Personality Psychology Compass*, and the *Journal of Personality and Social Psychology*. Dr. Robinson's research focuses on the areas of personality, cognition, and emotion.

Edward R. Watkins, PhD, is Full Professor of Experimental and Applied Clinical Psychology at the University of Exeter, United Kingdom. He is a recipient of the British Psychological Society's May Davidson Award for significant early-career contributions to clinical psychology. Dr. Watkins is a consulting editor for *Journal of Abnormal Psychology*, *Behaviour Research and Therapy*, and *Cognition and Emotion*.

Eddie Harmon-Jones, PhD, is Professor of Psychology at the University of New South Wales, Australia. A recipient of the Award for Distinguished Early Career Contributions to Psychophysiology from the Society for Psychophysiological Research, he is associate editor of *Emotion*. Dr. Harmon-Jones's research focuses on emotions and motivations, their implications for cognitive and social processes and behaviors, and their underlying neural circuits.

Contributors

Lyn Y. Abramson, PhD, Department of Psychology, University of Wisconsin–Madison, Madison, Wisconsin

Lauren B. Alloy, PhD, Department of Psychology, Temple University, Philadelphia, Pennsylvania

Adam A Augustine, PhD, Department of Clinical and Social Sciences in Psychology, University of Rochester, Rochester, New York

Frank Baeyens, PhD, Department of Psychology, University of Leuven, Leuven, Belgium

Stephanie Bagby-Stone, MD, Department of Psychiatry, School of Medicine, University of Missouri, Columbia, Missouri

Kirsten Barnicot, PhD, Unit for Social and Community Psychiatry, Department of Psychiatry, Wolfson Institute for Preventive Medicine, Queen Mary University of London, London, United Kingdom

Arielle R. Baskin-Sommers, MS, Department of Psychology, University of Wisconsin–Madison, Madison, Wisconsin

Elise Bausseron, MS, UQ Business School, University of Queensland, St. Lucia, Queensland, Australia

Christopher G. Beevers, PhD, Department of Psychology, University of Texas at Austin, Austin, Texas

Michelle Bertoli, MA, Department of Psychology, Yale University, New Haven, Connecticut

Shimrit K. Black, MA, Department of Psychology, Temple University, Philadelphia, Pennsylvania

Ryan Bogdan, PhD, Department of Psychology, Washington University in St. Louis, St. Louis, Missouri

Elaine M. Boland, MA, Department of Psychology, Temple University, Philadelphia, Pennsylvania

Marc A. Brackett, PhD, Department of Psychology, Yale University, New Haven, Connecticut

Ryan W. Carpenter, BA, Department of Psychology, University of Missouri, Columbia, Missouri

Charles S. Carver, PhD, Department of Psychology, University of Miami,
Coral Gables, Florida

Ruth Castillo, Faculty of Psychology, University of Malaga, Malaga, Spain

Patrick J. F. Clarke, PhD, School of Psychology, University of Western Australia,
Perth, Australia

Peter C. Clasen, BFA, Department of Psychology, University of Texas at Austin,
Austin, Texas

Seth G. Disner, BA, Department of Psychology, University of Texas at Austin,
Austin, Texas

Anke Ehlers, PhD, Department of Experimental Psychology, University of Oxford,
Oxford, United Kingdom

Thomas Ehring, PhD, Institute of Psychology, University of Münster, Münster, Germany

Nicole Elbertson, BS, Department of Psychology, Yale University,
New Haven, Connecticut

Jamie Ferri, MA, Department of Psychology, Stony Brook University,
Stony Brook, New York

Joseph P. Forgas, DPhil, DSc, School of Psychology, University of New South Wales,
Sydney, Australia

Philip A. Gable, PhD, Department of Psychology, University of Alabama,
Tuscaloosa, Alabama

Allison E. Gaffey, MA, Department of Psychology, University of Notre Dame,
Notre Dame, Indiana

Kim E. Goldstein, MA, Department of Psychology, Temple University,
Philadelphia, Pennsylvania

Dina Gordon, MA, Department of Psychology, Temple University,
Philadelphia, Pennsylvania

William G. Graziano, PhD, Department of Psychological Sciences, Purdue University,
West Lafayette, Indiana

Leslie S. Greenberg, PhD, Department of Psychology, York University, Toronto,
Ontario, Canada

James J. Gross, PhD, Department of Psychology, Stanford University, Stanford, California

Greg Hajcak, PhD, Department of Psychology, Stony Brook University,
Stony Brook, New York

Ahmad R. Hariri, PhD, Department of Psychology and Neuroscience, Duke University,
Durham, North Carolina

Cindy Harmon-Jones, PhD, School of Psychology, University of New South Wales,
Sydney, Australia

Eddie Harmon-Jones, PhD, School of Psychology, University of New South Wales,
Sydney, Australia

Richard G. Heimberg, PhD, Department of Psychology, Temple University,
Philadelphia, Pennsylvania

Dirk Hermans, PhD, Department of Psychology, University of Leuven, Leuven, Belgium

Alisha C. Holland, PhD, Department of Psychology, Boston College, Boston, Massachusetts

Michael Inzlicht, PhD, Department of Psychology, University of Toronto, Toronto, Ontario, Canada

Abigail L. Jenkins, MA, Department of Psychology, Temple University, Philadelphia, Pennsylvania

Liam C. Kavanagh, MA, Department of Psychology, University of California, San Diego, San Diego, California

Elizabeth A. Kensinger, PhD, Department of Psychology, Boston College, Boston, Massachusetts

Birgit Kleim, PhD, Department of Clinical Psychology and Psychotherapy, University of Zurich, Zurich, Switzerland

Alex S. Koch, DplPsych, Department of General Psychology, University of Cologne, Cologne, Germany

Ernst H. W. Koster, PhD, Department of Experimental Clinical and Health Psychology, University of Ghent, Ghent, Belgium

Denise R. LaBelle, MA, Department of Psychology, Temple University, Philadelphia, Pennsylvania

Randy J. Larsen, PhD, Department of Psychology, Washington University in St. Louis, St. Louis, Missouri

Hwaryung Lee, MA, Department of Psychology, Washington University in St. Louis, St. Louis, Missouri

Colin MacLeod, DPhil, School of Psychology, University of Western Australia, Perth, Australia

Ashleigh R. Molz, MA, Department of Psychology, Temple University, Philadelphia, Pennsylvania

Agnes Moors, PhD, Department of Experimental Clinical and Health Psychology, Ghent University, Ghent, Belgium; Swiss Center for Affective Sciences, University of Geneva, Geneva, Switzerland

Amanda S. Morrison, MA, Department of Psychology, Temple University, Philadelphia, Pennsylvania

Brendan D. Murray, MA, Department of Psychology, Boston College, Boston, Massachusetts

Joseph P. Newman, PhD, Department of Psychology, University of Wisconsin–Madison, Madison, Wisconsin

Yuliya S. Nikolova, BA, Department of Psychology and Neuroscience, Duke University, Durham, North Carolina

Olga V. Obraztsova, MA, Department of Psychology, Temple University, Philadelphia, Pennsylvania

Mirtes G. Pereira, PhD, Department of Physiology and Pharmacology, Fluminense Federal University, Niterói, Brazil

Luiz Pessoa, PhD, Department of Psychology, University of Maryland,
College Park, Maryland

Carly K. Peterson, PhD, Minneapolis VA Health Care System, Minneapolis, Minnesota

Tom F. Price, PhD, School of Psychology, University of New South Wales,
Sydney, Australia

Michael D. Robinson, PhD, Department of Psychology, North Dakota State University,
Fargo, North Dakota

Peter Salovey, PhD, Department of Psychology, Yale University, New Haven, Connecticut

Michael F. Scheier, PhD, Department of Psychology, Carnegie Mellon University,
Pittsburgh, Pennsylvania

Klaus R. Scherer, PhD, Swiss Center for Affective Sciences, University of Geneva,
Geneva, Switzerland

Brandon J. Schmeichel, PhD, Department of Psychology, Texas A&M University,
College Station, Texas

Benjamin G. Shapero, MA, Department of Psychology, Temple University,
Philadelphia, Pennsylvania

Gal Sheppes, PhD, Department of Psychology, Tel Aviv University, Tel Aviv, Israel

Paul Slovic, PhD, Decision Research, Eugene, Oregon; Department of Psychology,
University of Oregon, Eugene, Oregon

Gaurav Suri, MA, Department of Psychology, Stanford University, Stanford, California

Ross A. Thompson, PhD, Department of Psychology, University of California, Davis,
Davis, California

Renée M. Tobin, PhD, Department of Psychology, Illinois State University,
Normal, Illinois

Timothy J. Trull, PhD, Department of Psychological Sciences, University of Missouri,
Columbia, Missouri

Daniel Västfjäll, PhD, Decision Research, Eugene, Oregon; Department of Psychology,
Linköping University, Linköping, Sweden

Bram Vervliet, PhD, Department of Psychology, University of Leuven, Leuven, Belgium

Edward R. Watkins, PhD, School of Psychology, University of Exeter,
Exeter, United Kingdom

Anna Weinberg, MA, Department of Psychology, Stony Brook University,
Stony Brook, New York

Abby C. Winer, AB, Department of Human and Community Development,
University of California, Davis, Davis, California

Piotr Winkielman, PhD, Department of Psychology, University of California, San Diego,
La Jolla, California

Michelle M. Wirth, PhD, Department of Psychology, University of Notre Dame,
Notre Dame, Indiana

Jenny Yiend, PhD, Department of Psychosis Studies, Institute of Psychiatry,
King's College London, London, United Kingdom

Contents

PART VI. PROBLEMS, DISORDERS, AND TREATMENT

PART I

OVERVIEW OF THIS VOLUME

CHAPTER 1

Cognition and Emotion

An Introduction

Michael D. Robinson, Edward R. Watkins, and Eddie Harmon-Jones

Our intrapsychic lives are dominated by two sorts of phenomena: thoughts (more formally, cognition) and feelings (more formally, emotion). Both are internal events that cannot be directly observed by others and, in this important sense, are subjective or at least particular to a person (Chalmers, 2007). Both are partially dependent on events in the environment, but partially independent of them as well (Klinger, 1999). Indeed, an important reason that we have thoughts and feelings is presumably to decouple stimulus and response and therefore allow for greater flexibility in behavior (Scherer, 1984). Yet, there appear to be important differences between thoughts and feelings. Thoughts lend themselves to words or propositional content, whereas feelings seem to lack this propositional content (Izard, 2009; Pinker, 2007). Thoughts often seem to follow an orderly chain of reasoning, whereas feelings seem to operate in ways that sometimes do not make logical sense (Epstein, 1994).

In fact, Greek philosophers made a sharp distinction between thoughts and feelings (Lyons, 1999). They suggested that thoughts are the source of rationality and proper conduct, whereas following feelings could often get us into trouble. The idea that thoughts and feelings are distinct sources of influence in fact pervades many of the major literary works of Western civilization. From Plato to St. Augustine to Shakespeare, the head (the presumed locus of rationality) and the heart (the presumed locus of emotionality) suggest different courses of action and often conflict (Swan, 2009). Typically, but perhaps not in all realms (e.g., courtship), it is deemed more functional to follow the head rather than the heart (Solomon, 1976).

In the 1990s, three books by prominent neuroscientists questioned this conventional wisdom. LeDoux (1996) reviewed evidence for the idea that purported emotional areas of the brain (and particularly the amygdala) can react more quickly and perhaps more decisively to physical threats to the organism than can cortical (more thought-based) pathways. Panksepp (1998) contended that cortical lesions in animals—preserving the emotional areas of the brain—often result in behaviors that make more sense from a functional biological perspective. Damasio (1994) extended this analysis to human beings. Primarily on the basis of case studies involving brain-damaged individuals, it was concluded that damage to emotion-processing regions of the brain, even in the context of intact cognitive capacities, results in problematic decision making and impulsive, reckless interpersonal behaviors.

The present volume does not generally focus on the question of whether thoughts (cognition) or feelings (emotion) are more functional. Rather, this introductory material is sufficient to make the case that, typically, thoughts and feelings are seen to be distinct entities with distinct effects (e.g., Epstein, 1994). Yet, it has become increasingly apparent that cognition and emotion often interact and are perhaps not isolated entities. Before outlining the content of this handbook, we consider some important statements in the literature on cognition and emotion and comment on them in light of the present contributions.

Prominent Theoretical Statements on Cognition and Emotion

There are strong, but often conflicting, theoretical statements on cognition and emotion in the psychology literature. These statements have been influential, and all likely contain a grain of truth. However, and in light of the present contributions, all such statements are likely too strong given the evidence. Accordingly, in each case, we favor a more moderate position. Table 1.1 provides a graphic overview of the theoretical statements and our rejoinders.

Do Cognition and Emotion Operate Independently?

An important book by LeDoux (1996) reviewed numerous results from rodent work favoring an independence of cognition and emotion in neural terms. Following but refining earlier suggestions (MacLean, 1973), it was suggested that the amygdala is a key brain structure mediating emotional reactions to potential threats that are not cognitively mediated. Consistent with this point, the amygdala plays an important role in very basic reactions to potential threats such as fight or flight (Fanselow, 1994). On the basis of such data, LeDoux (1996) generally seemed to favor distinct processing routes for cognition and emotion. However, he also reviews evidence for nonindepen-

dence. Indeed, there is considerable cross talk between the brain structures typically considered more cognitive versus more emotional (Ochsner & Gross, 2005). In addition, Pessoa and Pereira (Chapter 4, this volume) review evidence that cognitive resources are often necessary for the amygdala to recognize and respond to threatening stimuli.

Pursuing this theme of independence, there are cases in which cognition and emotion, or at least rationality and emotion, seem to be at cross-purposes. For example, Mischel, Shoda, and Rodriguez (1989) pitted rationality and emotionality against each other in a classic delay of gratification task in which eating a single marshmallow now (which the emotional system would presumably favor) will preclude having two marshmallows later (which the rational system would presumably favor). This simple test has been shown to predict individual differences in self-control in adolescence and adulthood (Mischel & Ayduk, 2011). Some moral dilemmas also appear to effectively pit the rational and emotional systems against each other. For example, people often react adversely to having to kill another person even if doing so is rationally the best solution to the dilemma (McClure, Botvinick, Yeung, Greene, & Cohen, 2007).

Yet, there are also numerous results challenging the idea that cognition and emotion always operate independently (Davidson, 2003; Izard, 2009). For example, there are many constructs—such as stress, worry, depression, and anxiety—that possess both cognitive and emotional features working in concert. Worry, for example, is a hybrid of negative affect and repetitive, future-oriented thinking (Watkins, Chapter 21, this volume). Perhaps more directly, manipulations related to cognitive interpretation, whether involving appraisal (Lazarus, 1991) or reappraisal (Ochsner & Gross, 2005), have a profound effect on emotional reactions to stimuli and situations. Also, there is considerable evidence for the idea that manipulations of emotion impact cognition, memory, and judgment in ways that are systematic and robust (Forgas & Koch, Chapter 13, this volume; Murray, Holland, & Kensinger, Chapter 9, this volume). Such results could not occur if cognition and emotion were entirely independent, encapsulated entities. In answer to the question of whether cognition and emotion operate independently, then, we suggest that the answer is perhaps *sometimes*, but definitely not always.

Is Cognition Necessary for Emotion?

Lazarus (1984) suggested that cognition is necessary for emotion. By this, he meant that we cannot react emotionally to a situation until we interpret its personal significance. For example, we cannot react with sadness to a loss until we interpret it is such. There is certainly evidence that we can predict people's emotional responses to situations by knowing their interpretations of them (Smith & Ellsworth, 1985). On the other hand, consider the potentially important results of Reisenzein and Hofmann (1993). They presented people with scenarios, measured interpretations of them in a comprehensive manner, and also assessed emotional reactions to the scenarios. If interpretations of situations were necessary to understand their impact on emotional reactions, then controlling for interpretations should eliminate the impact of them in predicting emotional reactions. In essence, and consistent with Lazarus's (1991) view, interpretations or appraisals would fully mediate and explain the emotional impact of emotion-relevant situations. This was simply not the case. Situations predicted emotional reactions even after controlling for a host of relevant appraisals. In other words, and consistent with LeDoux's (1996) analysis, there are probably some noncognitive determinants of people's reactions to emotional stimuli (also see Berkowitz & Harmon-Jones, 2004).

Lazarus's (1984) cognitive appraisal view of emotions resulted in a body of research showing that there are systematic relations between self-reported cognitive appraisals and self-reported emotional reactions (e.g., Smith & Ellsworth, 1985). Such results, however, are essentially correlational in nature, and a nearly exclusive reliance on self-reported measures is now deemed limiting (Smith & Kirby, 2001), even by Lazarus (1995) himself. Fortunately, there is a handful of appraisal investigators conducting groundbreaking experimental work in the

area; this work is reviewed by Moors and Scherer (Chapter 8, this volume). Among other points, they suggest that it is an intractable task to show that every emotional reaction is cognitively mediated. The doctrinaire position of Lazarus (1984) has therefore been replaced by one in which there is greater nuance in understanding when, how, and why cognition plays an important role in understanding emotional reactions. Cognition, too, is now defined in broader terms. For example, MacLeod and Clarke (Chapter 29, this volume) review evidence for the idea that manipulations of selective attention, independent of cognitive appraisal, have a causal influence on the extent to which people will experience anxiety when encountering a stressor.

Does Affect Precede Cognition?

Primarily on the basis of results involving the mere exposure effect, Zajonc (1980) suggested that affective responses to a stimulus precede a cognitive interpretation of that stimulus. The *mere exposure effect* is one in which repeated presentations of a stimulus result in greater liking for it (Zajonc, 1998). Studies have shown that mere exposure effects can be obtained when stimuli are presented subliminally (Kunst-Wilson & Zajonc, 1980). There are also studies showing that subliminal presentations of affective stimuli can bias evaluations of subsequent neutral targets (Murphy & Zajonc, 1993) and trigger skin conductance responses (Öhman & Soares, 1998), facial muscle activity (Dimberg, Thunberg, & Elmehed, 2000), and brain activity in the amygdala (Morris, Öhman, & Dolan, 1998).

This line of research surely establishes that subliminal presentations can influence emotional responding, but does it show that the affect precedes cognition? No, it does not. Equating cognition with conscious awareness is problematic because subliminal presentations also alter many cognitive processes, including those related to semantic priming (Kemp-Wheeler & Hill, 1988), response preparation (Eimer & Schlaghecken, 1998), and judgments that are primarily of a cognitive type (Bevan, 1964). In other words, it is not warranted to equate unconscious processes with those that are particularly affective in nature (Merikle, 2007). Doing so is too heavily influenced by a Freudian model that has been shown to be incorrect (Kihlstrom, Mulvaney, Tobias, & Tobis, 2000).

Building on the analysis of Rolls (1999), Storbeck, Robinson, and McCourt (2006) suggested that a certain basic form of cognition—namely, stimulus identification—is necessary for understanding the affective reactions of individuals. Yet, other results in the literature suggest that, in certain cases and in certain paradigms, affect may be available before such stimulus identification processes (e.g., Draine & Greenwald, 1998; Peyk, Schupp, Elbert, & Junghöfer, 2008). Ultimately, then, we suggest that it is wrong to insist on a doctrinaire position in which affect necessarily precedes cognition, though we do allow for the possibility that this is sometimes true (Berridge & Winkielman, 2003; Dixon, 1981; LeDoux, 1996).

Can Cognition and Emotion Be Distinguished?

Following considerable precedent (e.g., Panksepp, 1998), LeDoux (1996) suggested that some subcortical structures (most prominently, the amygdala, but also the insula and basal ganglia) specialize in emotional processing, whereas cortical brain structures (most prominently, the frontal cortex, but also the sensory cortices) specialize in cognitive processing. Questioning this idea, Duncan and Feldman Barrett (2007) suggested that such divisions of labor are not apparent and that the same brain structures appear to perform both cognitive and emotional tasks. For example, the amygdala responds to uncertain events of multiple types (Whalen, 1998), regions of the visual cortex response to emotional arousal (Peyk et al., 2008), and the frontal cortex is also surprisingly responsive to emotional stimuli and tasks (Canli et al., 2001).

What are we to make of these overlapping activations? One response is to suggest that the same brain structures do respond to both cognitive and emotional events, but that different neuron groups are involved. In support of this idea, Bush, Luu, and Posner (2000) found, in their meta-analysis, that different regions of the anterior cingulate cortex respond to cognitive conflicts versus emotional inputs. The frontal cortex is heterogeneous as well, and there are reasons for thinking that different regions of the frontal cortex mediate emotional processing versus cognitive control or response inhibition (Eisenberger, Lieberman, & Satpute, 2005). Single-cell recording studies further support this separability of cognitive and emotional processing, in that particular neurons are tuned to cognitive versus emotional features of stimuli and tasks performed on them, even in cases in which such neurons are found in the same brain structures and indeed close together (Rolls, 1999).

Regardless, the cognitive (e.g., is it a table?) and emotional (e.g., is it positive or negative?) systems have very different tasks to perform—tasks that must necessarily recruit different, but partially overlapping, neural networks (Davidson, 2003; Rolls, 1999). In addition, many empirical results have suggested that these two systems can be dissociated in numerous paradigms—such as those involving priming effects (Storbeck & Robinson, 2004), effects on judgments (Murphy & Zajonc, 1993), lesion studies (Damasio, 1994), and moral decision making (McClure et al., 2007). Accordingly, our position is that cognition and emotion are different phenomena. Although the same regions of the brain (Pessoa & Pereira, Chapter 4, this volume) and the same indices of neural processing (Weinberg, Ferri, & Hajcak, Chapter 3, this volume) can be activated by both cognitive and emotional stimuli, the relevant processes and achievements need to be distinguished (Izard, 2009).

In Summary

Theorists often make strong claims about cognition and emotion. These have ranged from suggestions that cognition and emotion are independent, that cognition is necessary for emotion, that affective reactions to stimuli precede a cognitive analysis, and that cognition and emotion cannot be distinguished (more or less every possibility!). We suggest that each viewpoint has some merit some of the time, but cannot be considered to be true all of the time (see Table 1.1). Cognition and emotion, in our view, can be dis-

TABLE 1.1. Prominent Theoretical Statements on Cognition and Emotion and Rejoinders

Position	Example advocate	Our view
Independence	LeDoux (1996)	Sometimes, but not always
Cognition is necessary	Lazarus (1984)	Sometimes, but not always
Affective primacy	Zajonc (1980)	Sometimes, but not always
Equivalence	Duncan & Feldman Barrett (2007)	Sometimes, but not always

tinguished, but do nonetheless interact with each other in multiple ways (Izard, 2009), the nuances of which deserve a fuller treatment than available.

Audience for the Present Volume

This handbook occurs at an opportune time. The journal *Cognition and Emotion* was launched in 1987, and its impact factor has steadily climbed since then. The American Psychological Association journal *Emotion* was launched in 2001, and its impact factor is admirably high. The journal *Social Cognitive and Affective Neuroscience* was launched in 2006 to provide an outlet for emerging research in social-cognitive neuroscience, with cognition–emotion interactions as a primary focus. The journal *Emotion Review* was established in 2009. The journal *Social and Personality Psychology Compass* was established in 2007, with a motivation–emotion section as one of its core sections. Research on cognition and emotion is flourishing as never before.

No journals have included special issues or sections of the present type. Some edited books have sought to do so, however, and we discuss our handbook in light of these previous volumes. Dalgleish and Power (1999) published a *Handbook of Cognition and Emotion* many years ago. The volume is excellent, but its content is now outdated. Since 1999, many advances have been made in understanding cognition and emotion interactions, and the content of the present volume attests to this fact. Eich, Kihlstrom, Bower, Forgas, and Niedenthal (2000) published a book titled *Cognition and Emotion*, but its contents focused primarily on a particular theory (Bower, 1981) of mood

and cognition. Martin and Clore (2001) published *Theories of Mood and Cognition: A User's Guidebook*, focusing on mood effects on cognition in social psychology, a small portion of the present volume. More recently, De Houwer and Hermans (2010) published *Cognition and Emotion: Reviews of Current Research and Theories*, consisting of a relatively small number of chapters, none of which directly addresses personality processes or distinct forms of psychopathology. Overall, then, the present volume is more comprehensive than the latter three edited books and represents state-of-the-art research relative to an earlier handbook of the same name.

The primary audience for this handbook is graduate students and researchers whose work touches on, or centrally considers, the topic of emotion. Emotion is a hot topic in all areas of psychology, however, and cognitive-processing approaches to it are widespread. Thus, a diverse audience is targeted. The secondary audience for the handbook is students, researchers, clinicians, and professionals whose interests are in emotion and its applied ramifications. More or less, the foci here—for example, appraisals, social considerations, clinical manifestations—may resonate with a wider readership audience than that primarily targeted. The handbook is suited as a primary text for seminars on emotion or cognition and emotion. It is a primary rather than supplementary text, given its comprehensive nature, though chapters or sections may be used as supplementary material for seminars in neuroscience, cognitive psychology, social psychology, judgment and decision making, personality psychology, or clinical psychology.

What is special about the book is that it represents a comprehensive, up-to-date volume addressing relations between cognition and emotion. The editors represent multiple subdisciplines of psychology and so do the chapters. What should be highlighted is therefore the comprehensive, yet focused, nature of the handbook.

Sections, Topics, and Chapters

The typical psychology department consists of distinct subdisciplines—for example, cognitive neuroscience, social psychology, personality psychology, and clinical psychology. Emotion in general and cognition and emotion in particular cross such typical boundaries. There is a healthy body of research on the cognitive neuroscience of emotion (e.g., in relation to how the brain regulates its emotions); emotion figures prominently in many social phenomena (e.g., cognitive dissonance, mood effects); some of the most important personality traits are affective at their core (e.g., extraversion, neuroticism); and many clinical conditions are marked by experiences of negative emotion (e.g., anxiety, depression) or by apparent difficulties in regulating negative emotions (e.g., borderline personality disorder). Even in particular subdisciplines of psychology, the cognition–emotion interface crosses topics that are typically studied independently of each other. In clinical psychology, for example, people tend to specialize in particular disorders such as posttraumatic stress disorder, anxiety disorders, depression, borderline personality disorder, or psychopathy. A key goal of the present volume is to bridge distinct subdisciplines of psychology and distinct topics within particular subdisciplines. Such goals guided the topics selected and the contributors invited.

The volume is divided into six parts. The first is an introduction to the field of inquiry (the present chapter). The second considers cognition and emotion from a biological perspective. The third focuses on key cognitive processes in emotion, such as attention, learning, and memory. The fourth focuses on cognition and emotion in social psychology. The fifth focuses on several individual differences—such as emotional intelligence—that greatly benefit from considering the interplay of cognition and emotion. The sixth section focuses on clinical

phenomena, given the excellent work that has been conducted on cognition and emotion in the clinical literature. Here we briefly state the importance of each chapter topic and its scope.

Chapter 2: Neurogenetics

Dopamine and serotonin are neurotransmitters in the brain long thought to play an important role in emotion and emotional reactivity. Increasingly, neurotransmitter and genetic approaches to personality, emotion, and psychopathology have shown considerable merit. In their chapter, Nikolova, Bogdan, and Hariri focus primarily on four dopamine-related genes and their relevance in understanding human reward processing, though a broader scope of this research approach is also introduced.

Chapter 3: Electrophysiology

The brain used to be viewed as a "black box." Stimuli are presented and responses are made, but why responses are made to certain stimuli was largely a mystery. By recording brain activity recorded over the scalp and linking it to the stimuli presented (event-related potentials [ERPs]), we gain important knowledge concerning what the brain does in stimulus perception and response preparation. In their chapter, Weinberg, Ferri, and Hajcak compare and contrast attention- and emotion-related influences on the late positive potential. Among other conclusions, the authors suggest that this ERP component reflects the joint influences of cognition (attention) and emotion.

Chapter 4: Neuroimaging

Critical questions concerning cognition and emotion can be answered using neuroimaging methods (e.g., functional magnetic resonance imaging [fMRI]). Are there distinct brain structures devoted to cognition and emotion? In their chapter, Pessoa and Pereira indicate that some evidence from fMRI studies supports antagonistic relations between cognition and emotion, but that cognition and emotion also combine in complex ways to predict activation patterns in regions of the prefrontal cortex. Note that, overall, these findings favor neither an independence nor an equivalence view of cognition and emotion (see Table 1.1), but rather suggest that greater nuance is necessary to characterize how the brain processes cognitive and emotional inputs.

Chapter 5: Hormones

Hormones are often secreted in response to emotionally evocative situations. Understanding the factors that predict hormone release provides important information on cognition–emotion interactions. In their chapter, Wirth and Gaffey review what is known about stress hormones, neurosteroids, testosterone, and oxytocin in terms of factors that predict their release, consequences of such release, and the manner in which cognition and emotion play important, respective roles in understanding the link between hormones and social functioning.

Chapter 6: Attention

Attentional processes have played a key role in understanding the cognitive basis of emotional reactivity and emotional disorders. The first generation of such work sought to demonstrate this point across multiple attention-related paradigms. The second generation began to make distinctions among different aspects of attention (e.g., orienting vs. disengagement). In their chapter, Yiend, Barnicot, and Koster review different designs and attention tasks that can be used to understand cognition–emotion interactions from a selective attention perspective as well as the multiple findings that have accrued when doing so.

Chapter 7: Learning and Generalization

Learning is a cognitive process with considerable implications for understanding emotional phenomena. An important form of learning is affective in nature: People learn to like or dislike particular stimuli based on whether they have been paired with reward- or punishment-related events in the past. A question of great interest is whether such affective associations generalize to new stimuli that are different from the original stimuli encountered. For example, an original aversive learning experience (e.g., being bitten by a particular dog) might generalize to other stimuli that were not the source of the original aversive learning experience (e.g., other dogs, other animals, and so forth), setting the stage for the development of potential phobias or anxiety disorders. In their chapter, Hermans, Baeyens, and Vervliet review this literature and its potential applications to understanding anxiety disorders.

Chapter 8: Appraisal

Cognitive theories of emotion have long suggested that emotional reactions are dependent on how events are appraised or—in other words—interpreted. Much of the early evidence for appraisal views of emotion involved self-reports and cross-sectional designs. Major developments in favor of appraisal views of emotion have occurred since then. In their state-of-the-art chapter, Moors and Scherer review what we know so far concerning the role of appraisals in determining subsequent emotional reactions, discuss various designs and the inferences that can be drawn by using them, and offer insightful recommendations for future work in this area.

Chapter 9: Memory

Does emotion bias the memory system? Do memories play an important role in understanding emotional reactions? In their chapter, Murray, Holland, and Kensinger review both directions of influence, particularly from an episodic memory perspective. Episodic memories are particular to time and place and are more self-relevant than are most semantic (e.g., Australia is a continent) memories. Murray and colleagues highlight neural mechanisms and boundary conditions as well as suggest future directions of research that can be advocated in better understanding the emotion–memory interface.

Chapter 10: Goals

Goals can be conceptualized in cognitive terms and as precipitators of emotion. In thinking about their goals, individuals must ask themselves certain key questions, such as whether they are making sufficient progress toward them, whether redoubled efforts might be desirable, and whether certain goals might be best abandoned. All such goal-related processes are likely to have implications for understanding emotional reactions to goal-relevant events and, in fact, more general emotional phenomena such as rumination and depression. In their chapter, Carver and Scheier present a theoretical framework for understanding relations between goals and emotions, review findings from this area of enquiry, and highlight ways in which a goal-related perspective can greatly enrich our understanding of cognition–emotion interactions.

Chapter 11: Emotion Regulation

Human beings have unique capacities to regulate their emotions. To what extent do they do so and how can such emotion regulation processes be characterized? Are certain emotion regulation processes generally more beneficial than others? To regulate one's emotions, Suri, Sheppes, and Gross suggest, necessarily involves cognitive processes, yet the processes involved are different and include distracting oneself from an emotional stimulus, attempting to reappraise it as less emotional, and attempting to suppress one's overt manifestations of emotional reactivity (e.g., facial expressions of emotion). These different forms of emotion regulation have different consequences. Such evidence will be reviewed, with a particular emphasis on recent findings.

Chapter 12: Embodiment

A great deal of cognition and (to a lesser extent) emotion research seems to ignore the fact that people have bodies that function in particular ways. For example, we see things, we smell things, we touch things, and we often express our emotions in terms of muscle movements of the face. To what extent do such factors matter? In cognitive psychology, it has been increasingly suggested that our thoughts are *embodied*, which in part means that they arise because we have the particular bodies and sensory organs that we do. This should be true of our emotional reactions and processing as well. In their chapter, Winkielman and Kavanagh review theories of embodiment and relevant evidence in the emotion realm, including recent evidence for the idea that metaphors (e.g., to be physically clean is to be moral) seem to possess striking value in understanding emotional reactions and social judgments.

Chapter 13: Mood Effects

An important social cognition literature has sought to determine the manner in which our mood (or emotional) states affect our cognitions and behaviors. Although it is clear that they often do so, it is also clear that they do so through different mechanisms and different routes. For this reason, an integrated framework is necessary for understanding such effects. In their chapter, Forgas and Koch review evidence from this literature consistent with a multimechanism perspective of mood effects on cognition, social judgment, and behavior.

Chapter 14: Decision Making

Traditional models of decision making treat it as a rational, nonemotional process. Increasingly so, however, emotion has been shown to bias decision making in certain systematic manners. Great progress has been made in understanding such influences. In their chapter, Västfjäll and Slovic review classic work in the literature, make important distinctions between different types of affect and emotion, and review recent sources of data as well. They offer a comprehensive review of research in this decision-making area.

Chapter 15: Self-Control

Self-control is critical to successful functioning and involves overriding problematic tendencies or behaviors (e.g., to procrastinate, to eat fatty foods, to drink too much alcohol). Our emotions may play an important role in understanding self-control failures versus successes. For example, the clinical literature often suggests that negative emotional states undermine self-control (e.g., we might overeat when particularly stressed). In their chapter, Schmeichel and Inzlicht review this literature. In the first part of the chapter, they show that manipulated states of negative emotion, more so than manipulated states of positive emotion, result in subsequent self-control failures, and they also review relevant potential mechanisms for this effect. The second part of the chapter, however, suggests that low-intensity affective signals (i.e., not full-blown, intense emotions) may be critical to effective self-control. In other words, they present a nuanced perspective of when affect facilitates versus undermines self-control.

Chapter 16: Development

As infants age, they gain new cognitive skills and also new capacities to regulate their emotional states. A developmental perspective can reveal whether cognitive skills precede emotion regulation capacities, as is typically assumed, or whether there is a more complex relationship between developments in the cognition and emotion realms. In their chapter, Thompson and Winer review this developmental literature. They suggest that there are bidirectional relationships between developments in cognition and emotion and make a convincing case for the idea that this developmental analysis can inform and constrain how we think about adulthood relations between cognition and emotion as well.

Chapter 17: Extraversion and Neuroticism

Extraversion and neuroticism, respectively, predict positive and negative emotional states. Why do they do so? There is a general consensus that such relations cannot be due to differential exposure to positive (extraverts) versus negative (neurotics) events, but beyond this consensus, the mechanisms for such relations have been underexplored in the personality trait literature. In their chapter, Augustine, Larsen, and Lee consider cognitive approaches to understanding extraversion/positive emotion and neuroticism/negative emotion relations and conclude that such approaches possess considerable merit. Data related to attention, judgment, memory, and emotional reactivity are reviewed.

Chapter 18: Behavioral Approach and Inhibition Systems

To survive and thrive, we need to approach rewarding stimuli (e.g., food) and avoid threatening stimuli (e.g., hostile others). A prominent theory suggests that these two functions are subserved by two underlying motivational systems, one termed the behavioral approach system (BAS) and the other termed the behavioral inhibition system (BIS). In their chapter, Harmon-Jones, Price, Peterson, Gable, and Harmon-Jones review a substantial body of evidence linking individual differences in BAS and BIS to asymmetric brain activation, affect-modulated startle effects, event-related brain potentials, attention, memory, and learning. Among other phenomena, there is evidence that individuals high in BAS are more reactive to rewarding stimuli, whereas individuals high in BIS are more reactive to threatening stimuli.

Chapter 19: Agreeableness

Agreeableness is a major dimension of personality with implications for social functioning and emotions such as empathy and anger. In their chapter, Graziano and Tobin first review the emotional and behavioral correlates of agreeableness. They then review temperament-related evidence for the idea that agreeable individuals are better able to self-regulate their problematic thoughts and feelings relative to individuals low in agreeableness. Finally, they present a dual-process model of reactions to interpersonal conflict. Agreeableness can be conceptualized in terms of a motivation to maintain positive relations with others, which has major implications for why agreeable people are less prejudiced and more helpful in their interpersonal transactions. The model highlights processes related to personal distress and countervailing processes related to empathetic concern.

Chapter 20: Emotional Intelligence

Emotionally intelligent individuals are thought to better perceive, use, and manage emotions, both in the self and in relation to others. Controversy has surrounded the best ways of measuring emotional intelligence, whether it is distinct from other traits and abilities, and whether high levels of it are associated with higher levels of subjective and social well-being, as popular press has assumed. In their chapter, Brackett and colleagues review considerations in favor of an ability-related perspective of emotional intelligence, evidence in favor of its beneficial effects on emotional and social functioning, and its discriminant validity relative to other abilities such as general intelligence. Finally, the authors make a case that, like other abilities, emotional intelligence can be trained. Several innovative programs have sought to do so, and the results have shown considerable promise.

Chapter 21: Repetitive Thought

Experimental clinical researchers have highlighted a number of forms of repetitive thinking—for example, rumination, worry, reflection, intrusive thoughts, obsessions—that are likely to contribute to and exacerbate problematic emotional outcomes among vulnerable individuals. How can such processes be understood? Can they be mitigated? In his chapter, Watkins suggests that repetitive thought, per se, is not necessarily maladaptive and can sometimes support problem solving. However, when it occurs in combination with negative affect or depression, it often results in maladaptive outcomes. In addition, the author suggests that it is critical to distinguish between concrete and abstract forms of repetitive thinking. Although concrete forms of repetitive thinking may sometimes be functional, abstract forms of repetitive thinking appear less so, trapping some individuals into cycles of rumination and worry. Watkins also reviews evidence from recent psychotherapeutic approaches targeting repetitive thinking processes.

Chapter 22: Posttraumatic Stress Disorder

Stress is inevitable in daily living, but some individuals encounter major stressors (e.g., being physically assaulted) that challenge one's view of an effective self in a safe world. In relation to such major stressors, some people develop posttraumatic stress disorder (PTSD), which is marked by reliving the event involuntarily, elevated physiological arousal, avoidance, considerable anxiety and depression, exhaustion, and problems in work and relationship realms. In their chapter, Ehring, Kleim, and Ehlers consider the cognitive processes that are likely to maintain and exacerbate posttraumatic symptoms over time (e.g., poor memory integration, thought suppression, and rumination) and whether and how such processes combine to predict such symptoms. They call for future research in which cognition and emotion are jointly considered in models of PTSD.

Chapter 23: Anxiety Disorders

Anxiety disorders are particularly common. It is therefore important to understand how cognitive–processing tendencies contribute to such disorders. Questions include whether there is a common cognitive core to the anxiety disorders and whether research of a cognitive-emotional type has translational relevance to clinical practice. In their chapter, Morrison, Gordon, and Heimberg review multiple paradigms and sources of evidence for a cognitive perspective on anxiety disorders. Morrison and colleagues review cases in which the relevant cognitive biases converge, but are sometimes distinct. They also call for research examining how the various cognitive biases found in anxiety disorders relate to each other. Finally, they review studies in which anxiety-related cognitive biases have been examined as outcomes of effective psychotherapy and generally favor this line of inquiry in the future.

Chapter 24: Depression

Depression is also a common disorder and it is particularly debilitating to sufferers. In their chapter, Clasen, Disner, and Beevers review what is known about cognitive biases in depression. A number of different cognitive biases are reviewed, ranging from those related to attention to those related to rumination and emotion regulation. The authors also distinguish cognitive factors that predict the onset of depressive episodes versus those associated with the maintenance of depression over time. The cognitive factors involved are likely to be somewhat different, with distinct implications for psychotherapeutic interventions. In their Future Directions section, the authors review available data for the idea that depressogenic cognitive biases can be retrained, in turn alleviating suffering and perhaps even changing diagnostic status.

Chapter 25: Borderline Personality Disorder

Borderline personality disorder (BPD) is comorbid with many other psychiatric conditions. In addition, borderline patients are at high risk for self-harm and suicide. How can such symptoms be understood? In their chapter, Carpenter, Bagby-Stone, and Trull note that borderline personality is typically understood in terms of emotions. These individuals may have very high levels of negative emotion, may have unstable emotions over time, and may lack emotional awareness. In their review, Carpenter and colleagues suggest that there is a more fundamental problem: individuals with BPD, relative to controls, cannot regulate their attention effectively. The authors review evidence in support of this point across a wide variety of sources of data (e.g., comorbidity of BPD with other disorders) and detail the manner in which this attentional dysregulation view of BPD may have considerable untapped merit.

Chapter 26: Bipolar Spectrum Disorders

Bipolar spectrum disorders are marked by states of both mania and depression. Depression is often viewed in terms of high levels of negative emotion, but such depressive states may often result from unrealistic goals and failures to achieve them. In their chapter, Alloy and colleagues suggest that an overactive or oversensitive BAS may underlie this set of disorders. This perspective can account for both manic and depressive symptoms exhibited by such individuals and can account for comorbidity (particularly during manic states) with behavioral problems linked to an overactive BAS system (e.g., sexual promiscuity, gambling, and aggression). Importantly, Alloy et al. review evidence for the idea that especially high levels of BAS can predict bipolar symptoms at a later time. In addition, the authors consider implications of their findings for treatments of bipolar spectrum disorders.

Chapter 27: Psychopathy

Those diagnosed with antisocial personality disorder are impulsive in their behav-

iors. However, impulsivity is multiply determined. In their chapter, Baskin-Sommers and Newman contrast psychopathy with externalizing behaviors more broadly considered (e.g., delinquency, drug use, and aggression). On the basis of considerable data, they suggest that psychopathic individuals, relative to externalizers, have unique problems in regulating their attention at an early stage of processing, are less prone to executive-processing deficits, and exhibit less neural activation in response to threatening stimuli. Subsequently, Baskin-Sommers and Newman present an integrative model of psychopathy and highlight the importance of cognition–emotion interactions in understanding this unique form of antisocial behavior.

Chapter 28: Cognition and Emotion in Psychotherapy

Traditional views of psychotherapy seek to target dysfunctional cognitions with the idea that doing so should help to mitigate emotional problems. An alternative approach within psychotherapy seeks to target dysfunctional emotions rather than the cognitions that might underlie them. In his chapter, Greenberg contrasts the basis for these differential targets of psychotherapy and the rationale for seeking to alter emotions rather than cognitions. Emotion-focused psychotherapy has gained traction in areas in which the relevant disorders can be viewed as primarily emotion-related in nature. That the therapy often works is also consistent with the idea that there are bidirectional relations between emotion and cognition, a general theme of the present volume.

Chapter 29: Cognitive Bias Modification

It has long been known that anxiety and depression are associated with cognitive biases related to selective attention and interpretation. To the extent that such processing biases causally matter, experimental manipulations designed to reduce them should reduce distress. In their chapter, MacLeod and Clarke review a systematic body of work for this idea. For example, people can be trained to attend away from threatening information, and it has been shown that manipulations of this type in fact reduce experiences of distress in response to laboratory stressors. A more recent body of evidence suggests that prolonged training of this cognitive type can render diagnostically anxious individuals nonanxious, can do so over at least half a year, and can do so in relation to multiple diagnostic categories. Although there is considerable research to be done in the future, this line of research, as reviewed by MacLeod and Clarke, is unprecedented in its causal implications, scope, and demonstrations of clinical utility. Their chapter is therefore the last one of the handbook.

Conclusions

The Western philosophical tradition views cognition and emotion as inimical to each other (Lyons, 1999). We do not believe this to be always true, nor do we believe that cognition and emotion are necessarily independent, that cognition is necessary for emotion, that affect always precedes cognition, or that cognition and emotion are inseparable or equivalent. Instead, we suggest that relations between cognition and emotion need to be investigated rather than proposed a priori. The present handbook does so across many subdisciplines of psychology and particular topics. Facts were of interest to us. The most general statement that we can make on the basis of the chapters and findings reported is that cognition and emotion interact in complex ways that need to be appreciated in nuanced terms requiring the close analysis of context. Moreover, given the extensive range of interactions between cognition and emotion, we strongly argue that there is value in typically considering cognition and emotion together rather than in isolation. We hope that the present volume sufficiently makes this point and does so in multiple manners that will be informative to students of the field as well as to future researchers.

References

Berkowitz, L., & Harmon-Jones, E. (2004). Toward an understanding of the determinants of anger. *Emotion, 4*, 107–130.

Berridge, K. C., & Winkielman, P. (2003). What is an unconscious emotion? (The case for unconscious "liking"). *Cognition and Emotion, 17*, 181–211.

Bevan, W. (1964). Subliminal stimulation: A pervasive problem for psychology. *Psychological Bulletin, 61*, 81–99.

Bower, G. H. (1981). Mood and memory. *American Psychologist, 36*, 129–148.

Bush, G., Luu, P., & Posner, M. I. (2000). Cognitive and emotional influences in anterior cingulate cortex. *Trends in Cognitive Sciences, 4*, 215–222.

Canli, T., Zhao, Z., Desmond, J. E., Kang, E., Gross, J. J., & Gabrieli, J. D. E. (2001). An fMRI study of personality influences on brain reactivity to emotional stimuli. *Behavioral Neuroscience, 115*, 33–42.

Chalmers, D. (2007). The hard problem of consciousness. In M. Velmans & S. Schneider (Eds.), *The Blackwell companion to consciousness* (pp. 225–235). Malden, MA: Blackwell.

Dalgleish, T., & Power, M. J. (1999). *Handbook of cognition and emotion.* New York: Wiley.

Damasio, A. (1994). *Descartes' error.* New York: Grosset/Putnam.

Davidson, R. J. (2003). Seven sins in the study of emotion: Correctives from affective neuroscience. *Brain and Cognition, 52*, 129–132.

De Houwer, J., & Hermans, D. (2010). *Cognition and emotion: Reviews of current research and theories.* New York: Psychology Press.

Dimberg, U., Thunberg, M., & Elmehed, K. (2000). Unconscious facial reactions to emotional facial expressions. *Psychological Science, 11*, 86–89.

Dixon, N. F. (1981). *Preconscious processing.* New York: Wiley.

Draine, S. C., & Greenwald, A. G. (1998). Replicable unconscious semantic priming. *Journal of Experimental Psychology: General, 127*, 286–303.

Duncan, S., & Feldman Barrett, L. (2007). Affect is a form of cognition: A neurobiological analysis. *Cognition and Emotion, 21*, 1184–1211.

Eich, E., Kihlstrom, J. F., Bower, G. H., Forgas, J. P., & Niedenthal, P. M. (2000). *Cognition and emotion.* New York: Oxford University Press.

Eimer, M., & Schlaghecken, F. (1998). Effects of masked stimuli on motor activation: Behavioral and electrophysiological evidence. *Journal of Experimental Psychology: Human Perception and Performance, 24*, 1737–1747.

Eisenberger, N. I., Lieberman, M. D., & Satpute,

A. B. (2005). Personality from a controlled processing perspective: An fMRI study of neuroticism, extraversion, and self-consciousness. *Cognitive, Affective, and Behavioral Neuroscience, 5,* 169–181.

Epstein, S. (1994). Integration of the cognitive and the psychodynamic unconscious. *American Psychologist, 49,* 709–724.

Fanselow, M. S. (1994). Neural organization of the defensive behavior system responsible for fear. *Psychonomic Bulletin and Review, 1,* 429–438.

Izard, C. E. (2009). Emotion theory and research: Highlights, unanswered questions, and emerging issues. *Annual Review of Psychology, 60,* 1–25.

Kemp-Wheeler, S. M., & Hill, A. B. (1988). Semantic priming without awareness: Some methodological considerations and replications. *Quarterly Journal of Experimental Psychology A: Human Experimental Psychology, 40,* 671–692.

Kihlstrom, J. F., Mulvaney, S., Tobias, B. A., & Tobis, I. P. (2000). The emotional unconscious. In E. Eich, J. F. Kihlstrom, G. H. Bower, J. P. Forgas, & P. M. Niedenthal (Eds.), *Cognition and emotion* (pp. 30–86). New York: Oxford University Press.

Klinger, E. (1999). Thought flow: Properties and mechanisms underlying shifts in content. In J. A. Singer & P. Salovey (Eds.), *At play in the fields of consciousness: Essays in honor of Jerome L. Singer* (pp. 29–50). Mahwah, NJ: Erlbaum.

Kunst-Wilson, W. R., & Zajonc, R. B. (1980). Affective discrimination of stimuli that cannot be recognized. *Science, 207,* 557–558.

Lazarus, R. S. (1984). On the primacy of cognition. *American Psychologist, 39,* 124–129.

Lazarus, R. S. (1991). *Emotion and adaptation.* New York: Oxford University Press.

Lazarus, R. S. (1995). Vexing research problems inherent in cognitive-mediational theories of emotion—and some solutions. *Psychological Inquiry, 6,* 183–196.

LeDoux, J. E. (1996). *The emotional brain: The mysterious underpinnings of emotional life.* New York: Simon & Schuster.

Lyons, W. (1999). The philosophy of cognition and emotion. In T. Dalgleish & M. J. Power (Eds.), *Handbook of cognition and emotion* (pp. 21–44). New York: Wiley.

MacLean, P. D. (1973). *A triune concept of the brain and behaviour: Hincks memorial lecture.* Toronto: University of Toronto Press.

Martin, L. L., & Clore, G. L. (2001). *Theories of mood and cognition: A user's guidebook.* Mahwah, NJ: Erlbaum.

McClure, S. M., Botvinick, M. M., Yeung, N., Greene, J. D., & Cohen, J. D. (2007). Conflict monitoring in cognition–emotion competition. In J. J. Gross (Ed.), *Handbook of emotion regulation* (pp. 204–226). New York: Guilford Press.

Merikle, P. (2007). Preconscious processing. In M. Velmans & S. Schneider (Eds.), *The Blackwell companion to consciousness* (pp. 512–524). Malden, MA: Blackwell.

Mischel, W., & Ayduk, O. (2011). Willpower in a cognitive–affective processing system: The dynamics of delay of gratification. In K. D. Vohs & R. F. Baumeister (Eds.), *Handbook of self-regulation: Research, theory, and applications* (2nd ed., pp. 83–105). New York: Guilford Press.

Mischel, W., Shoda, Y., & Rodriguez, M. L. (1989). Delay of gratification in children. *Science, 244,* 933–938.

Morris, J. S., Öhman, A., & Dolan, R. J. (1998). Conscious and unconscious emotional learning in the human amygdala. *Nature, 393,* 467–470.

Murphy, S. T., & Zajonc, R. B. (1993). Affect, cognition, and awareness: Affective priming with optimal and suboptimal stimulus exposures. *Journal of Personality and Social Psychology, 64,* 723–739.

Ochsner, K. N., & Gross, J. J. (2005). The cognitive control of emotion. *Trends in Cognitive Sciences, 9,* 242–249.

Öhman, A., & Soares, J. J. F. (1998). Emotional conditioning to masked stimuli: Expectancies for aversive outcomes following nonrecognized fear-relevant stimuli. *Journal of Experimental Psychology: General, 127,* 69–82.

Panksepp, J. (1998). *Affective neuroscience: The foundations of human and animal emotions.* New York: Oxford University Press.

Peyk, P., Schupp, H. T., Elbert, T., & Junghöfer, M. (2008). Emotion processing in the visual brain: A MEG analysis. *Brain Topography, 20,* 205–215.

Pinker, S. (2007). *The stuff of thought: Language as a window into human nature.* New York: Viking Press.

Reisenzein, R., & Hofmann, T. (1993). Discriminating emotions from appraisal-relevant situational information: Baseline data for structural models of cognitive appraisals. *Cognition and Emotion, 7,* 271–293.

Rolls, E. T. (1999). *The brain and emotion.* New York: Oxford University Press.

Scherer, K. R. (1984). Emotion as a multicomponent process: A model and some cross-cultural data. *Review of Personality and Social Psychology, 5,* 37–63.

Smith, C. A., & Ellsworth, P. C. (1985). Patterns of cognitive appraisal in emotion. *Journal of Personality and Social Psychology, 48,* 813–838.

Smith, C. A., & Kirby, L. D. (2001). Toward delivering on the promise of appraisal theory. In K. R. Scherer, A. Schorr, & T. Johnstone (Eds.), *Appraisal processes in emotion: Theory, methods, research* (pp. 121–138). New York: Oxford University Press.

Solomon, R. C. (1976). *The passions: The myth and nature of human emotion.* Oxford, UK: Anchor.

Storbeck, J., & Robinson, M. D. (2004). Preferences and inferences in encoding visual objects: A systematic comparison of semantic and affective priming. *Personality and Social Psychology Bulletin, 30,* 81–93.

Storbeck, J., Robinson, M. D., & McCourt, M. E. (2006). Semantic processing precedes affect retrieval: The neurological case for cognitive primacy in visual processing. *Review of General Psychology, 10,* 41–55.

Swan, T. (2009). Metaphors of body and mind in the history of English. *English Studies, 90,* 460–475.

Whalen, P. J. (1998). Fear, vigilance, and ambiguity: Initial neuroimaging studies of the human amygdala. *Current Directions in Psychological Science, 7,* 177–188.

Zajonc, R. B. (1980). Feeling and thinking: Preferences need no inferences. *American Psychologist, 35,* 151–175.

Zajonc, R. B. (1998). Emotions. In D. T. Gilbert, S. T. Fiske, & G. Lindzey (Eds.), *The handbook of social psychology* (pp. 591–632). New York: McGraw-Hill.

PART II

BIOLOGICAL FACTORS AND CONSIDERATIONS

CHAPTER 2

Neurogenetics Approaches

Insights from Studies of Dopamine Signaling and Reward Processing

Yuliya S. Nikolova, Ryan Bogdan, and Ahmad R. Hariri

A substantial body of experimental psychology and neuroscience research has focused on uncovering the mechanisms underlying behavioral phenomena universal across individuals. Yet human behavior is characterized by remarkable diversity. Interindividual variability exists in almost every domain of psychological functioning, ranging from perception and cognition to affective processing and social behavior. Importantly, some of these individual differences can serve as predictors of vulnerability to neuropsychiatric disorders, such as depression, anxiety, and addiction. Understanding the biological underpinnings of this variability may thus help us not only better grasp the complexities of human behavior, but also identify individuals who may be susceptible to mental illness.

Recent advances in social, cognitive, and affective neuroscience have begun to shed light on the biological basis of human behavior, yielding particularly notable insights into the neural substrates of cognition, emotion, and their interactions (Dolan, 2002; Gray, Braver, & Raichle, 2002; Phelps, 2006). Building primarily upon research into the functional anatomy of neural circuits supporting analogous phenomena in nonhuman animal models, this progress has

also been critically dependent on the increasing sophistication of methodologies capable of measuring activity in the living human brain. Neuroimaging techniques producing indirect (e.g., glucose positron emission tomography [PET]; blood oxygen level–dependent functional magnetic resonance imaging [BOLD fMRI]) and direct (e.g., electroencephalography [EEG]) measures of activity within and across brain regions have helped begin to delineate the roles for specific brain structures and patterns of activity in generating cognition, emotion, and their interactions (e.g., Dolan, 2002). To gain further insight into the biological bases of these phenomena, the fields of neuropsychopharmacology, biological psychiatry, molecular imaging and, most recently, genetics have attempted to identify the neurochemistry that regulates behaviorally relevant neural circuitry.

In this context, a handful of recent studies has begun to link neurotransmitter function to complex brain activation patterns and, subsequently, behavior, using ligand PET imaging and/or pharmacological challenge paradigms alongside traditional MRI and behavioral measures (Bigos et al., 2008; Fisher et al., 2009; Kim et al., 2011; Santesso et al., 2009). Complementing these multimodal neuroscience studies, the relatively new field of imaging genetics has begun to examine how genetically driven variability in neurotransmitter action maps onto individual differences in brain function, structure, and behavior (Bigos & Weinberger, 2010; Egan et al., 2001; Hariri et al., 2002, 2009; Meyer-Lindenberg, 2010). By providing unprecedented insights into the origins of this vast interindividual variability, the advent of imaging genetics has fostered unique opportunities for progress into the neuroscience of human behavior (Hariri, 2009).

Neural and behavioral characteristics, or phenotypes, pertaining to cognition, emotion, and their interactions have quickly become a preferred study subject in imaging genetics research due to the increasingly detailed understanding of their underlying neurocircuitry (Haber & Knutson, 2010; LeDoux, 2000), as well as the demonstrated heritability of (1) disorders of emotion and cognition (e.g., depression: Kendler, Myers, Maes, & Keyes, 2011; schizophrenia: McGuffin, Farmer, Gottesman, Murray, & Reveley, 1984), and (2) normal-range variability in emotional and cognitive aspects of behavior (e.g., hedonic capacity and perceived stress: Bogdan & Pizzagalli, 2009; age-related cognitive decline: McGue & Christensen, 2001), which can subsequently be mapped onto individual differences in the functioning of neural circuits or the distribution of genetic variants.

Rather than presenting an exhaustive overview of the research on the neural and genetic basis of emotion, cognition, and their interactions, this chapter aims to review the basic principles of imaging genetics research as they pertain to a specific behavior, which exemplifies important aspects of the adaptive integration of emotion and cognition. The chapter focuses on reward processing—a behavioral and neural phenomenon whereby information regarding the appetitive value of stimuli in one's environment is collected, stored, and utilized to promote survival and well-being. This particular phenotype was chosen not only because of the increasingly sophisticated knowledge of the anatomy and physiology of its neurobiological substrates, but also because of its wide relevance to understanding both adaptive and maladaptive aspects of behavior: Individual differences in reward processing on the level of the brain have been linked to normal-range interindividual variability in personality constructs such as impulsivity and reward sensitivity (Forbes et al., 2009; Hariri et al., 2006), as well as to maladaptive extremes of behavior such as substance use disorders (Petry & Casarella, 1999) and depression (Steele, Kumar, & Ebmeier, 2007).

The Biological Basis of Reward Processing

Reward processing is subserved by a distributed mesocorticostriatal circuitry comprising a network of brain regions individually implicated in a number of affective and cognitive functions (Lawrence, Sahakian, & Robbins, 1998; Marchand & Yurgelun-Todd, 2010), whose signals are dynamically integrated into adaptive behavioral responses in accordance with environmental reward contingencies. This network is critically regulated by the neurotransmitter dopamine. Dopaminergic neurons residing in the ventral tegmental area (VTA) within the midbrain send axonal projections to the ventral portion of the striatum (VS), which receives additional input from cortical and limbic regions and serves as a hub for this distributed circuitry (Figure 2.1). Of particular relevance to the topic at hand, the VS also comprises the nucleus accumbens (NAcc)—a neural region that nonhuman animal research has implicated in various aspects of reward processing, ranging from core hedonic reactions to motivation to pursue appetitive stimuli (Berridge, Robinson, & Aldridge, 2009). Due to the limited resolution of human *in vivo* imaging, few imaging genetics studies have investigated the neuroanatomy and neurophysiology of the NAcc directly, with the majority of them focusing instead on the structural and functional properties of the VS more broadly (Forbes et al., 2009; Salvadore et al., 2009).

Research on the neural basis of reward processing has frequently focused on the VS, in large part due to its extensive connectivity, which places it in a position to continuously integrate a variety of inputs converging in the mesocorticostriatal system in order to dynamically and adaptively adjust complex

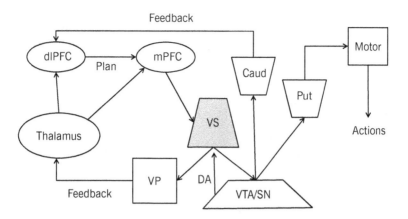

FIGURE 2.1. Schematic representation of key nodes and pathways within the reward system of the human brain. Caud, caudate; dlPFC, dorsolateral prefrontal cortex; Motor, motor cortex; mPFC, medial prefrontal cortex; Put, putamen; SN, substantia nigra; VP, ventral pallidum; VS, ventral striatum; VTA, ventral tegmental area.

behavioral responses according to changing environmental contingencies (Figure 2.1). In addition to the dopaminergic input from VTA neurons, the VS receives glutamatergic projections from the ventromedial prefrontal cortex (PFC). Importantly, these limbic cortical regions interface with more dorsal PFC regulatory regions supporting higher-order cognitive functions necessary for goal-directed behavior (Balleine & Dickinson, 1998; Miller, 2000), thus providing an indirect connection between those regions and the VS. Notably, however, these cortical areas also receive direct dopaminergic projections from the VTA (Bjorklund & Dunnett, 2007), providing an anatomical substrate for the direct involvement of dopamine in cognitive control, among other processes, as discussed later in this chapter.

Recent evidence suggests that reward processing is not a monolithic phenomenon, but can instead be parsed into distinct psychological, neuroanatomical, and neurochemical subcomponents such as "wanting" (anticipatory), "liking" (consummatory), and "learning" (prediction) (Berridge et al., 2009). Core hedonic or "liking" reactions have primarily been linked to opioid signaling within a subregion of the NAcc (the NAcc shell). Dopamine, in contrast, has been shown to play a primary role in mediating "wanting" and "learning" by regulating activity in other subcomponents of the NAcc (the NAcc core) and interconnected regions

of the extended mesocorticostriatal system. Given the relative inability of currently available research methodologies to fully parse these biological and behavioral components of reward processing in humans, as well as the large body of research investigating the role of dopamine in regulating VS reactivity, reward learning, and reward processing in general, this chapter focuses on the regulatory function of dopamine on mesocorticostriatal system reactivity and any aspects of reward processing this may affect.

Dopamine and Reward

Dopamine is a neurotransmitter involved in a variety of functions, ranging from lactation and movement to regulating crucial aspects of emotion and cognition. Of particular relevance to the topic of this chapter, within the mesocorticostriatal system, dopamine acts as a mediator of reward-related processes. Studies have demonstrated the existence of two types of dopaminergic activity of particular importance for this regulatory role: tonic and phasic. *Tonic activity* refers to a constant, slow "background" firing of dopaminergic neurons, whereas *phasic* refers to the quick bursts of action potentials that occur in response to specific environmental events (Grace, 1991).

Early studies linking dopamine to reward in nonhuman animal models did not dis-

criminate between tonic and phasic activity and have observed that both natural
and drug rewards result in a dopamine
surge in the NAcc (Hernandez & Hoebel,
1988). Conversely, pharmacological blockade of dopamine has been shown to result
in decreased reward seeking behavior (Yokel
& Wise, 1975). More recent studies have
begun to paint a more complex picture of
the involvement of this neurotransmitter in
reward processing by demonstrating that
dopamine release is not merely a correlate of
reward consumption or reward seeking, but
may instead be involved in coding complex
information about the appetitive stimuli in
one's environment. This research has demonstrated that spikes in phasic dopaminergic
activity in VTA neurons occur in response
to unexpectedly high rewards, whereas conversely, a dip in phasic activity occurs in
response to unexpectedly low rewards or the
absence of reward (Schultz, 2002). Furthermore, as reward-based learning progresses,
these phasic responses transition from the
reward itself to the stimulus predicting the
reward (Schultz, 2002). This transition, coupled with the adaptive modulation of dopamine phasic activity in response to changes
in reward contingencies (i.e., unexpectedly
high/low rewards), suggests that dopamine
may be specifically involved in reward learning and anticipation in addition to reward
responsiveness more generally.

Dopamine and Cognitive Control

In addition to regulating important aspects
of reward responsiveness and basic motivational drive, mesocorticostriatal dopamine
also plays a central role in mediating neural
processes pertaining to the cognitive control
of behavior. Early evidence for this modulatory effect comes from observations of
shared cognitive deficits across patients with
various disorders of dopamine signaling,
most notably Parkinson's disease (PD) and
schizophrenia (see Nieoullon, 2002, for a
review). Despite notable differences in overall symptomatology, both of these disorders
are associated with decreased working memory and executive function, as well as diminished mental flexibility in the face of changing environmental demands. Providing even
more direct support for the involvement of

PFC dopamine in cognitive function, studies
have shown that dopamine depletion in the
PFC of monkeys leads to a dramatic reduction in working memory task performance
(Brozoski, Brown, Rosvold, & Goldman,
1979), whereas a pharmacologically induced
increase in prefrontal dopamine signaling
results in improved cognitive flexibility in
both normal and dopamine-depleted nonhuman animals (Arnsten, Cai, Murphy, &
Goldman-Rakic, 1994; Tunbridge, Bannerman, Sharp, & Harrison, 2004). Similar
results have been obtained in neurologically
healthy humans, in whom pharmacological agents increasing prefrontal dopamine
transmission via diverse mechanisms lead to
enhancements in cognitive function (Apud
et al., 2007; Kimberg & D'Esposito, 2003;
Luciana, Depue, Arbisi, & Leon, 1992),
thus further corroborating the involvement
of prefrontal dopamine in cognitive control
and cognition more broadly.

It is important to note, however, that the
regulatory role of dopamine on PFC function
and top-down cognitive control processes
is not completely independent of its role in
regulating basic emotional drives. In fact,
there may be an inverse relationship between
dopamine signaling in the PFC and subcortical regions responsible for these more
basic drives. Specifically, theoretical models
backed by extensive empirical work suggest
that an overall increase in dopamine in the
PFC may raise tonic levels of dopaminergic
neuron firing subcortically and enhance baseline synaptic concentrations of dopamine in
regions such as the VS. These increased levels of tonic intrasynaptic dopamine may, in
turn, increase the threshold required to produce phasic spikes in dopaminergic activity
(Bilder, Volavka, Lachman, & Grace, 2004).
Conversely, reduced dopamine activity in
the PFC may result in a reactive increase in
subcortical phasic dopamine signaling. In
light of this reciprocal connection between
dopamine levels in the PFC and phasic dopaminergic signaling in subcortical regions, the
cognitive and behavioral deficits associated
with dopamine signaling abnormalities may
reflect dysfunction in both prefrontal and
striatal regions, including the VS (Cools,
2008). Thus, by virtue of its role in regulating mesocorticostriatal system reactivity,
dopamine is involved in modulating not only
bottom-up emotional drive pathways and

top-down cognitive control processes, but also the dynamic equilibrium between the two. Despite the interconnectedness of these top-down and bottom-up pathways, genetic polymorphisms (i.e., commonly occurring genetic variants), which differentially affect dopamine signaling in the PFC and VS, have allowed for an at least partial dissociation between the sets of processes each pathway mediates. Before we review these polymorphisms in depth, we consider the major steps involved in dopamine signaling and metabolism.

Dopamine Signaling and Metabolism

Within the mesocorticostriatal system, dopamine is synthesized in VTA neurons from the amino acid L-tyrosine (Figure 2.2). It is then packaged into vesicles and released into the synaptic cleft, where it acts on postsynaptic receptors located on striatal neurons or regulatory interneurons, as well as presynaptic dopaminergic autoreceptors. After its release into the synaptic cleft, dopamine is subject to reuptake into presynaptic neurons (primarily in the VS; Lewis et al., 2001) or extrasynaptic enzymatic degradation (primarily in the PFC; Chen et al.,

2004). Functional polymorphisms within genes involved in regulating each individual step of dopamine synthesis, signaling, and synaptic clearance can be mapped onto individual variability in mesocorticostriatal system reactivity and reward processing on the behavioral level. Genetic variants associated with relatively increased dopamine signaling, whether through decreased postrelease inactivation or decreased inhibition, have generally been associated with increased reactivity of the striatum and, in most cases, increased reward-related behaviors (Forbes et al., 2009). This chapter surveys several commonly studied functional genetic polymorphisms affecting dopamine signaling and discusses their effects on brain function and behavior. Thus, it presents several biological pathways through which dopamine signaling can be genetically up-regulated and demonstrates the remarkably convergent effects these diverse pathways have on reward system reactivity and, ultimately, reward-related behavior.

COMT Val[158]Met (rs4680)

The enzyme catechol-*O*-methyltransferase (COMT) catalyzes dopamine degradation and is expressed primarily in the PFC, with

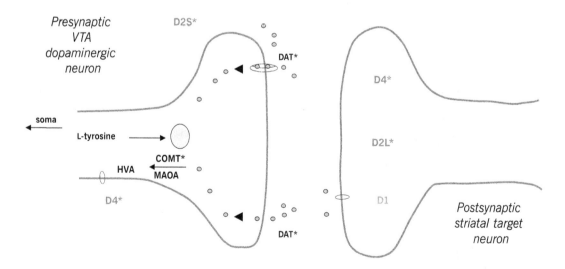

FIGURE 2.2. Schematic representation of a dopaminergic synapse. Items marked with an asterisk (*) are discussed in the chapter. COMT, catechol-*O*-methyltransferase; D1, D2, D3, D4, dopamine receptors; D2L, dopamine D2 receptor long (postsynaptic) isoform; D2S, dopamine D2 receptor short (presynaptic) isoform; DAT, dopamine transporter; HVA, homovanillic acid; MAOA, monoamine oxidase A.

much lower expression levels in the striatum (Chen et al., 2004; Gogos et al., 1998; Huotari et al., 2002). Genetic variants associated with reduced expression of COMT would presumably be associated with less efficient dopamine inactivation and an overall increase in dopamine signaling within COMT-expressing brain regions.

A common single nucleotide polymorphism (SNP) occurs within the *COMT* gene (rs4680). The SNP is an adenine to guanine substitution in the DNA sequence (i.e., a single letter change). This change in the DNA sequence is translated into two different amino acid sequences in the COMT protein: Adenine produces a valine (Val), but guanine produces a methionine (Met) at position 158 of the COMT protein amino acid chain (i.e., Val^{158}Met). The ^{158}Met allele is associated with up to three- to fourfold reduction in COMT enzymatic activity (Lotta et al., 1995), thus presumably slower dopamine breakdown and increased dopamine levels in the PFC (Chen et al., 2004). The Val^{158} allele, which is conversely associated with relatively low dopamine levels in the PFC, has been linked to diminished cognitive performance in healthy adults (Egan et al., 2001) as well as increased risk for schizophrenia, especially in interaction with adolescent cannabis use (Caspi et al., 2005). The role of the Val^{158}Met polymorphism in modulating cognition and schizophrenia risk has been reviewed extensively elsewhere (Dickinson & Elvevag, 2009; Savitz, Solms, & Ramesar, 2006; Tan, Callicott, & Weinberger, 2009). Here we focus on the relatively less studied effects of *COMT* Val-^{158}Met on reward-related brain function.

Even though COMT is expressed primarily in the PFC, with much lower expression levels in the striatum (Chen et al., 2004; Gogos et al., 1998; Huotari et al., 2002; Matsumoto et al., 2003), the *COMT* Val-^{158}Met polymorphism may affect striatal dopamine signaling indirectly. Consistent with the inhibitory effects of prefrontal dopamine on striatal dopamine transmission (Bilder et al., 2004; Cools, 2008), studies have shown that the Val^{158} allele, which presumably results in reduced prefrontal dopamine, is in fact associated with increased dopamine synthesis and release in subcortical regions such as the striatum (Akil et al., 2003; Meyer-Lindenberg et al.,

2005). Despite the associations between the Val^{158} allele and increased striatal dopamine synthesis, however, imaging genetics studies investigating the effects of *COMT* Val^{158}Met on striatal reactivity have not consistently linked this allele to increased striatal reactivity to reward, with some studies showing the opposite association.

Perhaps most notably, two independent BOLD fMRI studies have linked the ^{158}Met allele to relatively increased VS activation during reward anticipation in a gambling task (Dreher, Kohn, Kolachana, Weinberger, & Berman, 2009; Yacubian et al., 2007). Consistent with prior studies linking reward-related VS reactivity to increased impulsivity (Forbes et al., 2009), this association is borne out on the behavioral level: ^{158}Met allele carriers (i.e., individuals carrying at least one copy of the ^{158}Met allele) show higher delay discounting, compared to Val^{158} homozygotes (i.e., individuals carrying two copies of the Val^{158} allele; Paloyelis, Asherson, Mehta, Faraone, & Kuntsi, 2010). Delay discounting studies typically quantify an individual's preference for smaller rewards available immediately over rewards that are larger but delayed in time. Higher delay discounting is associated with increased reward sensitivity and behavioral impulsivity, typically seen in individuals with hyperactive reward systems (Forbes et al., 2009; Hariri et al., 2006). The association between the ^{158}Met allele and delay discounting is thus consistent with a heightened dopaminergic signaling phenotype.

Alongside these convergent neuroimaging and behavioral data suggesting that ^{158}Met is associated with heightened reward-related traits and behaviors, additional studies have suggested that the Val^{158} allele may in fact contribute to increases in other aspects of reward-related brain function. Specifically, Val^{158} homozygotes have been shown to exhibit relatively increased VS reactivity to unexpectedly high monetary gains in a gambling paradigm, in comparison with ^{158}Met homozygotes (Camara et al., 2010). In addition, another study has linked the Val^{158} allele to increased flexibility of decision making in the context of changing reward contingencies (Krugel, Biele, Mohr, Li, & Heekeren, 2009).

These seemingly conflicting results might in fact suggest a more fine-tuned genetic modulation of VS response to positive stimuli dependent on reward magnitude and predictability, whereby the [158]Met allele is associated with more robust reactivity to rewards in a stable environment, whereas the Val[158] allele is associated with more efficient reward learning in the context of changing reward contingencies (i.e., greater behavioral flexibility). This notion is at least partially consistent with the hypothesis put forward by Bilder and colleagues (2004) regarding the role of *COMT* Val[158]Met in phasic–tonic dopamine activity regulation. According to this hypothesis, the Val[158] allele, which is associated with lower prefrontal dopamine levels, is likely to be linked to decreased tonic and increased phasic striatal dopamine activity, relative to the [158]Met allele (Bilder et al., 2004). The link between the Val[158] allele and increased flexibility in the context of changing reward contingencies, as delineated by the above studies (Camara et al., 2010; Marco-Pallares et al., 2009), is thus consistent with the role of dopamine phasic bursts in reward learning, wherein phasic dopamine activity constitutes a reward prediction error that presumably triggers the encoding of new reward contingencies (Schultz, 2002).

Dopamine Transporter (DAT, *SLC6A3*)

Another protein with a key role in regulating dopamine neurotransmission is the dopamine transporter (DAT, coded by the gene *SLC6A3*). DAT binds dopamine after its release into the synaptic cleft and facilitates its reuptake into the presynaptic neuron. Thus, DAT helps regulate both the duration and intensity of postsynaptic responses to dopaminergic inputs and the available presynaptic pool of dopamine (via recycling). Unlike *COMT*, which regulates dopamine metabolism primarily in the PFC (Gogos et al., 1998; Huotari et al., 2002), DAT is expressed predominantly in the striatum, where it plays a crucial role in modulating dopamine signaling (Lewis et al., 2001; Sesack, Hawrylak, Matus, Guido, & Levey, 1998; Wayment, Schenk, & Sorg, 2001). Thus polymorphisms resulting in relatively reduced levels of DAT would be expected to result in less efficient dopamine reuptake and, consequently, relatively heightened

reward system reactivity and reward-related behaviors.

A 40 base pair (bp) sequence is repeated a variable number of times within the 3'-untranslated region (UTR) of the *SLC6A3* gene, resulting in a variable number tandem repeat (VNTR) polymorphism (DAT1) characterized by alleles of lengths ranging from 3 to 13 repeats. Among those, the 9- and 10-repeat alleles occur most frequently in the majority of world populations studied (Doucette-Stamm, Blakely, Tian, Mockus, & Mao, 1995; Kang, Palmatier, & Kidd, 1999; Mitchell et al., 2000). Even though the 3'UTR is outside of the main coding sequence of the gene, polymorphisms within this region may affect gene expression and function through altering the gene's interaction with various transcription inhibitors and enhancers, as well as by altering posttranscriptional modifications. Although not all studies have found an effect of DAT1 40-bp VNTR genotype on DAT expression (Martinez et al., 2001; Mill, Asherson, Craig, & D'Souza, 2005), several studies have linked the 9-repeat allele to reduced DAT availability *in vitro* (Arinami, Gao, Hamaguchi, & Toru, 1997; VanNess, Owens, & Kilts, 2005) and *in vivo* (Cheon, Ryu, Kim, & Cho, 2005; Heinz et al., 2000), which would presumably lead to less efficient dopamine reuptake and heightened mesocorticostriatal system reactivity through increased synaptic dopamine. Consistent with this notion, individuals carrying at least one copy of the low expressing 9-repeat allele have been shown to have increased VS reactivity to positive feedback in a number-guessing fMRI paradigm, relative to individuals homozygous for the 10-repeat allele (Forbes et al., 2009). Importantly, relatively increased VS reactivity, as measured by the same paradigm, has in turn been linked to higher dispositional impulsivity and steeper delay discounting (Forbes et al., 2009; Hariri et al., 2006).

In addition to modulating reward circuitry reactivity, the DAT1 40-bp VNTR has also been found to regulate important aspects of the neural interface between motivational and cognitive control (Aarts et al., 2010). In order to assess the effects of reward-related brain function on cognitive flexibility, alongside the further modulatory role of the DAT1 genotype, a recent study utilized an attentional task-switching fMRI paradigm wherein successful (i.e., fast enough and correct) responses received variable monetary rewards, the magnitude of which was presented in the beginning of each trial in order to induce reward anticipation. Carriers of the DAT1 9-repeat allele exhibited greater influence of anticipated reward on behavioral task-switching costs as well as heightened dorsomedial striatum activity during task switching in anticipation of a high, relative to low, reward. These results not only demonstrate the broader range of modulatory effects of the DAT1 genotype on reward circuitry, but also provide evidence of the involvement of striatal dopamine signaling in regulating higher-order flexible cognitive control processes sensitive to changes in motivational state (Aarts et al., 2010).

Dopamine Receptors

In addition to enzymatic degradation and reuptake mechanisms, dopamine signaling is also critically dependent on the properties of dopamine receptors. There are two major classes of dopamine receptors: D1-like receptors, which have primarily excitatory functions and include dopamine receptors D1 and D5; and D2-like receptors, which are primarily inhibitory and include dopamine receptors D2, D3, and D4 (Beaulieu & Gainetdinov, 2011). In light of these receptor properties, genetic variants associated with increased expression or function of D1-like or decreased expression or function of D2-like receptors would be expected to result in increased dopamine signaling. Receptors from the D2-like class have been studied more extensively in relation to both behavioral and neural phenotypes related to reward processing as well as to the molecular, cellular, neural, and behavioral effects of common polymorphisms in genes coding for these receptors. Thus, we focus on this class of dopamine receptors in our review.

Dopamine Receptor D2 (DRD2)

Dopamine D2 receptors, encoded by the DRD2 gene, are most densely expressed in the VS, where they are located both pre- and postsynaptically (Beaulieu & Gainetdinov, 2011). These receptors exist in two distinct isoforms, short (D2S) and long (D2L), which are expressed primarily pre- and postsynaptically, respectively (Giros et al., 1989; Monsma, McVittie, Gerfen, Mahan, & Sibley, 1989). The presynaptic D2S functions as an autoreceptor and is part of a negative feedback regulatory mechanism of dopamine signaling, whereas D2L mediates postsynaptic inhibition. Genetic knockout studies have shown that D2L may also act synergistically with the excitatory D1 receptor (Usiello et al., 2000). In light of evidence showing co-localization of D2 and D1 receptors on the same striatal neurons (Aizman et al., 2000; Surmeier, Song, & Yan, 1996), the observed synergism may result from intracellular mechanisms that allow for the interaction and cross-regulation of D1- and D2-activated signal transduction pathways.

Due to the multifaceted functionality and widespread expression of D2 receptors, human *in vivo* imaging studies have typically not afforded the capability to determine with sufficient certainty the *DRD2* isoform expressed as well as the specific cellular population that mediates any effects of *DRD2* on striatal functioning. Because of these limitations, imaging genetics studies into the effects of *DRD2* genetic variants on striatal function have sometimes yielded conflicting results. Nonetheless, useful insights can be gleaned from the sizeable body of research investigating these effects.

Consistent with the inhibitory effect of D2 receptor signaling on dopamine neurotransmission, some imaging genetics studies have linked polymorphisms resulting in relatively reduced *DRD2* expression to heightened VS reactivity. Specifically, the Deletion (Del) allele of a one-point insertion/deletion polymorphism (rs1799732) occurring within the 5'-UTR of *DRD2*, frequently termed *DRD2*-141C Ins/Del, has been associated with up to 78% reduction in striatal *DRD2* expression *in vitro* (Arinami et al., 1997) and increased VS reactivity to positive feedback in the same number-guessing BOLD fMRI paradigm that has linked the DAT1 9-repeat allele to increased reward-related reactivity (Forbes et al., 2009).

Another commonly studied *DRD2* polymorphism is the Taq1A (rs1800497), which is located in the adjacent ankyrin repeat and kinase domain containing one (*ANKK1*) gene and probably affects *DRD2* function only indirectly. Its two alleles, T (A1) and C (A2), have been linked to relatively decreased and increased D2 receptor availability, respectively (Jonsson et al., 1999; Pohjalainen et al., 1998). The C allele has been associated with increased striatal glucose metabolism (Noble, Gottschalk, Fallon, Ritchie, & Wu, 1997) and reactivity to reward (Stice, Spoor, Bohon, & Small, 2008). This pattern may reflect a specific effect of the *DRD2* Taq1A on postsynaptic D2 receptors localized on inhibitory gamma-aminobutyric acid (GABA) interneurons, which modulate striatal function by inhibiting glutamatergic medium spiny neurons. Thus, the C allele may result in increased dopamine-mediated inhibition of GABAergic interneurons, leading to disinhibition of excitatory medium spiny neurons and thus, ultimately, increased VS reactivity measured with fMRI. Alternatively, recent studies suggest that the *DRD2* Taq1A polymorphism may not itself affect dopamine signaling but rather "tag" (i.e., be physically linked to) two *DRD2* SNPs associated with differential expression of the D2S and D2L isoforms (Moyer et al., 2011; Zhang et al., 2007).

Interestingly, an imaging genetics study has shown that one of these SNPs (rs1076560) tagged by the Taq1A moderates the effects of striatal dopamine on PFC-mediated cognitive function (Bertolino et al., 2010). Specifically, the study demonstrated that participants homozygous for the more common G allele exhibited a positive relationship between PFC activation during a working memory task and striatal dopamine signaling, as indexed by a factor score taking into account the combined effects of D2S and D2L. Participants carrying one copy of the less common allele showed the opposite pattern, whereby higher striatal signaling was associated with reduced working memory–related PFC activation (Bertolino et al., 2010). As the authors themselves point out, the interpretation of these results on the circuit and systems level is compounded by the poor resolution of the imaging methodology they used (single-photon emission computed tomography; SPECT) and the intrinsic inability of any currently available human *in vivo* neuroimaging tools to discriminate between cellular populations. Although future studies com-

bining nonhuman animal model research with human neuroimaging are necessary to offer a precise neuroanatomical and physiological interpretation of these findings, these results indicate that D2 receptors are critical regulators of striatal dopamine and play an important role not only in reward processing, but also in broader cognitive processes.

Dopamine Receptor D4 *(DRD4)*

Similarly to the D2 receptor, the dopamine D4 receptor, encoded by the *DRD4* gene, mediates both autoreceptor regulation and postsynaptic inhibition of dopamine signaling. Unlike *DRD2*, however, *DRD4* exhibits relatively low expression in the striatum (Jaber, Robinson, Missale, & Caron, 1996) and the lowest expression levels in the brain of all dopamine receptors (Beaulieu & Gainetdinov, 2011; Rondou, Haegeman, & Van Craenenbroeck, 2010). Nonetheless, preliminary data suggest that the D4 receptor is expressed postsynaptically on striatal neurons, as well as presynaptically on glutamatergic afferents from the PFC to the striatum (Jaber et al., 1996; Missale, Nash, Robinson, Jaber, & Caron, 1998; Tarazi, Campbell, Yeghiayan, & Baldessarini, 1998). Thus, D4 receptor stimulation can inhibit striatal function either directly or indirectly, via one or both of these independent mechanisms. Based on these localization data, genetic variants associated with higher levels of D4 function are likely to result in greater dopamine-mediated inhibition of postsynaptic target neurons and reduced striatal reactivity.

A common 48-bp VNTR within exon 3 of *DRD4* results in alleles of different length (ranging from 2 to 11 repeats), associated with differential gene transcription and protein function (Asghari et al., 1995). Specifically, the 7-repeat allele has been linked to reduced D4 receptor sensitivity and reduced postsynaptic inhibition (Asghari et al., 1995). Consistent with the inhibitory role of D4 receptors on striatal dopamine, the 7-repeat allele has also been linked to higher VS reactivity to positive feedback (Forbes et al., 2009). Finally, in line with its putative neurochemical effects, the same allele has been associated with increased approach to reward on the behavioral level (Roussos, Giakoumaki, & Bitsios, 2010). Taken together, these findings demonstrate that, despite its relatively low expression levels in the striatum, *DRD4* plays an important role in regulating the reactivity of the mesocorticostriatal system and the behaviors associated therewith.

Summary and Future Directions

In recent years, the field of imaging genetics has effectively combined molecular genetics and neuroimaging tools to map genetically driven variability in brain chemistry onto individual differences in brain function and behavior (Hariri, 2009). Among imaging genetics studies of cognition and emotion, a sizeable body of research has been dedicated to uncovering the neurogenetic correlates of reward-related behaviors. The research on the neural basis of reward processing has widely relied upon biologically informed hypotheses regarding the role of dopamine on reward-related neural processes, formulated on the basis of findings from animal neurophysiology or laboratory *in vitro* studies (e.g., Arinami et al., 1997; Wang et al., 2004). Although there are notable exceptions, genetic variants resulting in increased dopamine signaling, either through relatively increased excitatory receptor function, reduced postsynaptic inhibition, or decreased enzymatic degradation or synaptic clearance, have generally been predicted, and found to, result in enhanced reward-related brain function and behavioral phenotypes consistent with increased reward sensitivity (Forbes et al., 2009; Nikolova, Ferrell, Manuck, & Hariri, 2011). Conversely, variants associated with reduced dopamine signaling generally correlate with a relative reduction in reward-related brain function and behaviors associated therewith.

The principles illustrated by the studies reviewed above can, and have been, widely applied to other neural and behavioral phenotypes pertaining to cognition and emotion. For example, genetic variants associated with increased serotonin (5-hydroxytryptamine [5-HT]) signaling have been linked to heightened amygdala reactivity to threat; a neural phenotype

robustly associated with trait anxiety; as well as the risk for, and pathophysiology of, mood and anxiety disorders (Fakra et al., 2009; Hariri et al., 2002). A genetic variant affecting the enzyme fatty acid amide hydroxylase (*FAAH* 385A, rs324420) and presumably resulting in increased endocannabinoid neurotransmission has been associated with decreased threat- but increased reward-related brain reactivity (Hariri et al., 2009), which is remarkably consistent with this polymorphism's association with risk for substance use disorders (Flanagan, Gerber, Cadet, Beutler, & Sipe, 2006; Sipe, Chiang, Gerber, Beutler, & Cravatt, 2002). Genetic variants associated with enhanced glutamate signaling have, independently or in interaction with genetic variants affecting other neurotransmitter systems, been linked to enhanced memory function (Jablensky et al., 2011; Tan et al., 2007). Importantly, and as evidenced by the above studies, the same neurotransmitter system frequently regulates more than one neural phenotype, and each neural phenotype is regulated by multiple neurotransmitter systems.

This multiplicity of effects across neurotransmitters and phenotypes is complemented by a multiplicity of genetic variants within each neurotransmitter system that can affect each individual phenotype. Although most genetic studies of reward processing conducted to date and surveyed herein focus on single genes or polymorphisms, like other complex behavioral phenomena, reward processing is shaped by a multitude of genetic influences, which act in concert to create specific neural and, ultimately, behavioral phenotypes. Although several studies have investigated epistatic interactions between two genetic loci and their effects on reward-related neural processes (Dreher et al., 2009; Yacubian et al., 2007), reward-related brain function is likely to be shaped by the simultaneous impact of many more genetic variants. In support of this notion, a recent study has demonstrated that a biologically founded genetic profile for dopamine signaling, based on five of the polymorphic loci reviewed herein (*COMT* Val[158]Met, DAT1 40-bp VNTR, *DRD4* 48-bp VNTR, *DRD2*-141C Ins/Del, and *DRD2* Taq1A), explains nearly 11% of variability in VS reactivity, whereas none of the loci taken individually explains any VS reactivity variance, after appropriate correction for multiple testing (Nikolova et al., 2011). This finding underscores the importance of taking the simultaneous impact of multiple loci into account when investigating the genetic correlates of complex neural and behavioral phenotypes.

Similar multilocus genetic profile approaches, especially if refined to include differential weights for polymorphisms of different effect sizes and interactions among different loci, as well as between loci and environmental factors, could greatly increase our power to detect smaller genetic effects on reward-related brain function, especially in larger samples. The identification of new functional polymorphic loci alongside the expansion of these profiling approaches to other neurotransmitter systems and neural phenotypes, together with the growing sophistication of neuroimaging techniques, holds promise to foster an increasingly nuanced understanding of how individual differences in brain function give rise to the vast interindividual variability in behavior and psychopathology risk.

In addition to providing insight into the origins of interindividual variability in neural and behavioral phenomena pertaining to cognition and emotion, genetics approaches are also likely to foster an improved mechanistic understanding of the basic biological underpinnings of these phenomena across individuals. Polymorphisms with effects specific to a neural region or function can be leveraged to allow for genetic dissection of the component processes of these complex phenotypes. For example, *COMT* Val158Met and DAT1 40-bp VNTR can be used to model the differential effects of dopamine on top-down and bottom-up components of reward processing, respectively. *COMT* Val158Met affects dopamine signaling directly only in the PFC, where dopamine transmission plays a central role in regulating top-down cognitive control processes. Accordingly, *COMT* Val158Met appears to be preferentially involved in the cognitive modulation of reward processing. Specifically, studies have shown that, unlike polymorphisms affecting striatal dopamine directly, *COMT* Val158Met genotype moderates the ability to flexibly adapt reward-based learning in the context of changing reward contingencies (Frank, Moustafa, Haughey, Curran, & Hutchison, 2007). The DAT1 40-bp VNTR, on the other hand, has specific effects on dopamine transmission only in the striatum and is thus likely to be more directly involved in regulating bottom-up emotional drive. Not surprisingly, the DAT1 40-bp VNTR has been shown to regulate VS reactivity patterns, which correlate with trait impulsivity and delay discounting (Forbes et al., 2009), but has not been linked directly to the cognitive modulation of these phenomena.

It is worth noting, however, that much like the effects of prefrontal and striatal dopamine signaling on reward processing, the dopamine transmission and reward processing effects attributable to *COMT* Val158Met and DAT1 40-bp VNTR are not completely dissociable. In fact, as reviewed earlier in the chapter, *COMT* Val158Met has been associated with differences in striatal reactivity (Dreher et al., 2009; Yacubian et al., 2007) and DAT1 40-bp VNTR has the capacity to modulate the neural interface between motivational and cognitive control (Aarts et al., 2010). Nonetheless, the partial genetic dissociation of these component pathways of reward processing has fostered a better understanding of the precise molecular mechanisms that underlie this complex neural and behavioral phenomenon.

As exemplified by the study of dopaminergic regulation of neural circuits for reward, emergent neurogenetics approaches have begun to map genetically driven variability in brain chemistry onto variability in brain function and, ultimately, behavioral traits, yielding insights into the origins of diversity in human behavior. Genes regulating various neurotransmitters have been implicated in numerous cognitive and affective functions, with multiple variants within these genes affecting variability in these same neural and behavioral phenotypes. In addition to facilitating progress into mechanisms of interindividual variability in behaviorally relevant brain function, neurogenetics approaches hold promise to further advance the treatment and possible prevention of psychopathology by identifying individual trajectories of risk that represent novel therapeutic targets.

References

Aarts, E., Roelofs, A., Franke, B., Rijpkema, M., Fernandez, G., Helmich, R. C., et al. (2010). Striatal dopamine mediates the interface between motivational and cognitive control in humans: evidence from genetic imaging. *Neuropsychopharmacology, 35*, 1943–1951.

Aizman, O., Brismar, H., Uhlen, P., Zettergren, E., Levey, A. I., Forssberg, H., et al. (2000). Anatomical and physiological evidence for D1 and D2 dopamine receptor colocalization in neostriatal neurons. *Nature Neuroscience, 3*, 226–230.

Akil, M., Kolachana, B. S., Rothmond, D. A., Hyde, T. M., Weinberger, D. R., & Kleinman, J. E. (2003). Catechol-O-methyltransferase genotype and dopamine regulation in the human brain. *Journal of Neuroscience, 23*, 2008–2013.

Apud, J. A., Mattay, V., Chen, J., Kolachana, B. S., Callicott, J. H., Rasetti, R., et al. (2007). Tolcapone improves cognition and cortical information processing in normal human subjects. *Neuropsychopharmacology, 32*, 1011–1020.

Arinami, T., Gao, M., Hamaguchi, H., & Toru, M. (1997). A functional polymorphism in the promoter region of the dopamine D2 receptor gene is associated with schizophrenia. *Human Molecular Genetics, 6*, 577–582.

Arnsten, A. F., Cai, J. X., Murphy, B. L., & Goldman-Rakic, P. S. (1994). Dopamine D1 receptor mechanisms in the cognitive performance of young adult and aged monkeys. *Psychopharmacology, 116*, 143–151.

Asghari, V., Sanyal, S., Buchwaldt, S., Paterson, A., Jovanovic, V., & Van Tol, H. H. (1995). Modulation of intracellular cyclic AMP levels by different human dopamine D4 receptor variants. *Journal of Neurochemistry, 65*, 1157–1165.

Balleine, B. W., & Dickinson, A. (1998). Goal-directed instrumental action: Contingency and incentive learning and their cortical substrates. *Neuropharmacology, 37*(4–5), 407–419.

Beaulieu, J. M., & Gainetdinov, R. R. (2011). The physiology, signaling, and pharmacology of dopamine receptors. *Pharmacological Reviews, 63*, 182–217.

Berridge, K. C., Robinson, T. E., & Aldridge, J. W. (2009). Dissecting components of reward: "Liking," "wanting," and learning. *Current Opinion in Pharmacology, 9*, 65–73.

Bertolino, A., Taurisano, P., Pisciotta, N. M., Blasi, G., Fazio, L., Romano, R., et al. (2010). Genetically determined measures of striatal D2 signaling predict prefrontal activity during working memory performance. *PLoS One, 5*, e9348.

Bigos, K. L., Pollock, B. G., Aizenstein, H. J., Fisher, P. M., Bies, R. R., & Hariri, A. R. (2008). Acute 5–HT reuptake blockade potentiates human amygdala reactivity. *Neuropsychopharmacology, 33*, 3221–3225.

Bigos, K. L., & Weinberger, D. R. (2010). Imaging genetics: Days of future past. *NeuroImage, 53*, 804–809.

Bilder, R. M., Volavka, J., Lachman, H. M., & Grace, A. A. (2004). The catechol-O-methyltransferase polymorphism: Relations to the tonic–phasic dopamine hypothesis and neuropsychiatric phenotypes. *Neuropsychopharmacology, 29*, 1943–1961.

Bjorklund, A., & Dunnett, S. B. (2007). Dopamine neuron systems in the brain: An update. *Trends in Neuroscience, 30*(5), 194–202.

Bogdan, R., & Pizzagalli, D. A. (2009). The heritability of hedonic capacity and perceived stress: A twin study evaluation of candidate depressive phenotypes. *Psychological Medicine, 39*, 211–218.

Brozoski, T. J., Brown, R. M., Rosvold, H. E., & Goldman, P. S. (1979). Cognitive deficit caused by regional depletion of dopamine in prefrontal cortex of rhesus monkey. *Science, 205*, 929–932.

Camara, E., Kramer, U. M., Cunillera, T., Marco-Pallares, J., Cucurell, D., Nager, W., et al. (2010). The effects of *COMT* (Val[108]/[158]Met) and *DRD4* (SNP-521) dopamine genotypes on brain activations related to valence and magnitude of rewards. *Cerebral Cortex, 20*, 1985–1996.

Caspi, A., Moffitt, T. E., Cannon, M., McClay, J., Murray, R., Harrington, H., et al. (2005). Moderation of the effect of adolescent-onset cannabis use on adult psychosis by a functional polymorphism in the catechol-O-methyltransferase gene: Longitudinal evidence of a gene × environment interaction. *Biological Psychiatry, 57*, 1117–1127.

Chen, J., Lipska, B. K., Halim, N., Ma, Q. D., Matsumoto, M., Melhem, S., et al. (2004). Functional analysis of genetic variation in catechol-O-methyltransferase (COMT): Effects on mRNA, protein, and enzyme activity in postmortem human brain. *American Journal of Human Genetics, 75*, 807–821.

Cheon, K. A., Ryu, Y. H., Kim, J. W., & Cho, D. Y. (2005). The homozygosity for 10–repeat allele at dopamine transporter gene and dopamine transporter density in Korean children with attention deficit hyperactivity disorder: Relating treatment response to methylphenidate. *European Neuropsychopharmacology, 15,* 95–101.

Cools, R. (2008). Role of dopamine in the motivational and cognitive control of behavior. *Neuroscientist, 14,* 381–395.

Dickinson, D., & Elvevag, B. (2009). Genes, cognition and brain through a COMT lens. *Neuroscience, 164,* 72–87.

Dolan, R. J. (2002). Emotion, cognition, and behavior. *Science, 298,* 1191–1194.

Doucette-Stamm, L. A., Blakely, D. J., Tian, J., Mockus, S., & Mao, J. I. (1995). Population genetic study of the human dopamine transporter gene (DAT1). *Genetic Epidemiology, 12,* 303–308.

Dreher, J. C., Kohn, P., Kolachana, B., Weinberger, D. R., & Berman, K. F. (2009). Variation in dopamine genes influences responsivity of the human reward system. *Proceedings of the National Academy of Sciences of the United States of America, 106,* 617–622.

Egan, M. F., Goldberg, T. E., Kolachana, B. S., Callicott, J. H., Mazzanti, C. M., Straub, R. E., et al. (2001). Effect of COMT Val^{108}/^{158}Met genotype on frontal lobe function and risk for schizophrenia. *Proceedings of the National Academy of Sciences of the United States of America, 98,* 6917–6922.

Fakra, E., Hyde, L. W., Gorka, A., Fisher, P. M., Munoz, K. E., Kimak, M., et al. (2009). Effects of HTR1A C(-1019)G on amygdala reactivity and trait anxiety. *Archives of General Psychiatry, 66,* 33–40.

Fisher, P. M., Meltzer, C. C., Price, J. C., Coleman, R. L., Ziolko, S. K., Becker, C., et al. (2009). Medial prefrontal cortex 5-HT(2A) density is correlated with amygdala reactivity, response habituation, and functional coupling. *Cerebral Cortex, 19,* 2499–2507.

Flanagan, J. M., Gerber, A. L., Cadet, J. L., Beutler, E., & Sipe, J. C. (2006). The fatty acid amide hydrolase 385 A/A (P129T) variant: Haplotype analysis of an ancient missense mutation and validation of risk for drug addiction. *Human Genetics, 120,* 581–588.

Forbes, E. E., Brown, S. M., Kimak, M., Ferrell, R. E., Manuck, S. B., & Hariri, A. R. (2009). Genetic variation in components of dopamine neurotransmission impacts ventral striatal reactivity associated with impulsivity. *Molecular Psychiatry, 14,* 60–70.

Frank, M. J., Moustafa, A. A., Haughey, H. M., Curran, T., & Hutchison, K. E. (2007). Genetic triple dissociation reveals multiple roles for dopamine in reinforcement learning. *Proceedings of the National Academy of Sciences of the United States of America, 104,* 16311–16316.

Giros, B., Sokoloff, P., Martres, M. P., Riou, J. F., Emorine, L. J., & Schwartz, J. C. (1989). Alternative splicing directs the expression of two D2 dopamine receptor isoforms. *Nature, 342,* 923–926.

Gogos, J. A., Morgan, M., Luine, V., Santha, M., Ogawa, S., Pfaff, D., et al. (1998). Catechol-O-methyltransferase-deficient mice exhibit sexually dimorphic changes in catecholamine levels and behavior. *Proceedings of the National Academy of Sciences of the United States of America, 95,* 9991–9996.

Grace, A. A. (1991). Phasic versus tonic dopamine release and the modulation of dopamine system responsivity: A hypothesis for the etiology of schizophrenia. *Neuroscience, 41,* 1–24.

Gray, J. R., Braver, T. S., & Raichle, M. E. (2002). Integration of emotion and cognition in the lateral prefrontal cortex. *Proceedings of the National Academy of Sciences of the United States of America, 99,* 4115–4120.

Haber, S. N., & Knutson, B. (2010). The reward circuit: Linking primate anatomy and human imaging. *Neuropsychopharmacology, 35,* 4–26.

Hariri, A. R. (2009). The neurobiology of individual differences in complex behavioral traits. *Annual Review of Neuroscience, 32,* 225–247.

Hariri, A. R., Brown, S. M., Williamson, D. E., Flory, J. D., de Wit, H., & Manuck, S. B. (2006). Preference for immediate over delayed rewards is associated with magnitude of ventral striatal activity. *Journal of Neuroscience, 26,* 13213–13217.

Hariri, A. R., Gorka, A., Hyde, L. W., Kimak, M., Halder, I., Ducci, F., et al. (2009). Divergent effects of genetic variation in endocannabinoid signaling on human threat- and reward-related brain function. *Biological Psychiatry, 66,* 9–16.

Hariri, A. R., Mattay, V. S., Tessitore, A., Kolachana, B., Fera, F., Goldman, D., et al. (2002). Serotonin transporter genetic variation and the response of the human amygdala. *Science, 297,* 400–403.

Heinz, A., Goldman, D., Jones, D. W., Palmour, R., Hommer, D., Gorey, J. G., et al. (2000). Genotype influences *in vivo* dopamine transporter availability in human striatum. *Neuropsychopharmacology, 22,* 133–139.

Hernandez, L., & Hoebel, B. G. (1988). Food reward and cocaine increase extracellular dopamine in the nucleus accumbens as measured by microdialysis. *Life Sciences, 42,* 1705–1712.

Huotari, M., Gogos, J. A., Karayiorgou, M., Koponen, O., Forsberg, M., Raasmaja, A., et al. (2002). Brain catecholamine metabolism in catechol-O-methyltransferase (COMT)-deficient mice. *European Journal of Neuroscience, 15,* 246–256.

Jaber, M., Robinson, S. W., Missale, C., & Caron, M. G. (1996). Dopamine receptors and brain function. *Neuropharmacology, 35,* 1503–1519.

Jablensky, A., Morar, B., Wiltshire, S., Carter, K., Dragovic, M., Badcock, J. C., et al. (2011). Polymorphisms associated with normal memory variation also affect memory impairment in schizophrenia. *Genes, Brain, and Behavior, 10,* 410–417.

Jonsson, E. G., Nothen, M. M., Grunhage, F., Farde, L., Nakashima, Y., Propping, P., et al. (1999). Polymorphisms in the dopamine D2 receptor gene and their relationships to striatal dopamine receptor density of healthy volunteers. *Molecular Psychiatry, 4,* 290–296.

Kang, A. M., Palmatier, M. A., & Kidd, K. K. (1999). Global variation of a 40–bp VNTR in the 3'-untranslated region of the dopamine transporter gene (SLC6A3). *Biological Psychiatry, 46,* 151–160.

Kendler, K. S., Myers, J. M., Maes, H. H., & Keyes, C. L. (2011). The relationship between the genetic and environmental influences on common internalizing psychiatric disorders and mental well-being. *Behavior Genetics, 41*(5), 641–650.

Kim, J. H., Son, Y. D., Kim, H. K., Lee, S. Y., Cho, S. E., Kim, Y. B., et al. (2011). Association of harm avoidance with dopamine D(2/3) receptor availability in striatal subdivisions: A high resolution PET study. *Biological Psychology, 87,* 164–167.

Kimberg, D. Y., & D'Esposito, M. (2003). Cognitive effects of the dopamine receptor agonist pergolide. *Neuropsychologia, 41,* 1020–1027.

Krugel, L. K., Biele, G., Mohr, P. N., Li, S. C., & Heekeren, H. R. (2009). Genetic variation in dopaminergic neuromodulation influences the ability to rapidly and flexibly adapt decisions. *Proceedings of the National Academy of Sciences of the United States of America, 106,* 17951–17956.

Lawrence, A. D., Sahakian, B. J., & Robbins, T. W. (1998). Cognitive functions and corticostriatal circuits: Insights from Huntington's disease. *Trends in Cognitive Science, 2*(10), 379–388.

LeDoux, J. E. (2000). Emotion circuits in the brain. *Annual Review of Neuroscience, 23,* 155–184.

Lewis, D. A., Melchitzky, D. S., Sesack, S. R., Whitehead, R. E., Auh, S., & Sampson, A. (2001). Dopamine transporter immunoreactivity in monkey cerebral cortex: Regional, laminar, and ultrastructural localization. *Journal of Comparative Neurology, 432,* 119–136.

Lotta, T., Vidgren, J., Tilgmann, C., Ulmanen, I., Melen, K., Julkunen, I., et al. (1995). Kinetics of human soluble and membrane-bound catechol-O-methyltransferase: A revised mechanism and description of the thermolabile variant of the enzyme. *Biochemistry, 34,* 4202–4210.

Luciana, M., Depue, R. A., Arbisi, P., & Leon, A. (1992). Facilitation of working memory in humans by a D2-dopamine receptor agonist. *Journal of Cognitive Neuroscience, 4,* 58–68.

Marchand, W. R., & Yurgelun-Todd, D. (2010). Striatal structure and function in mood disorders: A comprehensive review. *Bipolar Disorder, 12*(8), 764–785.

Marco-Pallares, J., Cucurell, D., Cunillera, T., Kramer, U. M., Camara, E., Nager, W., et al. (2009). Genetic variability in the dopamine system (dopamine receptor D4, catechol-O-methyltransferase) modulates neurophysiological responses to gains and losses. *Biological Psychiatry, 66,* 154–161.

Martinez, D., Gelernter, J., Abi-Dargham, A., van Dyck, C. H., Kegeles, L., Innis, R. B., et al. (2001). The variable number of tandem repeats polymorphism of the dopamine transporter gene is not associated with significant change in dopamine transporter phenotype in humans. *Neuropsychopharmacology, 24,* 553–560.

Matsumoto, M., Weickert, C. S., Akil, M., Lipska, B. K., Hyde, T. M., Herman, M. M., et al. (2003). Catechol-O-methyltransferase mRNA expression in human and rat brain: Evidence for a role in cortical neuronal function. *Neuroscience, 116,* 127–137.

McGue, M., & Christensen, K. (2001). The heritability of cognitive functioning in very old adults: Evidence from Danish twins aged 75 years and older. *Psychology and Aging, 16,* 272–280.

McGuffin, P., Farmer, A. E., Gottesman, I. I., Murray, R. M., & Reveley, A. M. (1984). Twin concordance for operationally defined schizophrenia: Confirmation of familiality and heritability. *Archives of General Psychiatry, 41,* 541–545.

Meyer-Lindenberg, A. (2010). Imaging genetics of schizophrenia. *Dialogues in Clinical Neuroscience, 12,* 449–456.

Meyer-Lindenberg, A., Kohn, P. D., Kolachana, B., Kippenhan, S., McInerney-Leo, A., Nussbaum, R., et al. (2005). Midbrain dopamine and prefrontal function in humans: Interaction and modulation by COMT genotype. *Nature Neuroscience, 8,* 594–596.

Mill, J., Asherson, P., Craig, I., & D'Souza, U. M. (2005). Transient expression analysis of allelic variants of a VNTR in the dopamine transporter gene (DAT1). *BMC Genetics, 6,* 3.

Miller, E. K. (2000). The prefrontal cortex and cognitive control. *Nature Reviews Neuroscience, 1*(1), 59–65.

Missale, C., Nash, S. R., Robinson, S. W., Jaber, M., & Caron, M. G. (1998). Dopamine receptors: From structure to function. *Physiological Reviews, 78,* 189–225.

Mitchell, R. J., Howlett, S., Earl, L., White, N. G., McComb, J., Schanfield, M. S., et al. (2000). Distribution of the 3' VNTR polymorphism in the human dopamine transporter gene in world populations. *Human Biology, 72,* 295–304.

Monsma, F. J., Jr., McVittie, L. D., Gerfen, C. R., Mahan, L. C., & Sibley, D. R. (1989). Multiple D2 dopamine receptors produced by alternative RNA splicing. *Nature, 342,* 926–929.

Moyer, R. A., Wang, D., Papp, A. C., Smith, R. M., Duque, L., Mash, D. C., et al. (2011). Intronic polymorphisms affecting alternative splicing of human dopamine D2 receptor are associated with cocaine abuse. *Neuropsychopharmacology, 36,* 753–762.

Nieoullon, A. (2002). Dopamine and the regulation of cognition and attention. *Progress in Neurobiology, 67,* 53–83.

Nikolova, Y. S., Ferrell, R. E., Manuck, S. B., & Hariri, A. R. (2011). Multilocus genetic profile for dopamine signaling predicts ventral striatum reactivity. *Neuropsychopharmacology, 36*(9), 1940–1947.

Noble, E. P., Gottschalk, L. A., Fallon, J. H., Ritchie, T. L., & Wu, J. C. (1997). D2 dopamine receptor polymorphism and brain regional glucose metabolism. *American Journal of Medical Genetics, 74,* 162–166.

Paloyelis, Y., Asherson, P., Mehta, M. A., Faraone, S. V., & Kuntsi, J. (2010). DAT1 and COMT effects on delay discounting and trait impulsivity in male adolescents with attention deficit/hyperactivity disorder and healthy controls. *Neuropsychopharmacology, 35,* 2414–2426.

Petry, N. M., & Casarella, T. (1999). Excessive discounting of delayed rewards in substance abusers with gambling problems. *Drug and Alcohol Dependence, 56,* 25–32.

Phelps, E. A. (2006). Emotion and cognition: Insights from studies of the human amygdala. *Annual Review of Psychology, 57,* 27–53.

Pohjalainen, T., Rinne, J. O., Nagren, K., Lehikoinen, P., Anttila, K., Syvalahti, E. K., et al. (1998). The A1 allele of the human D2 dopamine receptor gene predicts low D2 receptor availability in healthy volunteers. *Molecular Psychiatry, 3,* 256–260.

Rondou, P., Haegeman, G., & Van Craenenbroeck, K. (2010). The dopamine D4 receptor: Biochemical and signalling properties. *Cellular and Molecular Life Sciences, 67,* 1971–1986.

Roussos, P., Giakoumaki, S. G., & Bitsios, P. (2010). Cognitive and emotional processing associated with the season of birth and dopamine D4 receptor gene. *Neuropsychologia, 48,* 3926–3933.

Salvadore, G., Nugent, A. C., Chen, G., Akula, N., Yuan, P., Cannon, D. M., et al. (2009). Bcl-2 polymorphism influences gray matter volume in the ventral striatum in healthy humans. *Biological Psychiatry, 66*(8), 804–807.

Santesso, D. L., Evins, A. E., Frank, M. J., Schetter, E. C., Bogdan, R., & Pizzagalli, D. A. (2009). Single dose of a dopamine agonist impairs reinforcement learning in humans: Evidence from event-related potentials and computational modeling of striatal–cortical function. *Human Brain Mapping, 30,* 1963–1976.

Savitz, J., Solms, M., & Ramesar, R. (2006). The molecular genetics of cognition: Dopamine, COMT and BDNF. *Genes, Brain, and Behavior, 5,* 311–328.

Schultz, W. (2002). Getting formal with dopamine and reward. *Neuron, 36,* 241–263.

Sesack, S. R., Hawrylak, V. A., Matus, C., Guido, M. A., & Levey, A. I. (1998). Dopamine axon varicosities in the prelimbic division of the rat prefrontal cortex exhibit sparse immunoreactivity for the dopamine transporter. *Journal of Neuroscience, 18,* 2697–2708.

Sipe, J. C., Chiang, K., Gerber, A. L., Beutler, E., & Cravatt, B. F. (2002). A missense mutation in human fatty acid amide hydrolase associated with problem drug use. *Proceedings of the National Academy of Sciences of the United States of America, 99,* 8394–8399.

Steele, J. D., Kumar, P., & Ebmeier, K. P. (2007). Blunted response to feedback information in depressive illness. *Brain, 130,* 2367–2374.

Stice, E., Spoor, S., Bohon, C., & Small, D. M. (2008). Relation between obesity and blunted striatal response to food is moderated by TaqIA A1 allele. *Science, 322,* 449–452.

Surmeier, D. J., Song, W. J., & Yan, Z. (1996). Coordinated expression of dopamine receptors in neostriatal medium spiny neurons. *Journal of Neuroscience, 16,* 6579–6591.

Tan, H. Y., Callicott, J. H., & Weinberger, D. R. (2009). Prefrontal cognitive systems in schizophrenia: Towards human genetic brain mechanisms. *Cognitive Neuropsychiatry, 14,* 277–298.

Tan, H. Y., Chen, Q., Sust, S., Buckholtz, J. W., Meyers, J. D., Egan, M. F., et al. (2007). Epistasis between catechol-O-methyltransferase and type II metabotropic glutamate receptor 3 genes on working memory brain function. *Proceedings of the National Academy of Sciences of the United States of America, 104,* 12536–12541.

Tarazi, F. I., Campbell, A., Yeghiayan, S. K., & Baldessarini, R. J. (1998). Localization of dopamine receptor subtypes in corpus striatum and nucleus accumbens septi of rat brain: Comparison of D1-, D2-, and D4-like receptors. *Neuroscience, 83,* 169–176.

Tunbridge, E. M., Bannerman, D. M., Sharp, T., & Harrison, P. J. (2004). Catechol-O-methyltransferase inhibition improves set-shifting performance and elevates stimulated dopamine release in the rat prefrontal cortex. *Journal of Neuroscience, 24,* 5331–5335.

Usiello, A., Baik, J. H., Rouge-Pont, F., Picetti, R., Dierich, A., LeMeur, M., et al. (2000). Distinct functions of the two isoforms of dopamine D2 receptors. *Nature, 408,* 199–203.

VanNess, S. H., Owens, M. J., & Kilts, C. D. (2005). The variable number of tandem repeats element in DAT1 regulates *in vitro* dopamine transporter density. *BMC Genetics, 6,* 55.

Wang, E., Ding, Y. C., Flodman, P., Kidd, J. R., Kidd, K. K., Grady, D. L., et al. (2004). The genetic architecture of selection at the human dopamine receptor D4 *(DRD4)* gene locus. *American Journal of Human Genetics, 74,* 931–944.

Wayment, H. K., Schenk, J. O., & Sorg, B. A. (2001). Characterization of extracellular dopamine clearance in the medial prefrontal cortex: Role of monoamine uptake and monoamine oxidase inhibition. *Journal of Neuroscience, 21,* 35–44.

Yacubian, J., Sommer, T., Schroeder, K., Glascher, J., Kalisch, R., Leuenberger, B., et al. (2007). Gene–gene interaction associated with neural reward sensitivity. *Proceedings of the National Academy of Sciences of the United States of America, 104,* 8125–8130.

Yokel, R. A., & Wise, R. A. (1975). Increased lever pressing for amphetamine after pimozide in rats: Implications for a dopamine theory of reward. *Science, 187,* 547–549.

Zhang, Y., Bertolino, A., Fazio, L., Blasi, G., Rampino, A., Romano, R., et al. (2007). Polymorphisms in human dopamine D2 receptor gene affect gene expression, splicing, and neuronal activity during working memory. *Proceedings of the National Academy of Sciences of the United States of America, 104,* 20552–20557.

Interactions between Attention and Emotion

Insights from the Late Positive Potential

Anna Weinberg, Jamie Ferri, and Greg Hajcak

In the title of his now-famous essay from 1884, William James asked "What is an emotion?" Within the nascent field of psychology, James lamented, "the aesthetic sphere of the mind, its longings, its pleasures and pains, and its emotions, have been ignored" (p. 69). Yet, he wrote, "the emotional brain-processes not only resemble the ordinary . . . brain-processes, but in truth *are* nothing but such processes variously combined" (p. 69). Questions about the ways in which emotions may or may not be distinct from other cognitive processes—both philosophically and in terms of their physical instantiation—did not originate with James, of course, but began much earlier. For centuries, cool reason and untempered passion have been viewed as mutually antagonistic forces vying for control over human behaviors. However, though competition between ostensibly cognitive and emotional processes may exist, mutuality and interaction between the two may be far more common. In what follows, we discuss processes of competition and cooperation as they are reflected in the late positive potential (LPP), an event-related potential (ERP) component that indexes the sustained allocation of attention. There is increasing evidence that the LPP reflects the flexible and dynamic deployment of attention and, as such, represents an ideal vehicle for investigating interactions between emotional and cognitive processes.

Visual Attention and Emotion

At any given moment, the amount of information entering the human visual system far exceeds available processing resources (Anderson, Van Essen, & Olshausen, 2005; Driver, 2001; Parkhurst, Law, & Niebur, 2002; Rensink, O'Regan, & Clark, 1997; Treue, 2003). Only a small fraction of the information available in the visual field will be attended to, let alone encoded or remembered (Driver, 2001; Raichle, 2010; Rensink et al., 1997). In order to engage in the rapid and efficient selection process that determines which information is attended to, and which information falls by the wayside, the brain must have mechanisms in place to ensure that salient visual information is not lost (Driver, 2001; Vuilleumier, 2005).

Two major attentional mechanisms are thought to govern this selection process. Bottom-up, or exogenous, mechanisms of attention—which are presumed to be rapid and relatively obligatory—appear to be driven by the perceptual properties of visual stimuli (e.g., movement or color: Bacon & Egeth, 1994; Parkhurst et al., 2002; Theeuwes, 1994). Top-down, or endogenous, mechanisms are thought to reflect ongoing goals and intentions of the individual, and are relatively slower to capture or direct attention (Rock & Gutman, 1981; Tipper, Weaver, Jerreat, & Burak, 1994). However, the clear boundaries drawn between bottom-up and top-down processes may be more conceptually helpful than anatomically plausible. For example, despite the persistence of modular models of emotion that emphasize a predominance of limbic activity, recent evidence suggests an early and substantial role of the cortex in emotion processing (e.g., Pessoa & Adolphs, 2010). Likewise, emerging evidence suggests contributions from "emotional" limbic areas to top-down shifts in spatial attention (e.g., Mohanty, Egner, Monti, & Mesulam, 2009). As the field of cognitive neuroscience moves toward a more complex and nonhierarchical conceptualization of human neural activity that consists of ongoing, parallel, and iterative coactivation across multiple regions of the brain (Mesulam, 1998; Thielscher & Pessoa, 2007), evidence is emerging to suggest that top-down and bottom-up attentional processes act reciprocally and interactively (Mesulam, 1998; Mohanty et al., 2009; Pessoa, 2008, 2010; Pessoa & Adolphs, 2010; Raichle, 2010).

Emotional stimuli, or stimuli that relate to basic biological imperatives (e.g., to fight, flee, affiliate, feed, or mate), are prime examples of stimuli that appear to capture attention in a bottom-up fashion. Many have argued that, regardless of an individual's ongoing and idiosyncratic goals, emotional stimuli are *intrinsically* motivationally salient, not because of their perceptual properties, but because of their content (Bradley, Codispoti, Cuthbert, & Lang, 2001; Lang & Bradley, 2010; Lang, Bradley, & Cuthbert, 1998; Lang, Greenwald, Bradley, & Hamm, 1993; LeDoux, 1996). In other words, attention is commanded by motivational imperatives (Lang, Bradley, & Cuthbert, 1997). Consistent with this view, there is ample evidence that emotional stimuli are subject to prioritized processing. Compared to neutral stimuli, emotional cues are detected more easily (Fox et al., 2000; Öhman, Flykt, & Esteves, 2001), more effectively capture and hold attention (Lang et al., 1997; Mogg, Bradley, De Bono,

& Painter, 1997; Schupp et al., 2007; Vuilleumier, 2005), and are viewed for longer (Lang et al., 1993, 1997). Moreover, some have argued that the processing of emotional stimuli can occur independently of attention and awareness (e.g., Liu, Agam, Madsen, & Kreiman, 2009; Morris, DeGelder, Weiskrantz, & Dolan, 2001; Morris, Öhman, & Dolan, 1998; Whalen et al., 1998), suggesting some degree of automaticity.

However, the prioritization of attention to emotional stimuli may not always be adaptive. For example, task-irrelevant emotional stimuli can interfere with goal-directed behavior, slowing reaction times to target stimuli or decreasing accuracy (Blair et al., 2007; Buodo, Sarlo, & Palomba, 2002; MacNamara & Hajcak, 2009, 2010; Mitchell, Richell, Leonard, & Blair, 2006; Vuilleumier, Armony, Driver, & Dolan, 2001). Attention to task-irrelevant stimuli can even decrease the subsequent processing of task-relevant stimuli (Flaisch, Junghöfer, Bradley, Schupp, & Lang, 2008; Flaisch, Stockburger, & Schupp, 2008; Ihssen, Heim, & Keil, 2007; Most, Smith, Cooter, Levy, & Zald, 2007; Weinberg & Hajcak, 2011b).

In addition, though it may be prioritized, processing of emotional stimuli is not always obligatory or automatic (Bishop, Duncan, & Lawrence, 2004; Bishop, Jenkins, & Lawrence, 2007; Liberzon et al., 2000; Pessoa, McKenna, Gutierrez, & Ungerleider, 2002; Pessoa, Padmala, & Morland, 2005). Indeed, the impact of emotional stimuli depends critically on the availability of attentional resources. Engaging or challenging tasks that more effectively command attentional resources, for example, may interfere with the processing of emotional stimuli (Liberzon et al., 2000; MacNamara, Ferri, & Hajcak, 2011; Pessoa et al., 2002, 2005). Furthermore, emotional stimuli may be made more or less salient through manipulations of attention or by changing task demands (Beauregard, Levesque, & Bourgouin, 2001; Dunning & Hajcak, 2009; Hajcak & Nieuwenhuis, 2006; Lévesque et al., 2003; MacNamara, Foti, & Hajcak, 2009).

At the same time, top-down and bottom-up directives can work interactively to influence the allocation of attention—a topic that is a focus of this chapter. Furthermore, the competitive and cooperative nature of attention in the context of emotion unfolds over time, such that different directives may exert more or less influence over the time course of emotion processing. The study of these processes requires techniques with excellent temporal resolution that are capable of indexing dynamic processes.

In what follows, we discuss the ways in which ERPs may be modulated by emotional content. A comprehensive overview of ERP methodology is beyond the scope of this chapter, but briefly review the anatomical and electrical origins of ERP components and how they are suited to studies examining ongoing attentional deployment. The bulk of the chapter focuses on research related to the LPP, an ERP component that appears to reflect the confluence of bottom-up and top-down influences on sustained attention.

Anatomical Origins and Measurement of ERPs

The central nervous system runs on two main types of electrical activity: afferent action potentials and postsynaptic potentials (PSPs). When a neuron is activated by a neighboring cell, an action potential travels the length of the axon from the soma to the axon terminals, causing neurotransmitters to diffuse across the synaptic cleft. The binding of neurotransmitters to receptors on the postsynaptic cell generates an electrical potential: the PSP. Electrodes affixed to the scalp can record the rapidly fluctuating electrical activity evident in the ongoing electroencephalogram (EEG). ERPs reflect the activity of the EEG time-locked to specific events—such as the presentation of a stimulus or the generation of a motor response. These scalp-recorded ERPs are thought to reflect the summed activity of excitatory and inhibitory PSPs generated by large populations of pyramidal cortical neurons, which typically align such that they are parallel to one another and perpendicular to the cortical surface. The sustained duration of PSPs, along with the coherent orientation of the neurons, allows activity to summate and propagate to the surface of the scalp (Fabiani, Gratton, & Federmeier, 2007; Luck, 2005; Pizzagalli, 2007).

Because ERPs are bioelectrical signals conducted through the brain, meninges, skull, and scalp, they are subject to spread as the signal seeks paths of low resistance; precise identification of primary neural contributors is therefore often difficult. Furthermore, neural activity recorded from an electrode exterior to the skull reflects the simultaneous and summed activation of many, many thousands—even millions—of neurons (Luck, 2005). In addition, there is evidence that scalp-recorded ERPs can reflect large-scale neuronal synchronization across spatially distributed neuronal networks (e.g., see Pizzagalli, 2007 for more information). Nonetheless, mathematical solutions have been developed that are helpful in inferring neural sources of ERPs (reviewed in Pizzagalli, 2007). In short, the scalp-recorded ERP reflects the activity of a coordinated *network* of neurons, which in some instances may represent the activity of a single anatomical node, but which may also reflect dynamic exchanges between brain regions, as well as widespread neuromodulatory activity (de Rover et al., 2011; Hajcak, MacNamara, & Olvet, 2010). That is, it may be more fruitful to think about ERPs as indexing the activation of neural networks, rather than activity of a single and isolated region of the brain. Along these lines, ERP techniques may be ideal for measuring the activity of multiple areas working in concert, affording the ability to capture not just binary patterns of activation and rest, but also ongoing variation in neural activity as it unfolds over time (Hajcak, MacNamara, & Olvet, 2010; Hajcak, Weinberg, MacNamara, & Foti, 2012). Indeed, the speed of electrical conduction, which approaches the speed of light, affords an unparalleled level of temporal precision. Using ERPs, then, it may be possible to infer with great precision at what point in time bottom-up and top-down processes begin to exert their influence, and when and how these influences can be suppressive, additive, and interactive.

In terms of nomenclature and measurement, ERP components are commonly identified by their amplitude (measured in microvolts [μV]), polarity (positive or negative), latency (measured in milliseconds [ms]), and scalp topography (where on the scalp the component is maximal); at times, ERP components receive functionally descriptive names (e.g., the *error-related negativity* or *ERN*). *Amplitude* refers to the difference between activity occurring at some point following an event of interest and an average pre-event baseline period (e.g., 200 ms prior to stimulus onset); *latency* refers to the time from stimulus onset to some specific peak activity. Naming conventions then frequently reflect both the polarity and latency of the component.

In the literature we discuss, the "event" of interest is typically the onset of a picture—pleasant, neutral, or unpleasant. The bulk of the studies discussed below were conducted using the International Affective Picture System (IAPS: Lang, Bradley, & Cuthbert, 2005), a freely available and standardized stimulus set. In addition to the advantage of its size (the stimuli number in the hundreds) and the variety of content, normative ratings of valence and arousal have been collected from several hundred participants for each image, allowing researchers to systematically vary the content of their stimulus sets along dimensions of valence, arousal, or both. This variety is particularly useful for research interested in whether a particular physiological dependent variable is sensitive to the ways in which emotional stimuli (either pleasant or unpleasant) differ from neutral, or whether that measure is also sensitive to differences between pleasant and unpleasant valence.

Emotion and ERPs

Multiple ERP components are sensitive to emotional stimuli (see Hajcak et al., 2012, and Olofsson & Polich, 2007, for reviews). Indeed, the effects of both pleasant and unpleasant stimuli (compared to neutral) can be observed in ERP components occurring as early as 80 ms following stimulus onset (Mueller et al., 2009; Mühlberger et al., 2009; Olofsson & Polich, 2007) and can continue for several seconds, evident even after stimulus offset (Hajcak & Olvet, 2008). Despite this persistent influence of emotional content, there is increasing evidence that early, compared to late, components might index different cognitive–affective processes (Hajcak et al., 2012; Olofsson, Nordin, Sequeira, & Polich, 2008; Weinberg & Hajcak, 2011b). We briefly discuss evidence suggesting that comparatively early ERP components (i.e., components occurring prior

to 300 ms following stimulus onset) reflect the relatively obligatory capture of attention by emotional stimuli (Foti, Hajcak, & Dien, 2009; Hajcak et al., 2012; Olofsson et al., 2008; Weinberg & Hajcak, 2010, 2011b). However, our primary focus in this chapter is on the LPP, a positive-going slow wave that is thought to reflect more flexible and elaborated processing of emotional stimuli, and which affords an opportunity to index online manipulations of sustained attention.

Relatively Early ERPs Sensitive to Emotion

In passive viewing tasks, early visual ERP components are thought to be driven by bottom-up properties of the stimuli themselves (Olofsson et al., 2008), meaning amplitude fluctuates *primarily* as a function of perceptual stimulus features such as spatial frequency (Carretié, Hinojosa, López-Martín, & Tapia, 2007), color (Cano, Class, & Polich, 2009), complexity (Bradley, Hamby, Löw, & Lang, 2007), or size (Bradley et al., 2007; Cano et al., 2009; Carretié et al., 2007; De Cesarei & Codispoti, 2006). ERPs in this early time range appear to stem from areas of the visual cortex. However, there is also increasing evidence that ERPs in this time range may be sensitive to emotional content as well as physical properties of the stimuli themselves. Among the earliest components to index attention to emotion is the P1, which has been reported to be maximal at both occipital (Carretié, Hinojosa, Martín Loeches, Mercado, & Tapia, 2004; Holmes, Nielsen, & Green, 2008; Mueller et al., 2009) and frontal sites (Codispoti, Ferrari, & Bradley, 2007) roughly 100 ms following stimulus presentation. The P1 is responsive to emotional content across visual stimulus types, including faces (Pourtois, Dan, Grandjean, Sander, & Vuilleumier, 2005; Santesso et al., 2008), images (Smith, Cacioppo, Larsen, & Chartrand, 2003), and words (Bernat, Bunce, & Shevrin, 2001). Furthermore, there is evidence for emotional modulation of the P1 by subliminally presented stimuli (Bernat et al., 2001) suggesting that conscious awareness may not be necessary to potentiate the P1.

Following the P1 is the N1, a centroparietal negativity peaking around 130 ms after stimulus presentation (Foti et al., 2009; Keil et al., 2002). Like the P1, the N1 is consistently larger in response to emotional (both pleasant and unpleasant) compared to neutral stimuli (Carretié et al., 2007; Keil et al., 2001; Weinberg & Hajcak, 2010). Both the P1 and the N1 are thought to reflect increased early attention to, and facilitated perceptual processing of, visual information; these effects have been localized to visual processing areas such as the extrastriate cortex and the fusiform gyrus (Mueller et al., 2009; Pourtois et al., 2005). Figure 3.1a depicts the P1 as a positivity peaking roughly 100 ms following the presentation of fearful compared to neutral faces, along with scalp distribution for fearful minus neutral faces in the time range of the P1 *(right)*. Below this in Figure 3.1b are waveforms representing the N1 as a negative peak following the presentation of pleasant and unpleasant compared to neutral images along with scalp distributions for pleasant minus neutral and unpleasant minus neutral images in the time range of the N1 *(right)*.

Following the N1 is the P2, a positivity that is maximal at anterior and central sites approximately 200 ms after stimulus onset (Carretié et al., 2004; Carretié, Mercado, Tapia, & Hinojosa, 2001; Luck & Hillyard, 1994). The P2 is thought to reflect selective attention following initial visual perception, and has been localized to the anterior cingulate cortex as well as to visual areas (Carretié et al., 2004). Figure 3.1b depicts the P2 as a positive deflection elicited by pleasant and unpleasant compared to neutral images. As indicated, the P2 is larger (i.e., more positive) following emotional images.

The early posterior negativity (EPN) peaks roughly 200–300 ms after stimulus onset and presents either as a negative-going wave over temporal–occipital sites or as a positive deflection over frontal–central sites (Schupp, Flaisch, Stockburger, & Junghöfer, 2006; Schupp, Junghöfer, Weike, & Hamm, 2003b, 2004). The EPN is sensitive to both pleasant and unpleasant emotional content (De Cesarei & Codispoti, 2006; Junghöfer, Bradley, Elbert, & Lang, 2001; Schupp et al., 2006; Weinberg & Hajcak, 2010), though there is some evidence to suggest that the EPN is even larger following *pleasant* images compared to both neutral and unpleasant stimuli (Schupp et al., 2006; Schupp, Junghöfer, et al., 2004; Weinberg &

Hajcak, 2010). Emotional modulation of the EPN is generally consistent across stimulus presentation durations, stimulus types, and both passive viewing and active tasks (Herbert, Junghöfer, & Kissler, 2008; Junghöfer et al., 2001). Moreover, emotional modulation can be observed even when the task requires attention to be focused on nonemotional aspects of the stimuli (Kissler, Herbert, Winkler, & Junghöfer, 2009; Schupp, Junghöfer, Weike, & Hamm, 2003a). For example, when participants are asked to count the number of checkerboard images intermixed with task-irrelevant emotional pictures, emotional modulation of the EPN is still observed (Schupp et al., 2003a). In addition, some studies have shown that the EPN remains responsive to the emotional content of stimuli while the participant performs a secondary auditory task involving either low or high attentional demands (Schupp et al., 2008), indicating the persistence of the influence of emotion despite demanding concurrent tasks. Figure 3.1c depicts an enhanced EPN to both pleasant and unpleasant compared to neutral images, as well as scalp distributions for pleasant minus neutral and unpleasant minus neutral pictures in the time range of the EPN *(right)*.

The LPP

Following these earlier components is the LPP, a positive-going slow wave that is maximal at centroparietal sites beginning as early as 200 ms following stimulus onset and continuing for the duration of picture presentation (Cuthbert, Schupp, Bradley, Birbaumer, & Lang, 2000; Foti & Hajcak, 2008; Hajcak, Dunning, & Foti, 2007; Hajcak & Nieuwenhuis, 2006; Junghöfer et al., 2001; Lang et al., 1997). Recent research suggests that the LPP may consist of a series of overlapping positive deflections in the waveform (Foti et al., 2009; MacNamara et al., 2009; Weinberg & Hajcak, 2011b), the first of which is morphologically and temporally similar to the P300, a component that is among the most extensively researched in the ERP literature.

The P300 appears sensitive to the motivational salience of stimuli and is typically observed in nonaffective paradigms in which an infrequent target stimulus is presented in a context of frequent nontarget, or standard,

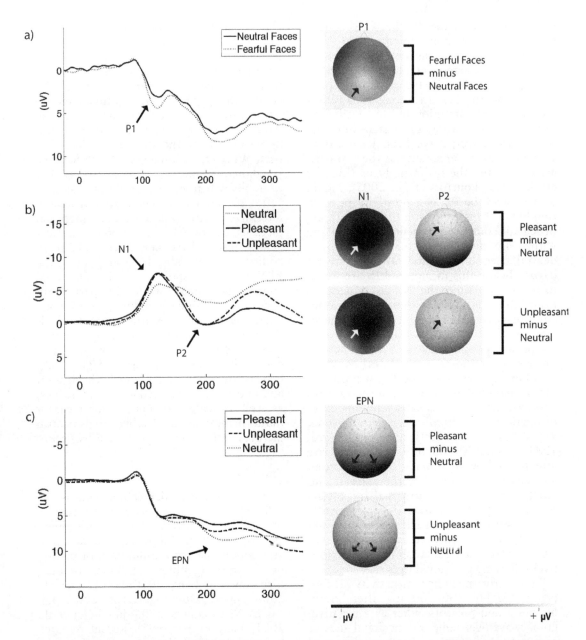

FIGURE 3.1. For each graph on the left, the *x*-axis represents time, and the *y*-axis represents voltage. Per ERP convention, positive voltage is plotted *down*. The waveforms presented are stimulus-locked to the onset of the stimulus at 0 ms. On the right are scalp topographies representing the difference between the conditions of interest (either emotional minus neutral faces, or emotional minus neutral IAPS images). (a) ERP data recorded at Oz from 46 subjects in a passive viewing task that included emotional and neutral faces. The P1 is labeled in the waveform, and is larger (more positive) for fearful compared to neutral faces. Data from Smith, Weinberg, Moran, and Hajcak (2012). (b) An example of the N1 and P2 components recorded at scalp site Cz from 64 subjects who passively viewed images in valence-specific blocks. The N1 and the P2 are each indicated in the waveform and are larger for unpleasant and pleasant compared to neutral images. Data from Weinberg and Hajcak, 2010. (c) The EPN recorded at scalp site Iz in a passive viewing task. The EPN is larger (more positive) for unpleasant and pleasant compared to neutral images. Data from Weinberg and Hajcak (2010). IAPS, International Affective Picture System.

stimuli (Polich, 2007, 2012). Yet the P300 is larger for targets even when targets and standards are equally probable, suggesting that task relevance or the instructed salience of the stimulus itself is sufficient to potentiate the P300 (Duncan Johnson & Donchin, 1977).

As discussed above, emotional stimuli may be intrinsically motivationally relevant, independent of task parameters, and may be thought of as "natural targets." Consistent with this, modulation of a P300-like component is also frequently observed for emotional (both pleasant and unpleasant) compared to neutral stimuli (Ferrari, Codispoti, Cardinale, & Bradley, 2008; Foti et al., 2009; Johnston, Miller, & Burleson, 1986; Lifshitz, 1966; Radilova, 1982; Weinberg & Hajcak, 2011b), suggesting that processes indexed by the P300 may be linked broadly to motivation. Though it is difficult to determine definitively whether two components derived under different experimental conditions are the same, similarities in terms of their topography, timing, and response to task parameters suggest that the P300 observed in nonaffective target detection tasks may reflect similar processes as the P300 observed in affective research. In order to distinguish between canonical P300 research and more recent affective research, however, we use *LPP* for the duration of the chapter to mean the sustained positive complex beginning in, and extending well beyond, the time range of the P300.

Like the prototypical P300, the LPP is larger following both pleasant and unpleasant compared to neutral stimuli (Cuthbert et al., 2000; Foti et al., 2009; Keil et al., 2002) and is sensitive to emotional images (Cuthbert et al., 2000; Foti et al., 2009; Pastor et al., 2008; Schupp et al., 2000), words (Fischler & Bradley, 2006; Kissler et al., 2009; Tacikowski & Nowicka, 2010), and even emotional hand gestures (Flaisch, Häcker, Renner, & Schupp, 2011). Furthermore, there is some evidence that the magnitude of the LPP is correlated with skin conductance and self-reported affective arousal in response to individual pictures (Cuthbert et al., 2000), though as we discuss below, the relationship with arousal may differ for specific picture types (e.g., see Briggs & Martin, 2009; Schupp, Cuthbert, et al., 2004; Weinberg & Hajcak, 2010). There is evidence that

the sustained positivity elicited by emotional compared to neutral images can persist well beyond picture offset (Codispoti, Mazzetti, & Bradley, 2009; Hajcak, MacNamara, & Olvet, 2010; Hajcak & Olvet, 2008) and that it may shift in distribution over the course of affective picture processing, progressing from an early parietal distribution to a more centrally maximal distribution (Foti et al., 2009; MacNamara et al., 2009).

Unlike earlier ERP components, which appear to index the relatively gross discrimination of emotional from nonemotional processes, the LPP can reflect more fine-grained distinctions within emotional categories such that emotional modulation of the LPP is enhanced for those stimuli most directly relevant to biological imperatives, irrespective of arousal ratings (e.g., threat, mutilation, and erotic images: Briggs & Martin, 2009; Schupp, Cuthbert, et al., 2004; Weinberg & Hajcak, 2010). For example, erotic images within the pleasant category elicit a larger electrocortical response than neutral images of objects, which are also rated as less arousing. But the LPP elicited by erotica is also larger than that elicited by "exciting" images (e.g., content related to sports, cars, or feats of daring), though both erotic and exciting images are rated as highly arousing and pleasant (Weinberg & Hajcak, 2010). This is presumably because exciting images have little direct bearing on survival or reproduction (Briggs & Martin, 2009) and as such, may not necessitate the same degree of sustained attention. Figure 3.2 *(top)* depicts a typical LPP in response to emotional compared to neutral images.

The LPP also appears to be *functionally* distinct from other ERP components that are sensitive to emotion. For example, in one study from our lab, participants were asked to identify a target—either a circle or a square—which was both preceded and followed by task-irrelevant pleasant, neutral, or unpleasant IAPS images. Consistent with previous research (Mitchell et al., 2006, 2008), responses to imperative targets were slowed by the presence of the task-irrelevant emotional images (Weinberg & Hajcak, 2011b). Although multiple ERP components were enhanced by the task-irrelevant emotional stimuli (i.e., EPN, P300), only the LPP predicted the degree of behavioral slowing: The larger the LPP, the slower the

Passive Viewing Paradigm

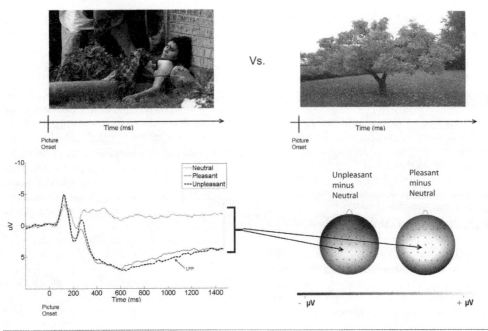

Directed Viewing Paradigm

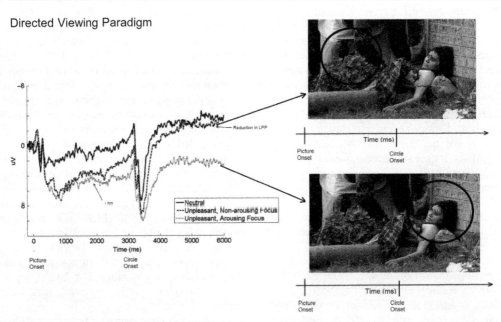

FIGURE 3.2. *Top:* An example of the LPP recorded in a passive viewing paradigm. The waveforms presented are averaged over five centroparietal sites (Pz, CPz, Cz, CP1, and CP2) for unpleasant, pleasant, and neutral images. These data (from Weinberg & Hajcak, 2010) were recorded from 64 participants engaged in a passive affective viewing task in which images were presented in valence-specific blocks. The LPP is larger for both pleasant and unpleasant compared to neutral images. Also shown *(top right)* are scalp topographies representing the difference between unpleasant and neutral and pleasant and neutral images in the time frame of the LPP. *Bottom:* An example of the LPP recorded in a directed viewing task. Participants passively viewed IAPS images of varying emotional content for 3 seconds. At the end of 3 seconds, a circle would appear on the screen, directing attention to a nonarousing or an arousing portion of the image. When attention was directed toward a nonarousing portion of aversive images, emotional modulation of the LPP was reduced. Data from Dunning and Hajcak (2009).

response to targets. This was true between participants, such that individuals with an enhanced LPP to task-irrelevant images were also slower to respond to targets. But it was also true within participants, in that, for each individual, slower trials tended to be preceded by pictures that elicited a larger LPP. Additionally, the LPP predicted variation in neural activity elicited by the targets: A larger LPP to task-irrelevant IAPS images was related to a reduction in the magnitude of the P300 elicited by targets. These results suggest that the continued elaboration and encoding indexed by the LPP uniquely relates to subsequently slower response times and reduced P300s to targets in this task.

Unlike the majority of peripheral and central measures sensitive to emotional stimuli, emotional modulation of the LPP is highly stable. Although skin conductance, heart rate, facial muscle activity, and neural activation measured using functional magnetic resonance imaging (fMRI; Codispoti & De Cesarei, 2007; Codispoti, Ferrari, & Bradley, 2006; Phan, Liberzon, Welsh, Britton, & Taylor, 2003) habituate over repeated presentations of stimuli, emotional modulation of the LPP does not (Codispoti et al., 2006, 2007; Olofsson & Polich, 2007). Furthermore, emotional modulation of the LPP appears insensitive to some forms of pharmacological blockade (Franken, Nijs, & Pepplinkhuizen, 2008; Olofsson, Gospic, Petrovic, Ingvar, & Wiens, 2011). Finally, affective enhancement of the LPP is evident across the lifespan, in children as young as 5 (Dennis & Hajcak, 2009; Hajcak & Dennis, 2009; Kujawa, Hajcak, Torpey, Kim, & Klein, 2012) and adults as old as 81 (Kisley, Wood, & Burrows, 2007; Langeslag & Van Strien, 2010). Combined, this research suggests that the LPP is a valuable tool for measuring sustained attention to emotional content across multiple populations and paradigms.

Anatomical Sources of the LPP

A number of features of the LPP make source localization difficult. For instance, the sustained LPP has a broad spatial distribution and may reflect a series of neural responses overlapping closely in time and space (Foti et al., 2009; MacNamara et al., 2009; Weinberg & Hajcak, 2011b). Furthermore, the shift in the distribution of the LPP over time from a relatively focal posterior distribution to a broader and more anterior distribution (Foti et al., 2009; Hajcak, MacNamara, & Olvet, 2010; MacNamara et al., 2009) suggests that processing of emotional images may engage multiple neural networks over the course of picture viewing. This is consistent with fMRI research suggesting that affective visual information traverses multiple processing stages and sites, from early visual to prefrontal areas (Thielscher & Pessoa, 2007).

Nonetheless, recent work has attempted to identify neural generators of the LPP. Two studies implicate areas of the visual cortex as likely generators of the LPP. For example, using minimum norm source localization methods, Keil and colleagues (2002) estimated the neural sources of the LPP to lie in the occipital and posterior parietal cortices. This is consistent with evidence from fMRI (Bradley et al., 2003; Lang et al., 1998) suggesting that emotional pictures trigger increased activation in secondary visual processing sites in the lateral occipital cortex, extending up the dorsal stream to the parietal cortex. Variation in the LPP has also been related to neural activity in occipital, parietal, and inferotemporal regions of the brain in a study that combined EEG and fMRI measures from the same participants (Sabatinelli, Lang, Keil, & Bradley, 2007). Though direct contributions from the amygdala to the magnitude of the LPP have not been identified, some have suggested, based on detailed animal models, that the LPP might reflect reentrant projections from the amygdala to multiple areas of the visual cortex (e.g., Lang & Bradley, 2010). Finally, based on theoretical explanations of the P300 (Nieuwenhuis, Aston-Jones, & Cohen, 2005), some have also proposed that variation in the LPP may reflect neuromodulatory activity of the locus coeruleus norepinepherine system (de Rover et al., 2012; Hajcak, MacNamara, & Olvet, 2010). This body of research is consistent with the notion that the magnitude of the LPP derives from ongoing communication among multiple brain regions. Though this highlights the spatial imprecision of the component (and the ERP technique), it also points to the LPP's utility as an online index of concerted neural efforts to direct and maintain visual attention.

Bottom-Up and Top-Down Interactions Evident in the LPP

Motivational salience can be determined in multiple ways. For example, the LPP is sensitive to target status as well as emotional content (Azizian, Freitas, Parvaz, & Squires, 2006; Chong et al., 2008; Ferrari, Bradley, Codispoti, & Lang, 2010; Ferrari et al., 2008; Luck & Hillyard, 2000; Weinberg, Hilgard, Bartholow, & Hajcak, 2012), and evidence suggests that bottom-up and top-down manipulations can work additively to determine allocation of attention when targets are emotional (Ferrari et al., 2010; Weinberg et al., 2012). *Personally salient* stimuli (e.g., photographs of relatives or one's own name and face) also appear to elicit an LPP that is larger than even familiar celebrity faces (Grasso & Simons, 2010; Tacikowski & Nowicka, 2010). Additionally, food deprivation appears to specifically enhance the magnitude of the LPP elicited by food images compared to flower images (Stockburger, Schmälzle, Flaisch, Bublatzky, & Schupp, 2009). Combined, these findings suggest that motivational salience can be determined through complex interactions of context, the individual, and stimulus properties. Next, we discuss the impact of several specific manipulations of salience and attention on the processing of emotional stimuli as reflected in the LPP.

Concurrent Task Difficulty

Evidence suggesting that emotional stimuli are prioritized in attentional and perceptual processes does not imply that processing of emotional stimuli is obligatory or automatic (e.g., Bishop et al., 2004, 2007; Liberzon et al., 2000; Pessoa et al., 2002, 2005). In fact, several studies have found that when attentional resources are consumed by a nonaffective foreground task, the magnitude of the LPP is reduced. However, this effect may depend on both the attentional demands of the task and the salience of the stimuli.

For example, simple arithmetic tasks can be completed with little-to-no impact on emotional modulation of the LPP by simultaneously presented images (Hajcak et al., 2007), indicating that attention to emotional images may be prioritized in the context of some types of competition. Similarly, in a recent study manipulating perceptual load during picture viewing, centrally presented, but task-irrelevant, IAPS images of spiders and mushrooms were shown to spider phobics and nonspider phobics. Participants were also asked to simultaneously perform a letter discrimination task consisting of the identification of either three or six letters presented in a circle outside of the images (Norberg, Peira, & Wiens, 2010). Although spider phobics showed larger LPPs to spider images than the nonphobic participants, emotional modulation of the LPP was not impacted by level of perceptual load, suggesting that sufficiently potent images presented in the center of the visual field may be resistant to the impact of some forms of competition.

Recent work examining working memory load and emotional picture viewing suggests that greater load (MacNamara, Ferri, & Hajcak, 2011; Wangelin, Löw, McTeague, Bradley, & Lang, 2011) can impact the overall magnitude of the LPP, though emotional modulation persists. For example, in MacNamara, Ferri, and Hajcak (2011) participants were given 5 seconds to memorize a string of consonants; an aversive or neutral task-irrelevant IAPS image was then presented in the retention interval for 2 seconds. At the end of each trial, participants were asked to type in the letters they had memorized. Working memory load was manipulated via the number of letters, such that on some trials participants were asked to memorize two letters, and on others they were asked to memorize six letters. The magnitude of the LPP decreased as a function of increasing working memory load: When participants were asked to memorize six letters, the LPP to both neutral and aversive images was attenuated. The effect appeared to be slightly—though nonsignificantly—stronger for aversive pictures. Likewise, though heavy working memory load may attenuate the overall LPP (i.e., the LPP elicited by both neutral and emotional images), emotional images continued to elicit a larger LPP than neutral. Though attention to task-irrelevant images overall was reduced by increased working memory load, emotional images continued to command increased processing resources compared to neutral.

Task Relevance

As discussed above, there is evidence that enhanced attention to task-irrelevant emotional images can compete with top-down imperatives to negatively impact performance on a task (e.g., Weinberg & Hajcak, 2011b). On the other hand, when the affective properties of emotional stimuli are made task-relevant, bottom-up and top-down processes may work *cooperatively* to enhance attention. For example, in a study from Hajcak, Moser, and Simons (2006), participants were asked to categorize IAPS images either along an affective dimension, indicating whether they were pleasant or unpleasant, or along a nonaffective dimension, indicating how many people were in each scene. Images for which the affective properties were relevant to the task elicited larger LPPs compared to when the same pictures were categorized along a nonaffective dimension (Hajcak et al., 2006), suggesting that top-down manipulations of attentional focus can further increase the magnitude of the LPP.

There is also reason to believe that bottom-up and top-down influences jointly influence the processing of emotional stimuli in a way that is relatively independent of one another. For example, a recent study in our lab utilized a variant of an "oddball" paradigm in which targets representing a given valence category (i.e., pleasant, neutral, or unpleasant) were presented infrequently within a stream of images from a different affective category (e.g., a single pleasant picture presented in a stream of unpleasant pictures; Weinberg et al., 2012). Thus, in this study, targets were identified by virtue of their valence (i.e., pleasant, neutral, unpleasant). Targets (whether emotional or neutral) and emotional stimuli (whether targets or nontargets) both were associated with an enhanced LPP in an earlier time window. These effects appeared additive, rather than interactive, such that emotional targets elicited the largest response of all, though target status enhanced both emotional and neutral images (see also Ferrari et al., 2008, 2010). In comparison, the later portion of the LPP appeared uniquely sensitive to target status (Weinberg et al., 2012), consistent with hypotheses that this later component reflects more flexible, sustained, and elaborative processes that might be more related

to task-relevant imperatives in this context (Foti & Hajcak, 2008; MacNamara, Ferri, & Hajcak, 2011; MacNamara, Ochsner, & Hajcak, 2011; MacNamara et al., 2009; Olofsson et al., 2008; Weinberg & Hajcak, 2011b).

Spatial Attention

Consistent with hypotheses that the effect of emotion depends critically on the availability of attentional resources, an emerging line of research suggests that affective stimuli presented in unattended spatial locations do not elicit increased ERPs (De Cesarei, Codispoti, & Schupp, 2009; Eimer, Holmes, & McGlone, 2003; Holmes, Vuilleumier, & Eimer, 2003; MacNamara & Hajcak, 2009, 2010). For instance, in a series of studies in our lab, participants viewed four briefly and simultaneously presented IAPS images: An image was located above, below, to the right, and to the left of fixation (MacNamara & Hajcak, 2009, 2010). On each trial, participants were instructed to attend only to two of the four pictures and to decide whether they were the same or different; the location of the target images was indicated prior to each trial. Thus, the remaining two images were distracters. Each of the image pairs could be either neutral or aversive. In this study, aversive targets elicited a larger LPP than neutral targets. However, there was no evidence of emotional modulation of the LPP by the unattended distracter images.

Likewise, online manipulations that direct attention within aversive stimuli can impact the amplitude of the LPP (Dunning & Hajcak, 2009; Hajcak, Dunning, & Foti, 2009). In a study from Dunning and Hajcak (2009; see Figure 3.2) participants passively viewed IAPS images for 3 seconds and demonstrated the typical emotional modulation of the LPP. After 3 seconds, a circle appeared on the screen and directed attention to either a nonarousing portion of the image (e.g., the pebbles surrounding a corpse) or an arousing portion of the image (e.g., the face of the corpse). When attention was directed to the arousing portion of the image, the magnitude of the LPP was unchanged relative to passive viewing. When participants were directed to attend to a nonarousing portion of aversive images, however, the magnitude of the LPP decreased such that it was comparable to the response to neutral images.

Thus it appears that spatial attention plays a critical role in the processing of emotional stimuli—at least as reflected in the magnitude of the LPP. Contrary to suggestions that emotional processing may occur outside of conscious awareness (e.g., Liu et al., 2009; Morris et al., 1998, 2001; Whalen et al., 1998), these data suggest awareness and attention critically impact neural activity indexed by the LPP. Further evidence for this comes from a study that systematically varied stimulus presentation times and used visual masks to obscure awareness of emotional images (Codispoti et al., 2009). Emotional stimuli masked after 25–40 ms failed to modulate the LPP or peripheral indices of affective processing. When the same stimuli were presented for 80 ms before the mask, the LPP was robustly potentiated. However, some participants were able to accurately report the valence and arousal of images shown for approximately 50 ms, suggesting that modulation of the LPP might depend on awareness. Indeed, those participants who were best able to accurately identify the valence and arousal of images masked after 50 ms ("discriminators") showed affective modulation of the LPP at this latency, whereas "non-discriminators" did not.

Stimulus Meaning

Although emotional stimuli may claim a privileged status in the competition for visual attention, the motivational value of these stimuli is not immutable. As reviewed above (Ferrari et al., 2010; Stockburger et al., 2009; Weinberg et al., 2012), the LPP not only tracks the intrinsic salience of stimuli based on content, but also reflects online and context-specific calculations of motivational salience. This is perhaps best demonstrated in emotion regulation studies that ask participants to modify their response to emotionally arousing stimuli. In our lab, we have tended to use techniques related to cognitive reappraisal, in which individuals are asked to change the way they think about emotional events or images (Gross & Thompson, 2007).

For example, a participant viewing a gory or gruesome image might tell him- or herself that the image is not real, that it is just a scene from a scary movie (e.g., Hajcak, Mac-Namara, & Olvet, 2010; Ochsner & Gross, 2005, 2007; for more on emotion regulation, see also Suri, Sheppes, & Gross, Chapter 11, this volume). Consistent with work suggesting that reappraisal alters emotional experience (Gross & Thompson, 2007; Ochsner, Bunge, Gross, & Gabrieli, 2002), reappraisal also impacts the magnitude of the LPP. For example, in one early study, participants were asked to either (1) attend to unpleasant pictures as they normally would, or (2) reinterpret the content to make it less negative (e.g., viewing an image of a man pointing a gun to his own head, the participant might tell himself, "This man ultimately decides not to commit suicide"; Hajcak & Nieuwenhuis, 2006). In this study, reappraisal appeared to impact both the subjective ratings of emotional response as well as the magnitude of the LPP; reappraised pictures elicited a smaller LPP. In subsequent years, the reduction in the magnitude of the LPP has been replicated in other studies using more open-ended emotion regulation techniques—in which participants are not directly instructed in how to change their emotional experience (Krompinger et al., 2008; Moser, Hajcak, Bukay, & Simons, 2006)—suggesting that modulation of stimulus meaning can impact attentional processes.

However, in such studies, it has not always been clear whether the reduction in the LPP was a result of cognitively driven changes in stimulus meaning, or whether variability in the LPP might instead be attributed to distraction or increased cognitive load. In several subsequent studies, participants were provided with either negative (e.g., "This plane was the target of a terrorist bomb") or neutral (e.g., "These people are boarding an early-morning flight") descriptions that preceded unpleasant and neutral pictures (Foti & Hajcak, 2008; MacNamara et al., 2009). Consistent with the notion that changes in stimulus meaning can impact neural response to emotional images, unpleasant and negatively described pictures elicited larger LPPs than neutral and neutrally described pictures, respectively. Self-report ratings of arousal and valence also appeared to follow this pattern; specifically, unpleasant pictures preceded by neutral descriptions were rated as less arousing and less negative by participants (Foti & Hajcak, 2008; MacNamara et al., 2009). Similarly, when task-irrelevant images are framed as fictitious depictions of emotionally arousing scenes prior to their presentation (e.g., participants are told that the images they are about to see are movie stills), the LPP is diminished, compared to the response to those same images presented as veridical depictions of life (Mocaiber et al., 2010). Finally, reappraisal appears to impact attention to emotional stimuli well after the manipulation has occurred. MacNamara, Ochsner, and Hajcak (2011) found that participants who listened to neutral descriptions of unpleasant images demonstrated a reduced LPP in response to these pictures when they were viewed again 30 minutes later, without the preceding descriptions.

Emotion regulation is often conceptualized as a process by which frontal areas of the brain down-regulate the activity of reflexive, affective regions of the brain (Beauregard et al., 2001; Ochsner et al., 2002; Phan et al., 2005). Consistent with this view is evidence that electrical stimulation of the dorsolateral prefrontal cortex (DLPFC) can attenuate the magnitude of the LPP elicited by unpleasant images, although it does not eliminate it (Hajcak, Anderson, et al., 2010). The Hajcak, Anderson, and colleagues (2010) paper on DLPFC stimulation was conducted in a small clinical sample of five chronically depressed individuals and should therefore be interpreted with care; however, the results suggest that activation of certain prefrontal areas may interrupt the ongoing elaborated processing of emotional stimuli. These results complement research indicating that working memory load can also reduce the LPP (e.g., MacNamara, Ferri, & Hajcak, 2011) insofar as there is evidence that working memory load reliably elicits activation of the DLPFC (Curtis & D'Esposito, 2003; D'Esposito, Postle, & Rypma, 2000) and that this activation increases as a function of the number of items held in memory (Manoach et al., 1997). These studies suggest that both mechanical and functional stimulation of the DLPFC might reduce the magnitude of the LPP.

Conclusion and Future Directions

Combined, evidence from ERPs suggests that attention to emotion is neither inflexible nor obligatory. Although activity reflected in early ERP components may indicate early preferential attentional capture, subsequent activity reflected in the LPP suggests that cognitive processes begin to interact with emotional processes within a few hundred milliseconds of stimulus presentation to determine the continued allocation of attention to emotional stimuli. We believe that the LPP will be useful for future work that considers interactions between cognitive and affective processes as they determine visual attention. Ongoing experimental work that manipulates salience—via task demands and stimulus value—will be critical to our understanding of how exogenous and endogenous attentional processes interact.

One promising application of this research will be in the study of individual differences. For example, in the working memory study mentioned above (MacNamara, Ferri, & Hajcak, 2011), greater memory load impacted the magnitude of the LPP. However, high levels of anxiety appeared to moderate the effect of load. Specifically, though there were no performance-related differences on the task, highly anxious individuals were characterized by less modulation of the LPP by working memory load—suggesting that individual differences may exert an influence on emotion–cognition interactions. A developing body of research further indicates differences in emotional modulation of the LPP as a function of anxiety (Flykt & Caldara, 2006; Holmes et al., 2008; MacNamara & Hajcak, 2009; Mühlberger et al., 2009; Weinberg & Hajcak, 2011a), depression (Foti, Olvet, Klein, & Hajcak, 2010; Williams et al., 2007), and schizophrenia (Horan, Wynn, Kring, Simons, & Green, 2010). The ways in which these individual differences interact with bottom-up or top-down manipulations of stimulus salience have not been fully explored. It is possible that attentional biases and deficits in sustained attention are driven by relatively circumscribed abnormalities in either bottom-up or top-down mechanisms. The inclusion of individuals and groups characterized by disordered emotional experience in studies examining the competition for attention might augment our understanding of these interactions.

Following from this direction, future studies might examine the predictive value of the LPP in prospective longitudinal studies. The literature presented in this review—and, to our knowledge, all of the extant literature examining the LPP—is concurrent and cross-sectional. Prospective studies might be helpful not only in enhancing the current body of knowledge as to what the LPP *is*—that is, what neural generators contribute—but also in clarifying what the LPP predicts in terms of attentional allocation and emotional response.

At present, the strength of ERP methodologies lies in their temporal precision and in their ability to reflect the communication between multiple regions of the brain. However, as discussed above, the neural generators of the LPP are far from fully determined. Combined fMRI and EEG research, as well as the continued improvement of source localization techniques within ERP methodologies, could help refine our understanding of which areas are recruited, and when, in the dynamic deployment of attention to emotion. In addition, although the ERP literature has traditionally emphasized deflections in the trial-averaged waveform (e.g., the LPP), single-trial EEG recordings consist of multiple sources of oscillatory activity—possibly emanating from distinct neural populations—which overlap in time and/or in frequency. Separation of this activity using time–frequency transforms could allow for richer representations of EEG activity, and might capture aspects of neural responding that are not evident in scalp-recorded ERP averages. Time–frequency approaches also allow for functional coherence analysis, which examines how activity in one region might impact—and be impacted by—other regions. Increasingly precise understanding of the anatomical and functional connections between brain regions will be critical in determining how and where bottom-up and top-down processes meet in the brain.

References

Anderson, C., Van Essen, D., & Olshausen, B. (2005). Directed visual attention and the dynamic control of information flow. In L. Itti, G. Rees, & J. Tsotsos (Eds.), *Encyclopedia of visual attention* (pp. 11–17). Cambridge, MA: MIT Press.

Azizian, A., Freitas, A., Parvaz, M., & Squires, N. (2006). Beware misleading cues: Perceptual similarity modulates the N2/P3 complex. *Psychophysiology, 43*(3), 253–260.

Bacon, W., & Egeth, H. (1994). Overriding stimulus-driven attentional capture. *Perception and Psychophysics, 55*(5), 485–496.

Beauregard, M., Levesque, J., & Bourgouin, P. (2001). Neural correlates of conscious self-regulation of emotion. *Journal of Neuroscience, 21*(18), 165.

Bernat, E., Bunce, S., & Shevrin, H. (2001). Event-related brain potentials differentiate positive and negative mood adjectives during both supraliminal and subliminal visual processing. *International Journal of Psychophysiology, 42*(1), 11–34.

Bishop, S., Duncan, J., & Lawrence, A. (2004). State anxiety modulation of the amygdala response to unattended threat-related stimuli. *Journal of Neuroscience, 24*(46), 10364–10368.

Bishop, S., Jenkins, R., & Lawrence, A. (2007). Neural processing of fearful faces: Effects of anxiety are gated by perceptual capacity limitations. *Cerebral Cortex, 17*(7), 1595–1603.

Blair, K., Smith, B., Mitchell, D., Morton, J., Vythilingam, M., Pessoa, L., et al. (2007). Modulation of emotion by cognition and cognition by emotion. *NeuroImage, 35*(1), 430–440.

Bradley, M., Codispoti, M., Cuthbert, B., & Lang, P. (2001). Emotion and motivation: I. Defensive and appetitive reactions in picture processing. *Emotion, 1*(3), 276–298.

Bradley, M., Hamby, S., Löw, A., & Lang, P. (2007). Brain potentials in perception: Picture complexity and emotional arousal. *Psychophysiology, 44*(3), 364–373.

Bradley, M., Sabatinelli, D., Lang, P., Fitzsimmons, J., King, W., & Desai, P. (2003). Activation of the visual cortex in motivated attention. *Behavioral Neuroscience, 117*(2), 369–380.

Briggs, K., & Martin, F. (2009). Affective picture processing and motivational relevance: Arousal and valence effects on ERPs in an oddball task. *International Journal of Psychophysiology, 72*(3), 299–306.

Buodo, G., Sarlo, M., & Palomba, D. (2002). Attentional resources measured by reaction times highlight differences within pleasant and unpleasant, high arousing stimuli. *Motivation and Emotion, 26*(2), 123–138.

Cano, M. E., Class, Q. A., & Polich, J. (2009). Affective valence, stimulus attributes, and P300: Color vs. black/white and normal vs.

scrambled images. *International Journal of Psychophysiology, 71*(1), 17–24.

Carretié, L., Hinojosa, J., López-Martín, S., & Tapia, M. (2007). An electrophysiological study on the interaction between emotional content and spatial frequency of visual stimuli. *Neuropsychologia, 45*(6), 1187–1195.

Carretié, L., Hinojosa, J., Martín Loeches, M., Mercado, F., & Tapia, M. (2004). Automatic attention to emotional stimuli: Neural correlates. *Human Brain Mapping, 22*(4), 290–299.

Carretié, L., Mercado, F., Tapia, M., & Hinojosa, J. (2001). Emotion, attention and the "negativity bias," studied through event-related potentials. *International Journal of Psychophysiology, 41*(1), 75–85.

Chong, H., Riis, J. L., McGinnis, S. M., Williams, D. M., Holcomb, P. J., & Daffner, K. R. (2008). To ignore or explore: Top-down modulation of novelty processing. *Journal of Cognitive Neuroscience, 20*(1), 120–134.

Codispoti, M., & De Cesarei, A. (2007). Arousal and attention: Picture size and emotional reactions. *Psychophysiology, 44*(5), 680–686.

Codispoti, M., Ferrari, V., & Bradley, M. (2006). Repetitive picture processing: Autonomic and cortical correlates. *Brain Research, 1068*(1), 213–220.

Codispoti, M., Ferrari, V., & Bradley, M. (2007). Repetition and event-related potentials: Distinguishing early and late processes in affective picture perception. *Journal of Cognitive Neuroscience, 19*(4), 577–586.

Codispoti, M., Mazzetti, M., & Bradley, M. (2009). Unmasking emotion: Exposure duration and emotional engagement. *Psychophysiology, 46*(4), 731–738.

Curtis, C. E., & D'Esposito, M. (2003). Persistent activity in the prefrontal cortex during working memory. *Trends in Cognitive Sciences, 7*(9), 415–423.

Cuthbert, B., Schupp, H., Bradley, M., Birbaumer, N., & Lang, P. (2000). Brain potentials in affective picture processing: Covariation with autonomic arousal and affective report. *Biological Psychology, 52*(2), 95–111.

De Cesarei, A., & Codispoti, M. (2006). When does size not matter?: Effects of stimulus size on affective modulation. *Psychophysiology, 43*(2), 207–215.

De Cesarei, A., Codispoti, M., & Schupp, H. (2009). Peripheral vision and preferential emotion processing. *NeuroReport, 20*(16), 1439–1443.

Dennis, T., & Hajcak, G. (2009). The late positive potential: A neurophysiological marker for emotion regulation in children. *Journal of Child Psychology and Psychiatry, 50*(11), 1373–1383.

de Rover, M., Brown, S., Boot, N., Hajcak, G., van Noorden, M., van der Wee, N., et al. (2012). Beta receptor-mediated modulation of the late positive potential in humans. *Psychopharmacology, 219*, 971"979.

D'Esposito, M., Postle, B. R., & Rypma, B. (2000). Prefrontal cortical contributions to working memory: Evidence from event-related fMRI studies. *Experimental Brain Research, 133*(1), 3–11.

Driver, J. (2001). A selective review of selective attention research from the past century. *British Journal of Psychology, 92*(1), 53–78.

Duncan Johnson, C. C., & Donchin, E. (1977). On quantifying surprise: The variation of event related potentials with subjective probability. *Psychophysiology, 14*(5), 456–467.

Dunning, J., & Hajcak, G. (2009). See no evil: Directing visual attention within unpleasant images modulates the electrocortical response. *Psychophysiology, 46*(1), 28–33.

Eimer, M., Holmes, A., & McGlone, F. (2003). The role of spatial attention in the processing of facial expression: An ERP study of rapid brain responses to six basic emotions. *Cognitive, Affective, and Behavioral Neuroscience, 3*(2), 97–110.

Fabiani, M., Gratton, G., & Federmeier, K. (2007). Event-related brain potentials: Methods, theory, and applications. In J. Cacioppo, L. Tassinary, & G. Bernston (Eds.), *Handbook of psychophysiology* (pp. 85–119). New York: Cambridge University Press.

Ferrari, V., Bradley, M., Codispoti, M., & Lang, P. (2010). Detecting novelty and significance. *Journal of Cognitive Neuroscience, 22*(2), 404–411.

Ferrari, V., Codispoti, M., Cardinale, R., & Bradley, M. (2008). Directed and motivated attention during processing of natural scenes. *Journal of Cognitive Neuroscience, 20*, 1753–1761.

Fischler, I., & Bradley, M. (2006). Event-related potential studies of language and emotion: Words, phrases, and task effects. *Progress in Brain Research, 156*, 185–203.

Flaisch, T., Häcker, F., Renner, B., & Schupp, H. (2011). Emotion and the processing of symbolic gestures: An event-related brain potential study. *Social Cognitive and Affective Neuroscience, 6*(1), 109–118.

Flaisch, T., Junghöfer, M., Bradley, M., Schupp, H., & Lang, P. (2008). Rapid picture processing: Affective primes and targets. *Psychophysiology, 45*(1), 1–10.

Flaisch, T., Stockburger, J., & Schupp, H. (2008). Affective prime and target picture processing: An ERP analysis of early and late interference effects. *Brain Topography, 20*(4), 183–191.

Flykt, A., & Caldara, R. (2006). Tracking fear in snake and spider fearful participants during visual search: A multi-response domain study. *Cognition and Emotion, 20*(8), 1075–1091.

Foti, D., & Hajcak, G. (2008). Deconstructing reappraisal: Descriptions preceding arousing pictures modulate the subsequent neural response. *Journal of Cognitive Neuroscience, 20*(6), 977–988.

Foti, D., Hajcak, G., & Dien, J. (2009). Differentiating neural responses to emotional pictures: Evidence from temporal–spatial PCA. *Psychophysiology, 46*(3), 521–530.

Foti, D., Olvet, D., Klein, D., & Hajcak, G. (2010). Reduced electrocortical response to threatening faces in major depressive disorder. *Depression and Anxiety, 27*, 813–820.

Fox, E., Lester, V., Russo, R., Bowles, R. J., Pichler, A., & Dutton, K. (2000). Facial expressions of emotion: Are angry faces detected more efficiently? *Cognition and Emotion, 14*(1), 61–92.

Franken, I. H. A., Nijs, I., & Pepplinkhuizen, L. (2008). Effects of dopaminergic modulation on electrophysiological brain response to affective stimuli. *Psychopharmacology, 195*(4), 537–546.

Grasso, D. J., & Simons, R. F. (2010). Perceived parental support predicts enhanced late positive event-related brain potentials to parent faces. *Biological Psychology, 86*, 26–30.

Gross, J. J., & Thompson, R. A. (2007). Emotion regulation: Conceptual foundations. In J. J. Gross (Ed.), *Handbook of emotion regulation* (pp. 3–24). New York: Guilford Press

Hajcak, G., Anderson, B., Arana, A., Borckardt, J., Takacs, I., George, M., et al. (2010). Dorsolateral prefrontal cortex stimulation modulates electrocortical measures of visual attention: Evidence from direct bilateral epidural cortical stimulation in treatment-resistant mood disorder. *Neuroscience, 170*, 281–288.

Hajcak, G., & Dennis, T. (2009). Brain potentials during affective picture processing in children. *Biological Psychology, 80*(3), 333–338.

Hajcak, G., Dunning, J., & Foti, D. (2007). Neural response to emotional pictures is unaffected by concurrent task difficulty: An event-related potential study. *Behavioral Neuroscience, 121*(6), 1156–1162.

Hajcak, G., Dunning, J., & Foti, D. (2009). Motivated and controlled attention to emotion: Time-course of the late positive potential. *Clinical Neurophysiology, 120*, 505–510.

Hajcak, G., MacNamara, A., & Olvet, D. (2010). Event-related potentials, emotion, and emotion regulation: An integrative review. *Developmental Neuropsychology, 35*(2), 129–155.

Hajcak, G., Moser, J., & Simons, R. (2006). Attending to affect: Appraisal strategies modulate the electrocortical response to arousing pictures. *Emotion, 6*(3), 517–522.

Hajcak, G., & Nieuwenhuis, S. (2006). Reappraisal modulates the electrocortical response to unpleasant pictures. *Cognitive, Affective, and Behavioral Neuroscience, 6*, 291–297.

Hajcak, G., & Olvet, D. (2008). The persistence of attention to emotion: Brain potentials during and after picture presentation. *Emotion, 8*(2), 250–255.

Hajcak, G., Weinberg, A., MacNamara, A., & Foti, D. (2012). ERPs and the study of emotion. In S. Luck & E. Kappenman (Eds.), *Handbook of event-related potential components* (pp. 441–474). New York: Oxford University Press.

Herbert, C., Junghöfer, M., & Kissler, J. (2008). Event related potentials to emotional adjectives during reading. *Psychophysiology, 45*(3), 487–498.

Holmes, A., Nielsen, M., & Green, S. (2008). Effects of anxiety on the processing of fearful and happy faces: An event-related potential study. *Biological Psychology, 77*(2), 159–173.

Holmes, A., Vuilleumier, P., & Eimer, M. (2003). The processing of emotional facial expression is gated by spatial attention: Evidence from event-related brain potentials. *Cognitive Brain Research, 16*(2), 174–184.

Horan, W. P., Wynn, J. K., Kring, A. M., Simons, R. F., & Green, M. F. (2010). Electrophysiological correlates of emotional responding in schizophrenia. *Journal of Abnormal Psychology, 119*(1), 18–30.

Ihssen, N., Heim, S., & Keil, A. (2007). The costs of emotional attention: Affective processing inhibits subsequent lexico-semantic analysis. *Journal of Cognitive Neuroscience, 19*(12), 1932–1949.

James, W. (1884). What is an emotion? In R. C. Solomon (Ed.), *What is an emotion?: Classic and contemporary readings* (pp. 66–76). New York: Oxford University Press.

Johnston, V., Miller, D., & Burleson, M. (1986). Multiple P3s to emotional stimuli and their theoretical significance. *Psychophysiology, 23*(6), 684–694.

Junghöfer, M., Bradley, M., Elbert, T., & Lang, P. (2001). Fleeting images: A new look at early emotion discrimination. *Psychophysiology, 38*(2), 175–178.

Keil, A., Bradley, M., Hauk, O., Rockstroh, B., Elbert, T., & Lang, P. (2002). Large-scale neural correlates of affective picture processing. *Psychophysiology, 39*(5), 641–649.

Keil, A., Müller, M., Gruber, T., Wienbruch, C., Stolarova, M., & Elbert, T. (2001). Effects of emotional arousal in the cerebral hemispheres: A study of oscillatory brain activity and event-related potentials. *Clinical Neurophysiology, 112*(11), 2057–2068.

Kisley, M. A., Wood, S., & Burrows, C. L. (2007). Looking at the sunny side of life. *Psychological Science, 18*(9), 838–843.

Kissler, J., Herbert, C., Winkler, I., & Junghöfer, M. (2009). Emotion and attention in visual word processing: An ERP study. *Biological Psychology, 80*(1), 75–83.

Krompinger, J., Moser, J., & Simons, R. (2008). Modulations of the electrophysiological response to pleasant stimuli by cognitive reappraisal. *Emotion, 8*(1), 132–137.

Kujawa, A., Hajcak, G., Torpey, D., Kim, J., & Klein, D. (2012). Electrocortical reactivity to emotional faces in young children and associations with maternal and paternal depression. *Journal of Child Psychiatry and Psychology, 53*(2), 207–215.

Lang, P., & Bradley, M. (2010). Emotion and the motivational brain. *Biological Psychology, 84*(3), 437–450.

Lang, P., Bradley, M., & Cuthbert, B. (1997). Motivated attention: Affect, activation, and action. In P. J. Lang, R. F. Simons, & M. Balaban (Eds.), *Attention and orienting: Sensory and motivational processes* (pp. 97–135). Mahwah, NJ: Erlbaum.

Lang, P., Bradley, M., & Cuthbert, B. (1998). Emotion, motivation, and anxiety: Brain mechanisms and psychophysiology. *Biological Psychiatry, 44*(12), 1248–1263.

Lang, P., Bradley, M., & Cuthbert, B. (2005). *International Affective Picture System (IAPS): Affective ratings of pictures and instruction manual.* Gainesville: University of Florida.

Lang, P., Greenwald, M., Bradley, M., & Hamm, A. (1993). Looking at pictures: Affective, facial, visceral, and behavioral reactions. *Psychophysiology, 30*(3), 261–273.

Langeslag, S. J. E., & Van Strien, J. W. (2010). Comparable modulation of the late positive potential by emotion regulation in younger and older adults. *Journal of Psychophysiology, 24*(3), 186–197.

LeDoux, J. (1996). *The emotional brain: The mysterious underpinnings of emotional life.* New York: Simon & Schuster.

Lévesque, J., Eugene, F., Joanette, Y., Paquette, V., Mensour, B., Beaudoin, G., et al. (2003). Neural circuitry underlying voluntary suppression of sadness. *Biological Psychiatry, 53*(6), 502–510.

Liberzon, I., Taylor, S., Fig, L., Decker, L., Koeppe, R., & Minoshima, S. (2000). Limbic activation and psychophysiologic responses to aversive visual stimuli: Interaction with cognitive task. *Neuropsychopharmacology, 23*(5), 508–516.

Lifshitz, K. (1966). The averaged evoked cortical response to complex visual stimuli. *Psychophysiology, 3*(1), 55–68.

Liu, H., Agam, Y., Madsen, J. R., & Kreiman, G. (2009). Timing, timing, timing: Fast decoding of object information from intracranial field potentials in human visual cortex. *Neuron, 62*(2), 281–290.

Luck, S. J. (2005). *An introduction to the event-related potential technique.* Cambridge, MA: MIT Press.

Luck, S. J., & Hillyard, S. A. (1994). Electrophysiological correlates of feature analysis during visual search. *Psychophysiology, 31*(3), 291–308.

Luck, S. J., & Hillyard, S. A. (2000). The operation of selective attention at multiple stages of processing: Evidence from human and monkey electrophysiology. In M. S. Gazzaniga (Ed.), *The new cognitive neurosciences* (2nd ed., pp. 687–700). Cambridge, MA: MIT Press.

MacNamara, A., Ferri, J., & Hajcak, G. (2011). Working memory load reduces the LPP and anxiety attenuates this effect. *Cognitive, Affective, and Behavioral Neuroscience, 11,* 321–331.

MacNamara, A., Foti, D., & Hajcak, G. (2009). Tell me about it: Neural activity elicited by emotional stimuli and preceding descriptions. *Emotion, 9*(4), 531–543.

MacNamara, A., & Hajcak, G. (2009). Anxiety and spatial attention moderate the electrocortical response to aversive pictures. *Neuropsychologia, 47*(13), 2975–2980.

MacNamara, A., & Hajcak, G. (2010). Distinct electrocortical and behavioral evidence for increased attention to threat in generalized anxiety disorder. *Depression and Anxiety, 27*(3), 234–243.

MacNamara, A., Ochsner, K., & Hajcak, G. (2011). Previously reappraised: The lasting effect of description type on picture-elicited electrocortical activity. *Social Cognitive and Affective Neuroscience, 6*(3), 348–358.

Manoach, D. S., Schlaug, G., Siewert, B., Darby, D. G., Bly, B. M., Benfield, A., et al. (1997). Prefrontal cortex fMRI signal changes are correlated with working memory load. *NeuroReport, 8*(2), 545–549.

Mesulam, M. M. (1998). From sensation to cognition. *Brain, 121*(6), 1013–1052.

Mitchell, D., Luo, Q., Mondillo, K., Vythilingam, M., Finger, E., & Blair, R. (2008). The interference of operant task performance by emotional distracters: An antagonistic relationship between the amygdala and frontoparietal cortices. *NeuroImage, 40*(2), 859–868.

Mitchell, D., Richell, R., Leonard, A., & Blair, R. (2006). Emotion at the expense of cognition: Psychopathic individuals outperform controls on an operant response task. *Journal of Abnormal Psychology, 115*(3), 559–566.

Mocaiber, I., Pereira, M. G., Erthal, F. S., Machado-Pinheiro, W., David, I. A., Cagy, M., et al. (2010). Fact or fiction?: An event-related potential study of implicit emotion regulation. *Neuroscience Letters, 476*(2), 84–88.

Mogg, K., Bradley, B., De Bono, J., & Painter, M. (1997). Time course of attentional bias for threat information in non-clinical anxiety. *Behaviour Research and Therapy, 35*(4), 297–303.

Mohanty, A., Egner, T., Monti, J., & Mesulam, M. (2009). Search for a threatening target triggers limbic guidance of spatial attention. *Journal of Neuroscience, 29*(34), 10563–10572.

Morris, J. S., DeGelder, B., Weiskrantz, L., & Dolan, R. J. (2001). Differential extragenicu-lostriate and amygdala responses to presentation of emotional faces in a cortically blind field. *Brain, 124*(6), 1241–1252.

Morris, J. S., Öhman, A., & Dolan, R. J. (1998). Conscious and unconscious emotional learning in the human amygdala. *Nature, 393*(6684), 467–470.

Moser, J., Hajcak, G., Bukay, E., & Simons, R. (2006). Intentional modulation of emotional responding to unpleasant pictures: An ERP study. *Psychophysiology, 43*(3), 292–296.

Most, S., Smith, S., Cooter, A., Levy, B., & Zald, D. (2007). The naked truth: Positive, arousing distractors impair rapid target perception. *Cognition and Emotion, 21*(5), 964–981.

Mueller, E., Hofmann, S., Santesso, D., Meuret, A., Bitran, S., & Pizzagalli, D. (2009). Electrophysiological evidence of attentional biases in social anxiety disorder. *Psychological Medicine, 39*(7), 1141–1152.

Mühlberger, A., Wieser, M. J., Herrmann, M. J., Weyers, P., Tröger, C., & Pauli, P. (2009). Early cortical processing of natural and artificial emotional faces differs between lower and higher socially anxious persons. *Journal of Neural Transmission, 116*(6), 735–746.

Nieuwenhuis, S., Aston-Jones, G., & Cohen, J. D. (2005). Decision making, the P3, and the locus coeruleus–norepinephrine system. *Psychological Bulletin, 131*(4), 510–532.

Norberg, J., Peira, N., & Wiens, S. (2010). Never mind the spider: Late positive potentials to phobic threat at fixation are unaffected by perceptual load. *Psychophysiology, 47*, 1151–1158.

Ochsner, K., Bunge, S., Gross, J., & Gabrieli, J. (2002). Rethinking feelings: An fMRI study of the cognitive regulation of emotion. *Journal of Cognitive Neuroscience, 14*(8), 1215–1229.

Ochsner, K., & Gross, J. (2005). The cognitive control of emotion. *Trends in Cognitive Sciences, 9*(5), 242–249.

Ochsner, K. N., & Gross, J. J. (2007). The neural architecture of emotion regulation. In J. J. Gross (Ed.), *Handbook of emotion regulation* (pp. 87–109). New York: Guilford Press.

Öhman, A., Flykt, A., & Esteves, F. (2001). Emotion drives attention: Detecting the snake in the grass. *Journal of Experimental Psychology General, 130*(3), 466–478.

Olofsson, J., Gospic, K., Petrovic, P., Ingvar, M., & Wiens, S. (2011). Effects of oxazepam on affective perception, recognition, and event-related potentials. *Psychopharmacology, 215*, 301–309.

Olofsson, J., Nordin, S., Sequeira, H., & Polich, J. (2008). Affective picture processing: An integrative review of ERP findings. *Biological Psychology, 77*(3), 247–265.

Olofsson, J., & Polich, J. (2007). Affective visual event-related potentials: Arousal, repetition, and time-on-task. *Biological Psychology, 75*(1), 101–108.

Parkhurst, D., Law, K., & Niebur, E. (2002).

Modeling the role of salience in the allocation of overt visual attention. *Vision Research, 42*(1), 107–123.

Pastor, M., Bradley, M., Löw, A., Versace, F., Moltó, J., & Lang, P. (2008). Affective picture perception: Emotion, context, and the late positive potential. *Brain Research, 1189,* 145–151.

Pessoa, L. (2008). On the relationship between emotion and cognition. *Nature Reviews Neuroscience, 9*(2), 148–158.

Pessoa, L. (2010). Emotion and attention effects: Is it all a matter of timing? Not yet. *Frontiers in Human Neuroscience, 4,* 1–5.

Pessoa, L., & Adolphs, R. (2010). Emotion processing and the amygdala: from a "low road" to "many roads" of evaluating biological significance. *Nature Reviews Neuroscience, 11*(11), 773–783.

Pessoa, L., McKenna, M., Gutierrez, E., & Ungerleider, L. (2002). Neural processing of emotional faces requires attention. *Proceedings of the National Academy of Sciences of the United States of America, 99*(17), 11458–11463.

Pessoa, L., Padmala, S., & Morland, T. (2005). Fate of unattended fearful faces in the amygdala is determined by both attentional resources and cognitive modulation. *NeuroImage, 28*(1), 249–255.

Phan, K., Fitzgerald, D., Nathan, P., Moore, G., Uhde, T., & Tancer, M. (2005). Neural substrates for voluntary suppression of negative affect: A functional magnetic resonance imaging study. *Biological Psychiatry, 57*(3), 210–219.

Phan, K., Liberzon, I., Welsh, R., Britton, J., & Taylor, S. (2003). Habituation of rostral anterior cingulate cortex to repeated emotionally salient pictures. *Neuropsychopharmacology, 28*(7), 1344–1350.

Pizzagalli, D. (2007). Electroencephalography and high-density electrophysiological source localization. In J. Cacioppo, L. G. Tassinary, & G. Berntson (Eds.), *Handbook of psychophysiology* (pp. 56–84). New York: Cambridge University Press.

Polich, J. (2007). Updating P300: An integrative theory of P3a and P3b. *Clinical Neurophysiology, 118*(10), 2128–2148.

Polich, J. (2012). Neuropsychology of P300. In S. Luck & E. Kappenman (Eds.), *Handbook of event-related potential components* (pp. 159–188). New York: Oxford University Press.

Pourtois, G., Dan, E. S., Grandjean, D., Sander, D., & Vuilleumier, P. (2005). Enhanced extrastriate visual response to bandpass spatial frequency filtered fearful faces: Time course and topographic evoked-potentials mapping. *Human Brain Mapping, 26*(1), 65–79.

Radilova, J. (1982). The late positive component of visual evoked response sensitive to emotional factors. *Activitas Nervosa Superior, Suppl. 3*(Pt. 2), 334–337.

Raichle, M. E. (2010). Two views of brain function. *Trends in Cognitive Sciences, 14*(4), 180–190.

Rensink, R. A., O'Regan, J. K., & Clark, J. J. (1997). To see or not to see: The need for attention to perceive changes in scenes. *Psychological Science, 8*(5), 368–373.

Rock, I., & Gutman, D. (1981). The effect of inattention on form perception. *Journal of Experimental Psychology, 7*(2), 275–285.

Sabatinelli, D., Lang, P., Keil, A., & Bradley, M. (2007). Emotional perception: Correlation of functional MRI and event-related potentials. *Cerebral Cortex, 17*(5), 1085–1091.

Santesso, D., Meuret, A., Hofmann, S., Mueller, E., Ratner, K., Roesch, E., et al. (2008). Electrophysiological correlates of spatial orienting towards angry faces: A source localization study. *Neuropsychologia, 46*(5), 1338–1348.

Schupp, H., Cuthbert, B., Bradley, M., Cacioppo, J., Ito, T., & Lang, P. (2000). Affective picture processing: The late positive potential is modulated by motivational relevance. *Psychophysiology, 37*(2), 257–261.

Schupp, H., Cuthbert, B., Bradley, M., Hillman, C., Hamm, A., & Lang, P. (2004). Brain processes in emotional perception: Motivated attention. *Cognition and Emotion, 18*(5), 593–611.

Schupp, H., Flaisch, T., Stockburger, J., & Junghöfer, M. (2006). Emotion and attention: Event-related brain potential studies. *Progress in Brain Research, 156,* 31–51.

Schupp, H., Junghöfer, M., Weike, A., & Hamm, A. (2003a). Attention and emotion: An ERP analysis of facilitated emotional stimulus processing. *NeuroReport, 14*(8), 1107–1110.

Schupp, H., Junghöfer, M., Weike, A., & Hamm, A. (2003b). Emotional facilitation of sensory processing in the visual cortex. *Psychological Science, 14*(1), 7–13.

Schupp, H., Junghöfer, M., Weike, A., & Hamm, A. (2004). The selective processing of briefly presented affective pictures: An ERP analysis. *Psychophysiology, 41*(3), 441–449.

Schupp, H., Stockburger, J., Bublatzky, F., Jung-höfer, M., Weike, A., & Hamm, A. (2008). The selective processing of emotional visual stimuli while detecting auditory targets: An ERP analysis. *Brain Research, 1230*, 168–176.

Schupp, H., Stockburger, J., Codispoti, M., Jung-höfer, M., Weike, A., & Hamm, A. (2007). Selective visual attention to emotion. *Journal of Neuroscience, 27*(5), 1082–1089.

Smith, N., Cacioppo, J., Larsen, J., & Chartrand, T. (2003). May I have your attention, please: Electrocortical responses to positive and negative stimuli. *Neuropsychologia, 41*(2), 171–183.

Smith, E., Weinberg, A., Moran, T., & Hajcak, G. (2012). *Electrocortical responses to NIM-STIM facial expressions of emotion.* Manuscript submitted for publication.

Stockburger, J., Schmälzle, R., Flaisch, T., Bublatzky, F., & Schupp, H. T. (2009). The impact of hunger on food cue processing: An event-related brain potential study. *NeuroImage, 47*(4), 1819–1829.

Tacikowski, P., & Nowicka, A. (2010). Allocation of attention to self-name and self-face: An ERP study. *Biological Psychology, 84*(2), 318–324.

Theeuwes, J. (1994). Endogenous and exogenous control of visual selection. *Perception, 23*, 429–440.

Thielscher, A., & Pessoa, L. (2007). Neural correlates of perceptual choice and decision making during fear–disgust discrimination. *Journal of Neuroscience, 27*(11), 2908–2917.

Tipper, S., Weaver, B., Jerreat, L., & Burak, A. (1994). Object-based and environment-based inhibition of return of visual attention. *Journal of Experimental Psychology: Human Perception and Performance, 20*(3), 478–499.

Treue, S. (2003). Visual attention: The where, what, how and why of saliency. *Current Opinion in Neurobiology, 13*(4), 428–432.

Vuilleumier, P. (2005). How brains beware: Neural mechanisms of emotional attention. *Trends in Cognitive Sciences, 9*(12), 585–594.

Vuilleumier, P., Armony, J., Driver, J., & Dolan, R. (2001). Effects of attention and emotion on face processing in the human brain: An event-related fMRI study. *Neuron, 30*(3), 829–841.

Wangelin, B., Löw, A., McTeague, L., Bradley, M., & Lang, P. (2011). Aversive picture processing: Effects of a concurrent task on sustained defensive system engagement. *Psychophysiology, 48*,112–116.

Weinberg, A., & Hajcak, G. (2010). Beyond good and evil: The time-course of neural activity elicited by specific picture content *Emotion, 10*(6), 767–782.

Weinberg, A., & Hajcak, G. (2011a). Electrocortical evidence for vigilance–avoidance in Generalized Anxiety Disorder. *Psychophysiology, 48*(6), 842–851.

Weinberg, A., & Hajcak, G. (2011b). The late positive potential predicts subsequent interference with target processing. *Journal of Cognitive Neuroscience, 23*, 2994–3007.

Weinberg, A., Hilgard, J., Bartholow, B., & Hajcak, G. (2012). Emotional targets: Evaluative categorization as a function of context and content. *International Journal of Psychophysiology, 84*, 149–154.

Whalen, P., Rauch, S., Etcoff, N., McInerney, S., Lee, M., & Jenike, M. (1998). Masked presentations of emotional facial expressions modulate amygdala activity without explicit knowledge. *Journal of Neuroscience, 18*(1), 411–418

Williams, L. M., Kemp, A. H., Felmingham, K., Liddell, B. J., Palmer, D. M., & Bryant, R. A. (2007). Neural biases to covert and overt signals of fear: Dissociation by trait anxiety and depression. *Journal of Cognitive Neuroscience, 19*(10), 1595–1608.

CHAPTER 4

Cognition–Emotion Interactions

A Review of the Functional Magnetic Resonance Imaging Literature

Luiz Pessoa and Mirtes G. Pereira

In the past two decades, functional magnetic resonance imaging (fMRI) has contributed immensely to the study of the neural bases of cognition and emotion. The goal of this chapter is to review some of this work, focusing particularly on the interactions between the two. Given the size of this literature, it is not possible here to provide a comprehensive survey. Instead, we focus on a few aspects that we believe are particularly noteworthy. And, perforce, we must leave out a vast array of topics—notably, interactions involving emotion and memory are not reviewed here.

The central question that is addressed in our chapter is the following: How do emotion and cognition interact in the prefrontal cortex? The prefrontal cortex (PFC) is clearly critical for several key aspects of cognitive function. Its role in emotional processing is less well understood, but, as described in this chapter, fMRI studies are making important contributions to filling in the gaps in the knowledge base.

Cognition and emotion have been traditionally conceptualized as mutually antagonistic. As reviewed in the subsequent sections, some evidence from fMRI studies is consistent with this notion. At the same time, many interactions between emotion and cognition do not fit well into a simple antagonistic relationship. Instead, cognitive and emotional signals appear to be combined in complex ways in the PFC, such that both contribute to observed activity—and ensuing behavior.

Emotional Conflict

To explore the mechanisms involved in emotional conflict, the "emotional Stroop" paradigm has been extensively investigated in behavioral and neuroimaging studies. In this task, participants are asked to identify the ink color of words that are either emotionally neutral (e.g., *apple*) or emotionally salient (e.g., *death*). Neuroimaging studies exploring brain regions involved in the emotional Stroop task have attempted to establish the correspondence of regions engaged in this form of interference relative to those in nonemotional response–interference paradigms.

For instance, Whalen and colleagues (1998) compared the counting Stroop task to an emotional version of the counting Stroop. Participants were asked to report the number of words on the screen. In the counting Stroop, the stimulus *one one* would constitute an incongruent stimulus and *two two* a congruent stimulus; in the emotional Stroop, stimuli containing negative words (e.g., *murder murder*) or neutral words (e.g., *bench bench*) were used. Behaviorally, both types of Stroop task were associated with increased reaction times (during incongruent and emotional conditions). During the counting Stroop, incongruent trials evoked greater responses relative to congruent ones in the dorsal and posterior portions of the medial PFC (Bush et al., 1998). During the emotional counting Stroop, emotional trials evoked greater responses relative to neutral ones in the anterior and ventral portion of the medial PFC.[1] These results support the proposal that the medial PFC is composed of subregions that are differentially involved in cognitive and emotional tasks, as discussed in greater depth below.

Further support for a dissociation of the neutral substrates of interference processing comes from studies from Etkin, Egner, and colleagues. In one study, they compared emotional and nonemotional conflict tasks (Egner, Etkin, Gale, & Hirsch, 2008). During the emotional conflict task participants categorized faces according to emotional expression (happy vs. fearful), while ignoring emotionally congruent or incongruent words (*HAPPY, FEAR*) written across the faces. During the nonemotional conflict task, participants performed a gender task, while ignoring gender words written across the faces. Based on the analysis of sequential effects (e.g., contrasting an incongruent trial that followed another incongruent vs. congruent trial), the authors proposed that the *resolution* of emotional conflict was handled by the ventromedial PFC, whereas the resolution of nonemotional conflict was handled by lateral PFC. In particular,

the former appeared to involve interactions with the amygdala; decreased activity in the amygdala was associated with increased activity in the ventromedial PFC (see also Etkin, Egner, Peraza, Kandel, & Hirsch, 2006). The authors also proposed that conflict *monitoring* engages dorsal aspects of the medial PFC for both emotional and nonemotional conditions. Together, their findings suggest that the neuroanatomical networks recruited to overcome distraction may vary with the nature of the con?ict, but a common mechanism for registering conflict is also at play.

Compton and colleagues also compared emotional and nonemotional versions of interference tasks to understand the extent to which neural circuits are shared between the two domains (Compton et al., 2003). They employed the traditional nonemotional color–word Stroop task and the emotional Stroop task in which the primary task was also to identify the ink color of a word, while the meaning of the distracter word was either neutral or emotional. Their results showed that activity increased in the left dorsolateral PFC during both incongruent color–word trials and negative trials, supporting the notion that this region is involved in maintaining attentional set whether or not the challenging task-irrelevant information is emotional.

In summary, whereas a body of studies has proposed a sharper segregation of the circuits involved in cognitive and emotional tasks, evidence for common neural substrates has accrued, too.

Emotional Distraction

Studies of emotional distraction have also contributed to our understanding of attentional control during the processing of affectively laden stimuli. A central question addressed by these studies is whether attentional control, when affective items are encountered, is qualitatively different from that of nonemotional control. Neuroimaging studies have thus investigated the extent to which activations observed in these two cases overlap. The distracting information employed is frequently of a visual nature, such as emotional pictures. Next, we review

---

[1]In the literature, what we refer here as *medial PFC* is frequently referred to as *anterior cingulate cortex*. But because the labeling of the anterior cingulate is fairly inconsistent, we favor the use of the more neutral term *medial PFC*. In addition, authors frequently label activation sites that are outside the cingulate gyrus itself (e.g., those in the presupplementary motor area) as *anterior cingulate cortex*, a practice that is both unfortunate and incorrect. Unless otherwise stated, *dorsomedial PFC* refers to cortical tissue that is both dorsal and posterior; *ventromedial PFC* refers to cortical tissue that is both ventral and anterior.

some of the studies that illustrate the effects of emotional distraction on brain responses.

Yamasaki, LaBar, and McCarthy (2002) investigated responses evoked by neutral and emotional distracters. Participants viewed a stream of square shapes of varying sizes and colors. Among this stream, both target stimuli (circles) and distracters (neutral and emotional pictures) were presented and required different button responses. Whereas dorsal PFC regions evoked greater responses to target stimuli than to neutral or emotional distracters (Figure 4.1A and B), inferior PFC regions evoked greater responses to emotional distracters than to both neutral distracters and target stimuli (Figure 4.1A and C). Interestingly, sites along the dorsomedial PFC exhibited equivalent responses to stimuli of greater behavioral relevance, namely target and emotional distracter stimuli.

The findings of several other studies are consistent with the dorsal–ventral separation described above. In a series of studies, Dolcos and colleagues investigated emotional distraction in the context of working memory tasks. Participants were shown sample stimuli that had to be remembered during a subsequent delay period. During the delay period, participants were shown distracting stimuli, including neutral and emotional pictures. The findings of one of the studies are illustrated in Figure 4.2 (Dolcos & McCarthy, 2006). During the delay period, responses in dorsolateral PFC (Figure 4.2B) were highest for the scrambled picture condition (i.e., digitally scrambled versions of the pictures were shown), intermediate for neutral distracters, and lowest for emotional distracters—a pattern of responses also observed in parietal cortex. In a parallel fashion, behavioral performance was best during the scrambled condition, intermediate for neutral distracters, and worst for emotional distracters. Both the dorsolateral PFC and the parietal site locations are similar to regions known to be robustly engaged during working memory tasks (Pessoa & Ungerleider, 2004). Notably, the magnitude of responses at similar sites is correlated with behavioral performance (Pessoa, Gutierrez, Bandettini, & Ungerleider, 2002). It therefore appears that viewing emotional distracters during the delay period interfered with the activity normally observed in

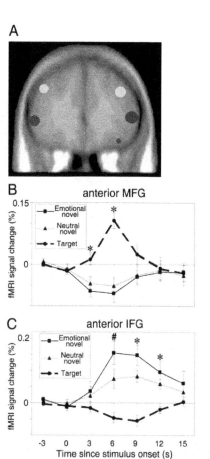

FIGURE 4.1. Emotional distraction during an oddball task. (A) Schematic illustration of dorsal (light gray) and ventral (dark gray) activation sites. Responses at the dorsal sites (B) were most sensitive to target stimuli, whereas those at the ventral sites (C) were most sensitive to emotional distractors. IFG, inferior frontal gyrus; MFG, middle frontal gyrus. Adapted from Yamasaki et al. (2002). Copyright 2002 by the National Academy of Sciences. Adapted by permission.

this area. Indeed, incorrect trials involving emotional distracters exhibited the weakest dorsolateral PFC responses during the delay period.

Responses in the ventrolateral PFC (Figure 4.2C) exhibited the opposite pattern as that observed in the dorsolateral PFC—the strongest responses were observed during the viewing of emotional distracters. What is the role of this region during the task? First, participants who showed greater activ-

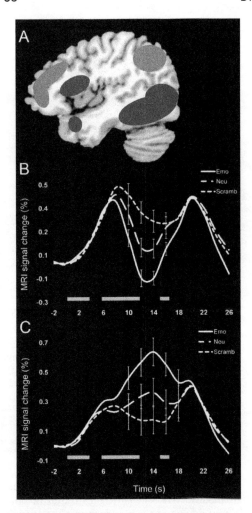

FIGURE 4.2. Emotional distraction during a working memory task (A) Schematic representation of differential responses. Light gray: scrambled > emotional; dark gray: emotional > scrambled. (B) Time course data for the dorsolateral PFC. (C) Time course data for the ventrolateral PFC. Adapted from Dolcos and McCarthy (2006). Copyright 2006 by the Society of Neuroscience. Adapted by permission.

tional pictures were viewed. Using a similar paradigm to investigate the effects of distraction during working memory, Anticevic and colleagues reported converging findings (Anticevic, Repovs, & Barch, 2010). In particular, when participants were faced with emotional distracters, ventrolateral PFC responses were stronger for correct versus incorrect trials. No differential responses were observed as a function of behavioral performance when neutral distracters were shown, suggesting that this region was especially important during emotional distraction.

When participants were shown negative distracters, Anticevic and colleagues (2010) observed a negative correlation between the strength of amygdala responses and behavioral performance (across participants). Notably, the same pattern was observed when both neutral pictures and other distracter stimuli (closely resembling to-be-remembered sample stimuli) were shown. These results suggest that amygdala responses may have reflected the behavioral relevance of the distracter stimulus and, more generally, are consistent with a broader role of the amygdala during cognitive performance (Schaefer et al., 2006)—a role that extends beyond the processing of emotion-laden items (Pessoa, 2008, 2010).

Attentional control has been studied extensively in the context of nonemotional information and, broadly speaking, two general frontal-parietal attention systems have been proposed: a dorsal system involved in controlling top-down attention and a more ventral system important in redirecting attention to behaviorally salient events (Corbetta & Shulman, 2002). The studies briefly reviewed above suggest that ventrolateral regions of the frontal cortex are engaged robustly during situations in which emotional stimuli act as distracters. It is thus possible that the frontal component of the ventral attentional system identified in nonemotional studies is particularly attuned to information with emotional content. In this regard, it is interesting to note that ventral aspects of the lateral PFC are more strongly interconnected with the amygdala than dorsal ones (although not as robustly as medial PFC areas) (Ghashghaei, Hilgetag, & Barbas, 2007); the ventrolateral PFC is also interconnected with the anterior insula

ity to emotional distracters in this region tended to rate emotional distracters as both less distracting and less emotional. Second, the larger the evoked responses, the better the performance during the working memory task. Together, these findings suggest that the ventrolateral PFC was involved in *inhibiting* the distracting effects of stimuli presented during the delay period, a function that was particularly needed when emo-

(Augustine, 1996), another structure that is important for valuation processes.

As noted, the ventrolateral PFC site observed in distraction studies appears to overlap areas of the ventral attentional system (the latter extends into the anterior insula). But here a possible contradiction is found. Whereas in the emotional distraction studies the ventrolateral PFC appears to counter the impact of distraction, its role in the reorienting network would be expected to be exactly the opposite. Namely, strong responses would signal the need to reorient attention toward the distracting object (contributing to the "interrupt" function described by Corbetta & Shulman, 2002). Given these opposite roles, at the scale of fMRI, the ventrolateral PFC may have spatially overlapping but separate neural populations that are engaged in these distinct situations.

An important question concerns the specificity of the engagement of the ventrolateral PFC during emotional distraction. Put another way, which dimensions of a stimulus are the most important: valence, arousal, or relevance? At the moment, the answer to this question remains unknown, and future studies are needed to fill in these gaps. It is possible, for instance, that the robust engagement of the ventrolateral PFC is related to the potency of the distraction—which is certainly a property of the emotional pictures employed in several studies—and not emotion per se.

Emotion Regulation

Emotion regulation involves processes that alter emotional experience. A body of work has documented the powerful ability that people have to regulate their emotions (Gross, 2007). Multiple regulation strategies exist, including "reappraisal" (e.g., reinterpreting the meaning of a stimulus), "cognitive distancing" (e.g., becoming a detached observer), and "behavioral suppression" (e.g., inhibiting external displays of emotion such as facial expression). Taken together, the corpus of studies suggests that the prefrontal cortex is broadly engaged during deliberative forms of emotion regulation (Figure 4.3), especially the ventrolateral PFC (Ochsner & Gross, 2005). In addition,

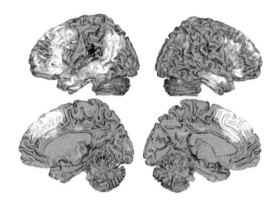

FIGURE 4.3. Emotional regulation. Regions in the lateral and medial frontal cortex that were more strongly engaged during reappraise versus maintain conditions in the study by Wager and colleagues. Adapted from Wager et al. (2008). Copyright 2008 by Cell Press. Adapted by permission.

about half of emotion regulation studies find activity in the dorsomedial prefrontal cortex (Berkman & Lieberman, 2009). Some studies also find activation in the dorsolateral prefrontal cortex, bilaterally. Furthermore, reappraisal also decreases activity in regions that are important for the evaluation of emotional significance, such as the amygdala, insula, and medial orbitofrontal cortex. Responses in these regions also increase when, in the laboratory, participants are instructed to enhance the emotional impact of a negative stimulus.

An important finding of the emotion regulation literature is that, not only are responses in the PFC increased and amygdala (as well as medial orbitofrontal cortex) responses decreased during emotional regulation but, across participants, these signals are inversely related (Kim & Hamann, 2007; Ochsner et al., 2004; Phan et al., 2005). For instance, activity in several areas of the frontal cortex, including dorsolateral, dorsomedial, and lateral orbital cortices, was reported to covary with amygdala activity during reappraisal, such that the strength of amygdala coupling with, for instance, the lateral orbitofrontal cortex and the dorsomedial prefrontal cortex predicted the extent of attenuation of negative affect following reappraisal (Figure 4.4) (Banks, Eddy, Angstadt, Nathan, & Phan,

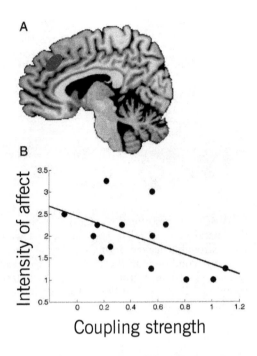

FIGURE 4.4. Emotional regulation. (A) Task-dependent coupling (reappraise > maintain) with the amygdala was observed in the dorsomedial prefrontal cortex (schematically shown in gray), as well as other regions (not shown). (B) The strength of the coupling was inversely related to the intensity of negative affect reported by participants. Adapted from Banks et al. (2007). Copyright 2007 by Oxford University Press. Adapted by permission.

2007). In other words, the greater the task-dependent coupling between the amygdala and these other regions, the more effective the reappraisal strategy, as noted by attenuated intensity of negative affect (see also Urry et al., 2006).

Although several studies have reported the negative coupling between the PFC and the amygdala during reappraisal, as discussed above, the relationship between these regions might be more context dependent. For instance, Wager, Davidson, Hughes, Lindquist, and Ochsner (2008) observed a positive (not negative) relationship between the ventrolateral PFC and the amygdala during reappraisal. Mediation analysis revealed a path through the ventral amygdala that predicted *reduced* reappraisal success (i.e., more negative emotion). In this case, successful reappraisal involved dampening, not

increasing, the (positive) coupling between the ventral PFC and the amygdala. Interestingly, Wager and colleagues observed a second path, involving the ventrolateral PFC through the nucleus accumbens, which predicted *greater* reappraisal success. Based on these results, Wager and colleagues proposed that two processes are engaged by the ventrolateral PFC: a negative appraisal process that leads to the generation of negative emotional responses to the stimuli and involves the amygdala, and a positive appraisal process that leads to positive reappraisal and involves the accumbens.

The findings by Wager and colleagues (2008) involving the amygdala stand in contrast to those described previously—the direction of the relationship with the PFC was positive, not negative. Whereas a clear reconciliation of these results is not straightforward, it is possible that particular regulation strategies play an important role in the observed interactions. In particular, Wager and colleagues asked their participants to produce a positive interpretation of the scene so as to reduce its emotional impact. In contrast, Banks and colleagues (2007), for example, asked participants to reinterpret the content of negative pictures so that they would no longer elicit a negative response. If indeed the precise instructions alter the associated regulatory circuits, this would indicate that the relationship between PFC regions engaged during reappraisal and the amygdala (and other regions) is malleable and context dependent.

In summary, deliberate emotion regulation is a process by which participants attempt to alter their experience while viewing emotional items. This process engages several prefrontal territories along lateral and medial aspects of the PFC, as well as dorsal and ventral sites. In parallel, in many cases, a set of regions whose function is linked to stimulus evaluation is also engaged, including the amygdala (as well as the medial orbitofrontal cortex and insula). Because the observed relationship between the PFC and evaluative regions is typically reciprocal, these interactions have frequently been described in terms of the "cognitive suppression of emotion." The study by Wager and colleagues (2008) reveals, however, that the coupling between PFC and other "regulated" regions may be context dependent, and multiple parallel circuits may operate to determine the fate of regulatory attempts. Finally, although the link between the PFC and the amygdala (or other regions) has been investigated across participants, an important goal for future research will be to establish this link on a trial-by-trial basis.[2] In other words, on a trial in which PFC response magnitude is stronger, one should observe decreased, say, amygdala activity, in conjunction with decreased negative affect. Such trial-by-trial relationship would help establish a stronger link between PFC and amygdala responses, on the one hand, and subjective experience, on the other.

Emotion–Cognition Push–Pull

In an influential paper, Drevets and Raichle (1998) noted that regional blood flow during attentionally demanding cognitive tasks *decreased* in regions such as the amygdala (see also (Shulman et al., 1997)), posteromedial orbitofrontal cortex, and ventromedial PFC—although blood flow *increased* in these regions during specific emotion-related tasks. Conversely, during experimentally induced and pathological emotional states blood flow *decreased* in regions such as the dorsomedial and dorsolateral prefrontal cortices—although blood flow *increased* in these regions during some cognitive tasks. These reciprocal patterns of activation suggested to Drevets and Raichle that emotion and cognition may engage in competitive interactions. In particular, they suggested that "deactivation of emotion-related areas may reflect a relative reduction in the processing resources devoted to emotional evaluation or experience in the control task relative to the experimental task" (p. 370). In addition, "during intense emotional responses to a threat, suppressing areas devoted to working memory and deep processing for visuospatial or semantic information may permit more rapid automatic responses to govern behaviour. Nevertheless, such deactivations may have associated 'costs' of reducing the functions of these areas" (p. 375). Following this initial study, the notion of a push–pull,

antagonistic organization between cognition and emotion has been probed in greater depth, as discussed in this section.

To explore the relationship between cognitive and emotional processing, Simpson and colleagues (Simpson et al., 2000) compared responses while participants viewed unpleasant images to the pattern that was known to be common to many effortful cognitive tasks—namely, decreases in activation in the medial PFC and other regions later suggested to be part of the so-called "task-negative" network (also called "default" or "resting-state" network), which is observed when participants lay passively in the scanner. When participants were asked to determine the number of humans in unpleasant pictures, an almost complete *absence of decreases* in activity in the medial PFC and the posterior cingulate was observed. In other words, during the processing of unpleasant pictures, reductions typically found during cognitive tasks were not observed, suggesting that emotional processing engages these regions—an engagement that is suppressed during cognitive processing. Together, the pattern of results suggested to the authors that some brain regions may be tonically active, and that their function "is necessary for the ongoing detection and evaluation of environmental and internal stimuli of relevance to the motivational state of the individual" (p. 166). Furthermore, an attenuation of this function takes place during the performance of tasks requiring focused attention.

To test the reciprocal nature of emotion and cognition, Goel and Dolan (2003) evaluated brain responses during "hot" and "cold" reasoning. Participants were asked to perform logical judgments about arguments that varied in emotional salience but that had the same general logical structure. Emotionally salient arguments involved terms such as *Nazis* and *child molesters*; neutral arguments involved terms such as *reptiles* and *mammals*. Participants were required to determine whether the conclusion followed logically from the premises. Cold reasoning trials resulted in *enhanced* activity in the dorsolateral PFC and *decreased* activity in the ventromedial PFC. By contrast, hot reasoning trials resulted in *enhanced* activation in the ventromedial PFC and *decreased* activation in the dorsolateral PFC.

---

[2]Although Eippert et al. (2007) attempted such an analysis, collinearity in their regressors precludes a clearer interpretation of the results.

In other words, a reciprocal relationship was observed in dorsal and ventral PFC regions that reflected the degree to which reasoning was "hot" or "cold."

A push–pull relationship has also been reported in the context of amygdala responses. For instance, Van Dillen and colleagues had participants engage in easy or difficult arithmetic problems that were presented immediately following unpleasant images (Van Dillen, Heslenfeld, & Koole, 2009). Whereas the more challenging problems produced greater responses than easier problems in the lateral PFC, the reverse pattern was observed in the amygdala: greater responses to emotional images during easy versus hard problems. Because of the sequential nature of their task, in which arithmetic operations followed the presentation of emotional images, their study was particularly well suited to reveal the dynamic nature of the evoked responses—such that performing a difficult task appeared to suppress amygdala responses (see Figure 4.5 for further details). A related push–pull finding was reported by Hsu and Pessoa (2007) during task conditions that, in fact, did not involve emotional stimuli. Amygdala responses during a difficult search task (searching for a target letter among distracter letters) were compared to responses during an easy search task (searching for a target letter among an array of O's). Decreased response was observed during difficult, relative to easy, search conditions, indicating that task load by itself impacts amygdala responses—that is, independently of its activation by emotional stimuli (see also Pessoa, Padmala, & Morland, 2005, for analogous findings in the absence of emotional stimuli).

The existence of a push–pull relationship between emotion and cognition has also been suggested in the context of clinical populations. For instance, Mayberg and colleagues (1999) reported that normal sadness, experienced following a mood induction procedure, was associated with increased blood flow in the subgenual cingulate cortex (Brodmann's area 25) and decreased blood flow in the right dorsolateral PFC. At the same time, remission of depression was associated with increased blood flow in the right dorsolateral prefrontal cortex and concomitant decreases in the subgenual cingulate cortex and mid- and posterior insula.

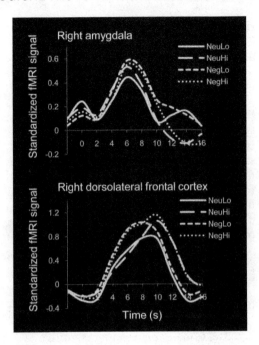

FIGURE 4.5. Cognition–emotional push–pull. Neutral/negative pictures were presented at $t = 0$ s and low–high load arithmetic problems were presented at $t = 4$ s. (A) In the right amygdala, responses were initially higher for negative versus neutral pictures (see values at 6–8 s). However, a high- versus low-load arithmetic problem considerably dampened responses (see values at 12–16 s). (B) This pattern should be contrasted to that observed in the right dorsolateral PFC, where the high-load arithmetic task increased evoked responses (see values at 10 s). The responses are consistent with a push–pull relationship in which the cognitive load in the PFC subsequently dampens responses in the amygdala. Adapted from Van Dillen et al. (2009). Copyright 2009 by Elsevier. Adapted by permission.

Mayberg and colleagues suggested that the experience of sadness results not only in ventromedial activation but also in the simultaneous deactivation of cortical regions known to mediate attentional processing.

A theme that emerges from many of the studies reviewed thus far in this chapter is that a dorsal–ventral distinction can be found in the sites that are sensitive to cognitive and emotional manipulations, respectively. A parallel development has focused on the organization of the medial PFC, which is a complex brain region involved in a host of functions, as indicated by neuropsychological and neuroimaging research, among other techniques. In a highly influential paper (surpassing 1,500 citations at the time of writing), Bush, Luu, and Posner (2000) proposed that the organization of the medial PFC can be understood in terms of anteroventral and posterodorsal sectors that are linked to emotional and cognitive processing, respectively (see also Devinsky, Morrell, & Vogt, 1995). The proposal was based on an informal meta-analysis of neuroimaging studies, as well as on data from lesion studies and anatomical connectivity. Although a *reciprocal* relationship between emotion and cognition was not emphasized, the framework was very prominent in highlighting an anatomical distinction between cognitive and emotional circuits that is based on a dorsal–ventral axis of organization.

Another approach to investigate dorsal and ventral circuits involves functional connectivity analysis, in which the pattern of correlations between brain regions is used as an indication of the strength of their "coupling" (which may involve indirect anatomical connections). A common procedure is to choose a specific "seed" region and characterize the region's interactions with the remainder of the brain during the so-called resting state. For instance, functional connectivity analysis during rest has revealed that signals in the amygdala are positively correlated with ventral brain regions such as the subgenual anterior cingulate cortex, orbitofrontal cortex, and insula (Anticevic et al., 2010; Roy et al., 2009). In contrast, activity in the amygdala is negatively correlated with responses in dorsal brain regions, including sites in the lateral PFC and parietal cortex.

Cognition–Emotion Interactions in the PFC

Although push–pull relationships between emotion and cognition at times exist in the brain, a broader review of the literature reveals several other types of interactions. In this section, a few representative studies are described to illustrate these interactions. In particular, we review experimental manipulations in which participants were asked to perform an executive function when they were faced with either neutral or emotional items, as well as other types of designs involving manipulations of emotion and cognition. We focus particularly on studies that revealed statistical interactions between emotion and cognition, both in terms of behavior and brain responses.

An important dimension of executive function is concerned with inhibiting and controlling behavior. Response inhibition, which involves processes required to cancel an intended action, engages several prefrontal regions, such as the dorsolateral PFC, inferior frontal cortex, and medial PFC (Aron, Robbins, & Poldrack, 2004; Rubia, Smith, Brammer, & Taylor, 2003). Response inhibition is often investigated by using so-called go/no-go tasks in which participants are asked to execute a motor response when shown the "go" stimulus (e.g., "Press a key as fast as possible when you see a letter stimulus"), but to withhold the response when shown the "no-go" stimulus (e.g., "Do not respond when you see the letter Y"). Typically, the go and no-go stimuli are shown as part of a rapid stream of stimuli (e.g., a sequence of letters). Goldstein and colleagues (2007) investigated the interaction between the processing of emotional words and response inhibition. Participants were asked to silently read every word in a rapid stream and to press a button to every word in regular font and to withhold responding to words that were italicized. Response inhibition when encountering negative words (e.g., *worthless*) engaged the dorsolateral PFC. Interestingly, this region was not recruited by negative valence or inhibitory task demands alone; instead, the dorsolateral PFC was sensitive to the explicit interaction between behavioral inhibition and the processing of negatively valenced words.

Evidence for cognition–emotion interactions comes from working memory studies, too. In the previous section "Emotional Distraction," we reviewed findings when emotional items are used as distracter stimuli. But what is the impact of the emotional content of to-be-remembered items on working memory maintenance? In one study, when participants were asked to keep in mind neutral or emotional pictures, maintenance-related activity in the dorsolateral PFC cortex was modulated by the valence of the picture, with pleasant pictures increasing activity and unpleasant pictures decreasing activity relative to neutral ones (Perlstein, Elbert, & Stenger, 2002). Interestingly, emotional pictures did not affect dorso-lateral responses in a second experimental condition, during which participants were *not* required to keep information in mind, indicating that the modulation of sustained activity by emotional valence was specific to the experimental context requiring active maintenance.

In another working memory study, participants watched short videos intended to induce emotional states, including clips from uplifting, sad, and neutral movies (Gray, Braver, & Raichle, 2002). After each video, participants were scanned while performing a "three-back" working memory task employing either word or face stimuli (participants were asked to press a target button if the stimulus currently on the screen was the same as the one seen three trials previously). Task-related activity in the lateral PFC in both hemispheres showed an emotional state-by-stimulus type of statistical interaction, with no main effects. For trials involving facial stimuli, evoked responses were strongest during the pleasant condition, weakest during the unpleasant, and intermediate for the neutral condition; for trials involving word stimuli, the reverse pattern of responses was observed. Notably, the crossover interaction activity pattern in the lateral PFC was correlated with behavioral performance across participants: Participants with a stronger effect of emotion behaviorally also exhibited stronger effects in terms of lateral PFC responses. In summary, lateral PFC activity in both hemispheres reflected equally the emotional and working memory task components, such that prefrontal activity did not stem from the cognitive task or the mood ensuing from the viewing of the video, but resulted from an interaction between emotion and cognition.

Cognition–emotion interactions also have been investigated during response conflict tasks (which were briefly reviewed in the section "Emotional Conflict"). In one study, Hart, Green, Casp, and Belger (2010) investigated the impact of viewing emotional pictures prior to performing the counting Stroop task. Both aversive and neutral images were employed. Stroop stimuli involved congruent (e.g., 22), incongruent *(222)*, and control (e.g., two star-shaped

geometrical shapes) conditions; as described previously, participants were asked to count the number of stimuli on the screen. Reaction times during incongruent trials were slower when participants viewed aversive compared to neutral stimuli (no effects of valence were observed during congruent or neutral trials). In terms of neuroimaging responses, the authors hypothesized that viewing aversive pictures would be associated with decreased responses in the dorsolateral PFC (due to a push–pull type of relationship). Whereas some reduction of evoked responses was observed during *congruent* trials that followed aversive pictures, decreased responses during *incongruent* trials were not detected. To further characterize brain responses, the authors investigated the relationship between reaction time during incongruent trials and differential responses. In several brain regions, including the middle and inferior frontal gyri in the lateral PFC, across participants, *faster* reaction times were associated with *greater* effects of aversive pictures (aversive > neutral). Thus, increased requirement for executive function during incongruent trials was linked to increased recruitment of lateral PFC regions—and such recruitment actually *improved* behavioral performance.

Finally, in a recent study we investigated cognition–emotion interactions in the context of a Stroop-like conflict task (Choi, Padmala, & Pessoa, 2012). We reasoned that shock anticipation would consume processing resources required for executive control (Pessoa, 2009) and thereby increase response conflict (but see Hu, Bauer, Padmala, & Pessoa, 2011). Trials started with the presentation of a cue stimulus that indicated trial type. During threat trials, participants received an unpleasant electrical stimulus in 30% of the trials (these shock trials were discarded from the main analyses); during safe trials no shock was administered. During the subsequent target phase (which occurred 2–6 seconds following the cue), participants were asked to indicate if images contained a house or building, while ignoring task-irrelevant words superimposed on the pictures. The strings *house*, *bldng*, and *xxxxx* were used to created congruent, incongruent, and neutral trials, respectively.

We focused our analyses on potential interference effects (incongruent vs. neutral), both behaviorally and in terms of brain responses. Behaviorally, a threat by congruency interaction was detected, such that interference *increased* during the threat condition. Moreover, this relationship was linearly related to state anxiety—larger interference for participants with higher anxiety scores. A threat-by-congruency interaction was not observed when brain responses were considered. However, interaction-related responses in the left anterior insula were correlated with state anxiety—larger interference-related responses occurred for participants with higher anxiety scores. Thus, the cognitive-emotional interaction was actually moderated by anxiety. In other words, an interaction pattern was observed for high-anxious individuals, but not for low-anxious individuals.

During the cue phase of the task (when participants were informed whether the trial was a threat or a safe one), differential responses (threat > safe) were observed in the dorsomedial PFC, in addition to the anterior insula and thalamus. Furthermore, differential responses in both dorsomedial PFC and thalamus were inversely related to state anxiety scores, such that larger differential responses were associated with lower anxiety scores, suggesting a potential role in regulating the impact of threat during our task. Notably, differential responses in the reverse direction (safe > threat) were quite extensive and overlapped quite distinctively with the task-negative network. Inspection of evoked responses in these areas suggested that threat produced a decrease in activation relative to safe.

As reviewed previously in the chapter, one type of interaction between emotion and cognition involves a push–pull relationship between more dorsal brain regions important for cognition and more ventral regions important for emotion. This type of interaction has been observed across several experimental paradigms, such as those involving emotional distraction and emotion regulation, among others. However, as illustrated in this section, cognition–emotion interactions take many forms that go beyond the simple antagonistic relationship often posited in the literature. Notably, the lateral PFC, including its dorsal aspects, which has well-documented roles in cognitive processing, appears to be an important convergence site for cognition–emotion interactions, as observed across several cognitive tasks, including attention, response inhibition, working memory, and conflict processing.

An important question concerning the role of the *lateral* PFC during cognition–emotion interactions is whether, during a cognitive task, emotional information decreases or enhances PFC responses. In a related fashion, what is the relationship between such responses and task performance—for example, do signal decreases impair performance? The studies by Dolcos and McCarthy (2006) as well as Anticevic and colleagues (2010) have clearly demonstrated instances during which emotional distracters lead to *decreased* dorsolateral PFC responses. However, decreased dorsolateral activation has not been observed universally. In particular, several studies with emotional distracters did not observe decreases in activation in the dorsolateral PFC (e.g., Hart et al., 2010; see also Blair et al., 2007). For instance, in the study by Hart and colleagues, across participants, *faster* reaction times during incongruent trials were associated with *greater* effects of aversive pictures (aversive > neutral) in the lateral PFC.

The relationship between dorsolateral PFC responses to emotional stimuli and task performance is complex as well. For instance, the working memory study by Dolcos and McCarthy (2006) showed that decreased responses were associated with impaired task performance. However, we argue that, more generally, it is not possible to uniquely interpret the functional significance of the direction of dorsolateral PFC engagement (i.e., increases vs. decreases) because it is unclear whether, for example, increased responses reflect greater capacity to utilize the regions functionally or, conversely, neural inefficiency (or increased effort).

The examples reviewed in this section highlight the notion that many of the effects of emotion on cognition (and vice versa) are best viewed not as a simple push–pull mechanism, but as interactions between the two, such that the resulting processes and signals are neither purely cognitive nor emotional. Instead, in several cases, the "cognitive" or "emotional" nature of the processes is blurred in a way that highlights the integration of these domains in the brain.

Conclusions

The goal of this chapter was to review key aspects of the current understanding of the neural substrates of cognition–emotion interactions based on the fMRI literature, with a particular emphasis on the PFC. The conflict between emotion and cognition naturally has a long history. This antagonism theme fits well with some of the results reviewed in this chapter. For instance, emotional distraction in the context of some working memory studies not only impaired performance but also exhibited a specific pattern of brain responses. More broadly, the theme is also clearly echoed in the reciprocal suppression relationship described by Drevets and Raichle (1998).

Nevertheless, cognition–emotion interactions are not limited to mutually suppressive ones. As discussed, the interactions are multifaceted and involve multiple cortical sites. An emerging theme is that the lateral PFC, including its dorsal aspects, is a focal point for cognition–emotion interactions; this relationship has been observed across a wide range of cognitive tasks. Notably, the direction of the interaction (increased vs. decreased activation) varies across studies. And the direction itself is not diagnostic with respect to the functional nature of the interaction—for instance, whether increased activation signifies more or less efficient engagement of the PFC.

Although space limitations preclude us from reviewing existing models of the organization of the PFC in terms of emotion, an interesting framework that goes beyond the cognition–emotion dichotomy is one proposing the existence of cognition–emotion gradients. For instance, Zelazo and Cunningham (2007) suggest that "rather than positing discrete systems for hot and cool EF [executive function], this model views hot–cool as a continuum that corresponds to the motivational significance of the problem to be solved" (p. 145).

Acknowledgments

The work of Luiz Pessoa is supported in part by a grant from the National Institute of Mental Health (No. MH071589). We would like to thank Florin Dolcos, Kevin LaBar, Luan Phan, Alexander Shackman, Lotte Van Dillen, and Tor Wager for assisting with figure preparation, and Srikanth Padmala for discussions.

References

Anticevic, A., Repovs, G., & Barch, D. M. (2010). Resisting emotional interference: Brain regions facilitating working memory performance during negative distraction. *Cognitive, Affective, and Behavioral Neuroscience, 10*(2), 159-73.

Aron, A. R., Robbins, T. W., & Poldrack, R. A. (2004). Inhibition and the right inferior frontal cortex. *Trends in Cognitive Sciences, 8*(4), 170–177.

Augustine, J. R. (1996). Circuitry and functional aspects of the insular lobe in primates including humans. *Brain Research Reviews, 22*(3), 229–244.

Banks, S. J., Eddy, K. T., Angstadt, M., Nathan, P. J., & Phan, K. L. (2007). Amygdala–frontal connectivity during emotion regulation. *Social Cognitive and Affective Neuroscience, 2*(4), 303–312.

Berkman, E. T., & Lieberman, M. D. (2009). Using neuroscience to broaden emotion regulation: Theoretical and methodological considerations. *Social and Personality Psychology Compass, 3*, 2–19.

Blair, K. S., Smith, B. W., Mitchell, D. G., Morton, J., Vythilingham, M., Pessoa, L., et al. (2007). Modulation of emotion by cognition and cognition by emotion. *NeuroImage, 35*(1), 430–440.

Bush, G., Luu, P., & Posner, M. I. (2000). Cognitive and emotional influences in anterior cingulate cortex. *Trends in Cognitive Sciences, 4*(6), 215–222.

Bush, G., Whalen, P. J., Rosen, B. R., Jenike, M. A., McInerney, S. C., & Rauch, S. L. (1998). The counting Stroop: An interference task specialized for functional neuroimaging—validation study with fMRI. *Human Brain Mapping, 6*(4), 270–282.

Choi, J. M., Padmala, S., & Pessoa, L. (2012). Impact of state anxiety on the interaction between threat monitoring and cognition. *NeuroImage, 59*, 1912–1923.

Compton, R. J., Banich, M. T., Mohanty, A., Milham, M. P., Herrington, J., Miller, G. A., et al. (2003). Paying attention to emotion: An fMRI investigation of cognitive and emotional Stroop tasks. *Cognitive, Affective, and Behavioral Neuroscience, 3*(2), 81–96.

Corbetta, M., & Shulman, G. L. (2002). Control of goal-directed and stimulus-driven attention in the brain. *Nature Reviews Neuroscience, 3*(3), 201–215.

Devinsky, O., Morrell, M. J., & Vogt, B. A. (1995). Contributions of anterior cingulate cortex to behaviour. *Brain, 118*(Pt. 1), 279–306.

Dolcos, F., & McCarthy, G. (2006). Brain systems mediating cognitive interference by emotional distraction. *Journal of Neuroscience, 26*(7), 2072–2079.

Drevets, W. C., & Raichle, M. E. (1998). Reciprocal suppression of regional cerebral blood flow during emotional versus higher cognitive processes: Implications for interactions between emotion and cognition. *Cognition and Emotion, 12*(3), 353–385.

Egner, T., Etkin, A., Gale, S., & Hirsch, J. (2008). Dissociable neural systems resolve conflict from emotional versus nonemotional distracters. *Cerebral Cortex, 18*(6), 1475–1484.

Eippert, F., Veit, R., Weiskopf, N., Erb, M., Birbaumer, N., & Anders, B. (2007). Regulation of emotional responses elicited by threat-related stimuli. *Human Brain Mapping, 28*(5), 409–423.

Etkin, A., Egner, T., Peraza, D. M., Kandel, E. R., & Hirsch, J. (2006). Resolving emotional conflict: A role for the rostral anterior cingulate cortex in modulating activity in the amygdala. *Neuron, 51*(6), 871–882.

Ghashghaei, H. T., Hilgetag, C. C., & Barbas, H. (2007). Sequence of information processing for emotions based on the anatomic dialogue between prefrontal cortex and amygdala. *NeuroImage, 34*(3), 905–923.

Goel, V. & Dolan, R. J. (2003). Reciprocal neural response within lateral and ventral medial prefrontal cortex during hot and cold reasoning. *NeuroImage, 20*(4), 2314–2321.

Goldstein, M., Brendel, G., Tuescher, O., Pan, H., Epstein, J., Beutel, M., et al. (2007). Neural substrates of the interaction of emotional stimulus processing and motor inhibitory control: An emotional linguistic go/no-go fMRI study. *NeuroImage, 36*(3), 1026–1040.

Gray, J. R., Braver, T. S., & Raichle, M. E. (2002). Integration of emotion and cognition in the lateral prefrontal cortex. *Proceedings of the National Academy of Sciences USA, 99*(6), 4115–4120.

Gross, J. J. (Ed.). (2007). *Handbook of emotion regulation.* New York: Guilford Press.

Hart, S. J., Green, S. R., Casp, M., & Belger, A. (2010). Emotional priming effects during Stroop task performance. *NeuroImage, 49*(3), 2662–2670.

Hsu, S. M., & Pessoa, L. (2007). Dissociable effects of bottom-up and top-down factors on the processing of unattended fearful faces. *Neuropsychologia, 45*(13), 3075–3086.

Hu, K., Bauer, A., Padmala, S., & Pessoa, L. (2011). Threat of bodily harm has opposing effects on cognition. *Emotion, 12,* 28–32.

Kim, S. H., & Hamann, S. (2007). Neural correlates of positive and negative emotion regulation. *Journal of Cognitive Neuroscience, 19*(5), 776–798.

Mayberg, H. S., Liotti, M., Brannan, S. K., McGinnis, S., Mahurin, R. K., Jerabek, P. A., et al. (1999). Reciprocal limbic-cortical function and negative mood: converging PET findings in depression and normal sadness. *American Journal of Psychiatry, 156*(5), 675–682.

Ochsner, K. N., & Gross, J. J. (2005). The cognitive control of emotion. *Trends in Cognitive Sciences, 9*(5), 242–249.

Ochsner, K. N., Ray, R. D., Cooper, J. C., Robertson, E. R., Chopra, S., Gabrieli, J. D., et al. (2004). For better or for worse: Neural systems supporting the cognitive down- and up-regulation of negative emotion. *NeuroImage, 23*(2), 483–499.

Perlstein, W. M., Elbert, T., & Stenger, V. A. (2002). Dissociation in human prefrontal cortex of affective influences on working memory-related activity. *Proceedings of the National Academy of Sciences USA, 99*(3), 1736–1741.

Pessoa, L. (2008). On the relationship between emotion and cognition. *National Reviews of Neuroscience, 9*(2), 148–1458.

Pessoa, L. (2009). How do emotion and motivation direct executive function? *Trends in Cognitive Sciences, 13*(4), 160–166.

Pessoa, L. (2010). Emotion and cognition and the amygdala: From what is it? to what's to be done? *Neuropsychologia, 48,* 3416–3429.

Pessoa, L., Gutierrez, E., Bandettini, P., & Ungerleider, L. (2002). Neural correlates of visual working memory: fMRI amplitude predicts task performance. *Neuron, 35,* 975–987.

Pessoa, L., Padmala, S., & Morland, T. (2005). Fate of unattended fearful faces in the amygdala is determined by both attentional resources and cognitive modulation. *NeuroImage, 28*(1), 249–255.

Pessoa, L. & Ungerleider, L. G. (2004). Top-down mechanisms for working memory and attentional processes. In M. S. Gazzaniga (Ed.), *The new cognitive neurosciences* (3rd ed., pp. 919–930). Cambridge, MA: MIT Press.

Phan, K. L., Fitzgerald, D. A., Nathan, P. J., Moore, G. J., Uhde, T. W., & Tancer, M. E. (2005). Neural substrates for voluntary suppression of negative affect: A functional magnetic resonance imaging study. *Biological Psychiatry, 57*(3), 210–219.

Roy, A. K., Shehzad, Z., Marqulies, D. S., Kelly, A. M., Uddin, L. Q., Gotimer, K., et al. (2009). Functional connectivity of the human amygdala using resting state fMRI. *NeuroImage, 45*(2), 614–626.

Rubia, K., Smith, A. B., Brammer, M. J., & Taylor, E. (2003). Right inferior prefrontal cortex mediates response inhibition while mesial prefrontal cortex is responsible for error detection. *NeuroImage, 20*(1), 351–358.

Schaefer, A., Braver, T. S., Reynolds, J. R., Burgess, G. C., Yarkoni, T., & Gray, J. R. (2006). Individual differences in amygdala activity predict response speed during working memory. *Journal of Neuroscience, 26*(40), 10120–10128.

Shulman, G. L., Fiez, J. A., Corbetta, M., Buckner, R. L., Miezin, F. M., Raichle, M. E., et al. (1997). Common blood flow changes across visual tasks: II. Decreases in cerebral cortex. *Journal of Cognitive Neuroscience, 9,* 648–663.

Simpson, J. R., Ongur, D., Akbudak, E., Conturo, T. E., Ollinger, J. M., Snyder, A. Z., et al. (2000). The emotional modulation of cognitive processing: An fMRI study. *Journal of Cognitive Neuroscience, 12*(Suppl. 2), 157–170.

Urry, H. L., van Reekum, C. M., Johnstone, T., Kalin, N. H., Thurow, M. E., Schaefer, H. S., et al. (2006). Amygdala and ventromedial prefrontal cortex are inversely coupled during regulation of negative affect and predict the diurnal pattern of cortisol secretion among older adults. *Journal of Neuroscience, 26,* 4415–4425.

Van Dillen, L. F., Heslenfeld, D. J., & Koole, S. L. (2009). Tuning down the emotional brain: An fMRI study of the effects of cognitive load on the processing of affective images. *NeuroImage, 45*(4), 1212–1219.

Wager, T. D., Davidson, M. L., Hughes, B. L., Lindquist, M. A., & Ochsner, K. N. (2008). Prefrontal–subcortical pathways mediating successful emotion regulation. *Neuron, 59*(6), 1037–1050.

Whalen, P. J., Bush, G., McNally, R. J., Wilhelm, S., McInerney, S. C., Jenike, M. A., et al. (1998). The emotional counting Stroop paradigm: A functional magnetic resonance imaging probe of the anterior cingulate affective division. *Biological Psychiatry, 44,* 1219–1228.

Yamasaki, H., LaBar, K. S., & McCarthy, G. (2002). Dissociable prefrontal brain systems for attention and emotion. *Proceedings of the National Academy of Sciences USA, 99,* 215–222.

Zelazo, P. D. & Cunningham, W. A. (2007). Executive function: Mechanisms underlying emotion regulation. In J. J. Gross (Ed.), *Handbook of emotion regulation* (pp. 135–158). New York: Guilford Press.

CHAPTER 5

Hormones and Emotion

Stress and Beyond

Michelle M. Wirth and Allison E. Gaffey

What Are Hormones and How Do They Work?

Our bodies produce a rich diversity of hormones that play roles in physiological functions from blood sugar storage (insulin) to thirst and salt–water balance (angiotensin II) to inhibition of neural firing (allopregnanolone). The brain coordinates hormone production, so levels of many hormones fluctuate during emotion. Hormones also affect the brain, which gives them the potential to influence emotion, cognition, and behavior.

Hormones are chemicals produced by glands without ducts, which exert effects on cells that can be distant from the glandular source (Nelson, 2005a). For example, estradiol produced by the ovary travels in the bloodstream and acts on cells in the cervix, breast tissue, and brain, among other organs. Hormones have effects on cells by binding to receptors on or in the cell; each hormone has specific receptors to which it binds in a "lock-and-key" fashion. Classic neurotransmitters (glutamate, gamma-aminobutyric acid [GABA], serotonin, acetylcholine, etc.) are not considered hormones because they are not produced by glands and tend to act only on nearby cells—that is, on other neurons in the vicinity of their release. However, some hormones in the bloodstream can enter the brain and exert neuromodu-

latory effects on neurons. Some hormones are even produced in the brain itself, such as *neurosteroids* (discussed later) and countless peptide hormones such as corticotropin-releasing hormone (CRH) and oxytocin. Such hormones can be considered both hormones and neuromodulators, depending on their source and target tissue.

The brain also controls the production of hormones in glands throughout the body (i.e., the endocrine system). Hormone production is orchestrated by the hypothalamus, a structure at the base of the brain, and the pituitary gland, a two-part "master gland" connected to the hypothalamus (Figure 5.1). There is a constant interchange of information between the brain and endocrine system: The brain sends signals to increase or decrease production of a given hormone, and hormones in turn exert effects on neurons. An example of this information exchange is *negative feedback*: A given hormone, traveling through the bloodstream and reaching the hypothalamus and pituitary, generally turns off the factors that lead to its own production. Negative feedback allows for regulation of hormone levels (Becker & Breedlove, 2002; Nelson, 2005a). In general, the bidirectional relationship between the brain and hormones means that cognition and behavior can affect hormone production, and vice versa, although both

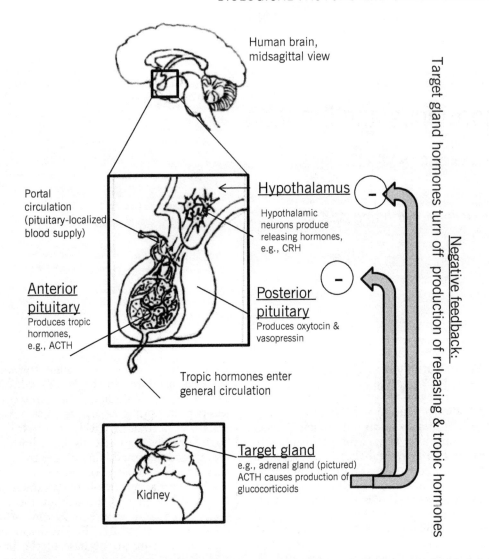

FIGURE 5.1. The hypothalamus and pituitary orchestrate hormone release from peripheral glands.

halves of the "loop" are not always considered. For example, we commonly think of stressful feelings causing increases in cortisol, but we don't always consider the effects of cortisol on cognition, including complex effects on memory (de Kloet, Oitzl, & Joels, 1999; Wolf, 2008). As another example, it is well known that testosterone can influence aggressive behavior (true in other animals and probably also in humans). However, it is less known that engaging in aggressive or competitive behaviors also causes increases in testosterone levels (Archer, 2006). Thus, the brain responds to various environmental and internal stimuli to regulate hypotha-

lamic signals that influence hormone production; hormones, in turn, affect the brain and thereby impact emotion, cognition, and behavior.

There are two main classes of hormones: peptide and steroid hormones. *Peptide hormones* are built out of amino acids, like all proteins. *Steroid hormones*, in contrast, are synthesized from cholesterol, and all share a similar four carbon-ring chemical structure. (See Table 5.1 for examples of steroid and peptide hormones.) One difference between these two classes of hormones is how they act on cells (Figure 5.2). Peptide hormones are large, hydrophilic (i.e., dissolve in water) molecules that cannot permeate the fatty membranes that surround cells. Thus, they act on receptors that are embedded in cells' membranes. Binding to the receptor causes a cascade of effects within the cell; the end result of this process depends on the hormone and the type of cell. For example, if the cell is a neuron, peptide hormones can influence neuronal excitability (Nelson, 2005a). Because peptide hormones cannot

traverse cell membranes, they cannot cross the blood–brain barrier except via transport molecules, levels of which can fluctuate. However, many peptide hormones are produced in the brain. Others, such as cholecystokinin, cause effects in the brain by stimulating the vagus nerve, which conveys parasympathetic input. There are also places in the brain where the blood–brain barrier can be bypassed (e.g., through the nasal epi-

TABLE 5.1. Some Examples of Peptide and Steroid Hormones

Hormones	Some functions
Peptide hormones	
Arginine vasopressin (AVP)	Blood pressure; aggression; HPA axis stress response
Oxytocin (OT)	Osmotic balance; smooth muscle contraction; social memory; affiliation and bonding
Insulin	Storage of blood glucose
Corticotropin-releasing hormone (CRH)	Hypothalamus: HPA axis stress response; elsewhere in brain: anxiety behavior
Adrenocorticotropic hormone (ACTH)	HPA axis stress response
Beta-endorphin	Stress-induced analgesia (i.e., reduction in pain sensitivity)
Ghrelin	Food intake/hunger; reduces anxiety and depression-like behavior in lab animals
Neuropeptide Y (NPY)	Food intake/hunger; reduces anxiety/anti–stress actions in lab animals
Steroid hormones[a]	
Cortisol (a glucocorticoid, or GC)	Increases energy availability; HPA axis regulation; affects learning and memory
Corticosterone (a GC)	Increases energy availability; HPA axis regulation; affects learning and memory
Estradiol	Behavioral estrus in lab animals; growth of tissues; learning
Testosterone (T)	Secondary sex characteristics; aggression; attention to challenge signals
Dihydrotestosterone (DHT)	Masculinization of genitals; male-pattern balding
Progesterone (P)	Uterine function; stress; antianxiety effects (via ALLO); affiliation/bonding?
Allopregnanolone (ALLO)	Neural inhibition; antianxiety; lower levels in depression; affilition/bonding?
Dihydroepiandrosterone (DHEA)	Possible stress-protection roles; preservation of cognitive function during stress?

[a]For an excellent chart showing synthesis of steroid hormones, see *http://en.wikipedia.org/wiki/File:Steroidogenesis.svg*.

Peptide hormones (+ some steroids)   Steroid hormones (classical mechanism)

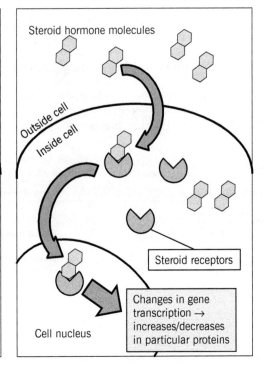

FIGURE 5.2. How peptide versus steroid hormones exert effects on cells.

thelium). Peptide hormones administered intranasally thus enter some parts of the brain (Born et al., 2002).

Steroid hormones are small, lipophilic (i.e., fatty molecules that do not dissolve in water) molecules that can pass through cell membranes. This means that they can cross the blood–brain barrier, although their entry also may be regulated by transport molecules. Because they are lipophilic, however, steroid hormones cannot easily dissolve in the bloodstream. In order to travel in blood, steroid molecules are generally bound to protein carrier molecules. At any given time, 5–10% of steroid hormone molecules in the blood are "free" or unbound to proteins. It is this portion that can enter the brain, and also the cells of salivary glands, which allows measurement of unbound steroid levels in saliva (Schultheiss & Stanton, 2009). After passing through cell membranes, steroid hormones exert their effects by binding to intracellular receptors. The hormone–receptor complex then migrates inside the cell's nucleus and affects gene transcription,

increasing or decreasing production of specific proteins (Figure 5.2). These effects on gene transcription can take hours or even days to build up. Such effects are too slow to change neuronal excitability on a moment-to-moment basis, though they can still have longer-term effects on behavior—for example, by restructuring neural connections (Nelson, 2005a).

However, researchers have discovered several ways in which steroid hormones can act on membrane-bound receptors and hence have "fast" effects on neuronal excitability. For example, there is evidence of membrane-bound androgen receptors in the mammalian brain (DonCarlos, Garcia-Ovejero, Sarkey, Garcia-Segura, & Azcoitia, 2003; Tabori et al., 2005). Glucocorticoid hormones have rapid effects on neurons, mediated by a type of receptor previously thought to be solely intracellular, which turns out to also be located in the cell membrane (de Kloet, Karst, & Joels, 2008). Also, some steroid hormones can bind to receptors for neurotransmitters. For example, allopregnanolone binds to GABA receptors and facilitates GABA binding (discussed below). Because GABA is an inhibitory neurotransmitter, allopregnanolone leads to inhibition of neuronal firing. Correspondingly, when administered to lab animals, certain steroid hormones exert effects on behavior that are too rapid to be explained by classical intracellular steroid receptors and changes in gene transcription (Dallman, 2005; de Kloet et al., 2008; Frye, 2001). Armed with knowledge of how hormones work, we can now explore specific hormones and how they both affect and are affected by emotion and cognition.

Stress Hormones and Cognition–Emotion Interactions

There are two primary stress-response systems. The *sympathetic nervous system* (SNS), a branch of the autonomic nervous system, exerts rapid (within seconds) effects on organs associated with "fight or flight" responses (e.g., pupil dilation, acceleration of heart rate, inhibition of salivation and digestive functions, and sweat response in the extremities). The SNS responds to an immediate threat, redirecting energy and blood flow to the limbs for any necessary fighting or fleeing (Nelson, 2005b; Sapolsky, 2002). The second major stress system in the body, and our focus, is the *hypothalamic–pituitary–adrenal axis* (HPA axis; Figure 5.1). The HPA axis is an evolutionarily old system that is very similar in all vertebrate animals and has strong interconnections with the immune system (Maier & Watkins, 1998). Neurons in the paraventricular nucleus (PVN) of the hypothalamus integrate challenge- or threat-related signals from elsewhere in the brain and respond by producing CRH, which travels to the pituitary and causes production of *adrenocorticotropic hormone* (ACTH). ACTH is released into the bloodstream and acts on the adrenal gland, causing production of *glucocorticoids* (GCs). GCs include cortisol (the primary glucocorticoid in primates, including humans) and corticosterone (the primary glucocorticoid in rodents). GCs affect cells via two intracellular receptors: the *mineralocorticoid receptor* (MR) and the *glucocorticoid receptor* (GR). These receptors

are ubiquitous throughout the body, including in the brain; GCs thus have widespread effects. A major function of GCs is to make more energy available to tissues throughout the body. For example, GCs mobilize glucose from the liver and stimulate the breakdown of proteins and fats (Nelson, 2005b).

Because the HPA axis and its production of GCs depends on hormones traveling through the bloodstream, this system responds much more slowly than the SNS, taking minutes to hours after stress onset for a full response. The HPA axis seems to function to replenish energy used after a short-lived fight or flight is over, or to continue to supply energy for sustained or chronic stressors (Nelson, 2005b). Often the SNS and HPA axis will both respond to a stressful stimulus, but one may predominate depending on the nature and duration of the stimulus. For example, hearing a startlingly loud noise or viewing an upsetting picture may generate an SNS response without an HPA axis response (Abercrombie, Kalin, Thurow, Rosenkranz, & Davidson, 2003; Wirth, Scherer, Hoks, & Abercrombie, 2011). On the other hand, impromptu public speaking—which is not only emotionally arousing but also involves a lack of control and an element of social-evaluative judgment (see below)—activates both SNS and HPA axis responses (Kirschbaum, Pirke, & Hellhammer, 1993). HPA axis hormones, in addition to responding to acute stressors, also show effects of chronic, long-term stress, such as effects of dominance hierarchies in many species (Sapolsky, 2005); and human-specific chronic stressors such as burnout (Pruessner, Hellhammer, & Kirschbaum, 1999), perceived work overload (Schlotz, Hellhammer, Schulz, & Stone, 2004), and material hardship (Ranjit, Young, & Kaplan, 2005).

HPA axis stress responses and resulting cortisol levels show considerable variability from person to person and from instance to instance. Early work by John Mason, a physician, identified three key characteristics of a situation that cause HPA axis responsivity in humans: *novelty, unpredictability*, and relative *lack of control* over the situation (Mason, 1975). Of course, these characteristics are subjective; what matters is whether one construes the situation as novel, unpredictable, etc. (Lupien, Maheu, Tu, Fiocco, & Schramek, 2007). In addition, a meta-analysis of studies using acute laboratory psychological stressors revealed that *social-evaluative judgment* is a key determinant of ACTH and cortisol increases (Dickerson & Kemeny, 2004). Thus, HPA axis activity seems most increased by situations in which other people are watching and judging one's actions—which perhaps makes evolutionary sense considering the hypersociality of our species and the extreme survival importance of being accepted into one's social group.

Several additional factors determine the degree of HPA axis response to stress. One factor is time of day of testing; high variability in HPA axis hormones in the morning hours, due to circadian factors, means that stressors have larger effect sizes on ACTH and cortisol if the study sessions took place in the late afternoon or evening (Dickerson & Kemeny, 2004). Another factor is sex; men typically have greater cortisol increases in response to lab stressors than women, despite the fact that women report the same or greater increases in negative emotions during the stressors (Kudielka & Kirschbaum, 2005). Why men's HPA axes respond more to speech stressors in the laboratory is unknown.

Early experiences have lifelong impacts on responses to stress. Rat pups that receive less maternal care (licking and grooming) exhibit elevated HPA stress responses in adulthood (Liu et al., 1997). Less maternal care causes a lifelong decrease in the expression of the gene for the GR (Meaney, 2001). Lower numbers of GR in the brain mean that the brain is less sensitive to GCs, and thus has reduced efficiency of negative feedback, resulting in larger and more prolonged GC responses to stress. There is evidence that these mechanisms may be at work in humans as well: A study of postmortem brains of suicide victims revealed that those with a history of childhood abuse also showed down-regulation of GR in the hippocampus (McGowan et al., 2009). Interestingly, mild early-life stressors may have beneficial effects. In a squirrel monkey model, moderate stressors postweaning led to smaller HPA responses to stress later in life, less distress in response to novelty, and enhanced performance on a prefrontal cortex–dependent inhibition task (Lyons, Parker, Katz, & Schatzberg, 2009).

Apart from early life experiences, other individual differences can affect HPA axis responsivity. How an individual construes a stressful situation can impact the magnitude of a cortisol response. For example, for people who are not accustomed to winning, winning a contest may be a more uncontrollable and/or novel experience to them, thus activating the HPA axis. In one study, implicit power motivation—a personality trait capturing a person's implicit desire to exert impact on others—moderated cortisol responses to winning or losing a (secretly rigged) contest: Those high in power motivation who "lost" the contest had increases in cortisol across the study session, whereas those low in power motivation who "won" (but not those who "lost") also appeared to have an increase in cortisol (Wirth, Welsh, & Schultheiss, 2006). A recent study of social identity threat provides another example of how individual differences and context interact to determine HPA axis responses. Women were rejected by a male confederate in a mock job interview for potentially sexist reasons; only those with higher chronic perceptions of sexism had increased cortisol in response to this situation. In groups rejected for merit-based reasons, the relationship was not found (Townsend, Major, Gangi, & Mendes, 2011).

Construal of a situation can also be manipulated in the lab, with subsequent effects on HPA axis responses. In one study, healthy participants were injected with pentagastrin, a substance that induces panic attacks and robust HPA axis activation. Significantly lower cortisol responses were seen in participants who were allowed to believe that they had control over the pentagastrin administration (that they could slow the infusion with controls on the pump), as well as in participants that received more detailed descriptions of expected symptoms of pentagastrin along with encouragement to attribute any symptoms experienced to the drug (Abelson, Khan, Liberzon, Erickson, & Young, 2008). So, brief interventions to reduce novelty and/or give people a greater sense of control over a situation can reduce the hormonal response to stress.

What is the relationship, if any, between cortisol and emotional experience? Negative affect is usually a component of "psychological" stress. However, negative affect is not always accompanied by HPA axis activation and cortisol secretion—for example, during a negative emotion that does not involve novelty, social-evaluative judgment, or high energetic demands. Because the primary role of GCs in the body is to increase availability of energy, a variety of physiological and psychological challenges, such as illness, waking up in the morning (Fries, Dettenborn, & Kirschbaum, 2009), and strenuous exercise (Kirschbaum, Wust, Faig, & Hellhammer, 1992), can increase cortisol without increasing negative affect. Some emotional events are accompanied by both changes in affect and HPA axis activation, which makes sense considering that the neural circuitry involved in processing emotional events (e.g., the amygdala and frontal cortex regions) provides input to CRH-producing neurons in the hypothalamus. One study reported a time lag between subjective emotional responses and cortisol reactivity, which makes sense given the cascade of neural and hormonal signals that must occur before cortisol levels rise in the bloodstream. When the time lag was taken into account, subjective emotional distress was found to positively predict ACTH and cortisol responses (Schlotz et al., 2008). Importantly, however, a meta-analysis of hormonal responses to laboratory stressors found, overall, no relationships between HPA axis hormones and self-reported mood (Dickerson & Kemeny, 2004). Thus, HPA axis activity and cortisol increases accompany some, but not all, emotional experiences—an example of (emotion-related) brain activity impacting hormone production.

HPA axis hormones also impact the brain and can therefore affect emotion and cognition. MR and GR are particularly densely expressed (i.e., more receptors per unit of tissue) in regions involved in emotion and learning, such as the amygdala, hippocampus, and prefrontal cortex (Joels & Krugers, 2007; Lupien et al., 2007). This helps explain why patients with abnormally high levels of cortisol commonly have affective symptoms as well as cognitive impairments (Haskett, 1985). Similarly, long-term treatment with drugs that activate GC receptors, such as prednisone or dexamethasone, is associated with mood changes (early mania

and later depression) as well as impaired declarative and working memory (Brown, 2009). However, chronic treatment with GC drugs does not produce the same effects as normal, physiological levels or acute treatment.

How does short-term (acute) manipulation of cortisol impact mood? In several double-blind, placebo-controlled studies, administration of GCs did not yield effects on mood, emotional arousal, or anxiety levels (Buchanan, Brechtel, Sollers, & Lovallo, 2001; Soravia, de Quervain, & Heinrichs, 2009; Wachtel & de Wit, 2001; Wolf et al., 2001). However, in other studies, GC administration had nuanced effects on emotional processing. For example, Buchanan and colleagues (2001) found that a lower dose of cortisol increased and a higher dose decreased the startle eyeblink response, without affecting emotional modulation of startle. Abercrombie, Kalin, and Davidson (2005) found that men given oral hydrocortisone (synthetic cortisol), compared to placebo controls, subsequently rated objectively neutral (vs. unpleasant) words and pictures as more emotionally arousing. In addition, studies have found decreased negative affect following acute GC administration. For example, oral cortisone decreased fear in people with spider phobias exposed to a phobic stimulus (Soravia et al., 2006). In other studies, healthy participants' affective responses to a laboratory stressor were decreased following acute cortisol treatment compared to placebo (Het & Wolf, 2007), and intravenous hydrocortisone appeared to decrease the effect of highly unpleasant pictures on negative affect, but only after prior exposure to the testing context and pictures (Wirth et al., 2011). Another group found evidence that cortisol administration shifts attention away from threat-related information: Cortisol abolished an emotional Stroop effect for fear faces (Putman, Hermans, Koppeschaar, van Schijndel, & van Honk, 2007) and reduced preferential processing of fearful faces in a spatial working memory task (Putman, Hermans, & van Honk, 2007). Thus, whereas chronically elevated GC levels may cause mood and memory dysfunction, acute GC elevations generally have no effect on mood or cause decreases in negative emotions.

We might better understand these effects on emotion in the context of the profound effects stress and GCs have on learning and memory. Depending on the dose, the material to be learned, emotional arousal, and the phase of learning (i.e., consolidation or retrieval), stress hormones may enhance or impair memory consolidation. GCs affect memory by enhancing or suppressing long-term potentiation (LTP), a neural mechanism that underlies learning, in the hippocampus and amygdala (Joels & Krugers, 2007). Corroborating animal research, human fMRI studies provide evidence that increases in amygdala activity induced via emotional arousal signals the hippocampus to enhance memory consolidation (Canli, Zhao, Brewer, Gabrieli, & Cahill, 2000; LaBar & Cabeza, 2006). Since GCs tend to increase amygdala activity (Duvarci & Pare, 2007), this is one pathway by which GCs can affect memory consolidation. Accordingly, exogenous or stress-related elevations in GCs seem to particularly enhance consolidation of emotional material, or material learned in an emotional context. Relatedly, GCs affect memory only in the presence of elevated norepinephrine (NE) in the amygdala, a marker of emotional arousal (Roozendaal, Okuda, de Quervain, & McGaugh, 2006; van Stegeren et al., 2007). How can the impact of GCs on memory explain the mixed findings regarding affect? In nonemotional contexts, GCs may boost amygdala activity and thereby enhance measures of emotional arousal (Abercrombie et al., 2005), whereas in emotionally arousing contexts GCs may enhance habituation or extinction learning processes (i.e., strengthen the association between the arousing stimulus and safety) and thereby cause a reduction in negative affect. This could help explain the fear-reducing effect of GCs in people with spider phobias (Soravia et al., 2006). Another possible explanation is that GCs interfere with consolidation of emotional aspects of the experience, causing decreased ratings of negative affect at a later time point (Het & Wolf, 2007; Wirth et al., 2011).

The effect of GCs on memory follows an inverted-U-shaped dose–response curve: Moderate GC elevations enhance consolidation and related neural processes (i.e., LTP), whereas very low and very high levels inhibit these processes (Joels & Krugers, 2007).

Optimal memory consolidation is achieved when most of the higher-affinity MRs in the brain are occupied by GC molecules, and an intermediate proportion of the lower-affinity GR are occupied. This is likely the case with mild or moderate stress. In humans, moderate doses of GCs facilitate, whereas high GC doses or too little GCs impair, declarative memory. For example, administration of metyrapone, a drug that blocks cortisol production, impaired memory (Lupien et al., 2002). Similarly, stress or a GC injection in the morning (when endogenous GC levels were already high) impaired memory, whereas stress or a GC injection in the afternoon left memory performance unchanged and decreased reaction times on a recognition memory task (Lupien et al., 2002; Maheu, Collicutt, Kornik, Moszkowski, & Lupien, 2005). These findings are consistent with animal research in which very low (not enough MR occupancy) or very high GC levels (too much GR occupancy) are associated with impaired memory consolidation.

As mentioned before, the effects of GCs on memory consolidation depend on emotional arousal and emotional qualities of the material being learned; one possible mechanism for these effects is the NE-dependent nature of the effects of GCs on memory. As an example, corticosterone injections enhanced object recognition in rats when the learning environment was novel (and thus emotionally arousing), but not in rats that had been habituated to the learning context (Okuda, Roozendaal, & McGaugh, 2004). In humans, GCs seem to particularly enhance memory for emotional material (Buchanan & Lovallo, 2001; Payne et al., 2007) or in the presence of elevated negative affect (Abercrombie, Speck, & Monticelli, 2006). Some studies find that stress enhances memory for emotional material while impairing memory for neutral material (Jelici, Geraerts, Merckelbach, & Guerrieri, 2004; Payne et al., 2007). Similarly, in a study utilizing a dose of GCs expected to impair memory formation, memory of emotionally arousing story details was impaired, whereas memory of neutral story details was enhanced (Rimmele, Domes, Mathiak, & Hautzinger, 2003).

In contrast with the sometimes-enhancing effects of GC on memory consolidation, GCs generally suppress memory retrieval and working memory. If stress or GCs are administered to lab animals or humans at the time of memory retrieval, memory is impaired (de Quervain, Aerni, Schelling, & Roozendaal, 2009; Smeets, Otgaar, Candel, & Wolf, 2008; Wolf, 2008). The effects of GCs on memory retrieval have been associated with decreased activity in medial temporal lobe structures such as the hippocampus and the superior frontal gyrus (Oei et al., 2007; Wolf, 2008). Working memory—the active, "online" manipulation of material in short-term storage—is also impaired by stress or GCs, particularly under high task load (Lupien et al., 2007; Oei, Everaerd, Elzinga, van Well, & Bermond, 2006). Working memory has been shown to depend on the dorsolateral prefrontal cortex. The prefrontal cortex is an area of particularly dense GR in the primate brain (Pryce, 2008; Sanchez, Young, Plotsky, & Insel, 2000); possibly GCs influence working memory by acting at receptors in this region. As with memory consolidation, the effects of GCs on memory retrieval and working memory also depend on elevated NE in the amygdala (Elzinga & Roelofs, 2005). GCs may affect other aspects of prefrontal-dependent executive functioning beyond working memory (Arnsten, 2009). Recent evidence in humans suggests that either stress or pharmacological elevations of GCs and NE cause shifts in performance from goal-directed behavior to habitual responding (Schwabe, Tegenthoff, Hoffken, & Wolf, 2010). These findings have implications for effects of stress and stress hormones on a variety of disorders (obsessive–compulsive disorder [OCD]; attention-deficit/hyperactivity disorder [ADHD]), executive functions, and behavioral flexibility.

Given the important roles of stress hormones in emotion and cognition, it is not surprising that psychopathology is sometimes accompanied by dysregulation in stress hormone systems (see Wolf, 2008, for a review). The largest and most consistent body of evidence for HPA axis dysregulation in psychopathology is with major depressive disorder. Researchers have found increased CRH levels in the cerebrospinal fluid and brain tissue of depressed patients (Bissette, Klimek, Pan, Stockmeier, & Ordway, 2003; Nemeroff et al., 1984), although increased CRH might be driven by early adverse experience (Carpenter et al., 2004). There is also ample evidence that HPA axis negative feedback is compromised in depressed patients (Abercrombie, 2009; Holsboer, 2001; Pariante, 2006). Impaired negative feedback is revealed by administering cortisol or drugs such as dexamethasone (a potent synthetic GC) to patients; depressed patients exhibit less suppression of ACTH levels than healthy controls. Impaired HPA axis negative feedback could, in turn, lead to elevated cortisol. Depression appears to involve lower sensitivity to GCs in the brain, whether by decreased numbers of GR or decreased transport of GCs into the brain (Pariante, Thomas, Lovestone, Makoff, & Kerwin, 2004). This lower sensitivity, or "glucocorticoid resistance," is thought to underlie the impaired negative feedback; the brain is less responsive to the GC signal that down-regulates HPA axis activity (Abercrombie, 2009; Pariante, 2006). It is still unclear whether this GR deficiency is a consequence or an antecedent of depression, or both. However, antidepressant medications decrease HPA axis activity, increase negative feedback, and lead to up-regulation of MR and GR in humans (Mason & Pariante, 2006). These findings suggest that HPA axis dysregulation could be a key contributing factor to depression. Importantly, though, HPA axis differences are not found in all depressed individuals. Signs of an overactive HPA axis are more often found in older patients and in inpatients versus outpatients (Gold & Chrousos, 2002; Stetler & Miller, 2011).

In contrast to depression, there is evidence that patients with posttraumatic stress disorder (PTSD) have lower cortisol levels and a more robust negative feedback response (i.e., greater suppression of plasma ACTH after administration of GCs) compared to controls (Yehuda, 2002; Yehuda, Yang, Buchsbaum, & Golier, 2006). Patients with PTSD may have greater densities of GR in the brain, causing increased sensitivity to GCs. Interestingly, low cortisol levels may predispose individuals to develop PTSD after trauma. Adults who later developed PTSD had lower cortisol and higher heart rate in the emergency room following their trauma compared to those who did not develop a disorder or those who developed depression (Yehuda, McFarlane, & Shalev, 1998). As heart rate is partly under SNS control, these data indicate that an imbalance between HPA axis and SNS responses to a traumatic event may predispose individuals to PTSD. A possible explanation for this is that low GCs coupled with high SNS activity/NE could lead to enhanced amygdala-driven memory traces of emotional aspects of the event, coupled with impaired hippocampal-driven spatial or episodic memory of the context of the emotional event (Wolf, 2008).

Given these findings, some suggest that GCs administered immediately after trauma might reduce the likelihood of an individual developing PTSD. In fact, GC administration during septic shock, intensive care unit treatment, or surgery reduces the incidence of posttreatment trauma symptoms (Schelling, Roozendaal, & De Quervain, 2004; Schelling et al., 2006). Even after the development of PTSD, chronic low-dose GC treatment appears to ameliorate symptoms (de Quervain & Margraf, 2008). GCs could become an important posttrauma preventive treatment option. Similarly, GC administration was found to be beneficial in people with phobias. This could be because GCs appear to facilitate extinction learning, or because GCs inhibit reconsolidation of fear memories (de Quervain & Margraf, 2008).

What is difficult to gauge in psychological conditions is whether "correcting" the observed HPA axis difference will help alleviate symptoms, and if so, how to go about correcting it. Interactions between the HPA axis, other hormonal systems, and the immune system mean that we must approach any pharmacological perturbations in stress hormones with caution. However, ongoing research on how the HPA axis regulates emotion and cognition promises to elucidate the workings of the healthy brain as well as the mechanisms involved in psychological disorders.

Beyond the HPA Axis: Neurosteroids in Stress, Affiliation, and Psychopathology

Stress involves a cascade of hormonal and neurochemical responses. In addition to the HPA axis and the SNS, many other hormones are produced during stress, including *neurosteroids* (Joels & Baram, 2009; Purdy, Morrow, Moore, & Paul, 1991). Neurosteroids are steroid hormones produced in the brain that affect neural activity by binding to membrane-bound receptors. This section explores the roles of progesterone-derived neurosteroids in emotional processes.

Progesterone (P) is best known for its role in mammalian reproduction, but P's broader role is underscored by its production in the adrenal glands and brain as well as in the gonads of both sexes (Magnaghi, 2007; Paul & Purdy, 1992). A number of other hormones are synthesized from P, including the neurosteroid allopregnanolone (ALLO). P-derived neurosteroids facilitate binding of the inhibitory neurotransmitter GABA to its receptors, a similar mechanism of action as benzodiazepine drugs such as diazepam (Valium) (Majewska, Harrison, Schwartz, Barker, & Paul, 1986; Paul & Purdy, 1992). Because ALLO reduces neural firing, administration of P or ALLO to rats causes reductions in anxiety behavior, or even sedation (Bitran, Shiekh, & McLeod, 1995; Paul & Purdy, 1992). P and ALLO levels also respond to stress; they increase in the blood and brain tissue of rats subjected to stressors such as forced swim or footshock (Barbaccia, Serra, Purdy, & Biggio, 2001; Purdy et al., 1991). Along with its effects on GABA binding, ALLO also was found to down-regulate HPA axis hormones such as CRH (Patchev, Shoaib, Holsboer, & Almeida, 1994), and ALLO administration causes antidepressant effects in rodents (Rodriguez-Landa, Contreras, Bernal-Morales, Gutierrez-Garcia, & Saavedra, 2007). It is thought that increases in P and ALLO during stress could function in part to help rein in the stress response.

In human clinical research, differences in P and/or ALLO levels have been found in a number of psychological disorders related to mood and emotion (Eser et al., 2006; Girdler & Klatzkin, 2007; van Broekhoven & Verkes, 2003). In particular, multiple studies have found decreased ALLO levels in depressed compared to healthy controls, in both blood and cerebrospinal fluid (which may reflect overall brain levels of ALLO) (Eser et al., 2006; van Broekhoven & Verkes, 2003). Intriguingly, the decreased ALLO levels seen in depression normalize with treatment by selective serotonin reuptake inhibitors (SSRIs) or other antidepressant drugs (Romeo et al., 1998; Uzunova et al., 1998), suggesting that lower ALLO levels might have relevance for the disease. However, ALLO levels do not change with effective nonpharmacological treatments for depression, such as sleep deprivation or electroconvulsive shock treatment (Baghai et al., 2005; Schule et al., 2004). The key question is: What is the import of lower ALLO levels in depression? As with HPA axis abnormalities in depression, it is unclear whether lower ALLO levels are part of the cause of depression, a consequence of depression, or both. An understanding of how P and ALLO function in stress, emotion, and cognition in healthy humans is needed.

Are P and ALLO stress-responsive in humans, as they appear to be in rodents? A handful of studies suggest that these hormones do in fact increase in humans under stress, along with other stress hormones such as cortisol. P and ALLO increase in response to pharmacological application of CRH or ACTH (Genazzani et al., 1998), and salivary P and cortisol are positively correlated and change together (Wirth, Meier, Fredrickson, & Schultheiss, 2007). These data suggest that HPA axis activation during stress causes the adrenal gland to produce P as well as cortisol. In more direct studies of the effect of stress on P and ALLO, plasma ALLO levels were increased during a real-life stressor (PhD examination) (Droogleever Fortuyn et al., 2004); another study found mixed support for P and ALLO increases during a standard speech stressor (Childs, Dlugos, & de Wit, 2010). Preliminary evidence shows salivary P increases in parallel with cortisol in response to venipuncture stress (Wirth, 2011). P also appears to increase during some social rejection stressors, which are discussed further below.

Does P or ALLO reduce stress and anxiety in humans? Findings so far are equivocal. Administration of P or ALLO causes mild increases in fatigue, confusion, and sedation in humans (Freeman, Purdy, Coutifaris, Rickels, & Paul, 1993; Timby et al., 2006). In a study of effects of P administration on stress, mixed effects were found on measures of stress physiology and subjective mood in men (Childs, Van Dam, & de Wit, 2010). These mixed findings could be explained in part if the effects of ALLO on mood followed an inverted-U-shaped dose–response pattern; that is, smaller increases in ALLO might have greater antianxiety

effects. In fact, some researchers argue that P and ALLO cause negative mood effects at lower doses (i.e., physiological levels) and reduce anxiety at higher (pharmacological) doses (Andreen et al., 2009). More research is needed to elucidate the roles of P and ALLO in mood and emotional processing. This area of research is especially important in order to understand whether the decreased ALLO in depression has any clinical significance.

Recent evidence suggests a role for P (and possibly ALLO) in affiliation and bonding. In rodents, these hormones increase the expression of social-affiliative behaviors (Frye et al., 2006). For example, ALLO administration increased the time that female rats spent in proximity to male rats; blocking ALLO had the reverse effect (Frye, Bayon, Pursnani, & Purdy, 1998). In one human study, arousal of affiliation motivation caused increases in P (Schultheiss, Wirth, & Stanton, 2004). In a follow-up study, priming abandonment and social rejection caused increases in P alongside cortisol; changes in P paralleled changes in affiliation motivation; and baseline affiliation motivation predicted change in P following the abandonment manipulation (Wirth & Schultheiss, 2006). These findings hint at a relationship between P and affiliation-related stress. Recent research also found P increases during social rejection in some cases (Maner, Miller, Schmidt, & Eckel, 2010), as well as during a manipulation designed to increase feelings of closeness and bonding between two same-sex study participants (Brown et al., 2009).

These results are reminiscent of those found for oxytocin, a hormone known for roles in affiliation and bonding (discussed below). Like oxytocin, P increases during stress and is possibly associated with the motivation to be close to others. Stress-induced oxytocin production was hypothesized to promote "tend and befriend" behaviors (Taylor et al., 2000); the same may be true of P. Importantly, relationships between P and human affiliation motivation may actually be mediated by ALLO and its GABAergic effects; this possibility remains to be studied (Wirth, 2011). Although further research is needed, findings so far suggest that stress-induced P and ALLO help reduce stress and anxiety not only by neural inhibition, mediated by GABA receptors, but also by promoting affiliative and bonding behaviors, which could have long-lasting stress-protective effects. Given the well-known protective effects of social support and relationship quality on health, and the severe health consequences of social isolation, a better understanding of the roles of P and ALLO in social-affiliative behaviors and motivation in humans remains a crucial piece of the puzzle in treating stress-related disease.

Androgens and the Brain: Testosterone's Influence on Development, Cognition, and Aggression

Androgens are a class of steroid hormones that include androstenedione, testosterone (T), and dihydrotestosterone (DHT). Our discussion focuses on T, one of the most potent and well-studied androgens. T has both anabolic (tissue growth) and androgenic (development of sex characteristics) effects on cells and tissues. T also affects the amygdala and other limbic structures containing T receptors. Most evidence regarding the effects of T on the brain draws on research in nonhuman species, so there is still much to learn about T's role in cognition and emotion in humans. Such research comes with many complications, including our current inability to measure androgen receptor occupancy in the living human brain.

T is produced in the ovaries, testes, and adrenal glands. Production in the gonads is controlled by the hypothalamus through the hypothalamic–pituitary–gonadal (HPG) axis, in a similar fashion to the HPA axis; in this case the hypothalamic hormone is gonadotropin-releasing hormone (GnRH), which stimulates the production of follicle-stimulating hormone (FSH) and lutenizing hormone (LH) from the pituitary. In turn, these pituitary hormones cause production of estradiol, P, and T from the gonads. Gonadal hormones generally exert negative feedback on the hypothalamus and pituitary to stop hormone production.

The HPA axis harnesses immediate energy for facing a stressor, whereas the HPG axis facilitates long-term functions inhibited by stress (e.g., growth and reproduction), so the two systems generally counteract one another. Gonadal hormones influence baseline and stress-reactive HPA axis hormone levels, as well as the effectiveness of HPA negative feedback (Viau, 2002). Higher T levels are sometimes associated with a decreased arousal response (Newman, Sellers, & Josephs, 2005). For example, anxiety-prone individuals who were administered T showed decreased skin conductance responses and reduced startle to aversive pictures (Hermans et al., 2007). T is also associated with greater attention captured by dominance- or threat-related social cues. One study found that for both males and females, endogenous T levels were correlated with feelings of anger and tension and selective attention to angry rather than neutral faces (van Honk et al., 1999). Further investigation revealed that individuals who unconsciously attended more to angry faces showed higher posttest cortisol and T (van Honk et al., 2000). Together, these results imply that T influences the relationship between HPA axis mechanisms and responses to social signals, and that effects are automatic rather than conscious. Another study provided further evidence that T levels correlate with attention paid to signals of challenge (i.e., angry facial expressions), as well as the reward value of those signals (Wirth & Schultheiss, 2007). T is often associated with dominance-seeking or status threat; T may promote approach or interaction with threatening individuals by reducing fear or stress.

T's influence on the brain and body begin very early. Prenatal T levels result in the development of male or female genitalia (Carlson, 2010). T's effects on the developing brain are shown in animal studies, revealing that abnormal prenatal androgen levels alter sexually dimorphic behavior such as play behavior patterns (Meaney & Stewart, 1981; Thornton, Zehr, & Loose, 2009). In rats, prenatal androgens and estrogens exert unique effects on hypothalamic organization (Isgor & Sengelaub, 1998). Therefore, prenatal androgens structure neural pathways that control sexually dimorphic behaviors later in life. Is this the case in humans as well? Some evidence comes from females with congenital adrenal hyperplasia (CAH), a disorder in which the adrenal gland produces extra androgens instead of cortisol.

This condition may result in more masculinized female brains, based on observed behavioral differences such as increased rough-and-tumble play and improved performance on spatial tasks (Carlson, 2010; Hines et al., 2003).

Androgens also affect a variety of cognitive functions in adulthood. T and DHT facilitate long-term memory and spatial and visuospatial memory in rodents. Researchers have indicated that the strength of associations between androgens and cognition in animal models is contingent on the type of cognitive task used in a given study as well as the type of T that is assessed: "free" T (not bound to proteins) versus "total" T (including protein-bound T) (Puts et al., 2010). Despite these reservations, T has been associated with improved spatial memory in humans (Aleman, Bronk, Kessels, Koppeschaar, & van Honk, 2004; Postma et al., 2000). Associations seem to be represented by an inverted-U-shaped curve: Women who have higher than average T for their sex, and men with lower T, both perform better at a spatial task (Moffat & Hampson, 1996), suggesting an optimal "medium" T level for spatial cognition. These studies must be assessed carefully, considering that T levels in humans are significantly influenced by a variety of inter- and intraindividual differences, including seasonal variation in men and the menstrual phase in women (Kimura & Hampson, 1994; Postma, Winkel, Tuiten, & van Honk, 1999). Though mechanisms for this effect are poorly understood, the hippocampus—a structure involved in spatial cognition—does contain high numbers of androgen receptors (Beyenburg et al., 2000).

Aggressive behavior is associated with androgens and with T in particular. Evidence is especially compelling in rodents, where T is necessary for full expression of maternal defense behaviors and male sexual behavior (Edinger & Frye, 2007). But social status moderates the effects of T (and alcohol) on aggression; a study in male squirrel monkeys showed that alcohol increases aggression only in the presence of high T and only in dominant males (Howell et al., 2007; Winslow & Miczek, 1985). The challenge hypothesis (Wingfield, Ball, Dufty, Hegner, & Rameofsky, 1987) suggests that T levels related to aggression are context-specific due to fluctuations in physiology (e.g., mating) and in response to other influences (e.g., the presence of a predator). In humans, T is hypothesized to increase in response to a challenge (causing more aggressive behavior) and decrease when an individual engages in parenting (Archer, 2006). Bidirectional relationships between T and behavior provide an important framework for examining social factors and endocrine responses in humans.

Although males typically exhibit more aggressive behavior, androgens are also associated with aggression in females (Cashdan, 2003; Pajer et al., 2006). One proposed pathway suggests that T may enhance the responsiveness of neural circuits of social aggression (Hermans, Ramsey, & van Honk, 2008). Another mechanism could be that T lowers inhibitions and increases risk taking, thereby lowering the threshold for acting on an aggressive impulse. Converging evidence links T to risk taking, including economic risk taking. One study showed that for both men and women, high endogenous T for their sex was associated with riskier behavior on a gambling task (Stanton, Liening, & Schultheiss, 2010). More recent research found that individuals with low or high T for their sex were risk-neutral, whereas individuals with moderate T were risk-averse, indicating another U-shaped dose–response curve (Stanton et al., 2011).

Studies using dominance contests have attempted to unpack the links between dominance, aggression, and T (Archer, 2006). Many studies that have investigated hormonal responses to competitions have revealed temporary increases in T after winning physical or mental contests. This can even be true if one identifies with an individual or group that won—such as a sports team or even a presidential candidate—rather than winning the contest oneself (Bernhardt, Dabbs, Fielden, & Lutter, 1998; Stanton, Beehner, Saini, Kuhn, & Labar, 2009). Although findings may be mediated by a number of factors such as the outcome of the particular contest, degree of social content, and the resources available to the individual (Salvador, 2005), these studies highlight the bidirectional nature of T–dominance relationships; baseline T or changes in T can interact with social status to affect the choice to engage in competition as well as hormone (cortisol, T, etc.) reactivity. Some research suggests that higher T levels are only associated with dominance/ status in those individuals with low cortisol levels, whereas higher T may be actually be associated with decreased dominance in high-cortisol individuals (Mehta & Josephs, 2010). Similar effects have been observed in nonhuman primates. Following a stressor, high-ranking baboons' T levels increased quickly, whereas low-ranking baboons' T levels decreased, an effect mediated by GCs (Sapolsky, 1985, 1986). These data indicate that the robust relationship between stress and T may be contingent on one's rank in the social hierarchy. Overall, T helps drive behaviors associated with dominant status, and status in turn promotes specific changes in T.

Oxytocin and Vasopressin: Hormones of Stress and Sociality

Oxytocin (OT) and arginine vasopressin (AVP) play key roles in modulating social behavior and stress. These two peptide hormones are very similar in structure, differing by only two amino acids, and are synthesized by magnocellular neurons in the PVN and supraoptic nucleus (SON) portions of the hypothalamus, in addition to the stria terminalis and medial amygdala, and some organs apart from the brain (Nelson, 2005a). OT and AVP produced by PVN and SON neurons are released from the posterior pituitary into the bloodstream (Figure 5.1). Other neurons elsewhere in the brain (e.g., amygdala) use OT and AVP as neuromodulators. Therefore, there are distinct "blood" and "brain" hormone systems. Structural similarities and the ability to bind to each other's receptors result in considerable overlap between OT and AVP functions. The most evolutionarily ancient purposes of these hormones include regulating blood osmolarity (salt–water balance) and smooth muscle contraction. In mammals, OT activates uterus contractions during birth and causes release of milk during lactation (Nelson, 2005a). From functions that evolved earlier, OT and AVP may have been incorporated into roles in parental relationships and pair bonding; they also play roles in aggression, sexual behavior, stress, and social cognition. Variations in OT levels

in the blood may also be associated with a predisposition to some forms of psychopathology (Campbell, 2010). Considerably less attention has been paid to the role of AVP in human behavior, though we do know that AVP is connected with managing vascular tone, stress, and mating-related behaviors in other animals (Goodson & Bass, 2001).

AVP and T interact in the brain, with T facilitating AVP synthesis and receptor binding in the hypothalamus. In rodents, AVP is associated with male social behaviors, including paternal behavior, pair bond formation, and the selective aggression involved in mate defense (Carter, Boone, Pournajafi-Nazarloo, & Bales, 2009). In prairie voles, OT and AVP have sex-specific roles; OT is essential for pair bonding in females, whereas AVP is essential for pair bonding in males (Carter, 1998; Lim & Young, 2006). Whether this is true in human males is largely unknown, though men have higher AVP levels than women, like in other mammals. Some researchers have suggested sex-specific roles for OT and AVP in social and stress regulation in humans (Donaldson & Young, 2008).

How do OT and AVP influence stress? First, these peptides increase during stress, along with other stress hormones (Bartz & Hollander, 2006; Carter & Altemus, 1997). Second, OT and AVP affect many aspects of the stress response. OT has stress-dampening effects such as lowering GC levels and anxiety (Blume et al., 2008; Uvnas-Moberg, 1998a). Mice missing the gene for OT or OT receptors display more anxiety, higher corticosterone, and higher markers of neural activity in stress-related brain regions after a stressor (Neumann, 2002). The stress reduction effect of OT in rodents has been localized to the central amygdala and the PVN (Blume et al., 2008). AVP plays a different role in stress systems. AVP is associated with SNS function and combines efforts with CRH to elicit pituitary ACTH secretion, increasing GC levels (Meaney et al., 1996). AVP is associated with anxiety behavior in rodents. Also, events during early rodent development, such as abnormal androgen levels and early life stress, may cause altered AVP levels (Carter, 2003; Plotsky & Meaney, 1993). Alterations in *V1aR* (one of the vasopressin receptors) gene expression and distribution results in decreased CRH and AVP in the PVN or increased coexpression of CRH and AVP, though effects appear to be species-specific (Hammock & Young, 2005; Walum et al., 2008). Furthermore, males seem more responsive to AVP than females (De Vries & Panzica, 2006; Winslow, Hastings, Carter, Harbaugh, & Insel, 1993).

OT and AVP may also exert differential effects on the physiological and behavioral outcomes of the human stress response (Neumann, 2008; Viviani & Stoop, 2008). OT administration causes decreased SNS activity and greater vagal nerve activity (part of the parasympathetic nervous system) (Higa, Mori, Viana, Morris, & Michelini, 2002). The connection of OT with social affiliation makes sense in terms of the hormone's anxiolytic properties; reductions in distress or anxiety may be necessary to enable affiliation or bonding to take place. In turn, the "tend and befriend" model of stress regulation hypothesizes that increases in OT during stress may promote greater nurturing activities and affiliation to protect against the negative effects of stress (Taylor et al., 2000). OT may be part of the biological mechanism by which positive social contact and social support buffer against stress.

OT and AVP are both vital to parent–offspring bonding (Carter, 2003). In sheep, OT is necessary for the ewes' recognition of and bonding with their newborn lambs; infant suckling triggers OT release in various brain regions in sheep and rodent mothers (Kendrick, Keverne, Chapman, & Baldwin, 1988; Nelson & Panksepp, 1998). AVP also contributes to parental bonding and maternal behavior. In many species, AVP levels increase during birthing and lactation (Bosch, 2011; Campbell, 2010). OT and AVP play roles in restructuring the maternal nervous system, forging a bond between parent and offspring. AVP also promotes maternal defensive aggression. In species where male animals also care for young, males experience hormonal changes when young are born, including increased OT/AVP gene expression in voles (Wynne-Edwards & Timonin, 2007). Furthermore, the affiliation-reinforcement properties of OT affect the offspring's maturational development. For example, rats that receive more maternal behavior (licking and grooming) as pups show greater OT and AVP receptor densities compared to those who received less maternal behavior. Early parental bonds may have lifelong effects, such that animals that receive different amounts of maternal attention may vary in their social aptitude (Francis, Young, Meaney, & Insel, 2002).

Considerably less research connects OT and AVP with human parental care. However, correlational studies have linked plasma OT levels with postpartum mother–infant interactions, including affect, touch, and vocalization (Feldman, Weller, Zagoory-Sharon, & Levine, 2007; Matthiesen, Ransjo-Arvidson, Nissen, & Uvnas-Moberg, 2001). Indirect evidence for OT's anxiolytic and antistress effects has also been found in nursing mothers, who have high OT levels and are more likely to describe positive mood states and decreased anxiety than nonlactating control mothers (Carter, Altemus, & Chrousos, 2001; Uvnas-Moberg, 1998b). The influence of AVP in human parental care might be related to aggression, vigilance, or protective behaviors (Heinrichs, Baumgartner, Kirschbaum, & Ehlert, 2003; Thompson, George, Walton, Orr, & Benson, 2006). Considering AVP's other roles in stress reactivity and social cognition, we can postulate that AVP may affect parental care similarly in humans as in animals, and might exert a greater influence on the parental behavior of human males.

OT and AVP also promote pair-bond formation. This relationship has been studied extensively in the prairie vole, a rodent species that exhibits pair-bonding and biparental care of young (Carter, DeVries, & Getz, 1995; Winslow et al., 1993). For prairie voles, these hormones are essential for forming selective partner preferences as well as for initiating parental behavior. During a pair's initial bouts of mating, their brains produce high levels of OT and AVP. The hormones bind to receptors in reward-related regions, such as the ventral pallidum, to facilitate the formation of new neural connections associating the partner's scent with reward/ reinforcement. These behaviors employ both AVP and OT receptors, though either may be sufficient to spur initial social contact (Cho, DeVries, Williams, & Carter, 1999; Young & Wang, 2004). Moreover, such effects are species-specific; AVP increases affiliation and bonding in social voles but does not affect nonsocial voles (Young, Nilsen, Waymire, McGregor, & Insel, 1999). This appears to be due to different distributions of V1aR (AVP receptors) in the brains of the two species (Lim et al., 2004).

Sexual interactions contribute to pair bonding. OT facilitates erectile function and male sexual behavior in many animals (Argiolas & Melis, 2004). In humans, OT levels increase during massage or warm social contact with a partner (Grewen, Girdler, Amico, & Light, 2005; Uvnas-Moberg, 1998a) and during orgasm in males and females (Carmichael et al., 1987). OT release during these behaviors could play a role in reinforcing bonding or attachment. In humans, OT and AVP may represent relationship quality biomarkers: OT is positively associated with marital distress in women, whereas higher AVP relates to higher relationship distress in men (Taylor, Saphire-Bernstein, & Seeman, 2010). These data suggest that OT and AVP play roles in bond-seeking (i.e., motivation) for relationship maintenance and repair. Some studies administering intranasal OT (vs. placebo) to humans have found increased social engagement, altruism, trusting behavior, and empathic concern, and decreased distress (Campbell, 2010). Though OT seems to influence a host of human affiliative and pair-bonding behaviors, similar to effects observed in animal models, these effects seem strongly moderated by individual differences and social context (Bartz, Zaki, Bolger, & Ochsner, 2011).

OT and AVP both influence learning and memory. In animals, OT serves a variety of cognitive functions, such as contributing to social cognition, reinforcement and reward learning, and spatial learning and memory (Bielsky & Young, 2004; de Wied, 1997). Numerous studies found that OT-knockout or OT-receptor-knockout mice have deficits in social recognition, though the mice retain normal nonsocial learning and memory abilities (Choleris et al., 2003; Ferguson et al., 2000; Takayanagi et al., 2005). In turn, OT administration in OT-deficient mice restores their social recognition capacities (Winslow & Insel, 2002). However, many of OT's other memory enhancement properties only seem to occur under specific conditions. In many rodent studies, OT generally inhibits memory, whereas AVP enhances it (Becker

& Breedlove, 2002; Engelmann, Wotjak, Neumann, Ludwig, & Landgraf, 1996). The effects of AVP on social memory have also been cited in animal models. For example, blocking AVP in the olfactory bulb impairs rats' social recognition abilities (Tobin et al., 2010). Therefore, AVP exerts unique effects on social memory and may aid OT's contribution to those processes.

What about social cognition in humans? As in other animals, OT appears to impair some types of memory and learning, such as recall performance, whereas AVP enhances those processes (Ebstein et al., 2009; Heinrichs, Meinlschmidt, Wippich, Ehlert, & Hellhammer, 2004). Intranasal OT administration has been reported to enhance interpretation and memory of social stimuli (Domes, Heinrichs, Michel, Berger, & Herpertz, 2007; Guastella, Mitchell, & Mathews, 2008; Savaskan, Ehrhardt, Schulz, Walter, & Schachinger, 2008), though others have shown that OT administration impairs memory, especially of nonsocial stimuli (Heinrichs et al., 2004). Intranasal AVP improves learning, including the encoding of happy and angry face stimuli, increased recall of sexual words, and improved verbal memory in males (Guastella et al., 2010; Perras, Droste, Born, Fehm, & Pietrowsky, 1997). AVP may also be connected to processing of dominance and aggression signals in humans (Zink, Stein, Kempf, Hakimi, & Meyer-Lindenberg, 2010). For example, AVP administration increased responses to threatening faces and increased feelings of anxiety (Thompson et al., 2006). Connections between OT, AVP, and memory may have important implications for psychological disorders characterized by social dysfunction. Intranasal OT seems to improve emotion recognition in individuals diagnosed with Asperger syndrome or autism (Guastella et al., 2010; Hollander et al., 2007). Whether OT or AVP administration could be part of treatments for such disorders warrants further investigation.

Conclusion

Hormones have nuanced and complex relationships with human emotion, cognition, and social behavior. Behavior and internal states exert effects on hormone levels via the brain; hormones, in turn, impact mood, memory, and a number of other cognitive and emotional functions. Hence, experiences interpreted by our brains as stressful increase our production of cortisol, oxytocin, progesterone, and other hormones; these hormones, in turn, exert actions on our brains that affect (1) our ability to make new associations and retrieve older memories; (2) our subjective feelings of negative affect and emotional arousal; and (3) perhaps even our propensities to compete with, spend time with, and trust other people. These bidirectional relationships between hormones and behavior have important implications for our understanding and treatment of a number of psychological disorders characterized by differences in cognitive and emotional function, as well as for our general understanding of the human mind and brain.

Acknowledgments

We thank Laura Carlson, Charles Crowell, and Oliver Schultheiss for feedback on an earlier draft of this chapter, and Kelsey Christoffel, Brandy Martinez, and Kelly Miller for proofreading and comments.

References

Abelson, J. L., Khan, S., Liberzon, I., Erickson, T. M., & Young, E. A. (2008). Effects of perceived control and cognitive coping on endocrine stress responses to pharmacological activation. *Biological Psychiatry, 64*(8), 701–707.

Abercrombie, H. C. (2009). Hypothalamic–pituitary–adrenal axis. In R. E. Ingram (Ed.), *The international encyclopedia of depression* (pp. 332–336). New York: Springer.

Abercrombie, H. C., Kalin, N. H., & Davidson, R. J. (2005). Acute cortisol elevations cause heightened arousal ratings of objectively nonarousing stimuli. *Emotion, 5*(3), 354–359.

Abercrombie, H. C., Kalin, N. H., Thurow, M. E., Rosenkranz, M. A., & Davidson, R. J. (2003). Cortisol variation in humans affects memory for emotionally laden and neutral information. *Behavioral Neuroscience, 117*(3), 505–516.

Abercrombie, H. C., Speck, N. S., & Monticelli, R. M. (2006). Endogenous cortisol elevations are related to memory facilitation only in individuals who are emotionally aroused. *Psychoneuroendocrinology, 31*(2), 187–196.

Aleman, A., Bronk, E., Kessels, R. P., Koppeschaar, H. P., & van Honk, J. (2004). A single administration of testosterone improves visuospatial ability in young women. *Psychoneuroendocrinology, 29*(5), 612–617.

Andreen, L., Nyberg, S., Turkmen, S., van Wingen, G., Fernandez, G., & Backstrom, T. (2009). Sex steroid induced negative mood may be explained by the paradoxical effect mediated by GABA$_A$ modulators. *Psychoneuroendocrinology, 34*(8), 1121–1132.

Archer, J. (2006). Testosterone and human aggression: An evaluation of the challenge hypothesis. *Neuroscience and Biobehavioral Reviews, 30*(3), 319–345.

Argiolas, A., & Melis, M. R. (2004). The role of oxytocin and the paraventricular nucleus in the sexual behaviour of male mammals. *Physiology & Behavior, 83*(2), 309–317.

Arnsten, A. F. (2009). Stress signalling pathways that impair prefrontal cortex structure and function. *Nature Reviews Neuroscience, 10*(6), 410–422.

Baghai, T. C., di Michele, F., Schule, C., Eser, D., Zwanzger, P., Pasini, A., et al. (2005). Plasma concentrations of neuroactive steroids before and after electroconvulsive therapy in major depression. *Neuropsychopharmacology, 30*(6), 1181–1186.

Barbaccia, M. L., Serra, M., Purdy, R. H., & Biggio, G. (2001). Stress and neuroactive steroids. *International Review of Neurobiology, 46*, 243–272.

Bartz, J. A., & Hollander, E. (2006). The neuroscience of affiliation: Forging links between basic and clinical research on neuropeptides and social behavior. *Hormones and Behavior, 50*(4), 518–528.

Bartz, J. A., Zaki, J., Bolger, N., & Ochsner, K. N. (2011). Social effects of oxytocin in humans: Context and person matter. *Trends in Cognitive Sciences, 15*(7), 301–309.

Becker, J. B., & Breedlove, S. M. (2002). Introduction to behavioral endocrinology. In J. B. Becker, S. M. Breedlove, D. Crews, & M. M. McCarthy (Eds.), *Behavioral endocrinology* (2nd ed., pp. 3–38). Cambridge, MA: MIT Press.

Bernhardt, P. C., Dabbs, J. M., Jr., Fielden, J. A., & Lutter, C. D. (1998). Testosterone changes during vicarious experiences of winning and losing among fans at sporting events. *Physiology & Behavior, 65*(1), 59–62.

Beyenburg, S., Watzka, M., Clusmann, H., Blumcke, I., Bidlingmaier, F., Elger, C. E., et al. (2000). Androgen receptor mRNA expression in the human hippocampus. *Neuroscience Letters, 294*(1), 25–28.

Bielsky, I. F., & Young, L. J. (2004). Oxytocin, vasopressin, and social recognition in mammals. *Peptides, 25*(9), 1565–1574.

Bissette, G., Klimek, V., Pan, J., Stockmeier, C., & Ordway, G. (2003). Elevated concentrations of CRF in the locus coeruleus of depressed subjects. *Neuropsychopharmacology, 28*(7), 1328–1335.

Bitran, D., Shiekh, M., & McLeod, M. (1995). Anxiolytic effect of progesterone is mediated by the neurosteroid allopregnanolone at brain GABAA receptors. *Journal of Neuroendocrinology, 7*(3), 171–177.

Blume, A., Bosch, O. J., Miklos, S., Torner, L., Wales, L., Waldherr, M., et al. (2008). Oxytocin reduces anxiety via ERK1/2 activation: Local effect within the rat hypothalamic paraventricular nucleus. *European Journal of Neuroscience, 27*(8), 1947–1956.

Born, J., Lange, T., Kern, W., McGregor, G. P., Bickel, U., & Fehm, H. L. (2002). Sniffing neuropeptides: A transnasal approach to the human brain. *Nature Neuroscience, 5*(6), 514–516.

Bosch, O. J. (2011). Maternal nurturing is dependent on her innate anxiety: The behavioral roles of brain oxytocin and vasopressin. *Hormones and Behavior, 59*(2), 202–212.

Brown, E. S. (2009). Effects of glucocorticoids on mood, memory, and the hippocampus. treatment and preventive therapy. *Annals of the New York Academy of Sciences, 1179,* 41–55.

Brown, S. L., Fredrickson, B. L., Wirth, M. M., Poulin, M. J., Meier, E. A., Heaphy, E. D., et al. (2009). Social closeness increases salivary progesterone in humans. *Hormones and Behavior, 56*(1), 108–111.

Buchanan, T. W., Brechtel, A., Sollers, J. J., & Lovallo, W. R. (2001). Exogenous cortisol exerts effects on the startle reflex independent of emotional modulation. *Pharmacology, Biochemistry, and Behavior, 68*(2), 203–210.

Buchanan, T. W., & Lovallo, W. R. (2001). Enhanced memory for emotional material following stress-level cortisol treatment in humans. *Psychoneuroendocrinology, 26*(3), 307–317.

Campbell, A. (2010). Oxytocin and human social behavior. *Personality and Social Psychology Review, 14*(3), 281–295.

Canli, T., Zhao, Z., Brewer, J., Gabrieli, J. D., & Cahill, L. (2000). Event-related activation in the human amygdala associates with later memory for individual emotional experience. *Journal of Neuroscience, 20*(19), RC99.

Carlson, N. R. (2010). *Physiology and behavior* (10th ed.). Boston: Allyn & Bacon.

Carmichael, M. S., Humbert, R., Dixen, J., Palmisano, G., Greenleaf, W., & Davidson, J. M. (1987). Plasma oxytocin increases in the human sexual response. *Journal of Clinical Endocrinology and Metabolism, 64*(1), 27–31.

Carpenter, L. L., Tyrka, A. R., McDougle, C. J., Malison, R. T., Owens, M. J., Nemeroff, C. B., et al. (2004). Cerebrospinal fluid corticotropin-releasing factor and perceived early-life stress in depressed patients and healthy control subjects. *Neuropsychopharmacology, 29*(4), 777–784.

Carter, C. S. (1998). Neuroendocrine perspectives on social attachment and love. *Psychoneuroendocrinology, 23*(8), 779–818.

Carter, C. S. (2003). Developmental consequences of oxytocin. *Physiology & Behavior, 79*(3), 383–397.

Carter, C. S., & Altemus, M. (1997). Integrative functions of lactational hormones in social behavior and stress management. In C. S. Cafter, I. I. Lederhendler, & B. Kirkpatrick (Eds.), *The integrative neurobiology of affiliation* (pp. 164–177). New York: New York Academy of Sciences.

Carter, C. S., Altemus, M., & Chrousos, G. P. (2001). Neuroendocrine and emotional changes in the post-partum period. *Progress in Brain Research, 133,* 241–249.

Carter, C. S., Boone, E. M., Pournajafi-Nazarloo, H., & Bales, K. L. (2009). Consequences of early experiences and exposure to oxytocin and vasopressin are sexually dimorphic. *Developmental Neuroscience, 31*(4), 332–341.

Carter, C. S., DeVries, A. C., & Getz, L. L. (1995). Physiological substrates of mammalian monogamy: The prairie vole model. *Neuroscience and Biobehavioral Reviews, 19*(2), 303–314.

Cashdan, E. (2003). Hormones and competitive aggression in women. *Aggressive Behavior, 29*(2), 107–115.

Childs, E., Dlugos, A., & de Wit, H. (2010). Cardiovascular, hormonal, and emotional responses to the TSST in relation to sex and menstrual cycle phase. *Psychophysiology, 47,* 550–559.

Childs, E., Van Dam, N. T., & de Wit, H. (2010). Effects of acute progesterone administration upon responses to acute psychosocial stress in men. *Experimental and Clinical Psychopharmacology, 18*(1), 78–86.

Cho, M. M., DeVries, A. C., Williams, J. R., & Carter, C. S. (1999). The effects of oxytocin and vasopressin on partner preferences in male and female prairie voles *(Microtus ochrogaster). Behavioral Neuroscience, 113*(5), 1071–1079.

Choleris, E., Gustafsson, J. A., Korach, K. S., Muglia, L. J., Pfaff, D. W., & Ogawa, S. (2003). An estrogen-dependent four-gene micronet regulating social recognition: A study with oxytocin and estrogen receptor-alpha and -beta knockout mice. *Proceedings of the National Academy of Sciences USA, 100*(10), 6192–6197.

Dallman, M. F. (2005). Fast glucocorticoid actions on brain: Back to the future. *Frontiers in Neuroendocrinology, 26*(3–4), 103–108.

de Kloet, E. R., Karst, H., & Joels, M. (2008). Corticosteroid hormones in the central stress response: Quick-and-slow. *Frontiers in Neuroendocrinology, 29*(2), 268–272.

de Kloet, E. R., Oitzl, M. S., & Joels, M. (1999). Stress and cognition: Are corticosteroids good or bad guys? *Trends in Neurosciences, 22*(10), 422–426.

de Quervain, D. J., Aerni, A., Schelling, G., & Roozendaal, B. (2009). Glucocorticoids and the regulation of memory in health and disease. *Frontiers in Neuroendocrinology, 30*(3), 358–370.

de Quervain, D. J., & Margraf, J. (2008). Glucocorticoids for the treatment of post-traumatic stress disorder and phobias: A novel therapeutic approach. *European Journal of Pharmacology, 583*(2–3), 365–371.

De Vries, G. J., & Panzica, G. C. (2006). Sexual differentiation of central vasopressin and vasotocin systems in vertebrates: Different mechanisms, similar endpoints. *Neuroscience, 138*(3), 947–955.

de Wied, D. (1997). Neuropeptides in learning and memory processes. *Behavioural Brain Research, 83*(1–2), 83–90.

Dickerson, S. S., & Kemeny, M. E. (2004). Acute stressors and cortisol responses: A theoretical integration and synthesis of laboratory research. *Psychological Bulletin, 130*(3), 355–391.

Domes, G., Heinrichs, M., Michel, A., Berger, C., & Herpertz, S. C. (2007). Oxytocin improves "mind-reading" in humans. *Biological Psychiatry, 61*(6), 731–733.

Donaldson, Z. R., & Young, L. J. (2008). Oxytocin, vasopressin, and the neurogenetics of sociality. *Science, 322,* 900–904.

DonCarlos, L. L., Garcia-Ovejero, D., Sarkey, S., Garcia-Segura, L. M., & Azcoitia, I. (2003). Androgen receptor immunoreactivity in forebrain axons and dendrites in the rat. *Endocrinology, 144*(8), 3632–3638.

Droogleever Fortuyn, H. A., van Broekhoven, F., Span, P. N., Backstrom, T., Zitman, F. G., & Verkes, R. J. (2004). Effects of PhD examination stress on allopregnanolone and cortisol plasma levels and peripheral benzodiazepine receptor density. *Psychoneuroendocrinology, 29*(10), 1341–1344.

Duvarci, S., & Pare, D. (2007). Glucocorticoids enhance the excitability of principal basolateral amygdala neurons. *Journal of Neuroscience, 27,* 4482–4491.

Ebstein, R. P., Israel, S., Lerer, E., Uzefovsky, F., Shalev, I., Gritsenko, I., et al. (2009). Arginine vasopressin and oxytocin modulate human social behavior. *Annals of the New York Academy of Sciences, 1167,* 87–102.

Edinger, K. L., & Frye, C. A. (2007). Androgens' effects to enhance learning may be mediated in part through actions at estrogen receptor-beta in the hippocampus. *Neurobiology of Learning and Memory, 87*(1), 78–85.

Elzinga, B. M., & Roelofs, K. (2005). Cortisol-induced impairments of working memory require acute sympathetic activation. *Behavioral Neuroscience, 119*(1), 98–103.

Engelmann, M., Wotjak, C. T., Neumann, I., Ludwig, M., & Landgraf, R. (1996). Behavioral consequences of intracerebral vasopressin and oxytocin: Focus on learning and memory. *Neuroscience and Biobehavioral Reviews, 20*(3), 341–358.

Eser, D., Romeo, E., Baghai, T. C., di Michele, F., Schule, C., Pasini, A., et al. (2006). Neuroactive steroids as modulators of depression and anxiety. *Neuroscience, 138*(3), 1041–1048.

Feldman, R., Weller, A., Zagoory-Sharon, O., & Levine, A. (2007). Evidence for a neuroendocrinological foundation of human affiliation: Plasma oxytocin levels across pregnancy and the postpartum period predict mother–infant bonding. *Psychological Science, 18*(11), 965–970.

Ferguson, J. N., Young, L. J., Hearn, E. F., Matzuk, M. M., Insel, T. R., & Winslow, J. T. (2000). Social amnesia in mice lacking the oxytocin gene. *Nature Genetics, 25*(3), 284–288.

Francis, D. D., Young, L. J., Meaney, M. J., & Insel, T. R. (2002). Naturally occurring differences in maternal care are associated with the expression of oxytocin and vasopressin (V1a) receptors: Gender differences. *Journal of Neuroendocrinology, 14*(5), 349–353.

Freeman, E. W., Purdy, R. H., Coutifaris, C., Rickels, K., & Paul, S. M. (1993). Anxiolytic metabolites of progesterone: Correlation with mood and performance measures following oral progesterone administration to healthy female volunteers. *Neuroendocrinology, 58*(4), 478–484.

Fries, E., Dettenborn, L., & Kirschbaum, C. (2009). The cortisol awakening response (CAR): Facts and future directions. *International Journal of Psychophysiology, 72*(1), 67–73.

Frye, C. A. (2001). The role of neurosteroids and non-genomic effects of progestins and androgens in mediating sexual receptivity of rodents. *Brain Research Reviews, 37*(1–3), 201–222.

Frye, C. A., Bayon, L. E., Pursnani, N. K., & Purdy, R. H. (1998). The neurosteroids, progesterone and 3alpha,5alpha-THP, enhance sexual motivation, receptivity, and proceptivity in female rats. *Brain Research, 808*(1), 72–83.

Frye, C. A., Rhodes, M. E., Petralia, S. M., Walf, A. A., Sumida, K., & Edinger, K. L. (2006). 3alpha-hydroxy-5alpha-pregnan-20–one in the midbrain ventral tegmental area mediates social, sexual, and affective behaviors. *Neuroscience, 138*(3), 1007–1014.

Genazzani, A. R., Petraglia, F., Bernardi, F., Casarosa, E., Salvestroni, C., Tonetti, A., et al. (1998). Circulating levels of allopregnanolone in humans: Gender, age, and endocrine influences. *Journal of Clinical Endocrinology and Metabolism, 83*(6), 2099–2103.

Girdler, S. S., & Klatzkin, R. (2007). Neurosteroids in the context of stress: Implications for depressive disorders. *Pharmacology and Therapeutics, 116*(1), 125–139.

Gold, P. W., & Chrousos, G. P. (2002). Organization of the stress system and its dysregulation in melancholic and atypical depression: High vs low CRH/NE states. *Molecular Psychiatry, 7*(3), 254–275.

Goodson, J. L., & Bass, A. H. (2001). Social behavior functions and related anatomical characteristics of vasotocin/vasopressin systems in vertebrates. *Brain Research Reviews, 35*(3), 246–265.

Grewen, K. M., Girdler, S. S., Amico, J., & Light, K. C. (2005). Effects of partner support on resting oxytocin, cortisol, norepinephrine, and blood pressure before and after warm partner contact. *Psychosomatic Medicine, 67*(4), 531–538.

Guastella, A. J., Einfeld, S. L., Gray, K. M., Rinehart, N. J., Tonge, B. J., Lambert, T. J., et al. (2010). Intranasal oxytocin improves emotion recognition for youth with autism spectrum disorders. *Biological Psychiatry, 67*(7), 692–694.

Guastella, A. J., Mitchell, P. B., & Mathews, F. (2008). Oxytocin enhances the encoding of positive social memories in humans. *Biological Psychiatry, 64*(3), 256–258.

Hammock, E. A., & Young, L. J. (2005). Microsatellite instability generates diversity in brain and sociobehavioral traits. *Science, 308*, 1630–1634.

Haskett, R. F. (1985). Diagnostic categorization of psychiatric disturbance in Cushing's syndrome. *American Journal of Psychiatry, 142*(8), 911–916.

Heinrichs, M., Baumgartner, T., Kirschbaum, C., & Ehlert, U. (2003). Social support and oxytocin interact to suppress cortisol and subjective responses to psychosocial stress. *Biological Psychiatry, 54*, 1389–1398.

Heinrichs, M., Meinlschmidt, G., Wippich, W., Ehlert, U., & Hellhammer, D. H. (2004). Selective amnesic effects of oxytocin on human memory. *Physiology & Behavior, 83*(1), 31–38.

Hermans, E. J., Putman, P., Baas, J. M., Gecks, N. M., Kenemans, J. L., & van Honk, J. (2007). Exogenous testosterone attenuates the integrated central stress response in healthy young women. *Psychoneuroendocrinology, 32*(8–10), 1052–1061.

Hermans, E. J., Ramsey, N. F., & van Honk, J. (2008). Exogenous testosterone enhances responsiveness to social threat in the neural circuitry of social aggression in humans. *Biological Psychiatry, 63*(3), 263–270.

Het, S., & Wolf, O. (2007). Mood changes in response to psychosocial stress in healthy young women: Effects of pretreatment with cortisol. *Behavioral Neuroscience, 121*(1), 11–20.

Higa, K. T., Mori, E., Viana, F. F., Morris, M., & Michelini, L. C. (2002). Baroreflex control of heart rate by oxytocin in the solitary-vagal complex. *American Journal of Physiology: Regulatory, Integrative and Comparative Physiology, 282*(2), R537–R545.

Hines, M., Fane, B. A., Pasterski, V. L., Mathews, G. A., Conway, G. S., & Brook, C. (2003). Spatial abilities following prenatal androgen abnormality: Targeting and mental rotations performance in individuals with congenital adrenal hyperplasia. *Psychoneuroendocrinology, 28*(8), 1010–1026.

Hollander, E., Bartz, J., Chaplin, W., Phillips, A., Sumner, J., Soorya, L., et al. (2007). Oxytocin increases retention of social cognition in autism. *Biological Psychiatry, 61*(4), 498–503.

Holsboer, F. (2001). Stress, hypercortisolism and corticosteroid receptors in depression: Implications for therapy. *Journal of Affective Disorders, 62*(1–2), 77–91.

Howell, S., Westergaard, G., Hoos, B., Chavanne, T. J., Shoaf, S. E., Cleveland, A., et al. (2007). Serotonergic influences on life-history outcomes in free-ranging male rhesus macaques. *American Journal of Primatology, 69*, 851–865.

Isgor, C., & Sengelaub, D. R. (1998). Prenatal gonadal steroids affect adult spatial behavior, CA1 and CA3 pyramidal cell morphology in rats. *Hormones and Behavior, 34*(2), 183–198.

Jelici, M., Geraerts, E., Merckelbach, H., & Guerrieri, R. (2004). Acute stress enhances memory for emotional words, but impairs memory for neutral words. *International Journal of Neuroscience, 114*(10), 1343–1351.

Joels, M., & Baram, T. Z. (2009). The neuro-symphony of stress. *Nature Reviews: Neuroscience, 10*(6), 459–466.

Joels, M., & Krugers, H. J. (2007). LTP after stress: Up or down? *Neural Plasticity, 2007*, 93202.

Kendrick, K. M., Keverne, E. B., Chapman, C., & Baldwin, B. A. (1988). Intracranial dialysis measurement of oxytocin, monoamine and uric acid release from the olfactory bulb and substantia nigra of sheep during parturition, suckling, separation from lambs and eating. *Brain Research, 439*(1–2), 1–10.

Kimura, D., & Hampson, E. (1994). Cognitive pattern in men and women is influenced by fluctuations in sex hormones. *Current Directions in Psychological Science, 3*(2), 57–61.

Kirschbaum, C., Pirke, K. M., & Hellhammer, D. H. (1993). The "Trier Social Stress Test"—A tool for investigating psychobiological stress responses in a laboratory setting. *Neuropsychobiology, 28*(1–2), 76–81.

Kirschbaum, C., Wust, S., Faig, H. G., & Hellhammer, D. H. (1992). Heritability of cortisol responses to human corticotropin-releasing hormone, ergometry, and psychological stress in humans. *Journal of Clinical Endocrinology and Metabolism, 75*(6), 1526–1530.

Kudielka, B. M., & Kirschbaum, C. (2005). Sex differences in HPA axis responses to stress: A review. *Biological Psychololgy, 69*(1), 113–132.

LaBar, K. S., & Cabeza, R. (2006). Cognitive neuroscience of emotional memory. *Nature Reviews: Neuroscience, 7*(1), 54–64.

Lim, M. M., Wang, Z., Olazabal, D. E., Ren, X., Terwilliger, E. F., & Young, L. J. (2004). Enhanced partner preference in a promiscuous species by manipulating the expression of a single gene. *Nature, 429*, 754–757.

Lim, M. M., & Young, L. J. (2006). Neuropeptidergic regulation of affiliative behavior and social bonding in animals. *Hormones and Behavior, 50*(4), 506–517.

Liu, D., Diorio, J., Tannenbaum, B., Caldji, C., Francis, D., Freedman, A., et al. (1997). Maternal care, hippocampal glucocorticoid receptors, and hypothalamic–pituitary–adrenal responses to stress. *Science, 277*, 1659–1662.

Lupien, S. J., Maheu, F., Tu, M., Fiocco, A., & Schramek, T. E. (2007). The effects of stress and stress hormones on human cognition: Implications for the field of brain and cognition. *Brain and Cognition, 65*(3), 209–237.

Lupien, S. J., Wilkinson, C. W., Briere, S., Menard, C., Ng Ying Kin, N. M., & Nair, N. P. (2002). The modulatory effects of corticosteroids on cognition: Studies in young human populations. *Psychoneuroendocrinology, 27*(3), 401–416.

Lyons, D. M., Parker, K. J., Katz, M., & Schatzberg, A. F. (2009). Developmental cascades linking stress inoculation, arousal regulation, and resilience. *Frontiers in Behavioral Neuroscience, 3*, 32.

Magnaghi, V. (2007). GABA and neuroactive steroid interactions in glia: New roles for old players? *Current Neuropharmacology, 5*(1), 47–64.

Maheu, F. S., Collicutt, P., Kornik, R., Moszkowski, R., & Lupien, S. J. (2005). The perfect time to be stressed: A differential modulation of human memory by stress applied in the morning or in the afternoon. *Progress in Neuro-Psychopharmacology and Biological Psychiatry, 29*(8), 1281–1288.

Maier, S. F., & Watkins, L. R. (1998). Cytokines for psychologists: Implications of bidirectional immune-to-brain communication for understanding behavior, mood, and cognition. *Psychological Review, 105*(1), 83–107.

Majewska, M. D., Harrison, N. L., Schwartz, R. D., Barker, J. L., & Paul, S. M. (1986). Steroid hormone metabolites are barbiturate-like modulators of the GABA receptor. *Science, 232*, 1004–1007.

Maner, J. K., Miller, S. L., Schmidt, N. B., & Eckel, L. A. (2010). The endocrinology of exclusion: Rejection elicits motivationally tuned changes in progesterone. *Psychological Science, 21*(4), 581–588.

Mason, B. L., & Pariante, C. M. (2006). The effects of antidepressants on the hypothalamic–pituitary–adrenal axis. *Drug News and Perspectives, 19*, 603–608.

Mason, J. W. (1975). Emotion as reflected in patterns of endocrine integration. In L. Levi (Ed.), *Emotions: Their parameters and measurement* (pp. 143–181). New York: Raven Press.

Matthiesen, A. S., Ransjo-Arvidson, A. B., Nissen, E., & Uvnas-Moberg, K. (2001). Postpartum maternal oxytocin release by newborns: Effects of infant hand massage and sucking *Birth, 28*(1), 13–19.

McGowan, P. O., Sasaki, A., D'Alessio, A. C., Dymov, S., Labonte, B., Szyf, M., et al. (2009). Epigenetic regulation of the glucocorticoid receptor in human brain associates with childhood abuse. *Nature Neuroscience, 12*(3), 342–348.

Meaney, M. J. (2001). Maternal care, gene expression, and the transmission of individual differences in stress reactivity across generations. *Annual Review of Neuroscience, 24*, 1161–1192.

Meaney, M. J., Diorio, J., Francis, D., Widdowson, J., LaPlante, P., Caldji, C., et al. (1996). Early environmental regulation of forebrain glucocorticoid receptor gene expression: Implications for adrenocortical responses to stress. *Developmental Neuroscience, 18*(1–2), 49–72.

Meaney, M. J., & Stewart, J. (1981). Neonatal-androgens influence the social play of prepubescent rats. *Hormones and Behavior, 15*(2), 197–213.

Mehta, P. H., & Josephs, R. A. (2010). Testosterone and cortisol jointly regulate dominance: Evidence for a dual-hormone hypothesis. *Hormones and Behavior, 58*(5), 898–906.

Moffat, S. D., & Hampson, E. (1996). A curvilinear relationship between testosterone and spatial cognition in humans: Possible influence of hand preference. *Psychoneuroendocrinology, 21*(3), 323–337.

Nelson, E. E., & Panksepp, J. (1998). Brain substrates of infant–mother attachment: Contributions of opioids, oxytocin, and norepinephrine. *Neuroscience and Biobehavioral Reviews, 22*(3), 437–452.

Nelson, R. J. (2005a). The endocrine system. In R. J. Nelson (Ed.), *An introduction to behavioral endocrinology* (3rd ed., pp. 41–107). Sunderland, MA: Sinauer.

Nelson, R. J. (2005b). Stress. In R. J. Nelson (Ed.), *An introduction to behavioral endocrinology* (3rd ed., pp. 669–720). Sunderland, MA: Sinauer.

Nemeroff, C. B., Widerlov, E., Bissette, G., Walleus, H., Karlsson, I., Eklund, K., et al. (1984). Elevated concentrations of CSF corticotropin-releasing factor-like immunoreactivity in depressed patients. *Science, 226*, 1342–1344.

Neumann, I. D. (2002). Involvement of the brain oxytocin system in stress coping: Interactions with the hypothalamo–pituitary–adrenal axis. *Progress in Brain Research, 139*, 147–162.

Neumann, I. D. (2008). Brain oxytocin: A key regulator of emotional and social behaviours in both females and males. *Journal of Neuroendocrinology, 20*(6), 858–865.

Newman, M. L., Sellers, J. G., & Josephs, R. A. (2005). Testosterone, cognition, and social status. *Hormones and Behavior, 47*(2), 205–211.

Oei, N. Y., Elzinga, B. M., Wolf, O. T., de Ruiter, M. B., Damoiseaux, J. S., Kuijer, J. P., et al. (2007). Glucocorticoids decrease hippocampal and prefrontal activation during declarative memory retrieval in young men. *Brain Imaging and Behavior, 1*(1–2), 31–41.

Oei, N. Y., Everaerd, W. T., Elzinga, B. M., van Well, S., & Bermond, B. (2006). Psychosocial stress impairs working memory at high loads: An association with cortisol levels and memory retrieval. *Stress, 9*(3), 133–141.

Okuda, S., Roozendaal, B., & McGaugh, J. L. (2004). Glucocorticoid effects on object recognition memory require training-associated emotional arousal. *Proceedings of the National Academy of Sciences USA, 101*(3), 853–858.

Pajer, K., Tabbah, R., Gardner, W., Rubin, R. T., Czambel, R. K., & Wang, Y. (2006). Adrenal androgen and gonadal hormone levels in adolescent girls with conduct disorder. *Psychoneuroendocrinology, 31*(10), 1245–1256.

Pariante, C. M. (2006). The glucocorticoid receptor: Part of the solution or part of the problem? *Journal of Psychopharmacology, 20*(4, Suppl.), 79–84.

Pariante, C. M., Thomas, S. A., Lovestone, S., Makoff, A., & Kerwin, R. W. (2004). Do antidepressants regulate how cortisol affects the brain? *Psychoneuroendocrinology, 29*(4), 423–447.

Patchev, V. K., Shoaib, M., Holsboer, F., & Almeida, O. F. (1994). The neurosteroid tetrahydroprogesterone counteracts corticotropin-releasing hormone-induced anxiety and alters the release and gene expression of corticotropin-releasing hormone in the rat hypothalamus. *Neuroscience, 62*(1), 265–271.

Paul, S. M., & Purdy, R. H. (1992). Neuroactive steroids. *FASEB Journal, 6*(6), 2311–2322.

Payne, J. D., Jackson, E. D., Hoscheidt, S., Ryan, L., Jacobs, W. J., & Nadel, L. (2007). Stress administered prior to encoding impairs neutral but enhances emotional long-term episodic memories. *Learning and Memory, 14*(12), 861–868.

Perras, B., Droste, C., Born, J., Fehm, H. L., & Pietrowsky, R. (1997). Verbal memory after three months of intranasal vasopressin in healthy old humans. *Psychoneuroendocrinology, 22*(6), 387–396.

Plotsky, P. M., & Meaney, M. J. (1993). Early, postnatal experience alters hypothalamic corticotropin-releasing factor (CRF) mRNA, median eminence CRF content and stress-induced release in adult rats. *Brain Research: Molecular Brain Research, 18*(3), 195–200.

Postma, A., Meyer, G., Tuiten, A., van Honk, J., Kessels, R. P., & Thijssen, J. (2000). Effects of testosterone administration on selective aspects of object-location memory in healthy young women. *Psychoneuroendocrinology, 25*(6), 563–575.

Postma, A., Winkel, J., Tuiten, A., & van Honk, J. (1999). Sex differences and menstrual cycle effects in human spatial memory. *Psychoneuroendocrinology, 24*(2), 175–192.

Pruessner, J. C., Hellhammer, D. H., & Kirschbaum, C. (1999). Burnout, perceived stress, and cortisol responses to awakening. *Psychosomatic Medicine, 61*(2), 197–204.

Pryce, C. R. (2008). Postnatal ontogeny of expression of the corticosteroid receptor genes in mammalian brains: Inter-species and intra-species differences. *Brain Research Reviews, 57*(2), 596–605.

Purdy, R. H., Morrow, A. L., Moore, P. H. Jr., & Paul, S. M. (1991). Stress-induced elevations of gamma-aminobutyric acid type A receptor-active steroids in the rat brain. *Proceedings of the National Academy of Sciences USA, 88,* 4553–4557.

Putman, P., Hermans, E. J., Koppeschaar, H., van Schijndel, A., & van Honk, J. (2007). A single administration of cortisol acutely reduces preconscious attention for fear in anxious young men. *Psychoneuroendocrinology, 32*(7), 793–802.

Putman, P., Hermans, E. J., & van Honk, J. (2007). Exogenous cortisol shifts a motivated bias from fear to anger in spatial working memory for facial expressions. *Psychoneuroendocrinology, 32*(1), 14–21.

Puts, D. A., Cardenas, R. A., Bailey, D. H., Burriss, R. P., Jordan, C. L., & Breedlove, S. M. (2010). Salivary testosterone does not predict mental rotation performance in men or women. *Hormones and Behavior, 58*(2), 282–289.

Ranjit, N., Young, E. A., & Kaplan, G. A. (2005). Material hardship alters the diurnal rhythm of salivary cortisol. *International Journal of Epidemiology, 34*(5), 1138–1143.

Rimmele, U., Domes, G., Mathiak, K., & Hautzinger, M. (2003). Cortisol has different effects on human memory for emotional and neutral stimuli. *NeuroReport, 14*(18), 2485–2488.

Rodriguez-Landa, J. F., Contreras, C. M., Bernal-Morales, B., Gutierrez-Garcia, A. G., & Saavedra, M. (2007). Allopregnanolone reduces immobility in the forced swimming test and increases the firing rate of lateral septal neurons through actions on the GABAA receptor in the rat. *Journal of Psychopharmacology, 21*(1), 76–84.

Romeo, E., Strohle, A., Spalletta, G., di Michele, F., Hermann, B., Holsboer, F., et al. (1998). Effects of antidepressant treatment on neuroactive steroids in major depression. *American Journal of Psychiatry, 155*(7), 910–3.

Roozendaal, B., Okuda, S., de Quervain, D. J., & McGaugh, J. L. (2006). Glucocorticoids interact with emotion-induced noradrenergic activation in influencing different memory functions. *Neuroscience, 138*(3), 901–910.

Salvador, A. (2005). Coping with competitive situations in humans. *Neuroscience and Biobehavioral Reviews, 29*(1), 195–205.

Sanchez, M. M., Young, L. J., Plotsky, P. M., & Insel, T. R. (2000). Distribution of corticosteroid receptors in the rhesus brain: Relative absence of glucocorticoid receptors in the hippocampal formation. *Journal of Neuroscience, 20*(12), 4657–4668.

Sapolsky, R. M. (1985). Stress-induced suppression of testicular function in the wild baboon: Role of glucocorticoids. *Endocrinology, 116*(6), 2273–2278.

Sapolsky, R. M. (1986). Stress-induced elevation of testosterone concentration in high ranking baboons: Role of catecholamines. *Endocrinology, 118*(4), 1630–1635.

Sapolsky, R. M. (2002). Endocrinology of the stress-response. In J. B. Becker, S. M. Breedlove, D. Crews, & M. M. McCarthy (Eds.), *Behavioral endocrinology* (2nd ed., pp. 409–450). Cambridge, MA: MIT Press.

Sapolsky, R. M. (2005). The influence of social hierarchy on primate health. *Science, 308,* 648–652.

Savaskan, E., Ehrhardt, R., Schulz, A., Walter, M., & Schachinger, H. (2008). Post-learning intranasal oxytocin modulates human memory for facial identity. *Psychoneuroendocrinology, 33*(3), 368–374.

Schelling, G., Roozendaal, B., & De Quervain, D. J. (2004). Can posttraumatic stress disorder be prevented with glucocorticoids? *Annals of the New York Academy of Sciences, 1032,* 158–166.

Schelling, G., Roozendaal, B., Krauseneck, T., Schmoelz, M., de Quervain, D., & Briegel, J. (2006). Efficacy of hydrocortisone in preventing posttraumatic stress disorder following critical illness and major surgery. *Annals of the New York Academy of Sciences, 1071,* 46–53.

Schlotz, W., Hellhammer, J., Schulz, P., & Stone, A. A. (2004). Perceived work overload and chronic worrying predict weekend–weekday differences in the cortisol awakening response. *Psychosomatic Medicine, 66*(2), 207–214.

Schlotz, W., Kumsta, R., Layes, I., Entringer, S., Jones, A., & Wust, S. (2008). Covariance between psychological and endocrine responses to pharmacological challenge and psychosocial stress: A question of timing. *Psychosomatic Medicine, 70*(7), 787–796.

Schule, C., Di Michele, F., Baghai, T., Romeo, E., Bernardi, G., Zwanzger, P., et al. (2004). Neuroactive steroids in responders and nonresponders to sleep deprivation. *Annals of the New York Academy of Sciences, 1032,* 216–223.

Schultheiss, O. C., & Stanton, S. J. (2009). Assessment of salivary hormones. In E. Harmon-Jones & J. S. Beer (Eds.), *Methods in social neuroscience* (pp. 17–44). New York: Guilford Press.

Schultheiss, O. C., Wirth, M. M., & Stanton, S. J. (2004). Effects of affiliation and power motivation arousal on salivary progesterone and testosterone. *Hormones and Behavior, 46*(5), 592–599.

Schwabe, L., Tegenthoff, M., Hoffken, O., & Wolf, O. T. (2010). Concurrent glucocorticoid and noradrenergic activity shifts instrumental behavior from goal-directed to habitual control. *Journal of Neuroscience, 30,* 8190–8196.

Smeets, T., Otgaar, H., Candel, I., & Wolf, O. T. (2008). True or false?: Memory is differentially affected by stress-induced cortisol elevations and sympathetic activity at consolidation and retrieval. *Psychoneuroendocrinology, 33,* 1378–1386.

Soravia, L. M., de Quervain, D. J., & Heinrichs, M. (2009). Glucocorticoids do not reduce subjective fear in healthy subjects exposed to social stress. *Biological Psychology, 81*(3), 184–188.

Soravia, L. M., Heinrichs, M., Aerni, A., Maroni, C., Schelling, G., Ehlert, U., et al. (2006). Glucocorticoids reduce phobic fear in humans. *Proceedings of the National Academy of Sciences USA, 103*(14), 5585–5590.

Stanton, S. J., Beehner, J. C., Saini, E. K., Kuhn, C. M., & Labar, K. S. (2009). Dominance, politics, and physiology: Voters' testosterone changes on the night of the 2008 United States presidential election. *PloS One, 4,* e7543.

Stanton, S. J., Liening, S. H., & Schultheiss, O. C. (2010). Testosterone is positively associated with risk taking in the Iowa Gambling Task. *Hormones and Behavior, 59,* 252–256.

Stanton, S. J., Mullette-Gillman, O. A., McLaurin, R. E., Kuhn, C. M., Labar, K. S., Platt, M. L., et al. (2011). Low- and high-testosterone individuals exhibit decreased aversion to economic risk. *Psychological Science, 22,* 447–453.

Stetler, C., & Miller, G. E. (2011). Depression and hypothalamic–pituitary–adrenal activation: A quantitative summary of four decades of research. *Psychosomatic Medicine, 73*(2), 114–126.

Tabori, N. E., Stewart, L. S., Znamensky, V., Romeo, R. D., Alves, S. E., McEwen, B. S., et al. (2005). Ultrastructural evidence that androgen receptors are located at extranuclear sites in the rat hippocampal formation. *Neuroscience, 130*(1), 151–163.

Takayanagi, Y., Yoshida, M., Bielsky, I. F., Ross, H. E., Kawamata, M., Onaka, T., et al. (2005). Pervasive social deficits, but normal parturition, in oxytocin receptor-deficient mice. *Proceedings of the National Academy of Sciences of the United States of America, 102*, 16096–16101.

Taylor, S. E., Klein, L. C., Lewis, B. P., Gruenewald, T. L., Gurung, R. A., & Updegraff, J. A. (2000). Biobehavioral responses to stress in females: Tend-and-befriend, not fight-or-flight. *Psychological Review, 107*(3), 411–429.

Taylor, S. E., Saphire-Bernstein, S., & Seeman, T. E. (2010). Are plasma oxytocin in women and plasma vasopressin in men biomarkers of distressed pair-bond relationships? *Psychological Science, 21*(1), 3–7.

Thompson, R. R., George, K., Walton, J. C., Orr, S. P., & Benson, J. (2006). Sex-specific influences of vasopressin on human social communication. *Proceedings of the National Academy of Sciences USA, 103*, 7889–7894.

Thornton, J., Zehr, J. L., & Loose, M. D. (2009). Effects of prenatal androgens on rhesus monkeys: A model system to explore the organizational hypothesis in primates. *Hormones and Behavior, 55*(5), 633–645.

Timby, E., Balgard, M., Nyberg, S., Spigset, O., Andersson, A., Porankiewicz-Asplund, J., et al. (2006). Pharmacokinetic and behavioral effects of allopregnanolone in healthy women. *Psychopharmacology, 186*(3), 414–424.

Tobin, V. A., Hashimoto, H., Wacker, D. W., Takayanagi, Y., Langnaese, K., Caquineau, C., et al. (2010). An intrinsic vasopressin system in the olfactory bulb is involved in social recognition. *Nature, 464*, 413–417.

Townsend, S. S., Major, B., Gangi, C. E., & Mendes, W. B. (2011). From "in the air" to "under the skin": Cortisol responses to social identity threat. *Personality and Social Psychology Bulletin, 37*(2), 151–164.

Uvnas-Moberg, K. (1998a). Antistress pattern induced by oxytocin. *News in Physiological Sciences, 13*, 22–25.

Uvnas-Moberg, K. (1998b). Oxytocin may mediate the benefits of positive social interaction and emotions. *Psychoneuroendocrinology, 23*(8), 819–835.

Uzunova, V., Sheline, Y., Davis, J. M., Rasmusson, A., Uzunov, D. P., Costa, E., et al. (1998). Increase in the cerebrospinal fluid content of neurosteroids in patients with unipolar major depression who are receiving fluoxetine or fluvoxamine. *Proceedings of the National Academy of Sciences USA, 95*(6), 3239–3244.

van Broekhoven, F., & Verkes, R. J. (2003). Neurosteroids in depression: A review. *Psychopharmacology, 165*(2), 97–110.

van Honk, J., Tuiten, A., van den Hout, M., Koppeschaar, H., Thijssen, J., de Haan, E., et al. (2000). Conscious and preconscious selective attention to social threat: Different neuroendocrine response patterns. *Psychoneuroendocrinology, 25*(6), 577–591.

van Honk, J., Tuiten, A., Verbaten, R., van den Hout, M., Koppeschaar, H., Thijssen, J., et al. (1999). Correlations among salivary testosterone, mood, and selective attention to threat in humans. *Hormones and Behavior, 36*(1), 17–24.

van Stegeren, A. H., Wolf, O. T., Everaerd, W., Scheltens, P., Barkhof, F., & Rombouts, S. A. (2007). Endogenous cortisol level interacts with noradrenergic activation in the human amygdala. *Neurobiology of Learning and Memory, 87*(1), 57–66.

Viau, V. (2002). Functional cross-talk between the hypothalamic–pituitary–gonadal and –adrenal axes. *Journal of Neuroendocrinology, 14*(6), 506–513.

Viviani, D., & Stoop, R. (2008). Opposite effects of oxytocin and vasopressin on the emotional expression of the fear response. *Progress in Brain Research, 170*, 207–218.

Wachtel, S. R., & de Wit, H. (2001). Lack of effect of intravenous hydrocortisone on mood in humans: A preliminary study. *Behavioural Pharmacology, 12*(5), 373–376.

Walum, H., Westberg, L., Henningsson, S., Neiderhiser, J. M., Reiss, D., Igl, W., et al. (2008). Genetic variation in the vasopressin receptor 1a gene *(AVPR1A)* associates with pair-bonding behavior in humans. *Proceedings of the National Academy of Sciences USA, 105*, 14153–14156.

Wingfield, J. C., Ball, G. F., Dufty, A. M., Hegner, R. E., & Rameofsky, M. (1987). Testosterone and aggression in birds. *American Scientist, 75*(6), 602–608.

Winslow, J. T., Hastings, N., Carter, C. S., Harbaugh, C. R., & Insel, T. R. (1993). A role for central vasopressin in pair bonding in monogamous prairie voles. *Nature, 365,* 545–548.

Winslow, J. T., & Insel, T. R. (2002). The social deficits of the oxytocin knockout mouse. *Neuropeptides, 36*(2–3), 221–229.

Winslow, J. T., & Miczek, K. A. (1985). Social status as determinants of alcohol effects on aggressive behavior in squirrel monkeys *(Saimiri sciureus). Psychopharmacology, 85,* 167–172.

Wirth, M. M. (2011). Beyond the HPA axis: Progesterone-derived neuroactive steroids in human stress and emotion. *Frontiers in Endocrinology, 2,* 19.

Wirth, M. M., Meier, E. A., Fredrickson, B. L., & Schultheiss, O. C. (2007). Relationship between salivary cortisol and progesterone levels in humans. *Biological Psychology, 74*(1), 104–107.

Wirth, M. M., Scherer, S. M., Hoks, R. M., & Abercrombie, H. C. (2011). The effect of cortisol on emotional responses depends on order of cortisol and placebo administration in a within-subjects design. *Psychoneuroendocrinology, 36,* 945–954.

Wirth, M. M., & Schultheiss, O. C. (2006). Effects of affiliation arousal (hope of closeness) and affiliation stress (fear of rejection) on progesterone and cortisol. *Hormones and Behavior, 50*(5), 786–795.

Wirth, M. M., & Schultheiss, O. C. (2007). Basal testosterone moderates responses to anger faces in humans. *Physiology & Behavior, 90*(2–3), 496–505.

Wirth, M. M., Welsh, K. M., & Schultheiss, O. C. (2006). Salivary cortisol changes in humans after winning or losing a dominance contest depend on implicit power motivation. *Hormones and Behavior, 49*(3), 346–352.

Wolf, O. T. (2008). The influence of stress hormones on emotional memory: Relevance for psychopathology. *Acta Psychologica, 127*(3), 513–531.

Wolf, O. T., Convit, A., McHugh, P. F., Kandil, E., Thorn, E. L., De Santi, S., et al. (2001). Cortisol differentially affects memory in young and elderly men. *Behavioral Neuroscience, 115*(5), 1002–1011.

Wynne-Edwards, K. E., & Timonin, M. E. (2007). Paternal care in rodents: Weakening support for hormonal regulation of the transition to behavioral fatherhood in rodent animal models of biparental care. *Hormones and Behavior, 52*(1), 114–121.

Yehuda, R. (2002). Current status of cortisol findings in post-traumatic stress disorder. *Psychiatric Clinics of North America, 25*(2), 341–368, vii.

Yehuda, R., McFarlane, A. C., & Shalev, A. Y. (1998). Predicting the development of post-traumatic stress disorder from the acute response to a traumatic event. *Biological Psychiatry, 44,* 1305–1313.

Yehuda, R., Yang, R. K., Buchsbaum, M. S., & Golier, J. A. (2006). Alterations in cortisol negative feedback inhibition as examined using the ACTH response to cortisol administration in PTSD. *Psychoneuroendocrinology, 31*(4), 447–451.

Young, L. J., Nilsen, R., Waymire, K. G., McGregor, G. R., & Insel, T. R. (1999). Increase affiliative response to vasopressin in mice expressing the vasopressin receptor from a monogamous vole. *Nature, 400,* 766–768.

Young, L. J., & Wang, Z. (2004). The neurobiology of pair bonding. *Nature Neuroscience, 7,* 1048–1054.

Zink, C. F., Stein, J. L., Kempf, L., Hakimi, S., & Meyer-Lindenberg, A. (2010). Vasopressin modulates medial prefrontal cortex-amygdala circuitry during emotion processing in humans. *Journal of Neuroscience, 30,* 7017–7022.

PART III

COGNITIVE PROCESSES IN EMOTION

CHAPTER 6

Attention and Emotion

Jenny Yiend, Kirsten Barnicot, and Ernst H. W. Koster

Contextualizing the Study of Emotional Attention

Attention has two major functions in our daily life. It is crucial in selecting and processing information that is relevant to current tasks, and it is important in processing novel, potentially relevant information (Allport, 1993). These two functions sometimes interfere with one another (e.g., for a student, attention to study materials may be interrupted by emotional thoughts about failing the exam). Arguably, the ability to switch flexibly between different stimuli in our environment is crucial to cope with such distracting thoughts and is important for healthy functioning and resilience. Conversely, impairments in the ability to regulate attention adaptively during processing of emotional information may contribute to stress vulnerability and the development of emotional disorders. This chapter considers emotion and attention in relation to normal functioning and, more specifically, in relation to emotional disorders. Selective processing of material relevant to a disorder is thought to play an important etiological role in maintaining that disorder. Within both sections, material is organized according to the experimental methodology involved. First, we define the topic, set it in its histori-

cal and current context, and introduce some key concepts.

The topic of this chapter concerns *emotional attention*, by which we mean the selective attentional processing of emotionally salient information. The study of emotional attention has a long history, with several early theorists proposing that emotional stimuli carry properties that strongly influence attentional processing. For instance, Easterbrook (1959) influentially claimed that highly negatively arousing stimuli or states narrow the focus of attention. Their influence on attentional breadth is of broad interest to social and clinical psychology today (e.g., Eysenck, 1992). Contemporary study of emotional attention originated in experimental psychopathology, where researchers studied attention to threat-relevant information in relation to anxiety (e.g., Mathews & MacLeod, 1985). Findings revealed that highly anxious individuals showed exaggerated attention to threat compared to those with low anxiety. These studies renewed interest in the investigation of basic attention and emotion interactions, and these two related fields continue as parallel research areas today, as reflected in the structure of this chapter.

It is important clarify some basic concepts that arise during our later detailed discussion of emotional attention. First, the attentional phenomena under consideration, almost without exception, involve *selective attention*. This term refers to the selection, by the cognitive system, of certain, more salient information over and above other less salient material. In empirical studies, this means that emotional information is presented under conditions of competition with other stimuli or with task demands. Much basic attention research has examined when and how this selection occurs and whether bottom-up characteristics (e.g., emotional properties of stimuli) and top-down factors (e.g., individuals' expectancies) influence selection (Desimone & Duncan, 1995). A further important concept within emotional attention is that of *automaticity*: the fast, efficient, preconscious and uncontrollable priority of access to further attentional processing that emotionally salient material appears to possess. Many of these features of automaticity (Moors & De Houwer, 2006) have been studied independently, and these facets of automaticity recur throughout the chapter. Finally, it is important to clarify at the outset that most studies have examined emotional attention through manipulation of the stimulus properties—the main focus of this chapter—rather than examining the *effects of specific mood states on attention*.

The Interaction between Attention and Emotion

In this section we review the study of emotional attention in the general population, according to the methodology used. Studies rely on paradigms from cognitive-experimental psychology, in which attention to emotional information can be inferred from performance indices such as reaction times, error rates, eye movements, and (most recently) patterns of neural activation. Most studies have investigated the visual–spatial domain, with notable exceptions including occasional studies of the auditory modality (Mathews & MacLeod, 1986) and cross-modal phenomena (e.g., Santangelo, Ho, & Spence, 2008). Studies either use emotional and nonemotional words or naturalistic stimuli such as faces or pictures. Research to date has not identified any systematic differences between such stimulus types (cf.

Bar-Haim, Lamy, Pergamin, Bakermans-Kranenburg, & van IJzendoorn, 2007)

The Emotional Stroop

The emotional Stroop is one of the earliest and best known experimental methods for demonstrating attentional bias effects. When color words (e.g., *blue*) are written in competing colored inks (e.g., in red ink), it takes longer to name the ink colors than when they are written in consistent colors (e.g., *blue* in blue ink, *red* in red ink). In the emotional version, longer color naming is found for emotional words (e.g., *cancer*) compared to neutral words, especially in those with emotional disorders or a vulnerability to them (MacLeod, 1991). In both cases, the inference made is that word meaning interferes with selective attention to the ink color, thereby slowing reaction times, and this interference is greater when word meaning is more salient to the task or the individual.

In a recent meta-analysis, Bar-Haim and colleagues (2007) found evidence of emotional Stroop interference, but only in blocked designs, in which trials of a particular valence were grouped together. This qualification, which has been reported elsewhere in unselected samples (McKenna & Sharma, 2004), may be due to the cumulative exposure to valenced stimuli that occurs across blocks. However, where the primary aim is to make inferences about *selective attention*, other methods are increasingly preferred, due to the inherent ambiguity of the inferences that can be made from Stroop interference. To give just one example, slowing of reaction times to name the color of emotional words could reflect inhibition rather than attentional selection. Rather than selectively attending to and processing word meaning, participants may instead be deploying attentional resources to actively inhibit the attentional processing of the salient, but irrelevant, word meaning. This too would consume attentional resources and lead to color-naming interference, making the two possibilities indistinguishable (see de Ruiter & Brosschot, 1994, for a full discussion of this problem). In the most recent example of the debate about the usefulness and meaning of this task, Algom, Chajut, and Lev (2004) argued that "the processes sustaining the classic and the emotional effects differ in a qualitative fashion" (p. 335). Although this remains a strong and contested claim (Dalgleish, 2005), it underlines what has been known for a long time: that the conclusions about emotion and attention, per se, from emotional Stroop studies are limited at best.

Visual Search

The largest literature on attention to emotion in the general population comes from visual search tasks. A target is presented among an array of distracters (typically 6–12; see Figure 6.1) and must be detected as quickly as possible. The current consensus suggests that negative information (especially related to anger and fear, but also to happy and sad—e.g., see Frischen, Eastwood, & Smilek, 2008) is both detected faster and is more distracting than neutral information (e.g., Öhman, Flykt, & Esteves, 2001; but see also Tipples, Young, Quinlan, Broks, & Ellis, 2002). Almost all studies use picture stimuli, such as different facial expressions or animals with matched, non-emotional objects (e.g., spiders, snakes, flowers, mushrooms). Better control over arbitrary perceptual differences is gained by using schematic faces (simple line drawings consisting of a circle, mouth, eyes, and sometimes eyebrows) or by using neutral stimuli that are associated with fear through conditioning (e.g., Batty, Cave, & Pauli, 2005). A very useful review of the literature on visual search to emotional information in the general population (and touching on individual differences in state) is that of Frischen and colleagues (2008). Focusing specifically on facial expressions, they conclude that preattentive visual search processes are sensitive to, and facilitated by, emotional information.

Visual search for "biologically relevant" stimuli has been a particular focus of interest in studies of normal volunteers because of the clear prediction that these stimuli should be especially effective in the competition for attentional selection. These stimuli are "biologically prepared" to be associated with fear, such as snakes and spiders, and are sometimes contrasted with stimuli whose relevance to fear must be learned, such as weapons. Fox, Griggs, and Mouchlianitis (2007) found neither class of threat

stimuli showed an advantage over the other, although both were more efficiently detected than neutral control pictures (e.g., mushrooms, flowers). Lipp and Waters (2007) showed enhanced attentional capture for spiders and snakes (regarded as biologically fear relevant) compared to similarly unpleasant animals that are not considered biologically prepared (e.g., cockroaches, lizards).

Varying the distracter array size during visual search allows researchers to assess the extent to which emotionally salient information is detected automatically (here meaning "in parallel" or "preattentive" as determined by near-zero additional cost from increasing the numbers of distracters). For example, Öhman and colleagues (2001), using pictures of snakes, spiders, mushrooms, and flowers, claimed that search for threat stimuli occurred in parallel because no slowing was found on a 3 × 3, compared to 2 × 2, array. Eastwood, Smilek, and Merikle (2001) used arrays of 7, 11, 15, and 19 schematic faces. Although search slopes were not flat, for negative targets they were shallower than for positive, suggesting a serial search that was faster in the former case. Angry faces appear to be particularly effective at promoting fast, efficient search (e.g., Calvo, Avero, & Lundqvist, 2006).

Attentional Cueing

A large behavioral literature draws on attentional cueing techniques, particularly the use of double cues (see Figure 6.1). Pairs of neutral–emotional stimuli are followed by a neutral target (e.g., a letter) that appears in one or other of the cued locations (emotional or neutral) and that must be identified as quickly as possible. Consistently speeded responses when targets occur in one location (e.g., emotional) imply an attentional preference for that type of stimulus. Double cueing (also called the *dot probe task* or the *attentional probe task*) is probably the most widely used technique to investigate attention to emotion. This is because (1) it allows the specific inference that selective attention to threat in preference to nonthreat occurred, and (2) it is not susceptible to many alternative interpretations that apply to other tasks, such as response bias (a neutral response to a neutral stimulus is required) or general performance impairments (detection is *speeded*

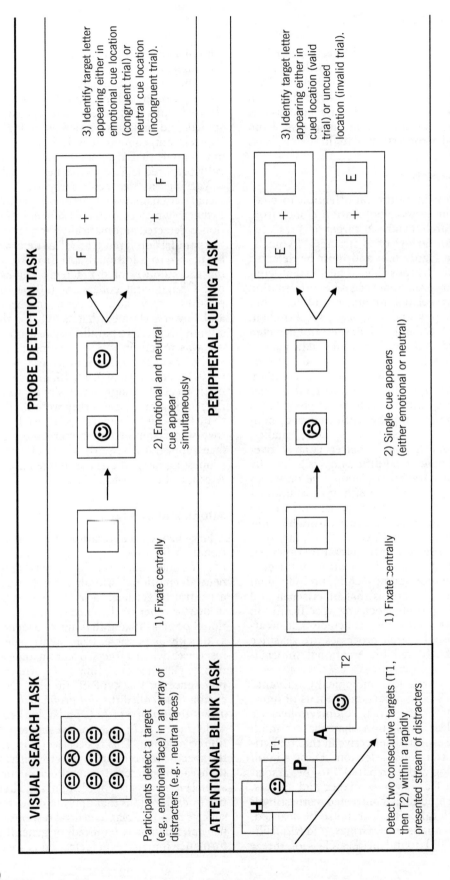

FIGURE 6.1. An illustration of four experimental paradigms commonly used to investigate the effect of emotional material on attentional deployment.

by threat). The overall pattern of data indicates that when specific stimulus material (severely threatening and/or biologically relevant) and short presentations (< 500 milliseconds [ms]) are used, selective attentional biases favoring negative information are evident.

Considering stimulus severity, two studies investigated the pattern of orienting to threat in low trait anxiety (Mogg et al., 2000; Wilson & MacLeod, 2003), with both reporting findings consistent with avoidance of minor threat and vigilance for high threat. In addition, in various individual difference studies, control participants have displayed attentional avoidance of mild threat (e.g., Bar-Haim et al., 2007; MacLeod et al., 1986; Yiend & Mathews, 2001). A working hypothesis (Mogg & Bradley, 1998), which has received empirical support, is that the general population shows adaptive avoidance of milder threat, but vigilance for severe threat. This pattern has an obvious evolutionarily adaptive function by allowing only serious survival challenges to interrupt the processing of current goals. As with visual search methods, biologically relevant stimuli have been a focus of interest. Lipp and Derakshan (2005) found an attentional bias toward snakes and spiders, compared to neutral stimuli, in healthy volunteers, and Beaver, Mogg, and Bradley (2005) reported that aversive conditioning increased selective attention to biologically relevant material.

One way of assessing whether biased selective attention occurs early or late in the processing stream is to vary the duration of the cue. In a normal sample, Cooper and Langton (2006) contrasted 100 ms and 500 ms cue durations, finding vigilance for threat faces compared to neutral (and neutral compared to happy) at the shorter duration. Short cue duration was also critical to demonstrating selective attention toward threat in Holmes, Green, and Vuilleumier's study (2005). They found attentional biases toward fearful compared to neutral faces, but only at 30 ms and 100 ms, not (in a later experiment) at 500 ms or 1,000 ms. Thus, although not yet extensive in number, the extant data suggest that normal individuals display a selective visual–spatial bias favoring threat, providing that attention is probed early enough.

Double-cueing studies provide little information about the likely attentional mechanisms underlying selective attentional effects. For example, are emotionally salient stimuli more effective at capturing attention *(engagement)*, or is it their ability to maintain attention *(disengagement* or *maintenance)*, or perhaps both, which produces the reaction time effects on double-cueing studies? Such questions prompted the development of the single-cueing paradigm (the original, nonemotional task was developed by Posner, 1980). Single cueing uses two critical comparisons to determine engagement and disengagement, respectively. On valid trials,[1] a neutral probe appears in the location of the preceding cue, and we can infer that, at least for short cue durations, the speed of performing this task reflects the speed of engagement to the cued location. Thus differences between valid emotional and neutral cued trials are taken to reflect differences in the engagement of attention to the emotional content of the cue. Conversely, on invalid trials, the probe appears in the opposite location to the cue, requiring disengagement of attention and reorienting toward the probed location. Thus, reaction time differences between different types of cues on invalid trials might reflect the relative ease of disengaging attention from the cues' respective location. As with any task, it is impossible to be sure that "process pure" measures are being taken, and this task is no exception. Possible interpretive problems, possible solutions, and ongoing current debates involving single-cueing techniques have arisen within the experimental psychopathology field. These are therefore considered in detail under the corresponding methodology of the next section.

The first studies presented peripheral cues for 500 ms on the assumption that this would be the optimally sensitive time to examine anxiety-related differences, given the previous literature. However, some reports of generally speeded reaction times to invalid compared to valid trials (e.g., Waters, Nitz, Craske, & Johnson, 2007) have suggested that attention may have already dis-

---

[1]Here the term *valid* or *invalid* denotes trials on which targets appear at cued or opposite-cued locations, irrespective of predictive validity (i.e., the overall ratio within the task of valid to invalid trials).

engaged the cued location by the time of probing at 500 ms (depending on the type of stimulus material used), and that inhibition of return[2] may be already taking effect. Shorter cue durations have therefore been preferred in later studies, so that effects can be attributed more unambiguously to early attentional cueing phenomena. Limited evidence from healthy samples to date suggests that both mechanisms, engagement and disengagement, are influenced by emotional salience. The studies of Stormark and colleagues (e.g., Stormark & Hugdahl, 1996) used classical conditioning to impart emotional salience to location cues and found faster reaction times to validly cued targets, but only for emotion word cues. Koster and colleagues (Koster, Crombez, Verschueve, & DeHouwer, 2004; Koster, Verschueve, Burssens, Custers, & Crombez, 2007) reported evidence for facilitated engagement and impaired disengagement from threat compared to neutral information using emotional images (2007) and aversive conditioning (2004). Consistent with double-cueing studies, selective attention to threat was limited to severe threat and short durations (100 ms, although not 28 ms, which was attributed to inherent processing limits involving complex scenes).

The Attentional Blink

In the attentional blink task, participants have to report two sequential targets in a rapid stream of stimuli (called *rapid serial visual presentation*: RSVP). If the targets (T1 presented first, followed by T2 presented second) are sufficiently close in presentation time to each other (typically a few hundred ms apart), then the second (T2) is often missed. The *attentional blink* refers to the finding that the efficiency of detecting T2 is modulated by the time interval (lag) between T1 and T2, which is often defined in terms of the number of intervening stimuli in the presentation stream (Raymond, Shap-

iro, & Arnell, 1992). When T2 detection is plotted against lag, a characteristic attenuation in T2 detection (or *blink* of attention) can be seen. This phenomenon is thought to stem from an overinvestment of attentional resources in stimulus processing (Olivers & Nieuwenhuis, 2006). Missing T2 is thought to occur because resources are still deployed in processing T1 and therefore insufficient are available at the time of T2 to allow it to be identified.

In emotional adaptations of this task, it is crucial to be clear about the precise nature of the emotional manipulation because predictions vary depending on when the emotional information is presented (e.g., at T1 or T2), and findings from extant studies differ markedly. The most typical adaptation is to look at the effect of neutral targets identified at T1 on emotional versus neutral targets identified at T2. Under these conditions, an attenuated attentional blink would be expected when T2 was emotional and therefore capable of commanding greater attentional resources. An alternative is to examine the differential effect of identifying emotional versus neutral targets at T1 on neutral T2 identification. If emotional information processing consumes additional capacity, as might be expected, the attentional blink should be enhanced when emotional information is processed at T1.

A few studies have examined the emotional attentional blink phenomenon in the general population. For example, Keil and Ihssen (2004) looked at the effect of pleasant, unpleasant, and neutral words presented at T2. Both emotional categories enhanced accuracy of T2 identification, especially at short lags, although not when emotional information rated low on arousal was used. Similarly, Anderson (2005) found that the attentional blink was reduced when emotional words were presented at T2, even when other factors related to differential distinctiveness were controlled. In the studies of Most and colleagues (e.g., Most, Smith, Cooter, Levy, & Zald, 2007), only one target had to be reported and the effects on detection accuracy when it was preceded by an emotional stimulus were compared to those of a preceding neutral stimulus. These researchers typically found reduced accuracy when targets appear after emotional, compared to nonemotional, images (Most,

---

[2]This term refers to the phenomenon identified by Posner (1980), such that cued locations lose their attentional advantage after a certain time has elapsed, becoming inhibited relative to uncued locations. The effect is thought to represent an adaptive attentional mechanism whereby novel locations are prioritized for attentional processing over recently attended ones.

Chun, Johnson, & Kiehl, 2006) and similar effects with arousing positive stimuli (Most et al., 2007) and stimuli made negative through aversive conditioning (Smith, Most, Newsome, & Zald, 2006).

Eye Movements

Using eye tracking to assess the number of times or the length of time for which participants fixate on stimuli can provide an insight into attentional processing beyond that provided by reaction times alone. Therefore, eye tracking is an increasingly popular methodology with which to examine visual attention for emotional information. Note that eye movements typically reflect *overt* attentional orienting, in contrast to *covert* attention, which is considered independent of eye movements and better indexed using the experimental techniques described above. Under normal circumstances, however, the two are closely coupled, with covert shifts of attention usually preceding corresponding eye movements (Jonides, 1981). Advantages of using eye movements to assess attentional biases include their rapid, naturalistic, and continuous nature. Typically, the registration of eye movements is performed during a cognitive-experimental task. The use of eye tracking provides a number of different indices, among others the location of initial fixation, the duration of fixations, and total time spent viewing a stimulus. Moreover, eye tracking can also be applied to examine attention under naturalistic viewing conditions wherein no task is required, but participants are simply asked to look at displays as they would normally do.

Studies examining eye movements toward emotional scenes presented concurrently with neutral scenes in the visual periphery are particularly interesting. In several of these, pairs of one emotional and one neutral scene were presented simultaneously for 3 seconds (s) in parafoveal vision (Calvo & Lang, 2004; Nummenmaa, Hyönä, & Calvo, 2006). These studies found that the probability of first fixation and the viewing time during the first 500 ms were greater for both pleasant and unpleasant scenes than for the paired neutral scenes. Moreover, Nummenmaa and colleagues (2006) found that the emotional picture of each pair was more likely to be fixated first even when the par-

ticipants were instructed to look first at the neutral picture. In contrast, after the first 650–700 ms, participants were able to control their gaze and comply with the instructions (i.e., look at the neutral picture, when requested) for the rest of the 3-s display time. This was interpreted as an early involuntary attentional capture by emotional content, which requires cognitive resources and time to be counteracted voluntarily. Further systematic research to exclude many potential visual confounds (e.g., luminance of stimuli, features) has shown that the initial saccades toward emotional scenes are driven in a reflexive manner (Nummenmaa, Hyönä, & Calvo, 2009).

In the area of emotional face processing, a number of interesting and systematic studies have been performed on rapid attentional orienting toward emotional versus neutral faces (e.g., Bannerman, Milders, & Sahraie, 2010). In these studies it was argued that the speed of the initial saccades toward emotional versus neutral expression may provide the most sensitive index of attentional capture by emotion. Indeed, using very brief face presentations (20 ms), it was found that individuals more rapidly made saccades toward fearful faces and were slower to move their eyes away from these faces (overt disengagement). Interestingly, manual response data only showed evidence of enhanced attentional orienting toward emotional faces with longer (e.g., 500 ms) cue presentations (Bannerman et al., 2010). These data corroborate the idea that emotional information can influence overt orienting by facilitating engagement of attention and delaying disengagement. In sum, studies using eye registration largely confirm the general findings of previous work using tasks that rely on manual responses.

Cognitive Neuroscience

Cognitive neuroscience methods have widely examined the processing of negative emotional information and issues concerning automaticity (specifically, its different features). Initial studies highlighted the role of the amygdala, which is known from animal work to be crucially involved in the fear response (see Freese & Amaral, 2009). The amygdala receives and integrates various inputs from external and internal sources and outputs to structures, such as the thalamus, involved in modulating autonomic, motor, and cognitive processes. As such, the amygdala is well positioned to exert a modulatory influence on cortical pathways that are involved in attentional orienting (see Vuilleumier, 2005). In much of this research, neural activity has been compared upon presentation of emotional versus nonemotional information under conditions of selective attention. Fearful faces are associated with enhanced activity in the amygdala as well as the extrastriate cortex, which is involved in sensory processing (Morris, Öhman, & Dolan, 1998). These studies are in line with the idea that sensory processing is enhanced for emotional information. In one example, Vuilleumier, Armony, Driver, and Dolan (2001) presented a pair of faces and a pair of houses on each trial. Participants had to attend to only one of the pairs and report whether stimuli were matching or mismatching. As hypothesized, the amount of activity in the fusiform cortex (a region known to be activated specifically by facial stimuli) was modulated by type of stimulus attended, but fearful faces activated the fusiform area even when presented in the unattended location (Vuilleumier et al., 2001).

In other work, it has been shown that even under conditions of *masked* presentation, fearful faces elicit stronger amygdala activity than neutral faces (e.g., Morris et al., 1998). In addition, in the study by Vuilleumier and colleagues (2001), the degree of amygdala activation during fearful face trials was independent of spatial attention. These findings suggest that processing of (particularly negative) emotional information is automatic in the sense that it does not require awareness, is highly efficient with dedicated and prioritized processing in the brain, and is, at early stages, independent of attentional resources. Further functional magnetic resonance imaging (fMRI) and neurological studies have led to suggestions of two separate neural pathways for emotional attention: a fast, subcortical, nonconscious "low road" and a slower, resource-dependent, cortical "high road" (LeDoux, 1995) that provides more detailed, contextualized information. However, this view is the subject of ongoing debate and has been challenged by the work of Pessoa and others (see Pessoa & Adolphs, 2010; also Pessoa and Pereira, Chapter 4, this volume).

Research has also extensively investigated the neural structures of attentional control in relation to emotion processing. Indeed, the allocation of attention has also been related to several higher-order cortical structures, such as the prefrontal cortex (PFC) and the anterior cingulate cortex (ACC), which can attenuate amygdala activity (Taylor & Fragopanagos, 2005). These brain regions are also crucial for the regulation of emotion, and can down-regulate (i.e., suppress) emotion-relevant limbic structures in a "top-down" manner (e.g., Ochsner & Gross, 2005). Interestingly, fMRI studies have shown remarkable similarity between the neural circuitry involved in successful emotion regulation and those that are implicated in attentional bias (e.g., the amygdala and dorsolateral PFC; see Bishop, 2007).

Emotional Disorders and Attention–Emotion Interactions

As we have seen, emotionally salient information typically attracts greater attention than neutral information. When studying attention–emotion interactions in emotional disorders, the specific type of emotional material is of particular interest. Usually it is the material most closely matched to symptom content that elicits important attentional effects different from those seen in healthy controls. These attentional effects in emotional disorders are commonly called *attentional biases* and are referred to as *emotion congruent*, reflecting the link between the emotional material that elicits the attentional effects and the disorder or vulnerability of the individual. Emotion-congruent attentional biases are important because of their demonstrated role in the cause and maintenance of the disorders with which they are associated. For example, longitudinal work shows biased processing predicts proxy symptoms (e.g., Pury, 2002), and "cognitive bias modification" research has shown that inducing biased processes elicits expected changes in mood, symptoms, and vulnerability (see MacLeod & Clarke, Chapter 29, this volume). In anxiety disorders, the effect would work as follows. An enhanced tendency to attend to threatening items (in preference to neutral) would lead to an artificially increased perception that such material is commonplace in one's immediate environment. This in turn is likely to fuel symptoms such as anxious mood (Mathews, 1990). There is a very large body of work, spanning three decades, that maps out the characteristics of selective attentional biases of emotionally salient information in those with emotional disorders. As before, we take a task-by-task approach to briefly review this literature, highlighting important conceptual issues along the way.

The Emotional Stroop

The emotional Stroop task has revealed selective, emotion congruent interference effects across a wide range of emotional disorders, including clinical anxiety (e.g., Mathews & MacLeod, 1985; Owens, Asmundson, Hadjistavropoulos, & Owens, 2004) and high-trait anxiety (e.g., Fox, 1993). A particularly good review of this extensive early literature is given in Williams, Mathews, and MacLeod (1996), and two more recent meta-analyses provide an update (Bar-Haim et al., 2007; Phaf & Kan, 2007). This body of work has addressed the issues of *stimulus specificity, psychopathology specificity*, and *awareness*. In terms of stimulus specificity, it seems that biases are greatest when the emotional stimuli match the specific concerns of clinical or subclinical participants (e.g., social threat words for social phobia patients: Hope, Rapee, Heimberg, & Dombeck, 1990). When investigating specificity of attentional bias to different emotional disorders *(psychopathology specificity)*, one is faced with the problematic confound of high comorbidity. This can be resolved statistically, using regression to partition the aspects of biased processing attributable to each psychopathology. Alternatively, it can be resolved by stringent selection of participants to eliminate or minimize the comorbid disorders themselves (e.g., anxious patients without comorbid depression). Several findings suggest that trait anxiety, relative to depression, is more strongly associated with biased attention toward congruently valenced information (e.g., Mathews & MacLeod, 1994; Wikstrom, Lundh, & Westerlund, 2003; Yovel & Mineka, 2005). However, this pattern may depend on the

duration of time allowed within the paradigm for attentional processing to occur (see below).

Attempts have been made to examine whether attentional biases occur below the level of awareness by reducing stimulus display durations until participants can no longer report the presence of the stimuli above chance level. This "subliminal presentation" usually requires stimulus displays of around 14–16 ms, followed by backward masking, and is often contrasted with a standard "supraliminal presentation" condition within one experiment. Many studies have reported subliminal emotional Stroop interference in anxiety (recent examples are Wikstrom et al., 2003; Yovel & Mineka, 2005). The broad consensus is that anxiety-related Stroop interference operates prior to attentional selection and below the level of conscious awareness. Recently, two meta-analyses have qualified this view. Phaf and Kan (2007) suggested that subliminal emotional biases are limited to blocked (as opposed to randomized) Stroop designs. Bar-Haim and colleagues (2007) found that subliminal Stroop effects in anxious groups had significantly smaller effect sizes than supraliminal effects.

Visual Search

Search tasks have been used in only a few studies relevant to emotional disorders. Mostly, these report clear between-group differences in specific phobias (Öhman et al., 2001), social anxiety (Eastwood et al., 2005), and panic (Eastwood et al., 2005). Byrne and Eysenck (1995) required high- and low-trait anxious individuals to detect a single happy or angry target face among an array of neutral faces. The groups performed equally for happy targets, but the high-anxious group was faster at detecting angry targets. Such results suggest that the *speed* of threat detection is faster for those with anxiety, implicating an initial attentional capture process similar to the "engage" mechanism inferred from single-cueing studies (see below; although probably contaminated by response bias effects). Consistent with the absence of depression-related effects on attention for emotion using other methods, Karparova, Kersting, and Suslow (2005) reported no differences for emotional information between major depression and controls.

Attentional Cueing

Many studies have used double cueing to confirm the presence of a spatial attentional bias favoring threat in both anxious patients (e.g., Horenstein & Segui, 1997) and high-trait anxious normals (e.g., Mogg, Bradley, De Bono, & Painter, 1997), with effects proving somewhat less reliable in subclinical groups. It seems that anxiety, in most of its forms, is associated with a preferential attentional bias toward negativity. Single (peripheral) cueing has revealed support for the impaired *disengagement* of attention as one contributory underlying mechanism for spatially selective attentional effects (e.g., Yiend & Mathews, 2001). Anxious individuals appear slower to disengage attention from threatening stimuli when required to do so in order to find a target located elsewhere. Effects have been replicated, but have also been criticized (see discussion at the end of this section).

Much work has been done using cueing to refine precisely the nature and characteristics of this bias, of which a few key issues are highlighted here. As mentioned previously, *severity* of negative emotion displayed in stimuli appears to be critical to whether, and in whom, attention is biased. It seems that stimuli of mild, rather than severe, emotional content is the most sensitive to displaying anxiety-related group differences (e.g., Koster et al., 2007), and theories have predicted this finding (e.g., Mogg & Bradley 1998). *Specificity* of biased attention across different disorders has been most extensively investigated using cueing. Initial findings in depression suggested that spatially selective attentional biases toward emotional information (as distinct from Stroop-like interference) were largely absent (e.g., MacLeod et al., 1986; Mathews & MacLeod, 1994), with some reporting a relative lack of bias toward positive stimuli (e.g., Mogg et al., 1991). This picture has now shifted considerably over recent years with several convergent findings of attentional bias in depression (e.g., Gotlib, Krasnoperova, Yue, & Joormann, 2004) under conditions allowing greater time for elaboration and encoding of stimulus material (usually by lengthened

presentation times). Some studies report findings carried mainly by effects on positive information (lack of a "normal" positive bias; e.g., Joorman & Gotlib, 2007), some on negative information (Donaldson, Lam, & Mathews, 2007), and some on both valences (Shane & Peterson, 2007). Further studies are likely to emerge in this active area of interest.

Investigation of *awareness*—that is, subliminal biased attention—has been widespread using cueing methods, with data clearly showing that attentional biases in anxiety operate at early automatic stages of processing (Hunt, Keogh, & French, 2006), even when the most stringent criteria for defining awareness are used (Cheeseman & Merikle, 1985). This conclusion has been confirmed by the meta-analysis of Bar-Haim and colleagues (2007), who reported that anxious participants showed biases with all exposure times using this paradigm, but that they were significantly larger for subliminal than supraliminal conditions when only cueing paradigms were considered. Biased attention in anxiety also appears to be *persistent* throughout the first second or so of stimulus presentation (e.g., Derryberry & Reed, 2002), although some evidence suggests it may wane somewhat as stimulus-onset asynchrony lengthens (Lee & Shafran, 2008).

There are important differences between mainstream attention researchers versus "attention in psychopathology" researchers in the interpretation and findings around time course effects. Mainstream attention researchers consider that "automatic" attentional processes occur within the first 50 ms of stimulus presentation and thereafter controlled processes are thought to be at work. In contrast, those working on attentional processes in psychopathology tend to assume a somewhat different timescale. For these researchers, "automatic" can imply anything up to 100 ms, and thereafter controlled processes continue to operate up to 1,000 ms or more. Studies from mainstream attention work report that endogenous effects seem to have dissipated well before these longer durations. The differences in findings (and assumptions) between the two fields may be due, in part, to the nature of the stimuli used. Those working on selective attention in psychopathology almost always use perceptually and semantically rich emotional material, whereas mainstream attention researchers tend to use simpler stimuli (e.g., lines or shapes differing only in a single feature such as orientation). The entire timescale of attentional phenomena may therefore be shifted later when more complex stimuli are involved.

The single cueing method to investigate mechanisms of attention to emotional material has generated much research interest since it was introduced. However, this has also highlighted an important weakness of the method. The critical effect can sometimes be confounded by a general interference effect, to which psychopathology groups are prone. Mogg, Holmes, Garner, and Bradley (2008) have explored this problem in some detail. Specifically, processing is usually slower and more error prone in the presence of emotionally negative information (e.g., Pereira et al., 2006), and psychopathology groups tend to show similar interference effects, but to a significantly greater degree than controls (e.g., Yiend & Mathews, 2001). Thus, if the psychopathology group is significantly slowed on all trials involving negative cues, then this generic slowdown may artificially enhance disengagement and reduce apparent engagement effects, respectively. There are currently several responses to this problem (see Yiend, 2010). The first is that not all studies find these generic interference group differences, thus bypassing the issue. The second is to treat the interference and spatial attentional effects as additive and to control for the former by subtraction (as discussed in Mogg et al., 2008). A third yet-to-be-specified solution is for researchers to devise a new experimental method for testing spatial orienting, which does not rely on selective reaction time impairments on negatively valenced trials. Although the examination of error rates rather than reaction times may hold promise, there appears to be an inherent limitation on the level of errors generated by cueing designs.

The Attentional Blink

The emotional variant of this task has now been used in several studies of emotional disorders. In one of the first, Rokke, Arnell, Koch, and Andrews (2002) investigated low,

mild, and severe dysphoria in a carefully controlled experiment. There were no group differences when reporting single targets, but with two targets separated by less than 500 ms, an attentional blink occurred and was significantly larger and longer for the severe dysphoric group. Although revealing mood-related attentional impairments, these data are not able to speak to emotion congruent effects because emotional information was not presented. However, Koster, De Raedt, Verschuere, Tibboel, & de Jong (2009) did use emotional words in selected high- and low-dysphoric groups. Within a 300-ms window, T2 identification was impaired by negative words presented at T1 in the people with high dysphoria, suggesting an enhanced attentional blink. This finding stands in contrast to work on depression and attention from other methods, given the relatively short time period available for stimulus processing.

The attentional blink has been examined more widely in relation to anxiety. Fox, Russo, and Georgiou (2005) manipulated the valence of T2 and found that low-trait and -state-anxious individuals showed a strong blink effect for fearful and happy faces, whereas in high-trait anxiety the blink was significantly reduced for fearful expressions. This is consistent with the general finding that threat stimuli elicit enhanced attentional processing in anxious individuals. The blink occurring at T2 reflects a reduction in the usual pattern of attentional processing established on previous trials. Therefore a reduction in the size of the blink associated with a given T2 stimulus suggests that the stimulus is especially attention-attracting (i.e., salient). In contrast, a more salient stimulus presented at T1 should enhance the blink (recall that the blink is thought to arise from the overuse of attentional resources when processing T1, leaving a deficit at T2 and therefore T2 targets being missed). Indeed this is what Barnard, Ramponi, Battye, and Mackintosh (2005) reported for state-anxious participants, who showed a larger blink than those who were nonanxious when threatening word distracters were presented at T1. Contrasting with these data, however, de Jong and Martens (2007) failed to find the predicted exacerbation of the attentional blink for happy and angry faces in selected high and low socially anxious participants. This is a further example of attentional effects in social anxiety not conforming to the wider anxiety literature. Finally, Trippe, Hewig, Heydel, Hecht, and Miltner (2007) examined the attentional blink in spider phobia using neutral T1 targets and varying the content of T2. All participants showed a reduced attentional blink for emotional (positive and negative) T2 targets. Individuals with spider phobias, however, showed a particularly attenuated blink for spider stimuli, detecting these at T2 more frequently than all other T2 targets.

Eye Movements

Recall that eye movement studies can be used to distinguish overt attentional engagement from disengagement, with increased fixation frequency suggesting increased attentional engagement and longer fixation durations suggesting difficulties disengaging. Under experimental conditions, anxious individuals fixate more frequently than controls on negatively valenced emotional stimuli such as angry faces (Kimbrell, 2010), indicating increased attentional engagement by fear-relevant stimuli. Others have found increased fixation frequency for both emotional and nonemotional stimuli (Gerdes, Alpers, & Pauli, 2008), indicating a more general hypervigilance. In contrast, Horley, Williams, Gonsalvez, and Gordon (2003) found that participants with social phobias were less likely than healthy controls to fixate on neutral or sad faces, perhaps indicating attentional avoidance. However, those with spider phobias have been found to fixate for longer on distracting spider stimuli than controls (Gerdes et al., 2008). Studies taking into account the occurrence of multiple saccades over time have shed light on these discrepancies. They suggest that anxious participants may initially show increased saccades and longer gaze durations toward fear-relevant stimuli, but then rapidly disengage visual attention and fixate elsewhere (e.g., Rinck & Becker, 2006)—in short, initial attentional capture followed by avoidance.

Depression studies have failed to find evidence of biased fixation frequency, suggesting that attention is not preferentially engaged by dysphoric material in depressed participants (e.g., Caseras, Garner, Bradley, & Mogg, 2007). By contrast, when gaze duration rather than frequency is examined, depressed participants consistently show longer fixation times on dysphoric material than controls (Caseras et al., 2007). This may indicate difficulties disengaging attention. Thus, as concluded by a recent review (De Raedt & Koster, 2010), findings from eye-tracking studies suggest that depression is characterized by normal engagement but difficulties disengaging attention from dysphorically themed material.

The antisaccade task can be used to distinguish between two other components of attentional performance: the accuracy versus the efficiency of attentional inhibition. In some trials participants are required to make a saccade from fixation toward a stimulus (a prosaccade), and on others to make a saccade away (an antisaccade). The *number of correct antisaccades* provides an index of ability to accurately inhibit and redirect overt attention, whereas the *latency of correct antisaccades* (i.e., the time between stimulus presentation and the onset of the antisaccade) indicates the extent of processing needed for attentional inhibition to (correctly) kick in. In an emotional antisaccade task in which participants were instructed to orient away from distracter stimuli, anxious participants were more likely than healthy controls to erroneously look at angry and fearful face distracters (Hardin et al., 2009), indicating that they were less able to override automatic capture of their attention by the faces. Other work suggests a more general difficulty inhibiting incorrect saccades to any stimuli in anxiety, whether emotionally or neutrally valenced (e.g., Wieser, Pauli, & Muhlberger, 2009). These findings are consistent with a more general hypervigliance in anxiety. However, some studies have found no difference in antisaccade accuracy between anxious and nonanxious participants (Derakshan, Ansari, Hansard, Shoker, & Eysenck, 2009).

In terms of efficiency, the latencies of anxious participants' correct antisaccades away from happy, sad, or threatening faces appear longer than those of controls, indicating that, even when managing to override overt attentional capture by the faces, anxious participants required more processing time to do so (Derakshan et al., 2009). However, it is not clear whether increased correct antisaccade latency indicates greater covert attentional capture by the faces or normal covert attentional capture but increased difficulty inhibiting capture.

Cognitive Neuroscience

Functional neuroimaging studies suggest that cognitive biases for emotional material in both anxiety and depression can be linked to abnormal activation of a network of limbic–cortical regions that play a crucial role in the attentional processing of emotional information. So far, most research has focused on the amygdala, the PFC, and the ACC. Both anxious and depressed samples show increased amygdala activation to threat-related stimuli, indicating hypervigilance relative to healthy controls (e.g., Fales et al., 2008). This amygdala hyperactivity could underlie the attentional biases found in these groups, and, consistent with this possibility, the degree of amygdala activation is correlated with behavioral attentional bias (van den Heuvel et al., 2005). However, it can also occur in the absence of behavioral evidence (Fales et al., 2008). One study (Mathews, Yiend, & Lawrence, 2004) indicates that task requirements may modulate the association between amygdala activation and trait anxiety. Individuals prone to anxiety showed greater amygdala activation to fear-related pictures than controls when the task required encoding of the emotional aspects of the images, but not when it required encoding of the nonemotional aspects.

The PFC and the ACC are considered higher-order structures involved in increasingly elaborative stages of attentional processing and in attentional control. They exert a top-down regulatory influence on the amygdala and other subcortical regions (Taylor & Fragopanagos, 2005). Thus, one may hypothesize that difficulties shown by anxious and depressed samples in disengaging attention from negative emotional material might be related to deficits in PFC and ACC function. Many studies have indeed found abnormal functioning of these structures in both anxiety (e.g., van den Heuvel et al., 2005) and depression (Beevers, Clasen, Stice, & Schnyer, 2010; Fales et al., 2008; Mannie et al., 2008; Mitterschiff-

thaler et al., 2007). However, the direction of effects varies between studies, with some finding hypo- and some hyperactivation of these regions. Underactivity of frontal regions could be related to a failure to down-regulate subcortical responses to emotional information, in the light of hyperreactive bottom-up emotional processing. Alternatively, overactivity could relate to the increased effort required by frontal areas to allocate attention appropriately for successful task completion, again in the light of hyperreactive bottom-up emotional processing. Furthermore, interpretation of imaging results in anxiety and depressive disorders is complicated by evidence of reduced PFC and ACC volume in depression (e.g., Cotter, Mackay, Landau, Kerwin, & Everall, 2001). It has been argued that failure to correct for reduced volume in these regions can sometimes give rise to misleading findings (Drevets, 2000).

Measurement of event-related potentials (ERPs) during emotional attention tasks (see Weinberg, Ferri, & Hajcak, Chapter 3, this volume) can provide a further indication of how brain activity may relate to attentional bias in anxiety and depression. It can also help to pinpoint the time frame of neural responding. For instance, some studies have found that anxiety disorders are associated with a greater P100 potential irrespective of stimulus content, during object identification, emotional Stroop, and passive viewing tasks (e.g., Michalowski et al., 2009). This may reflect a nonspecific early hypervigilance. Other studies have shown modulation of the P100 by threat relevance in anxious participants, suggesting threat-specific hypervigilance even at relatively early stages of information processing (Li, Zinbarg, & Paller, 2007).

Later ERPs, reflecting increasingly detailed processing, have consistently been found to be modulated by threat relevance. For instance, in an object identification task, participants with spider phobias showed larger P300 and P400 amplitudes in response to spiders than flowers—a difference not seen in the control group (Kolassa, Musial, Kolassa, & Miltner, 2006). Thus, threat-relevant stimuli may receive additional detailed attentional processing in anxious individuals, and may also be subject to greater elaboration at later information-processing stages accessible to conscious awareness. Furthermore, ERPs related to attentional control and response selection may be altered in anxious individuals. For instance, Taake, Jaspers-Fayer, and Liotti (2009) showed that delayed reaction times on threat trials in an emotional Stroop task were correlated with a decreased AN380 potential in a high-trait anxiety group, suggesting difficulties in attentional control.

ERP evidence in depression is more limited, but not dissimilar in nature. McNeeley, Lau, Christensen, and Alain (2008) found that, in an emotional Stroop task, participants with major depression showed a larger N450 potential over the parietal region for positive and negative words relative to neutral words, whereas the N450 was not modulated by emotional content in controls. There were also significant correlations between the degree of N450 modulation and the depressive symptom severity. The N450 potential is thought to reflect activity related to attentional control and inhibition of attention to irrelevant stimuli. Thus, these results, especially when viewed in the context of lack of behavioral differences between groups, may reflect the increased effort required to suppress attention to emotional stimuli in depressed participants.

It is interesting that both fMRI and ERP methodologies often reveal differential neural processing in psychological disorders even when behavioral differences are not apparent from reaction time data (Beevers et al., 2010; Fales et al., 2008; Kolassa et al., 2006; Li et al., 2007; Mannie et al., 2008; van den Heuvel et al., 2005). This suggests that such technologies can capture subtle differences not picked up in reaction time data. Further evaluation of the relationship between neural and behavioral data could enable a clearer understanding of the processes underlying biased attention in emotional disorders.

Summary

The Interaction between Emotion and Attention

Emotional attention—the selective attentional processing of emotionally salient information—has been widely investigated

as a phenomenon of general interest. The most copious literature in the behavioral domain uses visual search and shows that negative emotional information (emotional facial expressions and other stimuli of "biological relevance") is identified faster and more efficiently than neutral. Two notable features of emotional attention stand out from the research using attentional cueing methods. First, that its strongest effects occur very early in the processing stream (at around 100 ms poststimulus onset) and, second, that it is limited to emotional material at the highest levels of intensity. Added to this, there is evidence that facilitated engagement, and impaired disengagement, contribute to the effects of negative emotional material on orienting. Modulation of the attentional blink suggests that emotional information recruits extra attentional resources.

Eye movement data have strengthened many of the above conclusions, providing convergent evidence that is less susceptible to interpretive problems, such as response bias explanations. Furthermore, the speed of initial saccades appears to be particularly sensitive to early attentional modulation by emotional information. Cognitive neuroscience has provided important insights into the neural correlates of emotional attention, indicating that the amygdala plays a crucial role, although the details of precise pathways remain under debate. The combination of behavioral and neuroimaging data seems to offer particular promise in further constraining current theorizing about attention and emotion.

Emotional Disorders and Attention–Emotion Interactions

The selective attentional processing of emotionally salient information has been much studied in emotional disorders. The well-known emotional Stroop has fallen out of favor as a method to investigate *attentional* processes because its interpretation in this respect has proved ambiguous. Visual search studies, although few in number, suggest fast and efficient attentional selection of negative material, in general, and angry faces, in particular. The literature on emotional disorders is dominated by spatial attentional cueing studies, which have contributed much to our mechanistic understanding of emotional attention. Both facilitated engagement and impaired disengagement are implicated in anxiety. Although some work has argued that disengagement is the primary mechanism in both anxiety and depression, the interpretation of this has been challenged. The evidence regarding engagement remains equivocal, with few studies having used sufficiently short cue durations to allow optimal sensitivity to engagement differences. Furthermore, data from visual search appear to implicate processes more akin to speeded engagement, and this should not be ignored.

Eye movement measurement tells us about overt attention. Both naturalistic viewing and antisaccade tasks have confirmed that anxious individuals show enhanced overt attentional capture by emotional stimuli. There is some indication that anxious individuals avoid overtly attending to emotion at longer stimulus presentation times, but contrary to behavioral studies, eye movement data have not revealed overt disengagement effects. In the antisaccade task, the time required to correctly inhibit saccades to emotional material is longer than to neutral material, suggesting that successful overt inhibition incurs a reaction time cost. Further work exploring the interaction between covert and overt attention would be worthwhile. Cognitive neuroscience has added insights about mechanisms of top-down control and resource allocation and their neural substrates. Biases for emotional material in both anxiety and depression can be linked to abnormal activation of a network of limbic–cortical regions, including the amygdala, the PFC, and the ACC. The finding of increased amygdala activity in hypervigilance for emotional material appears clear. Abnormal activity in cortical regions can manifest as either hypo- or hyperactivation depending on context, suggesting that further work is needed to determine how stimulus type and task demands interact to determine cortical brain activity. The anatomical abnormalities found in clinical disorders must not be overlooked. ERP methods are the most time-sensitive, suited to fine-grained examination of the time course of emotional attention.

Concluding Remarks

We set out to consider emotional attention in general and more specifically in relation to emotional disorders, from the different perspectives of behavioral, eye movement, and cognitive neuroscience research. We have only been able to skim the surface of these topics, giving a concise overview, not exhaustive coverage. Emotionally salient information quite clearly attracts greater attention than neutral information, irrespective of the approach used to establish this. The important questions now revolve around understanding the mechanisms and moderators of emotional attention, how and when these apply in disorders, and their translational implications. Beyond this, several specific areas suggest themselves as potentially fruitful future topics.

One neglected but ecologically important issue is that of dynamic stimulus processing. Almost all work to date has used static displays of emotional information, when in real life the temporal unfolding of events is crucial in determining motivational relevance (compare a distant predator retreating with a close and approaching one). Stimulus modality is another understudied feature of emotional attention, since most work focuses exclusively on the visual–spatial domain. This is understandable, since the presentation of visual–spatial information can be controlled precisely and represents the primary sensory domain in humans. However, other modalities play an important role too, and few studies have investigated cross-modal integration (e.g., Santangelo et al., 2008), which would be an obvious new direction. An important emerging conceptual question is the influence of top-down control of emotional attention. Despite limited behavioral data, cognitive neuroscience is increasingly highlighting this question and revealing intriguing dissociations with corresponding behavioral indices of attentional control. More detailed consideration of top-down control of attention would help not only to explain interindividual differences, but would also be in line with current theorizing. Whatever future directions the field of emotional attention chooses to take, it will certainly remain an area of considerable research activity in both mainstream and clinical areas of psychology.

References

Algom, D., Chajut, E., & Lev, S. (2004). A rational look at the emotional Stroop phenomenon: A generic slowdown, not a Stroop effect. *Journal of Experimental Psychology: General 133*, 323–338.

Allport, A. (1993). Attention and control: Have we been asking the wrong questions? A critical-review of 25 years. *Attention and Performance, 14*, 183–218.

Anderson, A. K. (2005). Affective influences on the attentional dynamics supporting awareness. *Journal of Experimental Psychology: General 134*, 258–281.

Bannerman, R. L., Milders, M., & Sahraie, A. (2010). Attentional bias to brief threat-related faces revealed by saccadic eye movements. *Emotion, 10*, 733–738.

Bar-Haim, Y., Lamy, D., Pergamin, L., Bakermans-Kranenburg, M. J., & van IJzendoorn, M. H. (2007). Threat-related attentional bias in anxious and nonanxious individuals: A meta-analytic study. *Psychological Bulletin, 133*, 1–24.

Barnard, P. J., Ramponi, C., Battye, G., & Mackintosh, B. (2005). Anxiety and the deployment of visual attention over time. *Visual Cognition, 12*, 181–211.

Batty, M. J., Cave, K. R., & Pauli, P. (2005). Abstract stimuli associated with threat through conditioning cannot be detected preattentively. *Emotion, 5*, 418–430.

Beaver, J. D., Mogg, K., & Bradley, B. P. (2005). Emotional conditioning to masked stimuli and modulation of visuospatial attention. *Emotion, 5*, 67–79.

Beevers, C. G., Clasen, P., Stice, E., & Schnyer, D. (2010). Depression symptoms and cognitive control of emotion cues: A functional magnetic resonance imaging study. *Neuroscience, 167*, 97–103.

Bishop, S. J. (2007). Neurocognitive mechanisms of anxiety: An integrative account. *Trends in Cognitive Sciences, 11*(7), 307–316.

Byrne, A., & Eysenck, M. W. (1995). Trait anxiety, anxious mood and threat detection. *Cognition and Emotion, 9*, 549–562.

Calvo, M. G., Avero, P., & Lundqvist, D. (2006). Facilitated detection of angry faces: Initial orienting and processing efficiency. *Cognition and Emotion, 20*, 785–811.

Calvo, M. G., & Lang, P. J. (2004). Gaze patterns when looking at emotional pictures: Motivationally biased attention. *Motivation and Emotion, 28*, 221–243.

Caseras, X., Garner, M., Bradley, B. P., & Mogg, K. (2007). Biases in visual orienting to negative and positive scenes in dysphoria: An eye movement study. *Abnormal Psychology, 116*, 491–497.

Cheeseman, J., & Merikle, P. M. (1985). Word recognition and consciousness. In D. Besner, T. G. Waller, & G. E. MacKinnon (Eds.), *Reading research: Advances in theory and practice* (pp. 311–352). Orlando, FL: Academic Press.

Cooper, R. M., & Langton, S. R. (2006). Attentional bias to angry faces using the dot-probe task?: It depends when you look for it. *Behaviour Research and Therapy, 44*, 1321–1329.

Cotter, D., Mackay, D., Landau, S., Kerwin, R., & Everall, I. (2001). Reduced glial cell density and neuronal size in the anterior cingulate cortex in major depressive disorder. *Archives of General Psychiatry, 58*, 545–553.

Dalgleish, T. (2005). Putting some feeling into it—the conceptual and empirical relationships between the classic and emotional Stroop tasks: Comment on Algom, Chajut, and Lev (2004). *Journal of Experimental Psychology: General, 134*, 585–591.

de Jong, P. J., & Martens, S. (2007). Detection of emotional expressions in rapidly changing facial displays in high- and low-socially anxious women. *Behaviour Research and Therapy, 45*, 1285–1294.

De Raedt, R., & Koster, E. H. W. (2010). Understanding increasing vulnerability for depression from a cognitive neuroscience perspective: A reappraisal of attentional factors and a new conceptual framework. *Cognitive, Affective, and Behavioral Neuroscience, 10*, 50–70.

Derakshan, N., Ansari, T., Hansard, L., Shoker, L., & Eysenck, M. W. (2009). Anxiety inhibition efficiency and effectiveness. *Experimental Psychology, 56*, 48–55.

Derryberry, D., & Reed, M. A. (2002). Anxiety-related attentional biases and their regulation by attentional control. *Journal of Abnormal Psychology, 111*, 225–236.

de Ruiter, C., & Brosschot, J. F. (1994). The emotional Stroop effect in anxiety: Attentional bias or cognitive avoidance. *Behaviour Research and Therapy, 32*, 315–319.

Desimone, R., & Duncan, J. (1995). Neural mechanisms of selective visual attention. *Annual Review of Neuroscience, 18*, 193–222.

Donaldson, C., Lam, D., & Mathews, A. (2007). Rumination and attention in major depression. *Behaviour Research and Therapy, 45*, 2664–2678.

Drevets, W. C. (2000). Neuroimaging studies of mood disorders. *Biological Psychiatry, 48*(8), 813–829.

Easterbrook, J. (1959). The effect of emotion on cue utilization and the organization of behavior. *Psychological Review, 66*, 183–201.

Eastwood, J. D., Smilek, D., & Merikle, P. M. (2001). Differential attentional guidance by unattended faces expressing positive and negative emotion. *Perception and Psychophysics, 63*(6), 1004–1013.

Eastwood, J. D., Smilek, D., Oakman, J. M., Farvolden, P., van Ameringen, M., Mancini, C., et al. (2005). Individuals with social phobia are biased to become aware of negative faces. *Visual Cognition, 12*, 159–179.

Eysenck, M. W. (1992). *Anxiety: The cognitive perspective.* Hove, UK: Erlbaum.

Fales, C. L., Barch, D. M., Rundle, M. M., Mintun, M. A., Snyder, A. Z., Cohen, J. D., et al. (2008). Altered emotional interference processing in affective and cognitive-control brain circuitry in major depression. *Biological Psychiatry, 63*, 377–384.

Fox, E. (1993). Attentional bias in anxiety: Selective or not? *Behaviour Research and Therapy, 31*, 487–493.

Fox, E., Griggs, L., Mouchlianitis, E. (2007). The detection of fear-relevant stimuli: Are guns noticed as quickly as snakes? *Emotion, 7*, 691–696.

Fox, E., Russo, R., & Georgiou, G. A. (2005). Anxiety modulates the degree of attentive resources required to process emotional faces. *Cognitive, Affective, and Behavioral Neuroscience, 5*, 396–404.

Freese, J., & Amaral, D. G. (2009). Neuroanatomy of the primate amygdala. In P. J. Whalen & E. A. Phelps (Eds.), *The human amygdala* (pp. 3–42). New York: Guilford Press.

Frischen, A., Eastwood, J. D., & Smilek, D. (2008). Visual search for faces with emotional expressions. *Psychological Bulletin, 134*, 662–676.

Gerdes, A. B. M., Alpers, G. W., & Pauli, P. (2008). When spiders appear suddenly: Spider-phobic patients are distracted by task-irrelevant spiders. *Behaviour Research and Therapy, 46*, 174–187.

Gotlib, I. H., Krasnoperova, E., Yue, D. N., & Joormann, J. (2004). Attentional biases for negative interpersonal stimuli in clinical depression. *Journal of Abnormal Psychology, 113*, 127–135.

Hardin, M. G., Mandell, D., Mueller, S. C., Dahl, R. E., Pine, D. S., & Ernst, M. (2009). Inhibitory control in anxious and healthy adolescents is modulated by incentive and incidental affective stimuli. *Journal of Child Psychology and Psychiatry, 50*, 1550–1558.

Holmes, A., Green, S., & Vuilleumier, P. (2005). The involvement of distinct visual channels in rapid attention towards fearful facial expressions. *Cognition and Emotion, 19*, 899–922.

Hope, D. A., Rapee, R. M., Heimberg, R. G., & Dombeck, M. J. (1990). Representations of the self in social phobia: Vulnerability to social threat. *Cognitive Therapy and Research, 14*, 177–189.

Horenstein, M., & Segui, J. (1997). Chronometrics of attentional processes in anxiety disorders. *Psychopathology, 30*, 25–35.

Horley, K., Williams, L. M., Gonsalvez, C., & Gordon, E. (2003). Social phobics do not see eye to eye: A visual scanpath study of emotional expression processing. *Anxiety Disorders, 17*, 33–44.

Hunt, C., Keogh, E., & French, C. C. (2006). Anxiety sensitivity: The role of conscious awareness and selective attentional bias to physical threat. *Emotion, 6*, 418–428.

Jonides, J. (1981). Voluntary versus automatic control over the mind's eyes' movements. In J. Long & A. Baddeley (Eds.), *Attention and performance* (pp. 187–203). Hillsdale, NJ: Erlbaum.

Joormann, J., & Gotlib, I. H. (2007). Selective attention to emotional faces following recovery from depression. *Journal of Abnormal Psychology, 116*(1), 80–85.

Karparova, S. P., Kersting, A., & Suslow, T. (2005). Disengagement of attention from facial emotion in unipolar depression. *Psychiatry and Clinical Neurosciences, 59*, 723–729.

Keil, A., & Ihssen, N. (2004). Identification facilitation for emotionally arousing verbs during the attentional blink. *Emotion, 4*, 23–35.

Kimbrell, T. A. (2010). Attentional bias to angry faces in OEF/OIFF combat veterans using eye-tracking. *Biological Psychiatry, 67*(Suppl. 1), 213S.

Kindt, M., Bierman, D., & Brosschot, J. F. (1996). Stroop versus Stroop: Comparison of a card format and a single-trial format of the standard color–word Stroop task and the emotional Stroop task. *Personality and Individual Differences, 21,* 653–661.

Kolassa, I., Musial, F., Kolassa, S., & Miltner, W. H. R. (2006). Event-related potentials when identifying or color-naming threatening schematic stimuli in spider phobic and non-phobic individuals. *BMC Psychiatry, 6,* 38.

Koster, E. H. W., Crombez, G., Verschuere, B., & DeHouwer, J. (2004). Selective attention to threat in the dot probe paradigm: Differentiating vigilance and difficulty to disengage. *Behaviour Research and Therapy, 42,* 1183–1192.

Koster, E. H. W., De Raedt, R., Verschuere, B., Tibboel, H., & de Jong, P. J. (2009). Negative information enhances the attentional blink in dysphoria. *Depression and Anxiety, 26*(1), E16–E22.

Koster, E. H. W., Verschuere, B., Burssens, B., Custers, R., & Crombez, G. (2007). Attention for emotional faces under restricted awareness revisited: Do emotional faces automatically attract attention? *Emotion, 7,* 285–295.

LeDoux, J. E. (1995). Emotion: Clues from the brain. *Annual Review of Psychology, 46,* 209–235.

Lee, M., & Shafran, R. (2008). Processing biases in eating disorders: The impact of temporal factors. *International Journal of Eating Disorders, 41,* 372–375.

Li, W., Zinbarg, R. E., & Paller, K. A. (2007). Trait anxiety modulates supraliminal and subliminal threat: Brain potential evidence for early and late processing influences. *Cognitive, Affective, and Behavioral Neuroscience, 7,* 25–36.

Lipp, O. V., & Derakshan, N. (2005). Attentional bias to pictures of fear-relevant animals in a dot probe task. *Emotion, 5,* 365–369.

Lipp, O. V., & Waters, A. M. (2007). When danger lurks in the background: Attentional capture by animal fear-relevant distractors is specific and selectively enhanced by animal fear. *Emotion, 7,* 192–200.

MacLeod, C., Mathews, A., & Tata, P. (1986). Attentional bias in emotional disorders. *Journal of Abnormal Psychology, 95,* 15–20.

MacLeod, C. M. (1991). Half a century of research on the Stroop effect: An integrative review. *Psychological Bulletin, 109,* 163–203.

Mannie, Z. N., Norbury, R., Murphy, S. E., Inkster, B., Harmer, C. J., & Cowen, P. J. (2008). Affective modulation of anterior cingulate cortex in young people at increased familial risk of depression. *British Journal of Psychiatry, 192,* 356–361.

Mathews, A. (1990). Why worry?: The cognitive function of anxiety. *Behaviour Research and Therapy, 28,* 455–468.

Mathews, A., & MacLeod, C. (1985). Selective processing of threat cues in anxiety states. *Behaviour Research and Therapy, 23,* 563–569.

Mathews, A., & MacLeod, C. (1986). Discrimination of threat cues without awareness in anxiety states. *Journal of Abnormal Psychology, 95,* 131–138.

Mathews, A., & MacLeod, C. (1994). Cognitive approaches to emotion and emotional disorders. *Annual Review of Psychology, 45,* 25–50.

Mathews, A., Yiend, J., & Lawrence, A. D. (2004). Individual differences in the modulation of fear-related brain activation by attentional control. *Journal of Cognitive Neuroscience, 16,* 1683–1694.

McKenna, F. P., & Sharma, D. (2004). Reversing the emotional Stroop effect reveals that it is not what it seems: The role of fast and slow components. *Journal of Experimental Psychology: Learning, Memory, and Cognition, 30,* 382–392.

McNeeley, H. E., Lau, M. A., Christensen, B. K., & Alain, C. (2008). Neurophysiological evidence of cognitive inhibition anomalies in persons with major depressive disorder. *Clinical Neurophysiology, 119,* 1578–1589.

Michalowski, J. M., Melzig, C. A., Weike, A. I., Stockburger, J., Schupp, H. T., & Alfons, O. (2009). Brain dynamics in spider phobic individuals exposed to phobia-relevant and other emotional stimuli. *Emotion, 9,* 306–315.

Mitterschiffthaler, M. L., Williams, S. C. R., Walsh, N. D., Cleare, A. J., Donaldson, C., Scott, J., et al. (2008). Neural basis of the emotional Stroop interference effect in major depression. *Psychological Medicine, 38,* 247–256.

Mogg, K., & Bradley, B. P. (1998). A cognitive motivational analysis of anxiety. *Behaviour Research and Therapy, 36,* 809–848.

Mogg, K., Bradley, B. P., De Bono, J., & Painter, M. (1997). Time course of attentional bias for threat information in non-clinical anxiety. *Behaviour Research and Therapy, 35,* 297–303.

Mogg, K., Holmes, A., Garner, M., & Bradley, B. P. (2008). Effects of threat cues on attentional shifting, disengagement and response slowing in anxious individuals. *Behaviour Research and Therapy, 46,* 656–667.

Mogg, K., Mathews, A., May, J., Grove, M., Eysenck, M., & Weinman, J. (1991). Assessment of cognitive bias in anxiety and depression using a color perception task. *Cognition and Emotion, 5,* 221–238.

Mogg, K., McNamara, J., Powys, M., Rawlinson, H., Seiffer, A., & Bradley, B. P. (2000). Selective attention to threat: A test of two cognitive models of anxiety. *Cognition and Emotion, 14,* 375–399.

Moors, A., & De Houwer, J. (2006). Automaticity: A theoretical and conceptual analysis. *Psychological Bulletin, 132,* 297–326.

Morris, J. S., Öhman, A., & Dolan, R. J. (1998). Conscious and unconscious emotional learning in the human amygdala. *Nature, 393,* 467–470.

Most, S. B., Chun, M. M., Johnson, M. R., & Kiehl, K. A. (2006). Attentional modulation of the amygdala varies with personality. *NeuroImage, 31,* 934–944.

Most, S. B., Smith, S. D., Cooter, A. B., Levy, B. N., & Zald, D. H. (2007). The naked truth: Positive, arousing distractors impair rapid target perception. *Cognition and Emotion, 21,* 964–981.

Nummenmaa, L., Hyönä, J., & Calvo, M. G. (2006). Eye movement assessment of selective attentional capture by emotional pictures. *Emotion, 6,* 257–268.

Nummenmaa, L., Hyönä, J., & Calvo, M. G. (2009). Emotional scene content drives the saccade generation system reflexively. *Journal of Experimental Psychology: Human Perception and Performance, 35,* 305–323.

Ochsner, K. N., & Gross, J. J. (2005). The cognitive control of emotion. *Trends in Cognitive Sciences, 9,* 242–249.

Öhman, A., Flykt, A., & Esteves, F. (2001). Emotion drives attention: Detecting the snake in the grass. *Journal of Experimental Psychology: General, 130,* 466–478.

Olivers, C. N. L., & Nieuwenhuis, S. (2006). The beneficial effects of additional task load, positive affect, and instruction on the attentional blink. *Journal of Experimental Psychology: Human Perception and Performance, 32,* 364–379.

Owens, K. M. B., Asmundson, G. J. G., Hadjistavropoulos, T., & Owens, T. J. (2004). Attentional bias toward illness threat in individuals with elevated health anxiety. *Cognitive Therapy and Research, 28,* 57–66.

Pereira, M. G., Volchan, E., de Souza, G. G. L., Oliveira, L., Campagnoli, R. R., Pinheiro, W. M., et al. (2006). Sustained and transient modulation of performance induced by emotional picture viewing. *Emotion, 6,* 622–634.

Pessoa, L., & Adolphs, R. (2010). Emotion processing and the amygdala: From a "low road" to "many roads" of evaluating biological significance. *Nature Reviews Neuroscience, 11,* 773–782.

Phaf, R. H., & Kan, K.-J. (2007). The automaticity of emotional Stroop: A meta-analysis. *Journal of Behavior Therapy and Experimental Psychiatry, 38,* 184–199.

Posner, M. I. (1980). Orienting of attention. *Quarterly Journal of Experimental Psychology, 32,* 3–25

Pury, C. L. S. (2002). Information-processing predictors of emotional response to stress. *Cognition and Emotion, 16*(5), 667–683.

Raymond, J. E., Shapiro, K. L., & Arnell, K. M. (1992). Temporary suppression of visual processing in an RSVP task: An attentional blink? *Journal of Experimental Psychology: Human Perception and Performance, 18,* 849–860.

Rinck, M., & Becker, E. S. (2006). Spider fearful individuals attend to threat, then quickly avoid it: Evidence from eye movements. *Journal of Abnormal Psychology, 115,* 231–238.

Rokke, P. D., Arnell, K. M., Koch, M. D., & Andrews, J. T. (2002). Dual-task attention deficits in dysphoric mood. *Journal of Abnormal Psychology, 111,* 370–379.

Santangelo, V., Ho, C., & Spence, C. (2008). Capturing spatial attention with multisensory cues. *Psychonomic Bulletin and Review, 15,* 398–403.

Shane, M. S., & Peterson, J. B. (2007). An evaluation of early and late stage attentional processing of positive and negative information in dysphoria. *Cognition and Emotion, 21,* 789–815.

Smith, S. D., Most, S. B., Newsome, L. A., & Zald, D. H. (2006). An emotion-induced attentional blink elicited by aversively conditioned stimuli. *Emotion, 6,* 523–527.

Stormark, K. M., & Hugdahl, K. (1996). Peripheral cuing of covert spatial attention before and after emotional conditioning of the cue. *International Journal of Neuroscience, 86,* 225–240.

Taake, I., Jaspers-Fayer, F., & Liotti, M. (2009). Early frontal responses elicited by physical threat words in an emotional Stroop task: Modulation by anxiety sensitivity. *Biological Psychology, 81,* 48–57.

Taylor, J. G., & Fragopanagos, N. F. (2005). The interaction of attention and emotion. *Neural Networks, 18,* 353–369.

Tipples, J., Young, A. W., Quinlan, P., Broks, P., & Ellis, A. W. (2002). Searching for threat. *Quarterly Journal of Experimental Psychology Section A: Human Experimental Psychology, 55,* 1007–1026.

Trippe, R. H., Hewig, J., Heydel, C., Hecht, H., & Miltner, W. H. (2007). Attentional blink to emotional and threatening pictures in spider phobics: Electrophysiology and behavior. *Brain Research, 1148,* 149–160.

van den Heuvel, O. A., Veltman, D. J., Groenewegen, H. J., Witter, M. P., Merkelbach, J., Cath, D. C., et al. (2005). Disorder-specific neuroanatomical correlates of attentional bias in obsessive–compulsive disorder, panic disorder, and hypochondriasis. *Archives of General Psychiatry, 62,* 922–933.

Vuilleumier, P. (2005). How brains beware: Neural mechanisms of emotional attention. *Trends in Cognitive Sciences, 9,* 585–594.

Vuilleumier, P., Armony, J. L., Driver, J., & Dolan, R. J. (2001). Effects of attention and emotion on face processing in the human brain: An event-related fMRI study. *Neuron, 30,* 829–841.

Waters, A. M., Nitz, A. B., Craske, M. G., & Johnson, C. (2007). The effects of anxiety upon attention allocation to affective stimuli.

Behaviour Research and Therapy, 45(4), 763–774.

Wieser, M. J., Pauli, P., & Muhlberger, M. J. (2009). Probing the attentional control theory in social anxiety: An emotional saccade task. *Cognitive, Affective, and Behavioral Neuroscience, 9,* 314–322.

Wikstrom, J., Lundh, L. G., & Westerlund, J. (2003). Stroop effects for masked threat words: Pre-attentive bias or selective awareness? *Cognition and Emotion, 17,* 827–842.

Williams, J. M. G., Mathews, A., & MacLeod, C.(1996). The emotional Stroop task and psychopathology. *Psychological Bulletin, 120,* 3–24.

Wilson, E., & MacLeod, C. (2003). Contrasting two accounts of anxiety-linked attentional bias: Selective attention to varying levels of stimulus threat intensity. *Journal of Abnormal Psychology, 112*(2), 212–218.

Yiend, J., & Mathews, A. (2001). Anxiety and attention to threatening pictures. *Quarterly Journal of Experimental Psychology Section A: Human Experimental Psychology, 54,* 665–681.

Yiend, J. (2010). The effects of emotion on attention: A review of attentional processing of emotional information. *Cognition and Emotion, 24,* 3–47.

Yovel, I., & Mineka, S. (2005). Emotion-congruent attentional biases: The perspective of hierarchical models of emotional disorders. *Personality and Individual Differences, 38,* 785–795.

CHAPTER 7

Generalization of Acquired Emotional Responses

Dirk Hermans, Frank Baeyens, and Bram Vervliet

One of the core behavioral capacities of human and nonhuman animals is their ability to generalize on the basis of prior experiences. A bird that discovered energy-rich berries near a river will use this information on subsequent searches for food. Even though time and place may be different, the bird will take advantage of the previous experience and look for berries near streaming water. Generalization helps creatures to functionally adapt behavior in changing situations. It reduces the need to rediscover contingencies that were important in previous but similar circumstances. When a young child has learned, for instance, that a specific wooden object with four legs is referred to as a *table* by his or her mother, the child may successfully use this word for other, highly similar objects. After initial examples, the mother will no longer need to refer to each new table as *table*. The child now effectively generalizes on the basis of these previous experiences.

The topic of generalization has attracted much attention in the study of various domains of human functioning, including perception, reasoning, category, and language learning (see Banich & Caccamise, 2010). Within emotion research, however, the concept of generalization has received surprisingly less attention. Nevertheless, to the extent that one views emotions as adaptive and functional responses, it will be evident that generalization is a key process. Fear, for instance, can be most adaptive in relation to certain stimuli or situations (e.g., fear of deep and unprotected depths, such as ravines). Generalization of fear might then prevent the necessity of rediscovering the danger in every new (but comparable) situation. A parent, for example, who gets angry at the child when he or she recklessly tries to cross a busy street, hopes that the child will at least be a bit apprehensive in similar future traffic situations.

The present chapter focuses on the generalization of emotional responses, with a focal point on the generalization of (acquired) fear responses. After describing some of the core concepts of generalization research, we attempt to collate insights from various traditions in learning psychology that help us to understand this intriguing but underinvestigated phenomenon. Before doing so, and given the focus of this chapter, we first highlight some basic insights concerning the way in which fears are typically acquired.

Understanding (over)generalization significantly contributes to our understanding of emotional responses as well as of various forms of psychopathology, including anxiety disorders. Even though generalization is necessary for knowledge transfer across situations, some forms of overgeneralization are a basis for dysfunctional responding and pathology. Insights in this phenomenon will help to improve existing treatments and to devise new strategies of prevention and treatment. Even though we focus mostly on anxiety and its disorders, the study of generalization is also of relevance to other disorders such as depression or chronic pain. We briefly touch upon this issue in the discussion section.

The Acquisition of Fear Responses

The origin of fear is traditionally viewed from a learning perspective. Changes in emotional responding are assumed to result from learning experiences. One such type of experience concerns the co-occurrence between two stimuli/events. For instance, it can be observed that an originally neutral stimulus (CS; conditioned stimulus) that is presented in contingency with an aversive event (US; unconditioned stimulus) will elicit fear responses. At moment $t + 1$ the CS elicits fear responses that were not yet present at moment t. This change in emotional responding is attributed to the CS–US pairing that took place between t and $t + 1$. This is illustrated in the following case example:

During summer holidays, Suzy (now 9 years old) usually stays with her grandmother for several days. Often she can be found outside playing in the garden with the neighbor's dog. This German shepherd is good-natured and likes Suzy's attention. Two years ago, a sudden event must have startled the young animal; the dog got aroused and quite unexpectedly bit Suzy. The incident was quite severe, and Suzy was brought to the hospital for immediate medical care and had to stay overnight. Since that time Suzy fears the neighbor's dog. She avoids being in the garden and has expressed her concerns of being bitten again on a next occasion. Her parents and grandmother as well as the neighbor take care that such an incident would not happen again.

For Suzy, the crucial learning experience was the co-occurrence between the dog (CS) and the bite incident (US). Even though it is quite unlikely, it cannot be excluded that Suzy would also have started to fear the dog in the absence of this CS–US pairing. Natural situations do not allow for a strin-

gent control of alternative explanations, but in the lab this level of control is more easily accomplished. Most often, one CS (the CS+) is presented together with the US, whereas this is not the case for a second CS (the CS–). If increased fear responding is observed for the CS+ from moment t (pretest) to moment $t + 1$ (posttest), whereas no such change is observed for the CS–, one can conclude that this effect is due to the CS–US pairing.

This basic fear conditioning preparation has been well investigated and is considered a good laboratory model for the acquisition of human fears and phobias (Craske, Hermans, & Vansteenwegen, 2006). As a matter of fact, the classical conditioning model has proven to be a rich basis for understanding the complexity of human fears. Well-known phenomena such as blocking, extinction, renewal, and reinstatement have thoroughly impacted our understanding of how fears and phobias are acquired for some stimuli (and not for others), how they can be treated, and how apparently successfully treated fears sometimes reappear (e.g., Hermans, Craske, Mineka, & Lovibond, 2006; Vansteenwegen, Crombez, Baeyens, Hermans, & Eelen, 2006).

Generalized Fear Responding

One of the first examples of fear acquisition using conditioning principles is the well-known study of Little Albert described by John B. Watson and Rosalie Rayner in 1920. In this classic study, Watson conditioned an 11-month-old boy to fear white rats. In the actual experiment, a white rat (CS) was presented to the boy, and when Albert reached out to the animal a loud noise (US) was produced by striking a hammer upon a suspended steel bar. Previous tests at the age of 9 months had shown that this sound (the US) elicited clear fear responses in Albert. After repeated contingent presentations of the rat with this US, the originally neutral animal now elicited fear in the boy.

Even though a description of this study can be found in almost every psychology textbook, it is less known that John Watson was not only interested in the acquisition of fear, but also had a core interest in the generalization of acquired fear responses. His second research question was described as follows: "If such a conditioned emotional response can be established, will there be a transfer to other animals or other objects?" (Watson & Rayner, 1920, p. 3). Watson wondered by what mechanisms the limited emotional reaction patterns that are observed in infancy could develop into the complexity observed in adult responses. He reasoned that there "must be some simple method by means of which the range of stimuli which can call out these emotions and their compounds is greatly increased" (Watson & Rayner, 1920, p. 1). His investigation of how unconditioned responses (such as the fear response elicited by the loud noise) are transferred to originally neutral stimuli (such as the rat) and then further transferred to related stimuli was directly grounded in this more general developmental question. To directly study generalization of acquired fear, Watson presented a series of generalization stimuli before and after conditioning. These included a rabbit, a dog, a fur coat (seal), and cotton wool. After conditioning, not only the rat elicited fear responses, but this was also the case for the generalization stimuli, even in a context that differed from the original conditioning context. Based on these findings, Watson concluded, "From the above results it would seem that emotional transfers do take place. Furthermore it would seem that the number of transfers resulting from an experimentally produced conditioned emotional reaction may be very large" (Watson & Rayner, 1920, p. 10).

A similar type of generalization was observed for Suzy, the girl that was bitten by the neighbor's dog:

After the bite incident, and over a period of 2 years, Suzy's parents noticed that the event had a much stronger impact than originally thought. In addition to the immense fear of the German shepherd, Suzy developed fear of many other dogs, including small and objectively harmless ones. She started to avoid places where she could encounter dogs. Her fear extended to sounds of barking dogs and even to pictures of dogs or other graphic representations, which led her to almost completely abandon reading books and watching TV. There would always be a possibility that a dog would feature in the story, or a picture of a dog would be encountered when turning the page. More recently, her fears further broadened to other four-legged animals such as cats and

small goats. Together with this expansion, her usual day-to-day functioning got more and more hampered. At that stage her parents decided to seek professional help for her dog phobia.

The case examples of Suzy and Little Albert are somewhat anecdotal demonstrations of a phenomenon that is at the center of most, if not all, anxiety disorders. Many clients experience, at one or more stages, a gradual expansion of the stimuli that elicit the fear. The case example of Martha further illustrates this phenomenon:

Martha is 37 and was diagnosed with obsessive–compulsive disorder 3 years ago. Initially she feared pesticides and herbicides, but over the course of the first 6 months since the onset of the disorder her fears expanded to gasoline, household cleaning products, and even shoe polish and olive oil. Later on she started fearing unstubbed cigarettes, viral infections, knives, and other sharp objects. When her therapist asked her to make an inventory of the "discriminative stimuli" for her compulsive behaviors, she presented a list of almost two pages. These stimuli trigger a series of escape or avoidance behaviors, such as unstoppable washing of hands and repeated checking. The main reason why Martha sought treatment for her complaints is that the expansion in the number of fear-eliciting stimuli and the accompanying increase in compulsive behavior started to significantly impact her day-to-day functioning.

Usually the difference between "normal/adaptive" fears and pathological variations such as phobias is considered in terms of fear intensity: pathological fear is viewed as more intensive, or at least more intensive than one should reasonably expect. We believe, however, that a core characteristic of anxiety disorders is not only (or even, not so much) a more intensive fear, but rather its generalization. If Suzy had been afraid only of the neighbor's dog, this would not be considered as a clinical problem. The dog has proven to be dangerous, so it makes sense to be afraid of this specific dog. Even if her fear of this one dog had been extremely excessive, her functioning would probably not be hindered. As a matter of fact, it would not be too difficult to avoid the animal. Hence, the core of her dog phobia is not so much its intensity, but rather the fact that it did not remain restricted to this one particular animal but generalized to a broad set of stimuli, including other dogs, cats, and even pictures of dogs.

Given the clinical importance of the phenomenon of fear generalization, it is surprising that only limited research has been devoted to this subject. In spite of an apparent interest in generalization since Pavlov's work, empirical work in this area has clearly diminished since the 1970s. Moreover, most of the studies that were conducted before that time were directed at generalization of operant responses and/or used animal subjects (for an overview, see Honig & Urcuioli, 1981). Hence, it is quite surprising that almost no work has been done on *fear* generalization in *humans*. Only recently has such research been conducted (e.g., Lissek et al., 2008; Vervliet, Kindt, Vansteenwegen, & Hermans, 2010b). In addition, most of the existing studies have focused on perceptual forms of generalization, whereas (clinical) reality is probably more complex, as we argue later.

In the sections that follow, we illustrate a number of core concepts and findings using recent fear generalization studies in humans. We do not focus on relevant biological substrates. For recent findings in that context, we refer to work by Dunsmoor, Prince, Murty, Kragel, and LaBar (2011).

Generalization of Conditioned Fear in Humans: Generalization Gradient

One of the first demonstrations of generalization of conditioned fear was described by Lissek and colleagues (2008). They developed a simple but elegant paradigm in which circles of various sizes were used as conditioned stimuli (CS+; CS–) and generalization stimuli (GS). Comparable to animal studies, the procedure consisted of two crucial phases: a fear acquisition phase and a generalization test phase. During the fear acquisition phase, for half of the participants, the presentation of a small circle (CS+) was followed by an electric shock on 9 out of 12 presentations (75% reinforcement schedule), whereas the presentation of a large circle (CS–) was never followed by a shock. For the other half of the participants, the CS+ was the large circle and the CS– the small one. This procedure led to substantial differential

fear conditioning. Startle eyeblink responding (measured using facial electromyography [EMG] over the orbicularis oculi) to the CS+ was significantly augmented, as compared to the CS–. Also, after conditioning the CS+ was rated as more fear-provoking and arousing than the CS–. In the subsequent phase—the generalization test—the CS+ and CS– were presented again, but these trials were now intermixed with trials during which the generalization stimuli were presented. These were eight circles of intermediary size, ranging from slightly larger than the smallest of the two CSs to slightly smaller than the largest CS. These generalization stimuli were grouped in four classes of two stimuli and created a continuum of similarity from CS+ to CS–. Fear responses, as measured by startle EMG, were strongest for the CS+ and lowest for the CS–, with the classes of GSs at intermediary levels. For the GSs that were perceptually most similar to the CS+, fear responses were strongest, and these fear responses decreased in intensity with decreasing similarity between GS and CS+ (see Figure 7.1). This pattern of results is also known as the *generalization gradient*, which represents a curvilinearly shaped *generalization decrement*, or gradual decrease of response strength, with increasing CS–GS dissimilarity.

Generalization curves can have different slopes, which reflect the degree of stimulus generalization an organism exhibits. Gradient A in Figure 7.2 has a steep slope. Here, small differences with the original conditioning stimulus result in strong response decrements. The second slope (B) is shallow. Fear responding is high for stimuli that are rather dissimilar from the CS+.

The form of the generalization gradients provides important clinical and theoretical information. Let us assume for a moment that the two slopes represent two persons bitten by a dog. For client A, there is considerable fear for the dog that was involved in the bite incident, but other dogs, including those that highly resemble the CS+, elicit almost no fear responses. For client B, the situation is markedly different. Even though fear for the CS+ is somewhat lower, this person shows extensive generalization and now fears a broad range of dogs. Obvious objective perceptual differences between the CS+ and these other dogs seem to have less

Startle

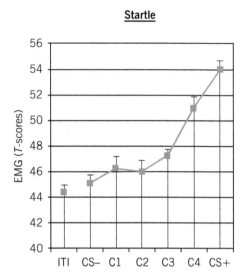

FIGURE 7.1. Generalization gradient of fear responses (startle EMG) to the CS+, CS−, and four classes of generalization stimuli. From Lissek et al. (2008). Copyright 2008. Reprinted with permission of Elsevier.

impact on the amount of fear. At present, not much is known about the factors that are responsible for individual differences in the form of generalization gradients. We do know, however, that these individual differences exist and can be manifest. Recent work by Lissek and colleagues (2010), for instance, showed more pronounced fear generalization in persons suffering from panic

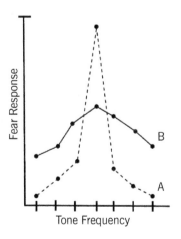

FIGURE 7.2. Example of a steep (A) and a shallow (B) generalization gradient.

disorder as compared to controls. This is an intriguing finding that opens a series of important new research questions. Is this proclivity toward fear overgeneralization in patients with panic disorder a "scar" of the disorder, or does it present a vulnerability factor that plays a causal role in the disorder's development? And if so, what is the origin of these individual differences in fear generalization?

Plasticity of the Generalization Gradient

A major route to investigate questions about individual differences in generalization and about the psychological mechanisms of generalization comprises a careful analysis of the variables that impact the form of the generalization curves (in terms of area, height, slope, and form). If, for instance, manipulation of variable x leads to sharpened or flattened curves, this would provide indications of the involvement of that variable in the mechanisms of generalization.

It is well known that generalization gradients are malleable and are impacted by different factors, including *procedural aspects of the training and testing situation*. A full discussion of these variables would lead us too far. We refer to Honig and Urcuioli (1981) for a more extensive overview and limit the discussion here to the previously discussed study of Lissek and colleagues (2008), which we present as a case example of how certain procedural variables can influence the generalization pattern.

As already mentioned, in this study, two stimuli were included in the acquisition and test session: one circle that was followed by the shock (CS+) and a second circle (CS−) that was never followed by a shock, and which thus can be considered as a safety signal. The two CSs were end points of a continuum of circles that varied in size. The generalization stimuli in the Lissek and colleagues (2008) study had sizes that were intermediate to those of the CS+ and CS−. Even though this is an elegant paradigm with which to investigate stimulus generalization, the choice of this particular procedure has certain implications of which one has to be aware. First of all, the generalization gradient is one-sided and flows from the CS+, over the GSs, to the CS−. For each participant, the generalization stimuli are either smaller or larger than the CS+, but do not contain both types of GSs. This is obviously different from the gradients in Figure 7.2, which are two-sided. These stem from a study in which a shock was first conditioned to a tone with a certain frequency, after which generalization stimuli were presented that were either lower or higher in frequency as compared to the CS+.

A second procedural element that is of importance is the inclusion of the CS–. Differential fear conditioning procedures always include a CS– as a control for nonassociative processes in acquisition. However, during tests of acquisition and generalization, the inclusion of this additional stimulus allows for mental comparisons, which would not be possible in the absence of a CS–. It is known that such comparisons can lead to sharpened gradients; in the absence of a comparison stimulus, greater generalization is expected. A second illustration of how adding a within-dimension comparison stimulus (CS–) can impact the gradient is the *peak shift phenomenon*. This term refers to the observation that when a comparison stimulus is part of acquisition and of the generalization test, the peak of the generalization curve shifts away from CS+ in a direction opposite to the comparison stimulus. For the gradients of Figure 7.2, this would mean that if an unreinforced comparison were included that was of somewhat higher tone frequency, the strongest fear response would not be observed in relation to the CS+, but to a tone that is of lower tone frequency than the CS+. The fact that fear responses may be more pronounced for one of the generalization stimuli than for the original conditioned response is also interesting from a clinical point of view.

A third element in the procedure of Lissek and colleagues (2008) is the fact that the CS– is not a mere comparison stimulus, but is most probably also an *inhibitory stimulus*. Because it was never followed by shock, it may have become a safety signal, indicating a period in which no US would be presented. It is known that, like excitation (a fear-inducing element in aversive learning), inhibition also generalizes. Hence, an intraclass gradient with CS+ and CS– as end points, like the one tested in the Lissek and colleagues study, might present a combination of generalization of excitation (departing from the CS+) and generalization of inhibition (departing from the CS–). Work from our lab has shown that there is an asymmetry between the two types of generalization, in that excitation generalizes more readily (Vervliet, Vansteenwegen, & Eelen, 2006). This is a theoretically as well as clinically important finding—for example, with respect to the generalization of extinction/exposure, which is basically an inhibitory phenomenon.

In conclusion, we can state that generalization curves are malleable and influenced by procedural variables (e.g., comparison stimuli). This knowledge enhances and clarifies our perspective on certain clinical phenomena. For instance, having an inhibitory stimulus in a stimulus dimension that was recently conditioned (e.g., a safe father figure for someone recently abused by an adult male) might make an important difference in the extent of generalization of negative emotions. In addition to the variables mentioned in this section, other procedural variables can impact the degree of generalization and the slope of the curve (e.g., the degree of original learning, schedules of reinforcement, time between acquisition and test). In addition, as we argue later, it is also impacted by a number of psychological processes such as attention, perception, and memory.

Generalization and Discrimination

We already noted that (having) the opportunity to discriminate between the CS+ and other stimuli can impact the amount of generalization. As a matter of fact, according to some theorists, generalization and discrimination are two sides of the same coin. If one has learned to fear a certain situation (maybe for good reasons), and one fails to discriminate this particular situation from other similar but harmless situations, there is a fair chance that these other situations will also elicit fear. In fact, Lashley and Wade (1946), who formulated one of the classic theories of generalization, proposed that generalization reflects a failure of subjects to discriminate differences between stimuli. They, for instance, note, " 'Stimulus generalization' is generalization only in the sense of failure to note distinguishing characteristics of the stimulus or to associate them with the conditioned reaction. A definite attribute of the stimulus is 'abstracted' and forms the basis of reaction; other attributes are either not sensed at all or are disregarded" (p. 81). At the core, their view presents a sort of "attentional model" of generalization. To the extent that the relevant dimension (to the experimenter!) has not received attention during conditioning, the subsequent testing of other stimuli differing on this dimension is expected to yield strong generalization. They illustrated their perspective as follows:

> If a monkey is trained to choose a large red circle and avoid a small green one, he will usually choose any red object and avoid any green but will make chance scores when like colored large and small circles are presented. There is no question of generalization here; the dimension of size is not seen as relevant to the situation. If, however, the monkey is trained with gray circles of unequal sizes, he not only differentiates the training objects but generalizes the reaction to size, as may be shown by transposition tests. (Lashley & Wade, 1946, p. 82)

Interestingly, a recent fear conditioning study followed exactly this proposal (Vervliet et al., 2010b). However, the "monkeys" were students at the University of Leuven, and instead of red and green circles, blue and yellow rectangles and triangles were used. For all participants in the study, a yellow triangle was coupled with an aversive shock during the acquisition phase. Successful fear conditioning was evidenced by heightened skin conductance responses and US-expectancy ratings to this CS+ as compared to a CS– (a black cross). After acquisition, participants were presented with two generalization stimuli. One was a yellow square and the other a blue triangle. Each GS thus carried one element of the original CS+ (color or shape). The crucial manipulation in this study was that participants had received preexperimental instructions saying that the shapes (or colors) of the stimuli were informative for the occurrence of shock (group Shape and group Color, respectively). This way, one dimension (and not the other) was made salient during fear learning. Interestingly, this manipulation had a strong effect on generalization. The results showed strongest generalization to the same shape stimu-

lus (blue triangle) in group Shape, versus the same color stimulus (yellow square) in group Color. Hence, the same learning experience can have opposite effects in terms of fear generalization, depending on the specific features or stimulus dimension to which attention was drawn during acquisition. More generally, these findings indicate that fear generalization may depend heavily on discrimination of stimulus features/dimensions.

If instances of fear generalization are indeed (at least partly) based on a failure to detect or attend to differences, it follows that discrimination training might be a way to prevent dysfunctional overgeneralization. Older studies have indeed shown that discrimination training leads to sharper generalization gradients (e.g., Doll & Thomas, 1967; Hanson, 1959). This finding may have important clinical implications. Clients may be trained to better discriminate between stimuli or situations that are indeed associated with danger and those that are not, or can even be regarded as safe. We return to this issue later when we discuss the clinical implications of fear generalization research.

Even though there are clear indications that generalization and discrimination are functionally related, this does not necessarily mean that all generalization is based on a failure to discriminate stimuli (or stimulus features). It is well possible that fear generalizes even though participants are well able to discriminate between the CS+ and the GSs. As a matter of fact, this has been one of the elements governing more theoretical discussions of the mechanisms of generalization.

Theoretical Models of Generalization

The concept of (fear) generalization can refer to three different constructs. Generalization can be viewed as a procedure, as a result, and as a process. Generalization as *procedure* refers to the basic laboratory paradigm, typically consisting of an acquisition phase, followed by a test phase during which responding to the CS+ and a series of generalization stimuli are compared. The term *generalization* can also refer to a *result*—that is, the observable outcome of the procedure. The following, classic definition of generalization by Kalish (1969) is an example of a description of the phenomenon of generalization as a *result*:

> Stimulus Generalization . . . occurs when responses conditioned to one stimulus can also be elicited by other stimuli on the same dimension. Under these circumstances a gradient of responses is usually obtained in which the amplitude or frequency of response decreases with increased differences (psychological or physical) between the CS and the test stimulus. (p. 209)

In addition to descriptions in terms of procedure and result, it is also possible to describe generalization as a *process*. The characterization of generalization as a failure to discriminate is such an example. Because processes, in contrast to procedures and results, are not directly observable, this is usually the level at which the theoretical debate is situated. The basic question is this: By what processes does a generalization procedure lead to behavioral generalization (as result)?

The first account of generalization can be found in the work of Pavlov (1927), who identified the concept of *irradiation*. According to Pavlov, sensory input activates corresponding points on the cerebral cortex, and this activation spreads slowly and with decrement to neighboring points. Because he assumed that any point in a cortical sensory field that is activated simultaneously with an unconditioned reaction becomes associated with that reaction, and because he believed that the strength of the resulting association is proportional to the degree of activation of that cortical point at the moment of conditioning, it is easy to see that Pavlov views the stimulus generalization phenomenon as the behavioral reflection of a speculated process of cortical irradiation.

Even though the specific neurological model of Pavlov has been discarded, it has been a source of inspiration for related models (e.g., Hull's [1943] neo-Pavlovian approach) as well as a basis for discussion (e.g., Lashley and Wade's [1946] model and their attack on the perspective taken by Pavlov and Hull). Also, in the years following this discussion, several models have been proposed to explain the generalization phenomenon. Examples are the common elements approach proposed by Mackin-

tosh (1974), Rescorla's (1976) elemental model of stimulus generalization, Bush and Mosteller's (1951) stimulus sampling theory of generalization, Wagner's replaced elements model (e.g., Brandon, Vogel, & Wagner, 2000), and Pearce's (1987) configural model.

Without going into too much detail, we believe that an approach in terms of stimulus similarity probably offers the most fruitful conceptualization of the generalization process. Stimulus similarity is a function of the intersection of the elements belonging to the CS and the GS (see Figure 7.3). It is merely assumed, then, that generalization is the result of associative connections originating from stimulus elements common to both the CS and the test stimulus (Kalish, 1969, p. 215). This account of stimulus similarity is subscribed by many authors (e.g., Blough, 1975; Bush & Mosteller, 1951; Pearce, 1987; Rescorla, 1976). Similarity can be defined as either the number of common elements (Rescorla, 1976), the proportion of common elements to the GS (Bush & Mosteller, 1951), or the product of the proportions of common elements to both stimuli (Pearce, 1987).

The models that were mentioned in this section all have a particular focus on the (associative) learning basis for generalization. However, an overarching model of (fear) generalization that does justice to the complexity of the phenomenon will require the theoretical input of additional elements. We already noted that *attention* might be a

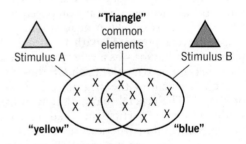

FIGURE 7.3. Stimuli can be viewed as sets of features. Some features are shared by two or more stimuli (common elements); stimulus A and B are both triangles. Other features are specific to a certain stimulus and are not shared (e.g., the color of the two triangles).

crucial concept in this respect. As a matter of fact, selective attention to certain (types of) features might influence what the organism exactly perceives as "common features" in a certain situation, and thus impacts the amount of generalization (see Mackintosh, 1965). Within our lab, we are currently exploring and empirically testing different aspects of a more general model of (fear) generalization. One example is a line of research that relates (fear) generalization to the study of human memory.

Generalization and Memory Specificity

An intriguing finding in the generalization literature is the observation that with passage of time between acquisition and test, generalization curves become flatter (e.g., Perkins & Weyant, 1958; Thomas & Lopez, 1962). This is illustrated by a recent fear conditioning study conducted by Wiltgen and Silva (2007). These authors conditioned mice to fear a specific context (the training cage) by presenting a foot shock (US) in that context (acquisition phase). Afterward, animals were tested in the same context or a different context (generalization test phase). The interval between fear learning and test was manipulated. Four groups of animals were tested, respectively, 1, 14, 28, or 36 days after acquisition. Results showed a systematic increase in generalization over this period. Initially, mice demonstrated more fear in the training context (as indexed by freezing behavior), but fear of the novel environment grew over time until animals eventually froze an equivalent amount in both contexts. Moreover, data from additional experiments showed that increased generalization at remote time points was due, at least in part, to forgetting specific features of the context.

Several studies now provide evidence for the idea that generalization gradients tend to flatten over time (see Land, Harrod, & Riccio, 1998). These observations fit in a model that was presented by Riccio and colleagues about two decades ago and that essentially views generalization as a memory phenomenon. More precisely, the model views generalization as the result of *forgetting of stimulus attributes* (Riccio, Ackil, & Burch-

Vernon, 1992). According to this model, a memory of a certain stimulus (e.g., a CS) is conceptualized as being composed of a complex of attributes (e.g., color, shape, texture). The combination of these attributes or features constitutes a holistic representation of that stimulus. Over time, some of these attributes are forgotten (Anderson & Riccio, 2005). To the extent that this results in a decrement in the discrimination between the original stimulus and novel stimuli (see "common elements" in previous section), the probability (or "capability") of these novel stimuli eliciting a conditioned response increases (i.e., generalization).

This memory perspective on (fear) generalization yields a number of interesting theoretical implications. If, for instance, generalization is indeed based on memory for specific "attributes" of (personal) learning events, an intriguing prediction would be that the amount of generalization might be a function of individual differences in memory specificity. During the last 25 years, there has been an ever-growing line of research on such differences in the specificity of autobiographical memory (e.g., Hermans, Raes, Philippot, & Kremers, 2006; Williams et al., 2007). Most studies have used the Autobiographical Memory Test (AMT) as a measure of memory specificity (Williams & Broadbent, 1986). In this task, participants are presented with a series of cue words (e.g., *happy, safe*), for which they are asked to generate a specific personal memory. A *specific memory* is defined as a memory for an event that occurred at a particular time and place and that lasted no longer than 1 day. Dozens of studies are now available that show that certain clinical conditions (e.g., depression, posttraumatic stress disorder) are characterized by reduced autobiographical memory specificity, also known as "overgeneral" autobiographical memory (e.g., Williams et al., 2007). For instance, when confronted with the cue word *happy*, depressed patients tend to come up with memories like "I feel happy every time I go to a concert," whereas a nonclinical control participant would rather produce a memory such as "Last Friday evening my friend Ted visited me, and we spent all evening watching tapes of when I was a kid." Depressed patients are prone to retrieve relatively less specific memories and more "categorical" memories, which are a kind of "summary" memory. What started off as a serendipitous finding has turned out to be central to a core pathological mechanism in depression. For instance, there is robust evidence that memory specificity is one of the better predictors for the course of depression (e.g., Hermans et al., 2008; for an overview, see Sumner, Griffith, & Mineka, 2010).

Against this theoretical background, we recently investigated whether lack of memory specificity is associated with more extensive generalization of conditioned responses (Lenaert et al., 2012). If participants fail to retrieve the specific attributes of the stimuli that were originally involved in the learning events (CS+, CS–) due to less specific autobiographical memory retrieval, one would predict, on the basis of Riccio's model, that stimuli that are (perceptually) similar to the original training stimuli would become increasingly capable of eliciting a conditioned response. Hence, more generalization (i.e., a shallower generalization gradient) is predicted for participants who are characterized by limited autobiographical memory specificity (or overgeneral memory) as compared to participants who are more specific in their autobiographical memories.

In this study, Lenaert and colleagues (2012) invited participants who scored high or low on memory specificity in a mass testing of the AMT. All participants took part in a conditioning study. The CS+ and CS– were pictures of a human face. Throughout acquisition, participants successfully learned that one picture predicted the US, whereas the other picture did not. During the test of generalization, the CS+ and CS– were presented again, as well as a series of six generalization stimuli, which were morphs of the two faces. Specialized software was employed to transform one CS into the other CS in six gradual steps. Results showed that memory specificity had no impact on acquisition, but did reliably influence the generalization gradient. In line with our predictions, more generalization was observed in participants who were less memory specific.

We believe that these results are important for several reasons. First, they demonstrate that generalization is a complex process in which not only associative processes, but also basic memory processes (in addition to perceptual and attentional mechanisms, probably), play a role. An overarching model of (fear) generalization thus needs to take into account these cognitive processes. Second, as mentioned before, not much is known about the basis for individual differences in generalization curves. This study provides a first answer to this probably more complex question.

Nonperceptual Generalization

In all studies thus far discussed, fear generalized over a perceptual dimension. Conditioned fear responses generalized from larger to smaller circles, from yellow to blue triangles, etc. These findings provide, without doubt, a valid laboratory model for the generalization of certain types of clinical fear. A good example is Suzy, who was bitten by a German shepherd, and was confronted with an expanding fear toward other dogs (other breeds, sizes) and other four-legged animals. Perceptual generalization can also be present in the person suffering from posttraumatic stress disorder who experiences intrusions of the trauma elicited by an ever-increasing set of odors (first the smell of burned rubber, later other burn smells, even later all kinds of pronounced smells). Another example would be the child who was bullied at school and whose fears extended from the wrongdoer to other older children, and later to people in general.

However, there are many clinical situations in which the dimension of generalization is obviously not a perceptual one. A good example was the case of Martha, introduced at the beginning of this chapter. Martha was diagnosed with obsessive–compulsive disorder. Initially, she feared pesticides and herbicides, but over the course of months and years she started to fear things such as gasoline, shoe polish, unstubbed cigarettes, viral infections, knives, and other sharp objects. The list of stimuli that fired her compulsions was almost two pages long. Many or even most of these CSs did not share strong perceptual similarity. The therapist whom she visited in an attempt to battle her fears did an extensive stimulus analysis as part of a larger functional analysis. One of his conclusions was that what was common to her obsessions and compulsions was an extensive fear of hurting or even killing her 3-year-old son.

Martha is a single mother who gave birth to her son about 3 years ago. As she was almost 34 at that time and had no steady partner, she feared that she would miss out on her chances of becoming a mother. A couple of weeks after another brief romantic relationship had ended, Martha found out that she was pregnant. The father had no interest in raising the child, so Martha decided to take the responsibility of being a single parent. This was not an easy decision because responsibilities had always been quite fear-provoking to her. Like many young mothers, she was a bit apprehensive of inflicting something bad on her child. This fear unexpectedly flared when one evening there was a news item about a young mother who was taken into custody after her young child died of drinking from a bottle of herbicide. Apparently, the bottle had been open and in reach of the child. The newsreader also stated that, according to a police investigation, there had been other hazardous situations in the house, and that a drama like this was bound to happen. The news item had aroused Martha, particularly when she discovered that there was a sort of herbicide in the kitchen. Even though it was out of reach for her son, she totally panicked and cursed herself for being such an irresponsible parent. Since that evening, contact (or even the possibility of contact) with herbicides (CS) elicited the idea that she would be responsible for the death of her son (US), which provoked enormous fears. Checking for these products in her environment and washing her hands to remove possible contamination of herbicides temporarily relieved her of her fears.

The functional analysis of the therapist made it clear that the generalization that was observed in Martha, starting from her initial fear of herbicides to the long list of stimuli she now avoided and escaped from, was in no way driven by a perceptual dimension. Rather, it became apparent that stimuli such as herbicides, gasoline, shoe polish, unstubbed cigarettes, viral infections, and knives were related through a *meaning dimension*, a semantic relatedness as stimuli that are considered potentially dangerous to her son's health. This type of generalization of clinical fear poses a challenge to researchers, as it does not seem to fit the perceptual generalization that is typically studied.

Nonperceptual Generalization: Mere Associations?

In clinical research, a concept that is often used is the idea of the "fear network" (e.g., Lang, 1985). Basically, this notion refers to the network of memory representations that are central to the anxiety problem of a given person. This network of representations contains information about the nature/identity of the stimuli that are crucial to the fears of that individual, their meaning, and the responses associated with these stimuli (verbal, physiological, motor responses). When the elements of this representational network are highly associated, activation of one element of the network (e.g., the perception of a dog or an odor) might be sufficient to activate the whole network and hence lead to the experience of fear or anxiety. From this perspective, generalization concerns the question of how stimuli that are related to the original CS are integrated into this associative network and thus acquire the potency to elicit the fear response. As we have seen, the answer to this question cannot be restricted to perceptually related elements alone.

One nonperceptual route might be merely associative. Would it be possible that fear travels through simple associative links? Let us do the following thought experiment. Imagine two unrelated neutral stimuli. In a first stage, these two neutral stimuli, A and B, are paired several times. Through these contingent pairings, the representations of A and B get associated in memory. After some time, one of the stimuli (B) is presented again, but now in the absence of A, and each presentation of B is terminated by an electric shock (US). As a result of this procedure, B starts to elicit fear. The core question is whether this fear would also generalize to A. If so, this would provide a straightforward example of nonperceptual, associative generalization: A and B only share a history of being associated in time and place.

Already more than 10 years ago, an experiment that followed such principles was conducted in our lab (Vansteenwegen et al., 2000). The procedure of this study is depicted in Figure 7.4. In a first phase, a pair of unrelated neutral stimuli, A and B, is repeatedly presented together. This procedure is also known as *sensory preconditioning*. During the second phase (acquisition), B was followed by an aversive electrocutaneous stimulus (B+). As an additional control, the study included a second set of neutral stimuli (C and D), which were likewise co-presented during the first phase. During the second phase, D was presented, but was never followed by shock. In the test phase, A and C were presented again (generalization test). If fear indeed spreads over mere associative paths (from B to A), it was predicted that A would elicit more fear than C. Indeed, even though A was never presented together with shock, A elicited significantly stronger skin conductance responses. Also, the presentation of A (as compared to C) induced a more active expectancy that a shock would actually appear. These findings provide an intriguing observation because they strongly suggest that fear can travel through associative pathways between otherwise arbitrary stimuli. This finding could also help to explain why it is sometimes difficult to retrieve the original conditioning experiences that are at the basis of some clinical fears.

A unique aspect of the procedure of this study, however, was that A always "preceded" B in the sensorial preconditioning phase. One could argue that the relation that is learned between A and B is more than a mere "association," as there is also a sequential relationship between the preconditioned stimulus (A) and the conditioned stimulus (B); A is not only associated with B, but it also precedes and predicts B. To investigate whether a precondition of this type is necessary, Vansteenwegen and colleagues (2000) added a second condition. In this condition, the preconditioned cues A and C were extinguished (i.e., repeatedly presented without being followed by the US) immediately after the preconditioning phase and before fear

acquisition. The extinction of the "sequential/predictive" relation did indeed impact the generalization effect for skin conductance responses. No generalization was observed for the extinguished condition.

A recent study is further relevant. Dunsmoor, White, and LaBar (2011) presented participants with a picture of a spider (A) or a wasp (C) that was followed by the presentation of a unrelated picture of an unrelated stimulus, such as a hospital corridor (B) or a waste drum (D). After this preconditioning phase, stimuli B and D entered a fear conditioning procedure in which B (CS+) but not D (CS–) was followed by an electric shock. Finally, the preconditioned stimuli A and C were tested. In line with the data of Vansteenwegen and colleagues (2000), stimulus A elicited more fear than stimulus C (i.e., higher skin conductance responses). Interestingly, the experimenters also included a condition in which A–B and C–D were conceptually related pictures: spider–web and wasp–wasp nest. For this condition, a sensory preconditioning effect was observed as well, and this was reliably stronger as compared to the unrelated condition (e.g., spider–hospital corridor). The authors reasoned that conceptual similarity might enhance generalization, possibly because "these objects have frequently co-occurred in the learning history of our participants, and thus participants have been 'preconditioned' prior to participation in this experiment. It is well known that experience shapes conceptual knowledge structures, so the effects observed likely include priors from both conceptual knowledge and direct learning history" (Dunsmoor et al., 2011, p. 158). An interesting finding of their study was also that the amount of generalization to preconditioned stimuli in the conceptually related condition was significantly associated with individual levels of trait anxiety. The more trait anxious the participant, the more fear generalization occurred.

Nonperceptual Generalization: Equivalence Relations

The findings of Dunsmoor and colleagues (2011) with respect to conceptually related stimuli are interesting in light of clinical observations. As exemplified by Martha's

Sensorial preconditioning	Acquisition	Test	Result
A–B	B+	A? C?	A > C
C–D	D–		

FIGURE 7.4. Procedure used in the control group of the study by Vansteenwegen, Crombez, Baeyens, Hermans, and Eelen (2000).

case, generalization sometimes seems to spread through classes of stimuli that are conceptually related (e.g., dirty objects, contexts that do not allow immediate escape). In these cases, there is more than a mere associative link; rather, stimuli share a symbolic or semantic relation. This opens the question of how such symbolic categories are formed and whether they are a vehicle for (fear) generalization.

At least two different research traditions in human and animal learning are highly relevant for an experimental study of such symbolic/semantic or functional generalization. Moreover, in both cases, there are recent data that demonstrate a particular relevance for the study of the generalization of acquired fear. The first domain pertains to (human) "matching-to-sample"-based *equivalence class learning* (and the creation of other types of *relational frames*; see below); the second pertains to (animal and human) *acquired equivalence learning based on common outcomes or antecedents of cues* ("many-to-one" or "one-to-many" relational learning; see also Hermans & Baeyens, 2013).

In the first of these—the domain of equivalence class learning—a procedure that is typically used is the matching-to-sample procedure, in which human participants are explicitly taught to relate arbitrary stimuli (e.g., nonsensical line drawings). On a given trial, a participant is shown a sample stimulus, perhaps a nonsensical line drawing like the one on top of the screen depicted in Figure 7.5. Below this sample (A1), three comparison stimuli are presented (B1, B2, B3). The participant is asked to select one of these comparisons, after which feedback is presented (*correct* or *wrong*). By trial and error, participants are taught to correctly match a series of comparison stimuli to the sample stimulus. In Figure 7.6, an example is given of two such sets of equivalence classes. According to this scheme, selecting C1 (among comparisons C1, C2, and C3) as a match for sample A1 would be correct. This response, however, would be incorrect when the sample was A2, in which case C2 would be the correct response. For participants, this is not a very easy task. Even though the two equivalence classes can easily be depicted, as in Figure 7.6, for the participant trials consist of a stream of sets

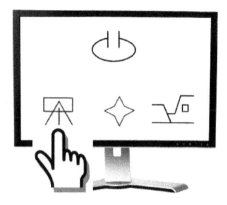

FIGURE 7.5. Matching-to-sample procedure. Stimuli used in study by Dougher et al. (1994).

of unfamiliar and completely arbitrary symbols. Moreover, designs can be elaborated such that participants learn longer strings of relations, such as X1 to Y1 and Y1 to Z1 (vs. X2 to Y2 and Y2 to Z2). If sufficiently trained with a procedure like this latter one, the subject will typically also relate X1 to X1 ("reflexive" responding), Y1 to X1 and Z1 to Y1 ("symmetrical" responding), X1 to Z1 ("transitive" responding), and finally Z1 to X1 ("equivalent" responding), *without any explicit training of these derived relations being necessary.*

For the training depicted in Figure 7.6, correct symmetrical responding would be to select A1 (and not A2 or A3) to sample B1. Equivalence would be evidenced, for instance, by selecting D1 (and not D2 or D3) to sample B1. It is important to note that when participants make correct responses in equivalence tests, this response is no direct function of previous training, as the D1–B1 pair was not trained, and D1 and B1 were actually never even presented together on the same trial. A real-world example would be the child who learns that a framed photograph of its mother on the mantel-

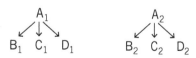

FIGURE 7.6. Two four-member equivalence classes.

piece (A) is conceptually similar to the auditory stimulus *Mama* (B), and independently learns that *Mama* (B) signifies the person who nourishes him (C). Symmetry would be evident when the photograph not only activates the representation of the noun *Mama* (A–B), but also vice versa (B–A). So, if upon presentation of the photograph, the child has learned to use the word *Mama* (A–B), symmetrical responding would be evidenced by the child now also pointing to the picture when he hears the word *Mama* (B–A), in the absence of specific B–A training. Transitivity would be evidenced by the child pointing to his mother (C) when shown the picture (A).

When these "emergent" relations (symmetry, transitivity, etc.) are demonstrated, an *equivalence class* is said to have been established (Sidman, 1994). *Stimulus equivalence* refers to the substitutability of one stimulus for another, given a certain context. For instance, even though the auditory percept of someone saying *fork*, the visual presentation of the four letters *f o r k*, a picture of a real metal fork, and a simple line drawing of the same object are perceptually completely different, they belong to the same class. For some functions or in certain contexts, they can be used as substitutes for each other. If I need a fork in a crowded environment, I can ask for it by saying the word, or by showing the fork of the person sitting next to me, or even by presenting a line drawing of a fork. The person I am addressing at that moment will probably understand each presented stimulus as a substitute of what I am requesting. In that respect, it has been argued that equivalence class formation may be at the origin of *symbol formation* in humans.

In addition to the performance on the *stimulus relatedness tests* (e.g., symmetry, transitivity), a second methodological criterion that is used to conclude that a set of stimuli functions as a category *(equivalence class)* is performance on response transfer tests (Adams, Fields, & Verhave, 1993). This *transfer* (or generalization) is evidenced by the observation that a behavioral function explicitly trained to one member of the class (A1) may *automatically transfer* (or be transformed) to all others members belonging to the class (B1 and C1), but not to the members of another class (A2, B2, C2).

To illustrate this transfer, and with direct relevance to the topic of this chapter, we briefly describe an interesting study by Dougher, Augustson, Markham, Greenway, and Wulfert (1994). They used a matching-to-sample procedure to teach their participants two four-member equivalence classes like those presented in Figure 7.6. Samples and comparisons were arbitrary pictorial stimuli like those presented in Figure 7.5. Participants learned six conditional stimulus relations (A1B1, A1C1, A1D1, A2B2, A2C2, and A2D2). A third set of stimuli (A3, B3, C3, D3) served only as incorrect comparisons during match-to-sample trials. Stimulus relatedness tests showed that all participants succeeded for symmetry and equivalence, which demonstrated the emergence of two four-member stimulus equivalence classes (A1, B1, C1, D1 vs. A2, B2, C2, D2). In a second phase of the experiment, one member of the first class (B1; CS+) was contingently followed by an unpleasant electric shock (US). This was never the case for a member of the second class (B2; CS–). In a final phase (*test for transfer*) all members of the two equivalence classes were presented again, and skin conductance responses were measured. Results showed that the conditioned responses "transferred" from B1 to the other members of that class (C1, D1), whereas this was not the case for the second class (C2, D2). These findings are of theoretical interest because they demonstrate generalization of conditioned fear responses to stimuli that were only symbolically associated with the CS+. From a clinical perspective, these findings suggest a route by which stimuli can acquire fear-inducing properties (1) without any direct relation with an aversive event, and (2) based on associations (e.g., B1–C1) that were never actually encountered (Hermans & Baeyens, 2013).

Other studies have focused on avoidance responding, which is an important behavioral response in the context of fear. For instance, Dymond and colleagues (2007, 2008) first created classes of functionally equivalent stimuli. In a subsequent phase, one stimulus (B1) of the A1, B1, C1 category signaled that a simple avoidance response cancelled a scheduled presentation of an aversive image and sound (US). At subsequent test of generalization, all participants who met criteria for conditioned avoidance also demonstrated derived avoidance by emitting the avoidance response in the presence of C1. An interesting feature of this study is that the relationships that were trained between A1, B1, and C1 were defined in terms of "sameness," whereas for a second series of stimuli (B2, C2) a relation of "oppositeness" was trained (e.g., Same: A1–B1; Same: A1–C1; Opposite: A1–B2; Opposite: A1–C2). In addition to the relation of sameness that is implied in traditional equivalence studies, *opposition* is one of several types of relational responding that can be trained (e.g., "difference," "more/less than," "bigger/smaller," "before/after"). These types of relations are central to the relational frame theory, a behavioral understanding of language and cognition (e.g., Törneke, 2010). In the studies of Dymond and colleagues, trained oppositeness resulted in a generalization of nonavoidance, which was evidenced by reduced avoidance in the presence of C2. Control participants who were not exposed to relational training and testing did not show derived avoidance. Studies in this context provide an excellent basis for analyzing and understanding nonperceptual generalization and its clinical implications.

In addition to the matching-to-sample-based equivalence class learning, there exists a relatively separate literature on *acquired equivalence learning based on common outcomes or antecedents of cues* (many-to-one or one-to-many relational learning). In a typical procedure, an organism learns that two or more stimuli are equivalent in terms of being mapped on the same outcome or response. For instance, two antecedents, A1 and A2, are followed by a common outcome (B1). This is not the case for antecedent stimulus A3. Subsequently, one of the antecedents is involved in an aversive conditioning procedure (e.g., A1-shock). Finally, responding to A2 is compared to A3. It is observed that conditioned fear responding to A2 is greater than to A3. The generalization from A1 to A2 is based on their "common outcome." An example of such a study in animals is provided by Honey and Hall (1989). Other studies have made use of a "common antecedent" procedure. We are currently employing these methodologies in our lab to study generalization (of fear) in humans (see Vervoort, Vervliet, Mutert, & Baeyens, 2011).

Discussion

Emotions are responses. These can be physiological, cognitive, or motor responses. Some emotions, such as fear and anxiety, are strongly characterized by physiological responding. Other emotions have a stronger cognitive component, such as guilt. More specifically, emotions are *responses* that are *elicited by stimuli*. These stimuli can be simple, like the presence of a certain fragrance, or can be more complex, like a social situation. As was argued by Watson and Rayner (1920), the newborn infant is characterized by a very limited set of stimuli that elicit emotions. Through processes of conditioning, more and more stimuli are endowed with a capacity to elicit combinations of cognitive, motoric, or physiological emotional responses. In this way, the emotional life of the child becomes richer and more differentiated, and toward adulthood it will reach levels of complexity that are in no way comparable to the simplicity of the limited set of innate reflexes expressed by the newborn.

An essential aspect of this developmental process is the fact that emotional responses can generalize toward related stimuli. This is a crucial and basically very adaptive characteristic. Because of generalization, the learning process does not need to be repeated for every new stimulus or situation. If, for instance, we have learned to be happy with a certain outcome, we can enjoy the fact that this emotion is elicited by (highly) similar situations. Likewise, fear, anger, or sadness can generalize toward (ranges of) other stimuli and events.

The fact that generalization has a central role in our emotional development (and the development of emotional pathologies) stands in marked contrast with a surprising paucity of research on this topic. Most research on emotional generalization has been conducted in the area of fear, which was the focus of this chapter. Predominantly animal studies have investigated the perceptual generalization of fear. Much of this research is already several decades old, and almost no work had been done on human participants. During the last decade, up-to-date procedures have been developed to study human fear generalization in the lab (Lissek et al., 2008; Vervliet et al., 2006, 2010a). Much more research is needed to start unveiling the preconditions and mechanisms of fear generalization. We believe that this work needs a multifaceted approach, in which not only perceptual, but also nonperceptual forms of generalization are studied, and in which the interaction with other (cognitive) mechanisms such as perception, attention, and memory are studied. Only in this way can we really get a firm grip on this phenomenon that hides layers of complexity behind a seemingly uncomplicated facade. In our lab, we are currently approaching the study of generalization from different empirical angles.

In addition to the study of the preconditions and processes, work also needs to be directed to the generality of these findings with respect to other emotions. To our knowledge, (almost) no work has been conducted on the generalization of other types of emotional responses (e.g., anger, elation). Similarly, there is no doubt that, from a clinical perspective, the relevance of (over)generalization cannot be limited to anxiety disorders. Beck (1976) already acknowledged the role of this process in the development and maintenance of depression. Some relevant work in this domain has been conducted by Carver and colleague (Carver, 1998; Carver & Ganellen, 1983). We are currently investigating mechanisms of generalization in depression, as well as in other domains (e.g., chronic pain). Finally, clinical implications of this work require empirical elaboration. Restricting and preventing dysfunctional overgeneralization will be a crucial focus of such research (e.g., Vervliet et al., 2010a).

Acknowledgments

Preparation of this chapter was supported by the KU Leuven Center of Excellence on Generalization Research (GRIP*TT; PF/10/005) and Grant No. GOA/2007/03 (KU Leuven).

References

Adams, B. J., Fields, L., & Verhave, T. (1993). Formation of generalized equivalence classes. *Psychological Record, 43*, 553–566.

Anderson, M. J., & Riccio, D. C. (2005). Ontogenetic forgetting of stimulus attributes. *Learning and Behavior, 33*, 444–453.

Banich, M., & Caccamise, D. (Eds.). (2010). *Generalization of knowledge: Multidisciplinary perspectives.* New York: Psychology Press.

Beck, A. T. (1976). *Cognitive therapy and emotional disorders.* New York: Meridian.

Blough, D. S. (1975). Steady state data and a quantitative model of operant generalization and discrimination. *Journal of Experimental Psychology: Animal Behavior Processes, 1*, 3–21.

Brandon, S. E., Vogel, E. H., & Wagner, A. R., (2000). A componential view of configural cues in generalization and discrimination in Pavlovian conditioning. *Behavioral Brain Research, 110*, 67–72.

Bush, R. R., & Mosteller, F. (1951). A mathematical model for simple learning. *Psychological Review, 58*, 313–323.

Carver, C. S. (1998). Generalization, adverse events, and development of depressive symptoms. *Journal of Personality, 66*, 609–620.

Carver, C. S., & Ganellen, R. J. (1983). Depression and components of self-punitiveness: High standards, self-criticism, and overgeneralization. *Journal of Abnormal Psychology, 92*, 330–337.

Craske, M. G., Hermans, D., & Vansteenwegen, D. (Eds.). (2006). *Fear and learning: From basic processes to clinical implications.* Washington, DC: American Psychological Association.

Doll, T. J., & Thomas, D. R. (1967). Effects of discrimination training on stimulus generalization for human subjects. *Journal of Experimental Psychology, 75*, 508–512.

Dougher, M. J., Augustson, E., Markham, M. R., Greenway, D. E., & Wulfert, E. (1994). The transfer of respondent eliciting and extinction functions through stimulus equivalence classes. *Journal of the Experimental Analysis of Behavior, 62*, 331–351.

Dunsmoor, J. E., Prince, S. E., Murty, V. P., Kragel, P. A., & LaBar, K. S. (2011). Neurobehavioral mechanisms of human fear generalization. *NeuroImage, 55*, 1878–1888.

Dunsmoor, J. E., White, A. J., LaBar, K. S. (2011). Conceptual similarity promotes generalization of higher-order fear learning. *Learning and Memory, 17*, 156–60.

Dymond, S., Roche, B., Forsyth, J. P., Whelan, R., & Rhoden, J. (2007). Transformation of avoidance response functions in accordance with the relational frames of same and opposite. *Journal of the Experimental Analysis of Behavior, 88*, 249–262.

Dymond, S., Roche, B., Forsyth, J. P., Whelan, R., & Rhoden, J. (2008). Derived avoidance learning: Transformation of avoidance response functions in accordance with same and opposite relational frames. *Psychological Record, 58*, 269–286.

Hanson, H. M. (1959). Effects of discrimination training on stimulus generalization. *Journal of Experimental Psychology, 58*, 321–334.

Hermans, D., & Baeyens, F. (2013). Generalization as a basis for emotional change: Perceptual and non-perceptual processes. In D. Hermans, B. Rimé, & B. Mesquita (Eds.), *Changing emotions* (pp. 67–73). Hove, UK: Psychology Press.

Hermans, D., Craske, M. G., Mineka, S., & Lovibond, P. F. (2006). Extinction in human fear conditioning. *Biological Psychiatry, 60*, 361–368.

Hermans, D., Raes, F., Philippot, P., & Kremers, I. (2006). Autobiographical memory-specificity and psychopathology. *Cognition and Emotion, 20*, 321–323.

Hermans, D., Vandromme, H., Debeer, E., Raes, F., Demyttenaere, K., Brunfaut, E., et al. (2008). Overgeneral autobiographical memory predicts diagnostic status in depression. *Behaviour Research and Therapy, 46*, 668–677.

Honey, R. C., & Hall, G. (1989). Acquired equivalence and distinctiveness of cues. *Journal of Experimental Psychology: Animal Behavior Processes, 15*, 338–346.

Honig, W. K., & Urcuioli, P. J. (1981). The legacy of Guttman and Kalish (1956): 25 years of research on stimulus generalization. *Journal of the Experimental Analysis of Behavior, 36*, 405–445.

Hull, C. L. (1943). *Principles of behavior.* New York: Appleton–Century–Crofts.

Kalish, H. (1969). Stimulus generalization. In M. Marx (Ed.), *Learning: Processes* (pp. 205–297). Oxford, UK: Macmillan.

Land, C., Harrod, S. B., & Riccio, D. C. (1998). The interval between the CS and the UCS as a determiner of generalization performance. *Psychonomic Bulletin and Review, 5*, 690–693.

Lang, P. J. (1985). Fear, anxiety and panic: Context, cognition and visceral arousal. In S. Rachman & J. D. Maser (Eds.), *Panic: Psychological perspectives* (pp. 219–236). Hillsdale, NJ: Erlbaum.

Lashley, K. S., & Wade, M. (1946). The Pavlovian theory of generalization. *Psychological Review, 53*, 72–87.

Lenaert, B., Claes, S., Raes, F., Boddez, Y., Joos, E., Vervliet, B., et al. (2012). Generalization of conditioned responding: Effects of autobiographical memory specificity. *Journal of Behavior Therapy and Experimental Psychiatry, 43*, S60–S66.

Lissek, S., Biggs, A. L., Rabin, S., Cornwell, B. R., Alvarez, R. P., Pine, D. S., et al. (2008). Generalization of conditioned fear-potentiated startle in humans: Experimental validation and clinical relevance. *Behaviour Research and Therapy, 46*, 678–687.

Lissek, S., Rabin, S. J., Heller, R. E., Luckenbaugh, D., Geraci, M., Pine, D. S., et al. (2010). Overgeneralization of conditioned fear as a pathogenic marker of panic disorder. *American Journal of Psychiatry, 167*, 47–55.

Mackintosh, N. J. (1965). Selective attention in animal discrimination learning. *Psychological Bulletin, 64*, 124–150.

Mackintosh, N. J. (1974). *The psychology of animal learning.* London: Academic Press.

Pavlov, I. (1927). *Conditioned reflexes.* London: Oxford University Press.

Pearce, J. M. (1987). A model for stimulus generalization in Pavlovian conditioning. *Psychological Review, 94*, 61–73.

Perkins, C. C., & Weyant, R. G. (1958). The interval between training and testing as determiner of the slope of generalization gradients. *Journal of Comparative and Physiological Psychology, 97*, 140–153.

Rescorla, A. R. (1976). Stimulus generalization: Some predictions from a model of Pavlovian conditioning. *Journal of Experimental Psychology: Animal Behavior Processes, 2*, 88–96.

Riccio, D. C., Ackil, J., & Burch-Vernon, A. (1992). Forgetting of stimulus attributes: Methodological implications for assessing associative phenomena. *Psychological Bulletin, 112*, 433–445.

Sidman, M. (1994). *Equivalence relations and behavior: A research story.* Boston: Authors Cooperative.

Sumner, J. A., Griffith, J. W., & Mineka, S. (2010). Overgeneral autobiographical memory as a predictor of the course of depression: A meta-analysis. *Behaviour Research and Therapy, 48*, 1–12.

Thomas, D. R., & Lopez, I. J. (1962). The effects of delayed testing on generalization slope.

Journal of Comparative and Physiological Psychology, 55, 541–544.

Törneke, N. (2010). *Learning RFT: An introduction to relational frame theory and its clinical applications.* Oakland, CA: New Harbinger.

Vansteenwegen, D., Crombez, G., Baeyens, F., Hermans, D., & Eelen, P. (2000). Preextinction of sensory preconditioned electrodermal activity. *Quarterly Journal of Experimental Psychology, Section B: Comparative and Physiological Psychology, 53B*, 359–371.

Vansteenwegen, D., Vervliet, B., Hermans, D., Beckers, T., Baeyens, F., & Eelen, P. (2006). Stronger renewal in human fear conditioning when tested with an acquisition retrieval cue than with an extinction retrieval cue. *Behaviour Research and Therapy, 44*, 1717–1725.

Vervliet, B., Kindt, M., Vansteenwegen, D., & Hermans, D. (2010a). Fear generalization in humans: Impact of prior non-fearful experiences. *Behaviour Research and Therapy, 48*, 1078–1084.

Vervliet, B., Kindt, M., Vansteenwegen, D., & Hermans, D. (2010b). Fear generalization in humans: Impact of verbal instructions. *Behaviour Research and Therapy, 48*, 38–43.

Vervliet, B., Vansteenwegen, D., & Eelen, P. (2006). Generalization gradients for acquisition and extinction in human contingency learning. *Experimental Psychology, 53*, 132–142.

Vervoort, E., Vervliet, B., Mutert, L., & Baeyens, F. (2011, May). *Non-perceptual generalization of fear acquisition and extinction.* Poster presented at the third European Meeting on Human Fear Conditioning, Affligem, Belgium.

Watson, J. B., & Rayner, R. (1920). Conditioned emotional reactions. *Journal of Experimental Psychology, 3*, 1–14.

Williams, J. M. G., Barnhofer, T., Crane, C., Hermans, D., Raes, F., Watkins, E., et al. (2007). Autobiographical memory specificity and emotional disorder. *Psychological Bulletin, 133*, 122–148.

Williams, J. M. G., & Broadbent, K. (1986). Autobiographical memory in suicide attempters. *Journal of Abnormal Psychology, 95*, 144–149.

Wiltgen, B. J., & Silva, A. J. (2007). Memory for context becomes less specific with time. *Learning and Memory, 14*, 313–317.

CHAPTER 8

The Role of Appraisal in Emotion

Agnes Moors and Klaus R. Scherer

The idea that appraisal plays a role in emotion can be traced back to Aristotle, Descartes, Spinoza, and Hume, who considered it self-evident that the states variously called *passions, affects,* or *emotions* are differentiated by the type of evaluation or judgment a person makes of the eliciting event. This shared conviction was shattered by James's (1884/1969) claim that "the bodily changes follow directly the perception of the exciting fact, and that our feeling of the same changes as they occur *is* the emotion" (p. 247). Although James meant *feeling* when he wrote *emotion* and later acknowledged that the nature of the bodily changes was determined by the overwhelming "idea" of the significance of a situation for well-being (e.g., the probability that the bear will kill us or that we will kill it; James, 1894, p. 518), a century of debate and misunderstanding was launched (Ellsworth, 1994). Appraisal did not play much of a role in this debate nor did it in the (biological versions of) basic emotion theories, pioneered by Tomkins (1962) and his disciples Ekman (1972) and Izard (1977), which dominated the emotion domain from the 1960s to the 1980s.

The term *appraisal* was first used in a technical sense by Arnold (1960) and Lazarus (1966). Detailed development of this notion only occurred in the early 1980s (Scherer, 1999; Schorr, 2001), leading to what is now referred to as *appraisal theories*. Theorists in this tradition propose that most, but not all, emotions are elicited and differentiated by people's evaluation of the significance of events for their well-being (Ellsworth & Scherer, 2003). Currently, many contemporary emotion theories mention appraisal. For instance, Ekman (2004, pp. 121–126) postulated "automatic appraisal mechanisms" as triggers of emotion. Feldman Barrett (2006) suggested that appraisal can play a role in the generation of core affect, and Russell (2003) suggested that appraisal may be one of several independent components of an emotion episode. Yet, not all theories that mention appraisal qualify as appraisal theories. In the present chapter, we propose two related criteria for a theory to count as an appraisal theory: (1) Appraisal theories consider appraisal as a typical cause of emotion (or of emotional components), and because of this, (2) appraisal is the core determinant of the content of feelings. Before addressing the relation between appraisal and emotion, we consider definitions of the terms *emotion* and *appraisal*. This is crucial because the definitions that one has of these concepts determine in part how one thinks of the relation between them. In addition to commonalities among appraisal theories, we also highlight their differences.

Definition of Emotion

The lack of an agreed-upon definition of the term *emotion* has led to serious misunderstandings. We need to briefly address this issue and mark our position. The set of emotions can be defined with an intensional definition. Such a definition lists the necessary and sufficient conditions or criteria for an emotion exemplar to belong to the set, and they demarcate the set from particular other sets such as moods, attitudes, reflexes, and personality traits. A first set of criteria that often turns up in the literature has to do with duration. Emotion theorists agree that emotions are episodes (i.e., phenomena with a beginning and an end) and not enduring states. Although these episodes vary in duration, they are usually short-lived. These criteria serve to distinguish emotions from personality traits and moods.

A second set of criteria is that emotions consist of multiple components, or better, changes in multiple components. Many theorists include a cognitive component, a motivational one, a somatic one, a motor one, and a subjective one. Components (or parts of them) have been linked to functions. The cognitive component consists of an appraisal process, whose function is to evaluate the implications of stimuli for well-being. The motivational component consists of action tendencies (e.g., to increase contact) and other forms of action readiness (e.g., passivity). The somatic component consists of physiological activity, both central (in the brain) and peripheral (outside the brain). The motivational and somatic components have the function to prepare and support behavior. In fact, the central part of the somatic component supports all components. The motor component consists of facial and vocal expressions and gross behavior (e.g., fleeing, fighting, repairing) and has the function to execute behavior. Finally, the subjective component consists of experience or feelings, and has been endowed with a monitoring function (and other functions associated with consciousness). Theorists differ in how many and which of these components (or parts of components) they require to be present and whether these need to be synchronized, in order to talk about an emotion. For instance, some authors (e.g.,

Mulligan & Scherer, 2012; Scherer, 1984) exclude gross behavior, considering it as a consequence of emotion. Some authors (e.g., Parrott, 2007) exclude central somatic activity because it is present, on a lower level of analysis, in all the other components. Some authors (e.g., Clore & Ortony, 2000) have added other cognitive processes in addition to appraisal, such as changes in attention and memory, and categorization and labeling of one's emotion. The presence of certain components serves to differentiate emotions from other phenomena, such as attitudes or preferences (these are said to lack the somatic and motor components) and reflexes (these are said to lack a cognitive component).

A third set of criteria involves the content or the properties of certain components. Appraisal theorists have argued that emotions occur when stimuli are appraised as goal relevant, goal congruent/incongruent, positive/negative, and novel and/or urgent (Frijda, 1986; Scherer, 2005). Some theorists (Ortony & Turner, 1990) have argued that the feeling component of emotions must have a positive or negative valence (excluding surprise and interest from the set of emotions). Others (Frijda, 2007) have argued that the action tendencies in emotions have control precedence: They demand priority over other action tendencies. A fourth criterion proposed by Scherer (2001, 2009) is that emotions are, more than other phenomena, characterized by a high degree of integration and synchronization among all components. A fifth criterion emphasized by philosophers (e.g., de Sousa, 1987; Solomon, 1984) is that emotions have the property of intentionality (in the philosophical sense of the term). This means that they are directed toward something beyond themselves, that they have an object (e.g., being angry at someone, or being afraid of something). This criterion differentiates emotions from purely physical sensations (e.g., pain) that are not about something.

Definition of Appraisal

Since Arnold (1960) first used the term *appraisal* in the context of emotion, there has been an evolution in the way in which theorists have used it. We therefore think it is important to present and justify our own definition of appraisal, which is neither limited to higher-order cognitive processes, nor overinclusive (to refute the most frequent criticisms of appraisal theories). The singular use (appraisal) refers to the appraisal process and the plural use (appraisals) to the values that form the output of this process. We discuss both below.

Appraisal Process

To arrive at an intensional definition of the appraisal process, we rely on Marr's (1982) proposal that any process can be described at three levels of analysis. At the functional level, a process is described as the relation between an input and an output. For example, the process of adding digits can be described as the relation between two digits and their sum. The conditions under which the process takes place, such as the presence or absence of consciousness, processing goals, attentional capacity, and time, can also be specified at this level. At the algorithmic level, the mechanisms and format of the representations (i.e., codes) that are involved in translating the input into the output are specified. Adding digits can be done by a rule-based process, such as counting the units in both digits, or it can be done by an associative process, that is, by retrieving a previously calculated and stored sum. The format of the representations can be verbal-like versus image-like and localist versus distributed. At the implementational level, the process is described in terms of areas or circuits of brain activity.

We propose an intensional definition of appraisal at the functional level (cf. Moors, 2010). That is, we demarcate the appraisal process from other processes on the basis of the content of its input and/or output. The appraisal process takes a stimulus (as its input) and produces (as its output) values for one or more appraisal factors (e.g., goal relevance, goal congruence, coping potential, expectancy). This definition is not all-inclusive. It does not include processes that produce a value for other factors than appraisal factors (e.g., size, length, gender, location, color).

A first implication of defining appraisal in terms of input and/or output is that appraisal is not confined to operate under a specific set of conditions. Appraisal theorists have argued from the very start (e.g., Arnold, 1960) that appraisal can and often does operate automatically. This means that it can operate in the absence of a conscious stimulus input, the absence of a goal to engage in the process, the absence of abundant attentional capacity, the absence of abundant time, and/or despite the presence of a goal to counteract the process.

A second implication of defining appraisal on the functional level is that we do not confine appraisal to one single mechanism or to one format of representations on the algorithmic level. Any mechanism that produces values for one or more appraisal factors is accepted as a valid mechanism underlying appraisal. Appraisal theorists have proposed two or three possible mechanisms: a rule-based mechanism, an associative mechanism, and sometimes also a sensory–motor mechanism (Clore & Ortony, 2000, 2008; Leventhal & Scherer, 1987; Smith & Kirby, 2000, 2001; Smith & Neumann, 2005; van Reekum & Scherer, 1997). The mechanisms may use and produce any possible format of representations. Representations can be verbal-like (propositional or conceptual) or image-like (perceptual or sensory). They can be localist and symbolic (one node refers to an appraisal value) or they can be distributed and subsymbolic (one appraisal value is represented as a pattern of activation over a set of nodes).

In sum, our intensional definition of appraisal at the functional level makes it clear that appraisal should not be narrowed down to a nonautomatic, rule-based mechanism that operates on verbal-like or symbolic codes, as is still too often assumed by critics of appraisal theories. Despite the fact that we allow the entire range of mechanisms and formats of representation to underlie appraisal and that we do not put a priori constraints on the conditions under which appraisal can operate, our definition of appraisal is not all-inclusive. This is because we reserve the term *appraisal* for only those processes that deal with specific types of information captured in the appraisal factors proposed by appraisal theories. Determining which factors do or do not qualify as real appraisal factors is a work in progress. At this point, the existing proposals can be considered as working hypotheses that require further empirical research.

Individual appraisal theorists agree about a core set of appraisal factors—goal relevance, goal congruence, expectancy or novelty, coping potential or control, agency, and intentionality—but they disagree about others, such as intrinsic valence (see Table 29.1 in Ellsworth & Scherer, 2003). Appraisal factors can be treated as categorical variables, with a discrete number of possible values (two or three), or as dimensional variables, with an infinite number of possible values. For example, in a categorical account, the factor *goal congruence* (i.e., whether a stimulus matches with goals or concerns) has two values (goal congruent, goal incongruent), whereas in the dimensional account, it has an infinite number of values ranging from totally goal incongruent to totally goal congruent. Some factors are necessarily categorical. For instance, agency (i.e., the cause of an event) has values such as self, other, and impersonal circumstances. Identifying a list of typical appraisal factors fits in a molecular approach toward appraisal. Lazarus and his collaborators (e.g., Lazarus, 1991; Smith & Lazarus, 1993) combined the molecular approach with a molar one. In a molar approach, appraisal is treated as a unitary factor with a number of discrete values such as danger, insult, and irrevocable loss ("core relational themes"). These molar values are often considered as summaries or gestalts of molecular values (Smith & Lazarus, 1993, p. 236).

Appraisal Output

As mentioned, the output of the appraisal process is a representation of one or more appraisal values (i.e., *appraisals*) that have specific effects on other components (motivational, somatic, motor, feeling). There are no a priori constraints on the format of this representation or the conditions under which it can exist. Representations of appraisal values are unconscious by default, but part of their content can become conscious. The part that does become conscious becomes part of the content of the feeling component (based on the idea that feelings are the reflection of the other components into consciousness; see below). Only part of this conscious part is available for verbal report (see Scherer, 2009).

Relations between Appraisal and Emotion or the Other Components

Emotion theorists have proposed various kinds of relations between appraisal and emotion or the other components of emotion (Ellsworth & Scherer, 2003; Frijda, 1993, 2007; Keltner, Ellsworth, & Edwards, 1993; Parkinson, 1997; Scherer, 2001, 2009). They have argued that appraisal (1) is a component of emotion (part–whole relation), (2) is a cause of the other components (causal relation), (3) is part of the content of the feeling component, (4) is a consequence of the other components (causal relation), (5) temporally co-occurs with the other components (contiguity relation), and (6) is part of the meaning of emotion labels (conceptual relation). We discuss each of these relations as well as the extent to which they are mutually compatible.

Appraisal as a Component of Emotion

In our componential definition of emotion, we presented appraisal as one of the components in an emotion. Appraisal in this sense is fairly uncontroversial (Frijda, 2007), but there may be disagreement about the proportion of emotions in which appraisal is a component. Theorists may think that appraisal is a component in (1) all, (2) most, or (3) some emotions. In other words, theorists may think that appraisal is a (1) necessary, (2) typical, or (3) occasional component of emotion. Most appraisal theorists side with the view that appraisal is a typical or even necessary component of emotion.

Appraisal as a Cause of the Other Components

Several appraisal theorists think that appraisal is not just a component of the emotion episode. They think it is also a cause of the other components. This means that appraisal comes first in the causal chain and that it drives the changes in action tendencies, physiological responses, expressive behavior, and feelings (see Figure 8.1 for an example of this approach). The word *first* should be nuanced because contemporary appraisal theorists build in the notions of recurrence and immediate efference. *Recurrence* means

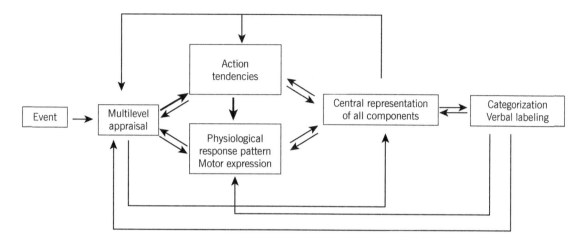

FIGURE 8.1. The causal, recursive relationship between emotion components, as suggested by the component process model. Adapted from Scherer (2009). Copyright 2009 by Taylor and Francis. Adapted by permission.

that changes in later components feed back to earlier components. Somatic and behavioral responses may produce a change of appraisal, either directly or indirectly (via a change in the stimulus). For example, an aggressive response may lead to an appraisal of high coping potential by making the person stronger (i.e., direct influence) or by making the opponent weaker (i.e., indirect influence). Because of recurrence, several emotional cycles may run in parallel. This is not incompatible with the idea that appraisal comes first, as long as appraisal comes first in each cycle. *Immediate efference* refers to the idea that the processes in early components can influence later components before they are entirely completed. Processes that are partially completed can influence other processes once they have produced a preliminary output.

Some theorists think appraisal causes the other components in all instances of emotions; they see appraisal as a necessary cause (e.g., Lazarus, 1991). Others think that appraisal causes the other components in most, but not all, instances of emotions; they see appraisal as a typical cause (e.g., Ellsworth & Scherer, 2003). This brings us to the first criterion that we propose for delineating the set of appraisal theories from other emotion theories: Appraisal theories consider appraisal to be at least a typical cause of the other components in emotions.

Appraisal as Part of the Content of the Feeling Component

Once a stimulus has produced changes in the components of appraisal, action tendencies, physiological responses, and behavior, an integrated representation of aspects of these changes surfaces into consciousness. Conscious aspects of appraisal are integrated with the representation of changes from other components (e.g., viscera-motor proprioception) and together they shape the content of the feeling component. What types of aspects contribute to the content of feelings? In the case of the appraisal component, Lambie and Marcel (2002) have argued that not the appraisal process itself but (part of) the output of the appraisal process surfaces into feelings. As explained above, the appraisal process produces an appraisal output, which is a representation of appraisal values. This representation is generally unconscious, but part of it can become conscious and hence contribute to the content of feelings. It may be noted, however, that the distinction between process and output is not so clear-cut when a process is considered on the functional level of analysis, that is, as the relation between an input and an output. Thus, it is possible that individuals are conscious of (1) the input (i.e., the stimulus), (2) the output of appraisal (i.e., appraisal values), and (3) the appraisal processes described on a functional level of analysis, as a relation between input and output (e.g., that a stimulus was appraised as goal incongruent and difficult to cope with). It is highly unlikely, however, that individuals have conscious access to processes described on the algorithmic or implementational levels of analysis (Moors & De Houwer, 2006).

As mentioned above, the content of feelings is not only determined by appraisal but also by the other components in the emotion episode. As a consequence, the relation between appraisal and feelings is not linear. Aspects of the appraisal component may blend in with the other components so that it is difficult to disentangle the aspects that come from appraisal and those that come from the other components. For example, when a person feels strong, this feeling may stem from an appraisal of high coping potential (appraisal component) or from the tendency to destroy (motivational component). Disentangling the sources of feelings is further complicated by possible causal influences among components. An appraisal of high coping potential may cause the tendency to fight (conform to the idea that appraisal causes the other components). Turning it around, the tendency to fight may cause a person to appraise his or her coping potential as high (conform to the idea of recurrence).

Individual components may differ with regard to the ease with which they are consciously accessed. It is important to keep in mind, however, that conscious access is not identical to ease of self-report. Some components (e.g., peripheral part of the somatic component) may be easy to feel but difficult to put into words.

If one accepts that appraisal is a component of emotion and that aspects of all components are integrated and reflected in the content of the feeling component, it clearly follows that appraisal determines part of the content of the feeling component. If one accepts that appraisal is also a cause of the other components (motivational, somatic, motor), it also determines the content of the feeling component via its influence on the other components. In that case, appraisal is not a minor contributing factor, but the core determinant of feelings. This is the second criterion that we propose for delin-

eating appraisal theories from other emotion theories. Appraisal theorists think of appraisal as the core determinant of feelings, at least in most emotion episodes, due to its direct and indirect impact. It may be noted that the notion of appraisal as part of the content of feelings is compatible but not redundant with the notion of appraisal as a component of emotion. This is because only part of appraisal is reflected in consciousness.

Appraisal as a Consequence of the Other Components

Some theorists have emphasized the role of appraisal as a consequence of emotion (or of the other components). For example, Berkowitz (1990; Berkowitz & Harmon-Jones, 2004) has argued that an appraisal of agency and/or intentionality may occur as a consequence of a feeling of anger. Anger encourages people to search for someone to blame (an intentional agent). Here too, there can be different opinions about whether appraisal is a consequence in all, most, or only some emotion episodes.

Theorists (e.g., Berkowitz, 1990) who emphasize the role of appraisal as a consequence of emotion have often treated it as an alternative to the role of appraisal as a cause of emotion. Yet, the roles of cause and consequence are not incompatible, as long as two separate appraisal processes are involved (or two phases in the same appraisal process). In a first step, one appraisal process (or phase) may cause the other components. In a second step, the other components may cause a new appraisal process (or phase) corresponding to what we called *recurrence*. Saying that appraisal is more often a consequence than a cause of emotion amounts to saying that the second step occurs more often than the first step. Several appraisal theorists have acknowledged that the first step often consists of a rudimentary form of appraisal (involving only the simplest appraisal factors or mechanisms), whereas the second step gives rise to a more complex form of appraisal (involving more sophisticated appraisal factors or mechanisms; Frijda, 1993). Even in these cases, appraisal does act as a cause and as a consequence of the other components.

Appraisal as Merely Temporally Co-Occurring with Other Components

All the relations discussed so far imply that appraisal occurs in close temporal proximity (i.e., before, after, or simultaneously) with the other components. For the sake of completeness, we mention the possibility that appraisal occurs in close temporal proximity with the other components without there being any causal relations among the components. In theory, appraisal can precede the other components without causing them and it can follow the other components without being caused by them. Even theorists who exclude appraisal as a component of emotion may still accept temporal co-occurrence between appraisal and the other components.

Appraisal as Part of the Meaning of Emotion Labels

Several authors (Frijda, 1993; Frijda & Zeelenberg, 2001; Parkinson, 1997) have drawn attention to the fact that appraisal and emotion are conceptually related. Appraisal values are part of the meaning of vernacular emotion labels. For example, danger is part of fear, loss is part of sadness, and high coping potential and other-agency are part of anger. Once a person establishes a relation between two concepts, it becomes a sort of knowledge. This knowledge may or may not be activated during an emotional episode, and it may or may not have an influence on the other components. This knowledge may also be activated outside an emotion episode. The conceptual relation between appraisal and emotion may stem originally from any of the relations between appraisal and emotion described above (part–whole, causal, temporal co-occurrence), but it may also have other sources (e.g., culturally transmitted stereotypic schemas). Hence, knowledge about appraisals and emotions may reflect the actual co-occurrence of appraisals and emotions at some point in time or it may reflect an imagined co-occurrence. Like the other relations described above, the conceptual relation between appraisal and emotion may be considered as being necessary, typical, or occasional (Parkinson, 1997).

Starting from the idea that the meaning of emotion words can be exhaustively described by profile values on all components (Scherer, 2005, pp. 709–712), Fontaine, Scherer, and Soriano (in press) conducted an intercultural and cross-linguistic study involving 35 datasets from 27 countries covering a total of 24 different languages. For 24 emotion words native speakers indicated the probability with which 144 features, representing all components, would apply to a person described as experiencing the respective emotion. Multiple discriminant analyses revealed that 31 appraisal features allowed the correct classification of 71% of the cases (after cross-validation). Adding features of the other components led to relatively small increases of the accuracy percentage: 40 action tendency features increased it to 75.4%, 18 bodily sensations and 26 motor expression features increased it to 80.9%, and 22 feeling features added nothing. The fact that appraisal explains the lion's share of the variance and that all other components explain a relatively small share aligns with appraisal theories' claim that appraisal drives changes in the other components.

To summarize, appraisal theories and other emotion theories attribute several roles to appraisal. We have put forward two criteria to demarcate appraisal theories from other theories: Appraisal theories argue that appraisal is a typical cause of the other components in emotions, and because of this, they argue that appraisal is the core determinant of the content of feelings. In the next section, we explore the first criterion (that appraisal is a typical cause of the other components) in further detail, using illustrations from causal appraisal theories. After that, we identify the kinds of evidence that would be needed to support the causal claim, and we review some of the existing empirical evidence. Given that the second claim (that appraisal is the core determinant of feelings) follows from the first claim, finding evidence for the first claim is essential for the second claim as well.

Exploration of the Causal Claim

The causal chain from stimulus to emotion can be split into two steps. The first step deals with the stimulus. In the second step, the output of the first step is translated into an emotion or the other emotional components. Appraisal theories have addressed both steps in the causal chain. The appraisal process takes place in the first step. Translation of the appraisal values into emotions or values of the other components takes place in the second step. The processes occurring in each of these steps can be considered at each of the three levels of analysis (functional, algorithmic, and implementational). In this chapter, we consider hypotheses about the functional level, the algorithmic level, and the relation between the two levels. So far, there has been little systematic work on the implementational level for appraisal and its relation to the other levels (but see Sander, Grandjean, & Scherer, 2005; Scherer & Peper, 2001).

Emotion Causation
at the Functional Level

At the functional level of analysis, appraisal theories propose hypotheses about the appraisal factors that are processed (first step) and about links between appraisal values and specific emotions or values of the other components (second step). Hypotheses about the first step are related to those about the second step because it is implicitly assumed that only those appraisal factors are processed (first step) that play a role in the causation of emotions or their components (second step). Hypotheses about the second step take appraisal values as the independent variables. These values may be of the molar (e.g., danger, loss, and insult) or the molecular kind (e.g., goal congruent, high coping potential, and other agency). The dependent variables can be the occurrence, the intensity, and the quality of (1) an emotion or of (2) each of the other components (action tendencies, somatic responses, motor responses, and/or feelings). Actually, each of these components can be treated in a molar or a molecular way (see Table 8.1).

Many appraisal theories propose hypotheses about links between molecular appraisal values and entire emotions. For example, they predict that a pattern consisting of the molecular appraisal values of goal incongruent, high coping potential, and other-agency leads to anger (Ellsworth & Scherer, 2003). Other appraisal theories have hypothesized links between molecular appraisal values

and the molar values of the other components. For instance, some theorists predict that a pattern consisting of the appraisal values of goal incongruent, high coping potential, and other-agency leads to the tendency to attack. Few appraisal theorists hypothesize links between molecular appraisal values and molecular values of other components. Roseman (2001), for example, predicts that goal congruence leads to action tendencies characterized by approach, and that low coping potential leads to action tendencies characterized by adjustment of the self to the environment. Scherer (2001, 2009) and Smith (1989) predict (and investigate) links between molecular appraisal values and molecular values of facial and vocal expressions and physiological responses (see Table 8.2 for examples).

Emotion Causation
at the Algorithmic Level

Appraisal theories have developed hypotheses about mechanisms and the format of the representations involved in (1) appraisal (first step) and in (2) the translation of appraisal values into emotions or values of the other components (second step). In addition, some appraisal theories (e.g., Scherer, 2009) present hypotheses about how to span the bridge between the functional and algorithmic levels.

With regard to the first step, most appraisal theorists adopt a dual- or triple-mode model, accepting rule-based, associative, and/or sensory–motor mechanisms as ones underlying appraisal. In a rule-based mechanism, a rule is applied to a stimulus and computation of the rule produces an appraisal value. These values may or may not be integrated in a pattern. The associative mechanism is sometimes described as the spreading of activation from the representation of the stimulus to a representation of a pattern of appraisal values, but not many appraisal theories have detailed hypotheses about the structure of the associations and the format of the representations involved. As in other research domains in which a dual- or triple-mode view is endorsed, it is often assumed that the rule-based mechanism operates on verbal-like representations and that it is flexible but nonautomatic, whereas the associative and sensory–motor mechanisms are

TABLE 8.1. Examples of Molar and Molecular Values for (Sub)components of Emotions

	Molar values	Molecular factors + values
Appraisal	Danger Irrevocable loss Demeaning offense	Goal congruence: congruent/incongruent Coping potential: low/high Agency: self/other/circumstances
Action tendencies	Tendency to fight Tendency to flee Tendency to give in	Level of activity: active versus passive Direction of movement: toward versus away from stimulus Direction of fit: fit stimulus to self versus fit self to stimulus Target: self versus not self
Peripheral physiological responses	Boiling Shivering Blushing	Heart rate Blood pressure Galvanic skin response Muscle tension
Central physiological responses	No examples	Activity in amygdala Activity in prefrontal cortex
Facial expressions	Smiling face Scowling face Fearful face Sad face	Facial activity in terms of: Action units: mouth corners pulled up, inner eyebrows raised, nose wrinkle Face muscles: zygomaticus major, orbicularis occuli, corrugator supercilii
Vocal expressions	Screaming Laughter	Pitch Tempo Rhythm Pausing Loudness Frequency perturbations
Gross behavior	Fleeing Fighting Protecting Repairing	Level of activity: active versus passive Direction of movement: toward versus away from stimulus Direction of fit: fit stimulus to self versus fit self to stimulus Target: self versus not self
Feelings	Anger Fear Sadness Happiness	Valence Arousal Values of all other components reflected in consciousness

thought to operate on image-like representations and are rigid but automatic. These assumptions, however, have not been tested empirically and may not necessarily hold (cf. Moors, 2010). It is possible that both rule-based and associative mechanisms can operate on all kinds of representations and that they can both take place in an automatic or a nonautomatic way.

Another remark is that within the three classes of mechanisms presented here, there is still room for a variety of detailed proposals. For example, Scherer's (2009) component process model (CPM) predicts that the appraisal factors are often processed sequentially, in a fixed order. To be precise, the CPM assumes that the processes operate in parallel, but that they achieve *preliminary closure* (i.e., a reasonably definitive output) in a sequential way. The sequence assumption is based on phylogenetic, ontogenetic, and microgenetic considerations (Scherer, 1984, pp. 313–314; Scherer, Zentner, & Stern, 2004) and received support from experiments using brain activity, peripheral measures, and expression patterns (cf. Scherer, 2009). Other appraisal theorists posit that appraisal factors are processed

TABLE 8.2. Predicted Effects of Molecular Appraisal Factors on Molecular Values of Other Emotion Components

Appraisal values	Examples of expected effects on AT, PR, and EB
Novel and goal relevant	AT: Orienting PR: Heart rate deceleration, pupillary dilatation EB: Eyebrows and lids raised, jaw drop, gaze-directed pausing of speech and action
Intrinsically positive	AT: Sensitization PR: Heart rate deceleration, salivation, pupillary dilatation EB: Lids up, open mouth and nostrils, lips part with corners pulled up increase in low frequency voice energy, soft speech, approach locomotion
Intrinsically negative	AT: Defense response PR: Heart rate acceleration EB: Brow lowering, nose wrinkling, upper lip rising, nostril compression, gaze aversion, avoidance locomotion
Goal congruent	AT: Relaxation PR: Decrease in respiration and heart rate decrease, decrease in general muscle tone EB: Voice pitch and loudness decrease
Goal incongruent	AT: Activation PR: Increase in respiration and heart rate, strong increase in muscle tension EB: Frowning, lids tightening, lips pressed together, chin raising, gaze-directed; high and loud voice
No or low control	AT: Adjustment/withdrawal PR: Decrease in respiration and heart rate, hypotonus of the musculature EB: Lip corner depression, lips parting, jaw drops, lids droop, inner brow raises and outer brow lowers, gaze aversion; low and loud voice; few and slowed movements, slumped posture
High control/high power	AT: Assertion/dominance PR: Strong increase in respiration rate and depth; slight heart rate decrease; increase in systolic and diastolic blood pressure; increased blood flow to head, chest, and hands (reddening, increased skin temperature in upper torso); pupillary constriction; balanced muscle tone; tension increase in head and neck EB: Eyebrows contract, lids tight, eyes narrow, lips tight and parted, bare teeth or lips tight, pressed together, nostril dilation, stare; low and loud voice; strong energy in entire frequency range; agonistic hand/arm movements; erect posture, body leaning forward, approach locomotion
Control possible/low power	AT: Protection/submission PR: Extreme, faster, and more irregular respiration; strong increase in heart rate; increase in pulse volume amplitude; vasoconstriction in skin (pallor, decreased skin temperature), gastrointestinal tract, and sexual organs; increase in blood flow to striped musculature; stomach upset, goose bumps, sweating, trembling EB: Brow and lid raising, mouth stretch and corner retraction, high-pitched voice, protective hand/arm movements, fast locomotion or freezing

Note. See also Table 8.1. AT, action tendencies; PR, physiological responses; EB, expressive behavior. Adapted from Table 5.3 in Scherer (2001). Copyright 2001 by Oxford University Press. Adapted by permission.

in a partially sequential way or simultaneously. Figure 8.2 gives a schematic overview of the predictions of the CPM. The horizontal panel, labeled *appraisal processes* (also called *appraisal checks*), shows the different groups of appraisal factors (with the individual appraisal factors within each respective group) organized in the predicted sequence (see Ellsworth & Scherer, 2003; Scherer, 2001, 2009) together with the respective cognitive faculties (attention, memory, motivation, reasoning, self) that are recruited in these appraisal processes. The downward arrows represent the input of the cognitive faculties into the appraisal process (e.g., memory retrieval based on similarity), and the upward arrows represent a modification of these structures by the appraisal results (e.g., redirection of attention by a relevance appraisal). It may be noted that the sequence assumption is most pertinent for rule-based appraisal. In the case of associative appraisal, the appraisal values may become available in sequence or all at once.

With regard to the second step in the stimulus-to-components chain, there are two broad proposals. According to a first proposal, the appraisal values are integrated in a pattern before affecting the ensuing emotion (Smith & Kirby, 2001). According to a second proposal (cf. Scherer, 2009), each appraisal value has a separate influence on each of the other components in the emotion. According to a variant of this proposal, the influence of each appraisal value on the other components is mediated by the motivational component. In the CPM, for example, each appraisal value triggers an action tendency value shaping the values of the somatic and expressive components. In Figure 8.2, the other components are presented in the horizontal panels below the appraisal

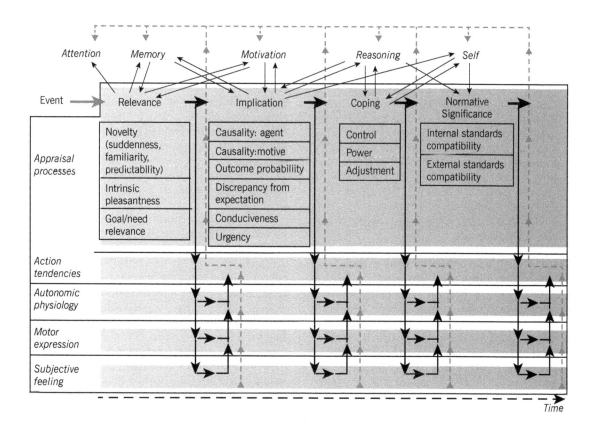

FIGURE 8.2. Predictions of the component process model on the sequential mechanisms involved in appraisal and their efferent effects on the various other components, highlighting the recursive and cumulative nature of the emotion episode. Adapted from Sander et al. (2005). Copyright 2005. Adapted with permission from Elsevier.

panel. The bold downward arrows illustrate the assumption that the appraisal values immediately, sequentially, and cumulatively influence the values of all other components. The feeling component integrates the changes in all the other components. Feelings correspond to representations of the multicomponential changes in the central nervous system. The dotted upward arrows represent the changes fed back to the appraisal process (and the cognitive structures subserving the appraisal process) where they may produce modifications of prior appraisals (i.e., reappraisal). This recursive feature of the model makes it radically dynamic.

The CPM clearly distinguishes between emotion episodes and the categorization or labeling of these episodes. The representation of the multicomponential changes triggered by certain appraisal outcomes in the central nervous system does not require, in and of itself, consciousness, categorization, or labeling. Rather, the latter processes are determined by many additional factors and the chosen category or label may represent only part of the emotion episode (see Scherer, 2009, pp. 1318–1323).

The first proposal (that all appraisal values need to be integrated in a pattern before influencing the other components) is compatible with a basic emotions view in which each basic emotion corresponds to a specific appraisal pattern. Moreover, such a proposal is not incompatible with a biological version of basic emotions theory, because each appraisal pattern may activate a brain circuit (i.e., affect program) dedicated to each basic emotion.

The second proposal (that each appraisal value independently influences the other components), on the other hand, is incompatible with a biological version of basic emotions theory (Moors, 2012; Scherer & Ellgring, 2007). Emotions are not latent constructs hardwired in our brains waiting to be triggered by the right appraisal pattern, like a lock that needs to be opened by the right key. They are emergent phenomena in the sense that their quality and intensity are shaped gradually with every additional piece of information resulting from each appraisal check. In line with this, the CPM does not assume the existence of a limited set of basic emotions, but considers the possibility of an infinite number of emotions (e.g., the generic

term *anger* may cover annoyance, exasperation, fury, gall, indignation, infuriation, irritation, outrage, petulance, rage, resentment, and vexation). Although other theories also accept the existence of "families" of emotions covering many shades, they do not explain how these shades come about. In contrast, appraisal theories explain the infinite variety by referring to the infinite number of possible appraisal configurations. We wish to note that the CPM does allow for so-called *modal* emotions (Scherer, 1994), such as anger and fear, that occur more frequently and engender more-or-less stereotypical responses to a frequently occurring type of event or stimulus (see Table 1 in Scherer, 2009).

Empirical Support for the Causal Claim

In this section, we examine the kind of empirical research that should be conducted to investigate the causal claim of appraisal theories. Before we do so, it is worth spending a few lines on what the term *causation* means. There are many approaches to causation. One approach that provides useful guidelines for the empirical study of causation is Mackie's (1974) proposal that a cause, C, of an effect, E, is an insufficient but necessary condition in a set of conditions that is itself unnecessary but sufficient for E. For example, dropping a lit cigarette in the woods is the cause of a fire if dropping the lit cigarette is, in itself, insufficient to cause the fire (other conditions are necessary, such as combustible material and oxygen), but it is a necessary part of a set of conditions (a set including the lit cigarette, the combustible material, and the oxygen) that is itself unnecessary (there may be other sets of conditions for fire, e.g., a set including a fire cracker, combustible material, and oxygen) but sufficient (when this set of conditions is present the fire is present as well). Appraisal is a cause of emotion when it is insufficient in itself for emotion (other conditions may be necessary, such as the condition that appraisal must have a certain output, e.g., goal relevant, goal congruent, goal incongruent, positive, negative, novel, or urgent), but it is a necessary part of a set of conditions that is itself unnecessary but sufficient for emotion. Based on this definition of causation, investigators who want to show that appraisal is a cause of emotion should find a set of conditions that is sufficient for emotion and demonstrate that appraisal is present in this set. In addition, they should demonstrate that the set is no longer sufficient when appraisal is eliminated from it.

We have argued that appraisal theories consider appraisal as a typical cause of emotion. Demonstrating that appraisal is a typical (let alone necessary) cause of emotion, however, is not a realistic aim of study. One cannot study most (let alone all) sets of conditions that are sufficient for emotion and demonstrate that appraisal is present in all these sets and that elimination of appraisal from these sets makes them insufficient. A more realistic aim is to demonstrate that appraisal is *a* cause of emotion (i.e., that there is one sufficient set of conditions in which appraisal is necessary), and preferably, to provide cumulative or converging evidence for this (i.e., that there are many sufficient sets of conditions in which appraisal is necessary). Emotion causation can be studied on all three levels of analysis. We focus here on ways to investigate emotion causation at the functional and algorithmic levels.

Testing Causal Hypotheses at the Functional Level of Analysis

The claim that appraisal causes emotion entails that appraisal not only determines the occurrence of emotions but also their intensity and quality. In addition to the general claim that appraisal determines the occurrence, intensity, and quality of emotions, appraisal theories also make specific claims about the specific appraisal factors involved in each of these effects (occurrence, intensity, and quality).

The general claim that appraisal causes emotions (with an intensity and quality) can be studied by comparing one set of conditions in which appraisal is present with another set in which appraisal is absent (independent variable) and by registering the presence or absence of emotion (dependent variable). To manipulate the presence or absence of appraisal, appraisal must be instantiated; that is, one must choose a certain pattern of appraisal values to be present or absent. Failure to find an effect does not, ipso facto, mean that appraisal does not

cause emotions. It may also mean that the wrong pattern of appraisal values was chosen.

The specific claims (about the specific appraisal factors involved in the occurrence, intensity, and quality of emotions) can be studied by manipulating the appraisal factors figuring in them and by measuring the presence or absence of emotions, their intensity, and their quality. Again, failure to find an effect of one of these appraisal factors means that the specific claim is false and requires adjustment, but not that the general claim is false as well. In the next sections, we discuss ways in which to manipulate appraisal processes and ways to measure the other components. For historical reasons, we first briefly review early studies in which appraisal was not manipulated but merely measured.

Measurement of Appraisal

Appraisals have been measured with self-report, based on the assumption that people have conscious access to appraisal on a functional level of analysis. In recall studies, participants are asked to recall emotion episodes (e.g., anger) and to rate the respective appraisals (e.g., who caused the event; Mauro, Sato, & Tucker, 1992; Roseman, Spindel, & Jose, 1990; Scherer, 1993; Scherer & Wallbott, 1994). A few studies measured appraisals in real-life situations. For instance, Smith and Ellsworth (1987) studied students' appraisals before and after taking an exam. Scherer and Ceschi (1997) measured appraisals of airline passengers immediately after having registered lost luggage. Although such self-report studies suggest the plausibility of the causal claim, experimental manipulation of appraisal is required to obtain empirical evidence.

Manipulation of Appraisal

Appraisal factors can be manipulated in a variety of ways: either (1) directly, with verbal stimuli that literally refer to appraisal values, or (2) indirectly, by manipulating stimuli in the expectation that participants will appraise them in a certain way, but without explicit verbal reference to appraisal values. In indirect methods, the to-be-appraised stimuli can be (1) really present (e.g., a real dog appears), or (2) externally represented in visual (e.g., picture of a dog) or verbal form (e.g., the word *dog*).

Examples of procedures in which real events are manipulated are experiments (1) presented as ability tests (Kreibig, Gendolla, & Scherer, 2010; Kulik & Brown, 1979; McGregor, Nash, & Inzlicht, 2009; Mikulincer, 1988; Smith & Kirby, 2009; Smith & Pope, 1992) or (2) construed as interactive games (e.g., ultimatum games; Harle & Sanfey, 2010; Yamagishi et al., 2009) in which participants compete with real (e.g., Bossuyt, Moors, & De Houwer, 2012; Cherek, Lane, & Pietras, 2003; McCloskey, Berman, & Coccaro, 2005) or virtual opponents (Johnstone, van Reekum, Hird, Kirsner, & Scherer, 2005; Kappas & Pecchinenda, 1999; Nelissen & Zeelenberg, 2009). In these experiments, participants encounter events that are (1) relevant or irrelevant for goals (Moors & De Houwer, 2001), (2) congruent or incongruent with goals (e.g., the goal to achieve, or to win a prize; Moors & De Houwer, 2001; Smith & Pope, 1992), (3) pleasant or unpleasant (e.g., words, pictures, sound blasts, electroshocks, tastes, virtual enemies; Geen, 1978; Johnstone et al., 2005; Roseman & Evdokas, 2004), (4) easy or difficult to cope with (e.g., Cherek, Spiga, Steinberg, & Kelly, 1990; Galinsky, Gruenfeld, & Magee, 2003; Geen, 1978; McCloskey et al., 2005), (5) certain or uncertain (e.g., Roseman & Evdokas, 2004), (6) caused by themselves or by others (Bossuyt et al., 2012), and (7) fair or unfair (e.g., Batson et al., 2007; Weiss, Suckow, & Cropanzano, 1999). In all these experiments, researchers expect participants to appraise the stimuli in the intended way.

Procedures in which the to-be-appraised stimuli or events are not really present but externally represented in verbal (words or stories) or visual form (pictures or films) are scenario studies and recall studies. In scenario studies (e.g., Kuppens, Van Mechelen, Smits, De Boeck, & Ceulemans, 2007; Robinson & Clore, 2001; Zeelenberg, van Dijk, & Manstead, 1998), participants are presented with fictitious events (verbal or visual) and instructed or expected to imagine that these events would happen to them. In recall studies, participants receive verbal instructions to retrieve events from their past. In both scenario and recall studies, appraisals

can be manipulated directly or indirectly. In the direct case, instructions literally refer to appraisal values (e.g., "Imagine that you have low power," Smith & Bargh, 2008; "Recall an event in which you had low power," Fast & Chen, 2009; Galinsky et al., 2003; Kuppens, Van Mechelen, Smits, & De Boeck, 2003; Lammers, Galinsky, Gordijn, & Otten, 2008). In the indirect case, events are described or depicted without explicit reference to appraisal values (e.g., de Hooge, Zeelenberg, & Breugelmans, 2010; Kuppens et al., 2007).

At least three issues are important to consider when choosing procedures for manipulating appraisal factors. A first issue is that of controlling for confounding variables. Procedures with real events in the laboratory allow for more control over confounding variables than those with imagined or recalled events. For instance, coping potential can be manipulated by leaving a door open or closed in a computer game or by telling participants that a door is open or closed in a verbal scenario. In the computer game, participants have no way to escape, whereas in the verbal scenario, they may imagine escape via a window. If we compare scenario procedures of the indirect (in which events are described in an appraisal-free manner) and direct type (in which events are described in appraisal terms), we argue that the former allows for more control over the confounding variables related to the concrete details of the events, whereas the latter allows for more control over confounding appraisal factors. For example, the scenario of hitting one's head against the kitchen cabinet (i.e., indirect type) allows the researcher to control the concrete features of the event, but not whether the person appraises the event merely as goal incongruent or as also caused by another agent (e.g., when the kitchen cabinet is treated as an agent for a split second). The scenario of appraising another person as the cause of a goal-incongruent event (i.e., direct type) allows less control over the concrete features of the event (many concrete events can be imagined that fit this appraisal pattern), but more control over the appraisal factors (the event is appraised as goal incongruent and caused by another person).

A second issue is the extent to which the processes induced by the manipulation resemble the processes induced by real emotion-eliciting events outside the laboratory. Compared to externally represented events, real events in the laboratory are more likely to induce the same processes as real events outside the laboratory. Many authors have suggested that externally represented events activate knowledge about the relation between appraisals and emotions, whereas real events induce real emotion-eliciting processes (e.g., Parkinson, 1997). The fact that externally represented events (e.g., films) can also elicit emotions raises the question of whether the activation of knowledge differs from so-called real emotion-eliciting processes, and as a consequence, whether the emotions elicited by externally represented events are of a special kind (e.g., Levinson, 1990; Radford, 1995). There is reason to believe that the activation of knowledge is especially likely when verbal material is used.

To summarize, the manipulation of real events has the advantage that there is control over confounding variables, but the disadvantage that one cannot be entirely sure that the participants appraise the events in the way the researcher expects them to. This is not always a problem and it can partly be met by adding a manipulation check. The manipulation of externally represented events that refer explicitly to appraisal factors allows one to have more control over the appraisal factors at stake, but runs the risk of inducing processes (e.g., the activation of conceptual knowledge) that are different from the ones induced by real events.

Measurement of Other Components

Measurement of the other components in the emotion episode can be done with a variety of procedures: objective and subjective ones and direct and indirect ones. Objective measures produce responses that are verifiable by others; subjective measures do not (cf. Muckler, 1992). Examples of objective measures are ones producing reaction times or other aspects of motor responses, electroencephalographic (EEG) signals, and skin conductance responses. Subjective measures rely on reports by internal (i.e., self-reports) or external observers, at least when the content of the reports is considered as the response (and not objective aspects such as reaction times). Subjective measures are suitable only

for constructs that are (to some extent) consciously accessible to the observer.

Following De Houwer and Moors (2010), we call a measure *direct* when the researcher uses the responses as a direct readout of the values of the to-be-measured variable. For example, self-reports of action tendencies (e.g., "I had the tendency to attack"; e.g., Frijda, Kuipers, & ter Schure, 1989) directly deliver the values of the to-be-measured variable of action tendencies. Likewise, a heart rate monitor directly delivers the values of the to-be-measured variable of heart rate. We call a measure *indirect* when the researcher derives the values of the to-be-measured variable from the values of another variable that is assumed to be influenced by the to-be-measured variable. For example, motor responses can be used as an indirect measure of action tendencies (e.g., Martinez, Zeelenberg, & Rijsman, 2011), based on the assumption that motor responses are influenced by action tendencies.

Components referring to overt responses, such as somatic and motor components, are preferably measured with direct measures, either objective ones (heart rate, blood pressure, skin conductance, overt behavior) or subjective ones (self-reports of somatic and motor responses). Components referring to internal constructs, such as action tendencies and feelings, cannot be measured with direct objective measures (they cannot be read out directly from responses that are verifiable by others). They can be measured with indirect objective measures (e.g., using behavior to infer the presence of action tendencies), direct subjective measures (e.g., self-reports of action tendencies and feelings; de Hooge et al., 2010; Frijda et al., 1989), and indirect subjective measures (e.g., using self-reports of behavior to infer the presence of action tendencies).

Testing Causal Hypotheses at the Algorithmic Level of Analysis

In addition to research about the functional level, there is also need to do research about the algorithmic level and about the link between both levels. In the present section, we consider empirical evidence for one specific hypothesis proposed by the CPM: that appraisal factors influence the other components in a sequential fashion. Various studies demonstrate that appraisal checks have a sequential influence on facial expressions and peripheral and central physiological activity. Lanctôt and Hess (2007) showed a sequential influence of intrinsic valence and goal congruence on zygomaticus and corrugator activity measured with electromyography (EMG). Aue, Flykt, and Scherer (2007) showed sequential effects of appraisals on heart rate and facial muscle innervations. Delplanque and colleagues (2009) showed that the appraisal of an odor as novel or familiar produces earlier effects on facial expressions (using EMG) and physiological reactions (using electrocardiogram and electrodermal activity) than the appraisal of the odor as positive or negative. Grandjean and Scherer (2008) and van Peer, Grandjean, and Scherer (2012) manipulated novelty, goal relevance, intrinsic valence, and goal congruence appraisals in visual stimuli and observed their sequential influence on EEG recordings (using topographical analyses of the event-related potentials and frequency bands). Gentsch, Grandjean, and Scherer (2013) extended this approach by showing that the coping potential check occurred after the goal congruence check. Empirical support for the sequence hypothesis strengthens the causal claim defended in this chapter. The observation that different appraisal factors affect the other components at different points in time suggests that they are supported by mechanisms with different latencies. This, in turn, suggests that appraisal is an intervening mental process and not merely a description of the stimulus situation.

Conclusion

There is now fair agreement among emotion theories that emotions are multicomponential episodes and that appraisal is a component in these episodes (Frijda, 2007; Moors, Ellsworth, Scherer, & Frijda, in press). The family of appraisal theories, however, goes beyond the facile inclusion of appraisal as one of many components in emotion episodes by arguing for a strong causal role of appraisal in determining the other components. As a consequence, appraisal is considered to be a major determinant of the content of feelings.

In a detailed exploration of the causal claim, we listed possible hypotheses about two steps in the stimulus-to-components chain (the step in which the stimulus is appraised and the step in which the output of appraisal influences the remaining components) at the functional and algorithmic levels of analysis.

We discussed methods to investigate hypotheses of appraisal theories formulated at the functional level of analysis. The general claim that appraisal is a typical cause of emotion is difficult if not impossible to prove in a definitive way. To support the plausibility of this claim, however, appraisal researchers are invited to provide cumulative support for it. The specific hypotheses about the specific appraisal factors that determine the presence, intensity, and quality of emotions or components are easier to study, relatively speaking. We listed ways to manipulate appraisals and ways to measure other emotional components. For the manipulation of appraisal, we distinguished between direct and indirect methods, and between methods using real events and externally represented events. For the measurement of emotions or emotional components, we distinguished between objective and subjective methods and between direct and indirect methods. Each method for the manipulation of appraisal can be combined with each method for measuring emotions or components. Contemporary appraisal researchers not only try to answer questions at the functional level of analysis, but also at the algorithmic level. To illustrate this, we discussed recent empirical support for the sequence hypothesis of the CPM (Scherer, 2009).

Central questions in emotion research concern how emotions come about and what factors determine their intensity and quality. Appraisal theories take up the challenge by proposing and testing hypotheses about the nature of these determinants (in the form of appraisal factors and values) and by specifying detailed links between these determinants and their effects (values on the other components). Appraisal is presented as a mental process that is specifically concerned with the postulated appraisal factors. Thus, the appraisal factors are more than descriptors of the situations that elicit emotions; they are the types of information that are somehow processed by the organism. The question of how they are processed is addressed in hypotheses about the underlying mechanisms and representations.

By defending the causal role of appraisal in emotions, appraisal theories put themselves in a vulnerable position. Empirical proof for causation is never definitive (even in experimental studies), and alternative explanations always lie in wait. Many appraisal theorists accept other processes than appraisal as possible causes of emotions, but only in marginal cases. The difficulty to prove that appraisal is a cause of emotions, let alone a typical cause, is not *in itself* a reason to reject it or to put forward other processes as typical causes. They too need to stand the test of causation. Unfortunately, many alternative emotion theories do not provide sufficiently precise hypotheses to allow rigorous empirical testing.

Acknowledgments

Preparation of this chapter was supported by Methusalem Grant (No. BOF09/01M00209) of Ghent University and an ERC Advanced Grant (No. PROPEREMO 230331) to Klaus R. Scherer.

References

Arnold, M. B. (1960). *Emotion and personality.* New York: Columbia University Press.

Aue, T., Flykt, A., & Scherer, K. R. (2007). First evidence for differential and sequential efferent effects of stimulus relevance and goal conduciveness appraisal. *Biological Psychology, 74,* 347–357.

Batson, C. D., Kennedy, C. L., Nord, L., Stocks, E. L., Fleming, D. A., Lisher, D. A., et al. (2007). Anger at unfairness: Is it moral outrage? *European Journal of Social Psychology, 37,* 1272–1285.

Berkowitz, L. (1990). On the formation and regulation of anger and aggression: A cognitive-neoassociationistic analysis. *American Psychologist, 45,* 494–503.

Berkowitz, L., & Harmon-Jones, E. (2004). Toward an understanding of the determinants of anger. *Emotion, 4,* 107–130.

Bossuyt, E., Moors, A., & De Houwer, J. (2012). *Experimentally studying the influence of appraisal on action tendencies: The case of the influence of agency on reparative and aggressive action tendencies.* Manuscript submitted for publication.

Cherek, D. R., Lane, S. D., & Pietras, C. J. (2003). Laboratory measures of aggression: Point subtraction aggression paradigm (PSAP). In E. F. Coccaro (Ed.), *Aggression: Assessment and treatment into the 21st century* (pp. 215–228). New York: Marcel Dekker.

Cherek, D. R., Spiga, R., Steinberg, J. L., & Kelly, T. H. (1990). Human aggressive responses maintained by escape or escape from point loss. *Journal of the Experimental Analysis of Behavior, 53,* 293–304.

Clore, G. L., & Ortony, A. (2000). Cognition in emotion: Always, sometimes, or never? In R. D. Lane & L. Nadel (Eds.), *Cognitive neuroscience of emotion* (pp. 24–61). New York: Oxford University Press.

Clore, G. L., & Ortony, A. (2008). Appraisal theories: How cognition shapes affect into emotion. In M. Lewis, J. M. Haviland-Jones, & L. Feldman Barrett (Eds.), *Handbook of emotions* (3rd ed., pp. 628–642). New York: Guilford Press.

de Hooge, I. E., Zeelenberg, M., & Breugelmans, S. M. (2010). Restore and protect motivations following shame. *Cognition and Emotion, 24,* 111–127.

De Houwer, J., & Moors, A. (2010). Implicit measures: Similarities and differences. In B. Gawronski & B. K. Payne (Eds.), *Handbook of implicit social cognition: Measurement, theory, and applications* (pp. 176–193). New York: Guilford Press.

Delplanque, S., Grandjean, D., Chrea, C., Copping, G., Aymard, L., Cayeux, L., et al., (2009). Sequential unfolding of novelty and pleasantness appraisals of odors: Evidence from facial electromyography and autonomic reaction. *Emotion, 9,* 316–328.

de Sousa, R. (1987). *The rationality of emotion.* Cambridge, MA: MIT Press.

Ekman, P. (1972). Universals and cultural differences in facial expression of emotion. In J. R. Cole (Ed.), *Nebraska Symposium on Motivation* (pp. 207–283). Lincoln: University of Nebraska Press.

Ekman, P. (2004). What we become emotional about. In A. S. R. Manstead, N. H. Frijda, & A. H. Fischer (Eds.), *Feelings and emotions: The Amsterdam symposium* (pp. 119–135). Cambridge, UK: Cambridge University Press.

Ellsworth, P. C. (1994). William James and emotion: Is a century of fame worth a century of misunderstanding? *Psychological Review, 101*, 222–229

Ellsworth, P. C., & Scherer, K. R. (2003). Appraisal processes in emotion. In R. J. Davidson, K. R. Scherer, & H. Goldsmith (Eds.), *Handbook of the affective sciences* (pp. 572–595). New York: Oxford University Press.

Fast, N. J., & Chen, S. (2009). When the boss feels inadequate: Power, incompetence, and aggression. *Psychological Science, 20*, 1406–1413.

Feldman Barrett, L. (2006). Solving the emotion paradox: Categorization and the experience of emotion. *Personality and Social Psychology Review, 10*, 20–46.

Fontaine, J. R. J., Scherer, K. R., & Soriano, C. (Eds.). (in press). *Components of emotional meaning: A sourcebook.* Oxford, UK: Oxford University Press.

Frijda, N. H. (1986). *The emotions.* New York: Cambridge University Press.

Frijda, N. H. (1993). The place of appraisal in emotion. *Cognition and Emotion, 7*, 357–387.

Frijda, N. H. (2007). *The laws of emotion.* Mahwah, NJ: Erlbaum.

Frijda, N. H., Kuipers, P., & ter Schure, L. (1989). Relations between emotion, appraisal, and emotional action readiness. *Journal of Personality and Social Psychology, 57*, 212–228.

Frijda, N. H., & Zeelenberg, M. (2001). What is the dependent? In K. R. Scherer, A. Schorr, & T. Johnstone (Eds.), *Appraisal processes in emotion* (pp. 141–155). New York: Oxford University Press.

Galinsky, A. D., Gruenfeld, D. H., & Magee, J. C. (2003). From power to action. *Journal of Personality and Social Psychology, 85*, 453–466.

Geen, R. G. (1978). Effects of attack and uncontrollable noise on aggression. *Journal of Research in Personality, 12*, 15–29.

Gentsch, K., Grandjean, D., & Scherer, K. R. (2013). *Temporal dynamics of event-related potentials related to goal conduciveness and coping potential appraisals.* Manuscript submitted for publication.

Grandjean, D., & Scherer, K. R. (2008). Unpacking the cognitive architecture of emotion processes. *Emotion, 8*, 341–351.

Harle, K. M., & Sanfey, A. G. (2010). Effects of approach and withdrawal motivation on interactive economic decisions. *Cognition and Emotion, 24*, 1456–1465.

Izard, C. E. (1977). *Human emotions.* New York: Plenum Press.

James, W. (1894). The physical basis of emotion. *Psychological Review, 1*, 516–529.

James, W. (1969). What is an emotion? In *William James: Collected essays and reviews* (pp. 244–280). New York: Russell & Russell. (Original work published 1884)

Johnstone, T., van Reekum, C. M., Hird, K., Kirsner, K., & Scherer, K. R. (2005). Affective speech elicited with a computer game. *Emotion, 5*, 513–518.

Kappas, A., & Pecchinenda, A. (1999). Don't wait for the monsters to get you: A video game task to manipulate appraisals in real time. *Cognition, 13*, 119–124.

Keltner, D., Ellsworth, P. C., & Edwards, K. (1993). Beyond simple pessimism: Effects of sadness and anger on social perception. *Journal of Personality and Social Psychology, 4*, 740–752.

Kreibig, S. D., Gendolla, G. H. E., & Scherer, K. R. (2010). Psychophysiological effects of emotional responding to goal attainment. *Biological Psychology, 84*, 474–487.

Kulik, J. A., & Brown, R. (1979). Frustration, attribution of blame, and aggression. *Journal of Experimental Social Psychology, 15*, 183–194.

Kuppens, P., Van Mechelen, I., Smits, D. J. M., & De Boeck, P. (2003). The appraisal basis of anger: Specificity, necessity, and sufficiency of components. *Emotion, 3*, 254–269.

Kuppens, P., Van Mechelen, I., Smits, D. J. M., De Boeck, P., & Ceulemans, E. (2007). Individual differences in patterns of appraisal and anger experience. *Cognition and Emotion, 21*, 689–713.

Lambie, J. A., & Marcel, A. J. (2002). Consciousness and emotion experience: A theoretical framework. *Psychological Review, 109*, 219–259.

Lammers, J., Galinsky, A. D., Gordijn, E. H., & Otten, S. (2008). Illegitimacy moderates the effects of power on approach. *Psychological Science, 19*, 558–564.

Lanctôt, N., & Hess, U. (2007). The timing of appraisals. *Emotion, 7*, 207–212.

Lazarus, R. S. (1966). *Psychological stress and the coping process.* New York: McGraw-Hill.

Lazarus, R. S. (1991). *Emotion and adaptation.* New York: Oxford University Press.

Leventhal, H., & Scherer, K. R. (1987). The relationship of emotion to cognition: A functional approach to a semantic controversy. *Cognition and Emotion, 1,* 3–28.

Levinson, J. (1990). The place of real emotion in response to fictions. *Journal of Aesthetics and Art Criticism, 48,* 79–80.

Mackie, J. L. (1974). *The cement of the universe: A study of causation.* Oxford, UK: Clarendon Press.

Marr, D. (Ed.). (1982). *Vision: A computational investigation into the human representation and processing of visual information.* New York: Freeman.

Martinez, L. M. F., Zeelenberg, M., & Rijsman, J. B. (2011). Behavioural consequences of regret and disappointment in social bargaining games. *Cognition and Emotion, 25,* 351–359.

Mauro, R., Sato, K., & Tucker, J. (1992). The role of appraisal in human emotions: A cross-cultural study. *Journal of Personality and Social Psychology, 62,* 301–317.

McCloskey, M. S., Berman, M. E., & Coccaro, E. F. (2005). Providing an escape option reduces retaliatory aggression. *Aggressive Behavior, 31,* 228–237.

McGregor, I., Nash, K. A., Inzlicht, M. (2009). Threat, high self-esteem, and reactive approach motivation: Electroencephalographic evidence. *Journal of Experimental Social Psychology, 45,* 1003–1007.

Mikulincer, M. (1988). Reactance and helplessness following exposure to unsolvable problems: The effects of attributional style. *Journal of Personality and Social Psychology, 54,* 679–686.

Moors, A. (2010). Automatic constructive appraisal as a candidate cause of emotion. *Emotion Review, 2,* 139–156.

Moors, A. (2012). Comparison of affect program theories, appraisal theories, and psychological construction theories. In P. Zachar & R. D. Ellis (Eds.), *Categorical versus dimensional models of affect: A seminar on the theories of Panksepp and Russell* (pp. 257–278). Amsterdam: John Benjamins.

Moors, A., & De Houwer, J. (2001). Automatic appraisal of motivational valence: Motivational affective priming and Simon effects. *Cognition and Emotion, 15,* 749–766.

Moors, A., & De Houwer, J. (2006). Automaticity: A theoretical and conceptual analysis. *Psychological Bulletin, 132,* 297–326.

Moors, A., Ellsworth, P., Scherer, K. R., & Frijda, N. H. (in press). Appraisal theories of emotion: State of the art and future development. *Emotion Review.*

Muckler, F. A. (1992). Selecting performance measures: "Objective" versus "subjective" measurement. *Human Factors, 34,* 441–455.

Mulligan, K., & Scherer, K. R. (2012). Toward a working definition of emotion. *Emotion Review, 4,* 345–357.

Nelissen, R. M. A., & Zeelenberg, M. (2009). When guilt evokes self-punishment: Evidence for the existence of a dobby effect. *Emotion, 9,* 118–122.

Ortony, A., & Turner, T. J. (1990). What's basic about basic emotions? *Psychological Review, 97,* 315–331.

Parkinson, B. (1997). Untangling the appraisal–emotion connection. *Personality and Social Psychology Review, 1,* 62–79.

Parrott, G. W. (2007). Components and the definition of emotion. *Social Science Information, 46,* 419–423.

Radford, C. (1995). Fiction, pity, fear, and jealousy. *Journal of Aesthetics and Art Criticism, 53,* 71–75.

Robinson, M. D., & Clore, G. L. (2001). Simulation, scenarios, and emotional appraisal: Testing the convergence of real and imagined reactions to emotional stimuli. *Personality and Social Psychology Bulletin, 27,* 1520–1532.

Roseman, I. J. (2001). A model of appraisal in the emotion system: Integrating theory, research, and applications. In K. R. Scherer, A. Schorr, & T. Johnstone (Eds.), *Appraisal processes in emotion: Theory, methods, research* (pp. 68–91). New York: Oxford University Press.

Roseman, I. J., & Evdokas, A. (2004). Appraisals cause experienced emotions: Experimental evidence. *Cognition and Emotion, 18,* 1–28.

Roseman, I. J., Spindel, M. S., & Jose, P. E. (1990). Appraisals of emotion-eliciting events: Testing a theory of discrete emotions. *Journal of Personality and Social Psychology, 59,* 899–915.

Russell, J. A. (2003). Core affect and the psychological construction of emotion. *Psychological Review, 110,* 145?172.

Sander, D., Grandjean, D., & Scherer, K. R. (2005). A systems approach to appraisal mechanisms in emotion. *Neural Networks, 18,* 317–352.

Scherer, K. R. (1984). On the nature and function of emotion: A component process approach. In K. R. Scherer & P. Ekman (Eds.), *Approaches to emotion* (pp. 293–317). Hillsdale, NJ: Erlbaum.

Scherer, K. R. (1993). Studying the emotion–antecedent appraisal process: An expert system approach. *Cognition and Emotion, 7,* 325–355.

Scherer, K. R. (1994). Toward a concept of "modal emotions." In P. Ekman & R. J. Davidson (Eds.), *The nature of emotion: Fundamental questions* (pp. 25–31). New York: Oxford University Press.

Scherer, K. R. (1999). Appraisal theories. In T. Dalgleish & M. Power (Eds.), *Handbook of cognition and emotion* (pp. 637–663). Chichester, UK: Wiley.

Scherer, K. R. (2001). Appraisal considered as a process of multilevel sequential checking. In K. R. Scherer, A. Schorr, & T. Johnstone (Eds.), *Appraisal processes in emotion* (pp. 92–120). New York: Oxford University Press.

Scherer, K. R. (2005). What are emotions? And how can they be measured? *Social Science Information, 44,* 693–727.

Scherer, K. R. (2009). The dynamic architecture of emotion: Evidence for the component process model. *Cognition and Emotion, 23,* 1307–1351.

Scherer, K. R., & Ceschi, G. (1997). Lost luggage: A field study of emotion–antecedent appraisal. *Motivation and Emotion, 21,* 211–235.

Scherer, K. R., & Ellgring, H. (2007). Are facial expressions of emotion produced by categorical affect programs or dynamically driven by appraisal? *Emotion, 7,* 113–130.

Scherer, K. R., & Peper, M. (2001). Psychological theories of emotion and neuropsychological research. In F. Boller & J. Grafman (Eds.), *Handbook of neuropsychology: Vol. 5. Emotional behavior and its disorders* (pp. 17–48). Amsterdam: Elsevier.

Scherer, K. R., & Wallbott, H. G. (1994). Evidence for universality and cultural variation of differential emotion response patterning. *Journal of Personality and Social Psychology, 66,* 310–328.

Scherer, K. R., Zentner, M. R., & Stern, D. (2004). Beyond surprise: The puzzle of infants' expressive reactions to expectancy violation. *Emotion, 4,* 389–402.

Schorr, A. (2001). Appraisal: The evolution of an idea. In K. R. Scherer, A. Schorr, & T. Johnstone (Eds.), *Appraisal processes in emotion: Theory, methods, research* (pp. 20–34). New York: Oxford University Press.

Smith, C. A. (1989). Dimensions of appraisal and physiological response in emotion. *Journal of Personality and Social Psychology, 56,* 339–353.

Smith, C. A., & Ellsworth, P. C. (1987). Patterns of appraisal and emotion related to taking an exam. *Journal of Personality and Social Psychology, 52,* 475–488.

Smith, C. A., & Kirby, L. D. (2000). Consequences require antecedents: Towards a process model of emotion elicitation. In J. P. Forgas (Ed.), *Feeling and thinking: The role of affect in social cognition* (pp. 83–106). Cambridge, UK: Cambridge University Press.

Smith, C. A., & Kirby, L. D. (2001). Toward delivering on the promise of appraisal theory. In K. R. Scherer, A. Schorr, & T. Johnstone (Eds.), *Appraisal processes in emotion* (pp. 121–138). New York: Oxford University Press.

Smith, C. A., & Kirby, L. D. (2009). Relational antecedents of appraised problem-focused coping potential and its associated emotions. *Cognition and Emotion, 23,* 481–503.

Smith, C. A., & Lazarus, R. S. (1993). Appraisal components, core relational themes, and the emotions. *Cognition and Emotion, 7,* 233–269.

Smith, C. A., & Pope, L. K. (1992). Appraisal and emotion: The interactional contributions of dispositional and situational factors. In M. S. Clark (Ed.), *Review of personality and social psychology: Vol. 14. Emotion and social behavior* (pp. 32–62). Newbury Park, CA: Sage.

Smith, E. R., & Neumann, R. (2005). Emotion processes considered from the perspective of dual-process models. In L. Feldman Barrett, P. M. Niedenthal, & P. Winkielman (Eds.), *Emotion and consciousness* (pp. 287–311). New York: Guilford Press.

Smith, P. K., & Bargh, J. A. (2008). Nonconscious effects of power on basic approach and avoidance tendencies. *Social Cognition, 26,* 1–24.

Solomon, R. C. (1984). *The passions: The myth and nature of human emotions.* New York: Doubleday.

Tomkins, S. S. (1962). *Affect, imagery, consciousness: Vol. 1. The positive affects.* New York: Springer.

van Peer, J., Grandjean, D., & Scherer, K. R. (2012). *Sequential unfolding and interactions of novelty and pleasantness appraisals: Evi-*

dence from electroencephalography. Manuscript submitted for publication.

van Reekum, C. M., & Scherer, K. R. (1997). Levels of processing for emotion–antecedent appraisal. In G. Matthews (Ed.), *Cognitive science perspectives on personality and emotion* (pp. 259–300). Amsterdam: Elsevier.

Weiss, H. M., Suckow, K., & Cropanzano, R. (1999). Effects of justice conditions on discrete emotions. *Journal of Applied Psychology, 84,* 786–794.

Yamagishi, T., Horita, Y., Takagishi, H., Shinada, M., Tanida, S., & Cook, K. S. (2009). The private rejection of unfair offers and emotional commitment. *Proceedings of the National Academy of Sciences of the United States of America, 106,* 11520–11523.

Zeelenberg, M., van Dijk, W. W., & Manstead, A. S. R. (1998). Reconsidering the relation between regret and responsibility. *Organizational Behavior and Human Decision Processes, 74,* 254–272.

CHAPTER 9

Episodic Memory and Emotion

Brendan D. Murray, Alisha C. Holland, and Elizabeth A. Kensinger

Memory is the ability to store, retain, and retrieve information, enabling experiences from the past to influence current behavior. These influences of the past can take many forms. They can be revealed in our acquisition of skills, in our accumulation of world knowledge, and in our reminiscences about our past. Although emotion is likely to interact with each of these aspects of memory, in this chapter we focus on its interactions with *episodic* memories, of specific events that have taken place in our past (Tulving, 1983). These events may be as circumscribed as the viewing of a particular picture within the context of a psychology experiment or as elongated as a spring break vacation. The critical commonality among these events is that we remember them as experiences from a particular time and place within our personal past.

In this chapter we discuss the reciprocal interactions between episodic memory and emotion. We first describe the way in which emotion can influence episodic memory, examining how the emotional content of an experience can influence the way in which the event is remembered. We then discuss how the retrieval of episodic memories can influence our affective state, discussing the ability for episodic retrieval to be used as

a means of affect regulation. We conclude with a discussion of some of the important variables that may moderate these interactions, including effects of age, anxiety level, and cognitive flexibility.

The Effect of Emotion on Episodic Memory

There has been a recent fascination with reports of individuals with "superior autobiographical memories," who seem to remember every event from their past (Parker, Cahill, & McGaugh, 2006). The completeness of their memory stores seems to stand in stark contrast to that of the average person, who can remember only a fraction of past experiences. For most of us, the segments we retain are those moments imbued with emotion (Hamann, 2001), and as Brown and Kulik (1977) reported in their seminal paper on "flashbulb memories," the details of these moments seem to stay with us over the long term. The effects of emotion on memory arise during multiple stages of memory: Emotion influences the way that information is initially processed and transformed into a memory (the step of *encoding*), affects the way that information is stabilized (the process of *consolidation*), and biases the way that we reexperience a memory (the act of *retrieval*).

The construct of "emotion" is typically divided along two dimensions in operational terms: how exciting or calming an emotional stimulus is ("arousal") and how pleasant or unpleasant it is ("valence"; Posner, Russell, & Peterson, 2005; Russell, 1980). Much of the extant research has focused on the role of arousal; however, we also examine evidence for an influence of valence on memory encoding. Because less research has focused on how memory is influenced by the particular feeling experienced (e.g., sadness or anger), we do not focus on that topic here, though we do note it to be an important direction for further research.

The Effect of Emotion on Memory Encoding

In much the same way that our keystrokes on a computer become transformed into a format that can appear on our screen, so must a set of cognitive and neural processes enable our processing of the world around us to be recorded. The initiation of these processes is referred to as *encoding*. Whether information is emotional in nature or not can affect these encoding processes in a variety of ways. The emotionality of information can direct our attention (see Pessoa, 2005; Vuilleumier & Driver, 2007), guide us to prioritize some details for processing over others (see Mather & Sutherland, 2011), and affect how we elaborate on information after attending to it (see Hamann, 2001; Talmi & Moscovitch, 2004).

Many of the effects of emotion on encoding seem to be due to the arousing nature of the stimuli (i.e., how calming or exciting a stimulus is) rather than to the valence of the stimuli (i.e., how positive or negative a stimulus is). Emotionally arousing information can serve as a powerful cue to direct our attention (Christianson & Loftus, 1991; Easterbrook, 1959; Öhman, Flykt, & Esteves, 2001; Reisberg & Heuer, 1992) and to guide our engagement of elaborative processes (Hamann, 2001). Easterbrook (1959) proposed that emotional arousal selectively narrows our attention on an arousing stimulus, allowing us to allocate resources to encode the emotionally salient (and therefore, presumably, biologically relevant) information and spare our cognitive resources from processing less relevant cues. One demonstration that emotional information can preferentially attract attention comes from Öhman and colleagues (2001). They presented participants with 2 × 2 or 3 × 3 grids of pictures, in which all pictures were different exemplars of the same semantic category (e.g., nine different mushrooms) or in which one item was from a discrepant category (e.g., eight different mushrooms and one flower). In those matrices containing a discrepant item, participants located the discrepant item significantly faster if it was negative and emotionally arousing (e.g., a spider or snake) than if it was nonemotional (e.g., a flower). Critically, detection time for the emotional targets was unaffected by the number of distracters present, consistent with an automatic "pop-out" effect, whereas detection time for neutral targets was related to the number of distracters, consistent with the engagement of an effortful search. Similar prioritization of attentional resources for emotional information has been demonstrated using a rapid serial visual presentation (RSVP) task to measure the "attentional blink" (Anderson, 2005; Anderson & Phelps, 2001), and this research has suggested that it is the high arousal of the information—regardless of its valence—that elicits the prioritization of attention (Anderson, 2005).

The selective attention and elaboration toward emotionally arousing information has been related to the "weapon-focus effect" (Loftus, 1979): Witnesses are more likely to recall emotionally arousing details of a crime (e.g., the shape and color of the perpetrator's gun), but to remember comparatively fewer nonemotional details (e.g., the details of the perpetrator's face or clothes). Laboratory studies have confirmed the presence of a "memory tradeoff," whereby memory for the neutral elements of a scene is "traded" in favor of memory for emotional aspects of the scene (reviewed by Levine & Edelstein, 2009; Reisberg & Heuer, 2004). This effect appears to be driven by the arousal level of the stimuli (Mickley Steinmetz & Kensinger, in press), and the memory tradeoff has been shown to occur when either positive or negative information is presented within a scene

(Mickley Steinmetz & Kensinger, in press; Waring & Kensinger, 2009). Although Easterbrook's (1959) original thesis refers to the narrowing of attention on negative information, memory tradeoff evidence suggests that the theory is not necessarily specific to negative emotion and occurs for both positive and negative information.

The emotional memory tradeoff often is revealed in studies that require participants to remember scenes containing emotional and neutral items set against neutral backgrounds. In one such study (Waring & Kensinger, 2009), participants viewed scenes containing an object that was positive, negative, or neutral against a neutral background. After a delay, recognition memory was tested separately for both the images and the backgrounds. Participants demonstrated enhanced memory for emotional objects, regardless of valence, relative to neutral items; this was true for both high- and low-arousal objects. Memory for backgrounds that were paired with highly arousing positive or negative items were remembered significantly below the baseline of memory for neutral backgrounds, consistent with proposals that attention can be narrowed during the experience of positive, high-approach motivations (Gable & Harmon-Jones, 2008) as well as negative emotions (Easterbrook, 1959). This reduction in memory for the context was less likely to occur if the items placed on the background were not arousing, and in fact the decrement was altogether absent for positive, low arousal stimuli, consistent with suggestions that positive, low-approach motivations may not narrow attention and in fact may lead to a broader and more flexible encoding of the environment (e.g., Fredrickson, 2001; Fredrickson & Branigan, 2005; Gable & Harmon-Jones, 2008).

At the neural level, the occurrence of this "tradeoff" is consistent with increasing evidence that amygdala engagement boosts the encoding of some, but not all, details present during an emotional event. In the case of complex scenes, amygdala engagement supports memory for the emotional item within the scene but not for the corresponding background (Waring & Kensinger, 2011). Even in the case of single emotional items, amygdala engagement corresponds with memory for visual features of those items but not for memory of other details, such as the item's location or order within a list (Kensinger, Addis, & Atapattu, 2011).

One interpretation of these findings is that an arousal response enhances memory for whatever is the current focus of a participant's attention (Mather & Sutherland, 2011). For instance, it has been proposed that the tradeoff occurs because people focus their visual attention on the emotional object and not on the other scene details. Indeed, participants first orient their attention and make more fixations to the arousing aspects of a complex visual scene than to the nonemotional aspects (Loftus, Loftus, & Messo, 1987; reviewed by Buchanan & Adolphs, 2002). However, recent research has suggested that looking time may not be related to whether people forget the background; a few studies have now suggested that whether nonemotional, peripheral information is remembered or forgotten is likely to have more to do with the post-encoding elaboration of that material than with the allocation of visual attention during the initial viewing of the information (Mickley Steinmetz & Kensinger, in press; Riggs, McQuiggan, Farb, Anderson, & Ryan, 2011). At the neural level, increased activity in the inferior frontal gyrus—thought to play a role in elaboration—is stronger when the nonemotional periphery is remembered along with the emotional items (see Figure 9.1; data from Waring & Kensinger, 2011), consistent with the interpretation that post-stimulus elaboration influences what information from the scene is retained or forgotten.

Although elaboration can play a role in memory for emotionally arousing information (Ritchey, LaBar, & Cabeza, 2011), it may be particularly important for explaining the mnemonic benefits conveyed by pleasant and unpleasant items that are not arousing (Fredrickson & Branigan, 2005; Kensinger & Corkin, 2003; Ochsner, 2000). Talmi and Moscovitch (2004) indicated that valenced words are more semantically relatable than neutral words, and may be more likely to be connected with one another or with related semantic information in memory (see Brainerd, Stein, Silveira, Rohenkohl, & Reyna, 2008, for evidence that this may be particularly true for negative information). The role of semantic elabora-

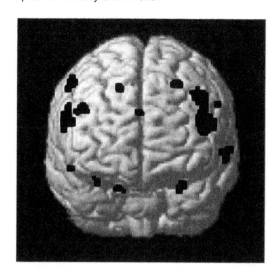

FIGURE 9.1. Prefrontal regions are dispropor-tionately recruited when all scene elements (not just the high-arousal item) will be remembered. Data from Waring and Kensinger (2011).

tion is further evidenced by the fact that the mnemonic benefit for valenced information is attenuated when valenced items and neu-tral items are matched on their number of semantic associates (Talmi & Moscovitch, 2004). Pleasant and unpleasant informa-tion may also lend itself more readily to autobiographical elaboration than neutral information. Being able to relate informa-tion to oneself makes that information more salient and memorable (Rogers, Kuiper, & Kirker, 1977; reviewed by Symons & John-son, 1997), and it is plausible that positive and negative stimuli (e.g., words such as *joy* and *failure*) are more easily relatable to the self than neutral stimuli (e.g., words such as *plastic* and *smooth*). Consistent with a role of semantic elaboration in the mnemonic benefit conveyed by nonarousing valenced information, Kensinger and Corkin (2004) found that activity in the inferior prefron-tal cortex—a region implicated in semantic elaboration—showed a stronger connection to the successful encoding of negative non-arousing information than of either neutral or negative arousing information. By con-trast, activity in the amygdala showed a stronger correspondence to the successful encoding of negative arousing information as compared to either neutral or negative nonarousing information, consistent with

extensive evidence for the role of the amyg-dala in enhancing the encoding of arousing information (e.g., Cahill et al., 1996, 2001; Canli, Zhao, Brewer, Gabrieli, & Cahill, 2000).

Although these studies distinguished valence and arousal by comparing nonar-ousing valenced information with arousing valenced information, the two dimensions can also be distinguished by investigating the processes that are shared for positive and negative arousing information versus the processes that differ based on valence. Neuroimaging studies have confirmed that amygdala and orbitofrontal engagement is high for positive and negative informa-tion, as long as that information is arous-ing (reviewed by Kensinger, 2009; LaBar & Cabeza, 2006). But there are some differ-ences in the neural activity engaged during the encoding of positive and negative infor-mation. For instance, regions of the ventral visual processing stream that are important for object recognition and visual encoding (e.g., Goodale & Milner, 1992; Mishkin & Ungerleider, 1982) tend to show a stronger link to the encoding of negative items than to positive ones (Mickley & Kensinger, 2008; Mickley Steinmetz & Kensinger, 2009). These temporal–occipital regions also show a stronger parametric relation to memory for episodic details of negative events than to positive ones (Kensinger et al., 2011). Additionally, the effects of arousal on neu-ral connectivity can differ depending on the emotional valence of information. For nega-tive information, connections to a number of regions—including the middle occipital gyrus—increase in strength when informa-tion is more arousing. For positive pictures, though, the strength of the amygdalar affer-ents decreases as the arousal of pictures increases (Mickley Steinmetz, Addis, & Kensinger, 2010). These findings are con-sistent with behavioral evidence that nega-tive information is more likely than positive information to be remembered with sensory detail (e.g., Kensinger & Choi, 2009) and that item-specific sensory processing may be prioritized for negative information (Sakaki, Gorlick, & Mather, 2011; Schmitz, De Rosa, & Anderson, 2009).

These results indicate that arousal and valence both must be considered when understanding how emotional information is encoded into memory. Arousing information tends to draw our attention, and the processing of that information is typically prioritized over the processing of less emotionally salient material. The prioritized attention and elaboration of arousing information is likely to lead to tradeoff effects in memory, whereby the information directly connected to the arousing item is remembered at the expense of other contextual information (see also Levine & Edelstein, 2009; Mather & Sutherland, 2011; Reisberg & Heuer, 2004). Yet arousal-based effects are not the whole story: information with negative valence is more likely to engage sensory processes during encoding, and this may lead to a more perceptually vivid memory representation for negative items.

The Effect of Emotion on Memory Consolidation

Just as the contents of an unsaved computer document can be erased when a computer crashes, so can the contents encoded into memory become lost if additional *consolidation* processes are not implemented to allow the stabilization of the memory trace after its initial acquisition (see Dudai, 2002; McGaugh, 2000, for reviews of consolidation). Consolidation processes are usually divided into those that happen at a molecular level and often within milliseconds of an event's occurrence and those that occur on a much grander spatial and temporal scale, involving large networks of brain areas and unfolding over hours, days, and years.

The proposal for a process of consolidation came at the turn of the 20th century, largely motivated by two sets of findings. First, in 1881, Théodule Ribot reported that there often is a temporal gradient to retrograde amnesia, with patients losing more recent memories than remote memories. Second, Müller and Pilzecker (1900) found that interference was particularly likely to impede the retrieval of recently learned information (see Lechner, Squire, & Byrne, 1999). These lines of evidence suggested that remote memories were more stable and less prone to disruption or disorganization than recent memories; these findings also implied that memories morphed into a more stable form with the passage of time.

Subsequent research has confirmed that consolidation processes occur to stabilize information over time, but these studies also have revealed that not all information is consolidated with equal efficiency. The consolidation of information is boosted when there is a release of the adrenal stress hormones, epinephrine and cortisol, as occurs during an emotionally arousing event (McGaugh, 2000). The amygdala is believed to mediate the effects of these hormones on memory (McGaugh, 2004). With regard to episodic memory, it is likely that this hormonal release and amygdala activation modulates hippocampal processes that boost episodic memory consolidation (Phelps & LeDoux, 2005).

Much of the research examining the effects of arousal on memory consolidation has used rodents as subjects and a shock as the emotional experience, but there is accumulating evidence that these findings generalize to the human experience of arousing events. First, there is an influence of arousal on a person's long-term retention: Although memory is often similar for arousing events and for neutral events just minutes after their occurrence, there is better retention of arousing events than of neutral ones over longer delays. Sometimes the emergence of this benefit represents an absolute increase in memory for the arousing information over time (Kleinsmith & Kaplan, 1963; Walker & Tarte, 1963), but more often it reflects a slower degradation of memory for the arousing event than for the neutral event (e.g., Pierce & Kensinger, 2011; Sharot & Yonelinas, 2008). In other words, memories of arousing experiences decay (Mahmood, Manier, & Hirst, 2004), but they do so at a slower rate than memories of neutral events, enabling arousing experiences to be better maintained over the long term than neutral experiences (but see Talarico & Rubin, 2003, for evidence that the rate of decay can also be similar for arousing and neutral events).

Second, the long-term effects of arousal require a functioning amygdala. Patients with amygdala damage are not amnesic, but they show no long-term memory benefit for arousing information (Hamann, Cahill, McGaugh, & Squire, 1997). They also do not show a disproportionate retention of arousing (vs. neutral) information over long delays (LaBar & Phelps, 1998).

Third, the time-dependent effects of arousal are dependent on the release of stress hormones: The administration of cortisol enhances the long-term recall of arousing information (Buchanan & Lovallo, 2001), whereas administration of beta-blockers (that block adrenergic transmission) eliminates the long-term memory enhancement for arousing information (Cahill, Babinsky, Markowitsch, & McGaugh, 1995). Critically, these effects seem to be limited to situations that induce arousal and do not generalize to experiences that are lower in arousal (see review by McIntyre & Roozendaal, 2007). Indeed, amygdala activation in the absence of an arousal response does not appear to be sufficient for inducing a hippocampal-mediated boost in memory (Anderson, Yamaguchi, Grabski, & Lacka, 2006; Kensinger & Corkin, 2004).

Fourth, as noted in the earlier section describing the effects of emotion on memory encoding, the amygdala and the hippocampus are often coactivated during the processing of emotional information, and their joint activity corresponds with the subsequent retention of arousing information (reviewed by LaBar & Cabeza, 2006; Strange & Dolan, 2006). Although it is impossible to know whether this contribution to subsequent memory is connected to processes implemented during initial memory encoding or to the effects of that coactivation on memory consolidation, or both, the findings are at least consistent with the proposed importance of amygdala–hippocampus interactions for the facilitated consolidation of emotional information.

Taken together, these studies suggest the recipe for enhanced consolidation: Have an arousal response, coupled with amygdala activation, which will trigger hippocampal consolidation processes. Recent research suggests that the optimal execution of this recipe may occur while the brain is "offline," during sleep. When sleep occurs soon after learning, the newly learned information is less susceptible to interference and decay (see review by Ellenbogen, Payne, & Stickgold, 2006). Slow wave sleep (SWS) may be particularly important for the consolidation of episodic memories; it has been proposed that the low acetylcholine levels present during SWS allow the brain to switch from an encoding-biased phase (in which

the neocortex inputs to the hippocampus) to a consolidation-biased phase (in which the hippocampus inputs to the neocortex; see Gais & Born, 2004; Hasselmo, 1999).

Although a period of sleep seems to be necessary for optimal consolidation of all episodic memories, the benefit may be particularly pronounced for emotional experiences. There still have not been many studies comparing the effects of sleep on memory for emotional versus nonemotional information, but the current evidence suggests that sleep provides particular benefits for emotional memory. For instance, Wagner, Hallschmid, Rasch, and Born (2006) asked participants to read emotional and neutral narratives. Some participants slept for 3 hours immediately after reading the narratives, whereas other participants remained awake. When memory was tested years later, it was found that the participants who slept after reading the narratives were more likely to remember the emotional narratives than were those who remained awake, whereas there was no effect of sleep on the likelihood of remembering the topics of the neutral narratives. Similar findings have been revealed when memory is tested after a short delay as well, with the benefit in memory for emotional information being exaggerated after a night of sleep but not after a day spent awake (e.g., Hu, Stylos-Allan, & Walker, 2006; Wagner, Gais, & Born, 2001; Wagner et al., 2006; Wagner, Kashyap, Diekelmann, & Born, 2007). Interestingly, some of these findings have been linked to the amount of time spent in rapid eye movement (REM)–rich sleep, rather than SWS (Wagner et al., 2001), raising an interesting question as to the roles of REM versus SWS in the consolidation of emotional memories.

Contrary to this evidence that information can become stabilized in memory over sleep-filled delays was a proposal that sleep may aid to flush out unwanted information from memory. Or, as Crick and Mitchison (1983) said, "We dream in order to forget." Although their proposal of "reverse learning" during sleep has not gained significant attention or corroboration (see Dudai, 2002, for discussion), recent evidence suggests that it may be worthwhile to think about the ultimate achievement of the processes carried out in the sleeping brain not as solidification but rather as selection (e.g., Saletin, Goldstein, & Walker, 2011). During sleep, there may be a selection of the components of past experiences that ought to be retained, while letting the rest of the information fall away.

It may be that emotional components of experiences are tagged as those that ought to be retained (see Payne & Kensinger, 2010, for a review). Suggestive evidence to support this conjecture comes from considering the results comparing memory for emotional and neutral information over sleep-filled delays. Although usually sleep provides a memory benefit for neutral information, when both emotional and neutral forms of information are studied, sleep benefits only the emotional memories and not the neutral ones (e.g., Wagner et al., 2006). One possible explanation for this finding is that the emotional information is preferentially targeted for consolidation.

To address this hypothesis, Payne, Stickgold, Swanberg, and Kensinger (2008) presented participants with low-arousal backgrounds (e.g., a forest, a lake, a road) that contained either a negative, arousing item (e.g., a snake, an injured person) or a neutral item (e.g., a chipmunk, a secretary). Later, participants viewed items separately from backgrounds and were asked to distinguish those that had been elements of the studied scenes from elements that had not been included. Participants performed this task after one of three delays: 30 minutes, 12 hours spent awake, or 12 hours including a night of sleep. The results revealed that daytime wakefulness led to forgetting of negative, arousing scenes in their entirety, with both items and backgrounds being recalled more poorly after 12 hours spent awake than after a delay of only 30 minutes. After the night of sleep, however, there was a selective preservation of memory for the negative items but not of their accompanying backgrounds. Memory for the negative, arousing items was just as good after a 12-hour delay including a night of sleep as it was after a 30-minute delay (compare gray bars in Figure 9.2), whereas memory for the backgrounds was just as poor after a night of sleep as it was after a day spent awake (compare gray slashed bars in Figure 9.2). This finding indicates that the processes that act during sleep do not unambiguously solidify memories of our past experiences; rather they select particular components

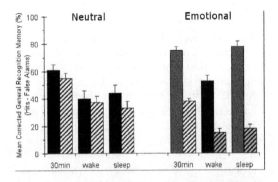

FIGURE 9.2. Participants show a "tradeoff" in memory for the components of emotional scenes, remembering items within emotional scenes (solid bars) better than the backgrounds presented with the items (slashed bars). A night of sleep exaggerates this tradeoff, selectively preserving memory for the emotional items. Adapted from Payne et al. (2008). Copyright 2008 by Sage Publications. Adapted by permission.

of past experiences for consolidation, possibly giving priority to the consolidation of emotionally salient elements (see also Lewis, Cairney, Manning, & Critchley, 2011, for evidence that sleep has different effects on memory for contextual details than on memory for emotional content).

This finding may help us to understand why memory for central, emotional information is often remembered at the expense of background details (Reisberg & Heuer, 2004). Although these tradeoffs have often been described in terms of attentional focus at encoding (Easterbrook, 1959), and having a visually evocative "attention magnet" in a scene can increase the likelihood that such tradeoffs occur (Reisberg & Heuer, 2004), recent evidence has suggested that visual capture of attention may not be sufficient to explain the effect (Mickley Steinmetz & Kensinger, in press). Instead, it may be necessary to consider postencoding processes—including those processes implemented during sleep—in order to understand this effect.

A recent functional magnetic resonance imaging (fMRI) study provided evidence that a single night of sleep is sufficient to provoke changes in the emotional memory circuitry, changes that could promote this type of tradeoff. In this study, participants studied the same types of scenes as described earlier, with either a neutral or a

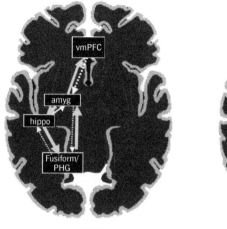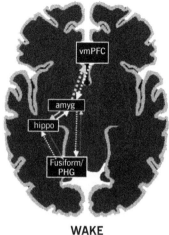

SLEEP   WAKE

FIGURE 9.3. During retrieval, participants had stronger connectivity between nodes of the emotional memory network after a night of sleep *(left)* than after a day spent awake *(right)*. vmPFC, ventromedial prefrontal cortex; amyg, amygdala; hippo, hippocampus; PHG, parahippocampal gyrus. Adapted from Payne and Kensinger (2011). Copyright 2011 by MIT Press. Adapted by permission.

negative item placed on a background. After a 12-hour delay, including either a night of sleep or a period of wakefulness, participants performed the recognition memory test while undergoing an fMRI scan. While successfully retrieving the negative items, participants who had slept showed stronger amygdala and ventromedial prefrontal cortex activity than did those who had been awake (see Figure 9.3), perhaps consistent with evidence that ventromedial prefrontal cortex activity may be connected to effective selection of relevant information (e.g., Nieuwenhuis & Takashima, 2011). The participants who had slept also showed strengthened connectivity between the amygdala and both the hippocampus and the ventromedial prefrontal cortex than did those who had been awake (Payne & Kensinger, 2011). This result suggests a possible mechanism by which sleep could intensify the selective nature of an emotional memory: By enhancing amygdala modulation of the emotional memory network, processes implemented during sleep may target the solidification of emotionally relevant aspects of an experience.

An important, open question for future research is to determine what aspects of an emotional experience trigger these prioritized consolidation processes. To date, most research has focused on memory for negative, arousing experiences, and so it is not clear how the valence and arousal dimensions, or the discrete emotions experienced, may contribute to the consolidation effects. As described earlier, there are many aspects of an emotional experience that influence the way it is encoded into memory, and so it seems likely that there may also be effects on consolidation that depend on the type of affect experienced.

The Effect of Emotion on Retrieval

Just as we need to be able to find and open a saved file on our computer, so must we be able to reaccess the information consolidated in memory, to use it at the moment when it is needed. This process of *retrieval* is often divided into a number of substeps, including memory search, memory recovery, and memory monitoring.

As compared to encoding and consolidation, relatively little investigation has been directed at how emotional content affects retrieval processes. Early neuroimaging investigations relied on block-designed studies, in which emotional and neutral materials were presented in separate test phases, and in which studied and nonstudied items could not be intermixed. Taylor and colleagues (1998) conducted one of the first neuroimaging investigations of the effects of emotion on memory retrieval, utilizing positron emission tomography (PET) technology and presenting participants with both neutral and emotional images. These authors found that the recognition of negative images engendered disproportionate activity in regions of the anterior cingulate cortex as well as the left lingual and middle frontal gyri. Also using a block design, Dolan, Lane, Chua, and Fletcher (2000) showed that the retrieval of emotional information was characterized by limbic activation—including regions such as the amygdala—over and above that seen for retrieving neutral information.

These studies suggest that the retrieval of emotional information does show some unique neural hallmarks. What these studies do not elucidate, however, is whether or not the different activity seen for retrieval of emotional information results from the retrieval process or simply reflects the processing of the emotional cue itself. Subsequent studies have aimed to tease these two possibilities apart by comparing the retrieval of neutral information studied in either a neutral or an emotional *context*.

In one such study, Maratos, Dolan, Morris, Henson, and Rugg (2001) asked participants to read sentences that had a positive, negative, or neutral connotation. Participants were later asked to recognize neutral words from each of the sentences while undergoing an fMRI scan. The authors found that when participants were asked to retrieve neutral words that had been featured in positive or negative sentences, there was significant activation of limbic regions (such as the amygdala) and other regions implicated in the processing of emotional information (such as the orbitofrontal cortex, in the case of positive contexts). These results clarify that it is not just the processing of an emotional cue that elicits different neural activity at retrieval, but rather retrieval of the emotional information itself. Using a similar design, Smith, Henson, Rugg, and Dolan (2005) asked participants to retrieve the context (emotional or neutral) in which a neutral object had been studied. The results revealed that accurate retrieval of the context was related to increased activity in the left amygdala and in regions throughout a frontal-temporal network.

More recent studies have returned to paradigms that use emotional information as a cue, attempting to distinguish memory effects from cue-processing effects by distinguishing accurate retrieval ("hits") from inaccurate retrieval ("misses"), with the emotionality of the cue being constant in both cases. For example, Dolcos, LaBar, and Cabeza (2005) subtracted neural activity during "miss" trials on a recognition task from activity during "hit" trials to isolate regions that showed a greater correspondence for retrieval success than failure. The results indicated that limbic regions showed a greater correspondence with retrieval success for emotional than for neutral items, indicating preferential involvement of the amygdala and the medial temporal lobe in the successful retrieval of emotional information.

As mentioned earlier, the entire retrieval process is understood to consist of a number of substeps, including search, recovery, and monitoring. It is possible that the emotionality of information could exert its influence at any or all of these substeps. A paper by Daselaar and others (2008) offered evidence that emotion can have a measurable influence on memory search. The authors asked participants to retrieve autobiographical memories while undergoing an fMRI. Participants received a memory cue and made a button press to indicate when a memory had been retrieved in response to that cue. The participant then continued to think about the retrieved content. This design allowed the authors to separate the neural processes recruited during memory search (prior to the button press) from those recruited during elaboration (from the button press until the end of the trial). The authors reported that participants' ratings of the emotional intensity of the memory were closely related to the amount of amygdala activity during the search, but not elaboration, phase of the trial. Such a result seems to indicate that emotion helps to guide the retrieval process, and that activity in the limbic regions is not necessarily due to the reprocessing or reliving of an emotional experience.

Not only can the emotional characteristics intrinsic to an event influence its retrieval, but one's current affective state can also guide retrieval. This influence is perhaps most evident in the case of mood-congruent memory, when individuals retrieve information that is congruent in valence with their current mood. This finding is robust in the case of both laboratory list-learning paradigms (see Matt, Vazquez, & Campbell, 1992, for a meta-analysis) and autobiographical retrieval (for reviews, see Blaney, 1986; Bower, 1981; Singer & Salovey, 1988), and it occurs under conditions of induced mood (e.g., Bower, 1981) and with naturally occurring moods such as depression (e.g., Blaney, 1986; Hertel, 2004). Indeed, mood-congruent memory may play an important role in affective disorders such as depression (see Gotlib & Joormann, 2010, for a review); easier access to negative memories may lead to the perpetuation of a negative mood state, leading to cyclical mood-congruent memory effects and the maintenance of depression (see also Teasdale, 1983, 1988).

Mood-congruent memory is often explained by the network theory of affect (Bower, 1981; Clark & Isen, 1982; see review by Holland & Kensinger, 2010). This theory suggests that emotions and events are stored as separate nodes in memory that become linked at encoding when an event elicits a particular affective response. One consequence is that when an "emotion" node becomes activated, such as in the case of mood, its associated events become easier to access at retrieval. Schema models of mood-congruent memory, including Beck's cognitive models of depression and anxiety (e.g., Beck, 1976; Beck & Clark, 1988), instead point to the existence of self-schemas that, once activated, can lead to schema-consistent cognitive processing. For example, if a depression-related schema is activated, individuals may have easier access to depression-related (i.e., mood-congruent) memories. However, as we elaborate below, these explanations of mood-congruent memory cannot account for the existence of mood-*incongruent* memory, when individuals are more likely to recall memories that are opposite in valence to their mood for the purposes of mood repair (e.g., Josephson, Singer, & Salovey, 1996; Parrott & Sabini, 1990). Other models of affective processing, such as Forgas's (1995) affect infusion model, make more specific predictions about the circumstances under which

mood-congruent memory occurs (see Rusting, 1998, for a similar discussion). For example, Forgas (1995) proposes multiple modes of information processing, including, on the one hand, heuristic ("shortcut") processing that results in mood-congruent memory and, on the other hand, motivated processing that allows for the existence of mood-incongruent memory in the service of mood regulation.

The Effect of Memory on Emotion

So far, we have discussed the way in which the emotional content of an experience or the affective state of an individual can influence the way in which it is remembered. But this is not the only direction of influence between emotion and memory. Not only does emotion influence the way an experience is remembered, but also the act of remembering an experience can influence our affective state. In this section we outline the influence of memory on affective states and the regulation of those affective states. In particular, we focus on the ways in which autobiographical memory retrieval can be used as an affect regulation technique, given that the bulk of the research in this domain has examined individuals' use of personally relevant past experiences to regulate their emotions.

The effect of recalling emotional information on current affective states is robust. Asking individuals to recall emotional autobiographical memories is one of the most effective ways that moods can be induced in a laboratory setting (Brewer, Doughtie, & Lubin, 1980; Westermann, Kordelia, Stahl, & Hesse, 1996). This is not to say, however, that we are passive recipients to the effects of memory on our current affective states. Rather, as we alluded to in the previous section, individuals can and do use memory recall to change their current affective state when motivated to do so. Emotion regulation, or the processes by which individuals influence the type and intensity of their experienced and expressed emotions (Gross, 1998), is cited by memory researchers as an important function of autobiographical memory retrieval (Bluck, Alea, Habermas, & Rubin, 2005); similarly, emotion regulation researchers cite memory recall as a potential emotion regulation strategy (Gross, 1998; Koole, 2009).

The constructive nature of autobiographical memory retrieval (e.g., Schacter & Addis, 2007) leaves its recall open to modulation by self-relevant goals, including those that are emotional in nature (Conway, 2005). Conway and colleagues have proposed that there exists a "working self" (analogous to the working memory system) that contains information about self-concept and short- and long-term goals that are actively being held in mind (e.g., Conway, 2005; Conway & Pleydell-Pearce, 2000). The working self can modulate access to goal-consistent memories or even distort the details constructed about a given event in a goal-consistent manner (Conway, 2005). As we describe below, the working self may include affect regulation goals that can influence memory recall via at least two possible routes: memory selection (e.g., which events are most likely or accessible to be recalled) and detail modulation (e.g., which details are most likely to be highlighted or even reappraised when a given event is being recalled).

Perhaps the best current evidence for the use of event selection as an affect regulation technique comes from the literature on mood-*incongruent* memory (e.g., Forgas, 2000; Isen, 1985). As we described in the section on memory retrieval, a number of papers have demonstrated that individuals are more likely to recall information that is congruent in valence to their current mood, a phenomenon termed *mood-congruent memory*. Although the first event recalled following a mood induction tends to demonstrate mood congruency, when participants are asked to recall additional events, the opposite effect occurs: Events are more likely to be opposite in valence to the induced mood (e.g., Josephson et al., 1996; but see Parrott & Sabini, 1990, for evidence of mood-incongruent recall in the first memory recalled). For example, Josephson and colleagues (1996) asked students to recall two autobiographical memories following a sad mood induction. They found that the students were more likely to recall negative events immediately following the induction (in line with a mood-congruent memory hypothesis), but that the memories recalled second in order were more likely to be positive. Participants were also likely to

cite mood repair as the reason for why they recalled the second positive event.

Although mood repair studies demonstrate how hedonic motivations can influence memory selection, it is important to note that individuals can also be motivated to recall negatively valenced memories when situationally appropriate to experience or display negative emotions. For instance, individuals who were told that they would play a confrontational video game demonstrated a preference to recall autobiographical memories of times when they felt angry, presumably to facilitate their performance on the video game (Tamir, Mitchell, & Gross, 2008).

There is also some evidence that affect regulation can occur via the specificity with which autobiographical events are recalled, though there is mixed evidence as to whether greater specificity is positively or negatively related to successful affect regulation. Autobiographical memories include broad lifetime themes ("When I was in college"), general events that are summaries of repeated events ("Going to English class every Tuesday"), and specific events that are unique to a particular time and place ("Taking my English midterm"; Conway & Pleydell-Pearce, 2000). Willfully retrieving specific events is presumably an effortful process that relies on executive functioning (Conway & Pleydell-Pearce, 2000). Individuals with a clinical diagnosis such as depression demonstrate a tendency to recall a greater proportion of general, repeated events when compared to healthy individuals (see Williams, 1996; Williams et al., 2007, for reviews). Three separate, but not mutually exclusive, mechanisms have been proposed for this so-called overgeneral memory effect (Williams et al., 2007): (1) reduced executive functioning capabilities that prevent successful retrieval of specific events (see Dalgleish et al., 2007), (2) rumination on past negative events that subsequently hinders the access of specific events (Watkins & Teasdale, 2001), and (3) the adoption of an overgeneral retrieval style based on the repeated avoidance of recalling specific, negative details (i.e., affect regulation; Williams et al., 2007).

Initially the affect regulation explanation of overgeneral memory garnered the most support based on evidence from clinical populations that had experienced childhood trauma and presumably as a result learned to functionally avoid the recall of specific, painful details (Williams, 1996; see similar discussion by Dalgleish et al., 2007). Indeed, healthy research participants subscribe to the belief that recalling events at a general level will lead to lower levels of emotional intensity (Philippot, Baeyens, & Douilliez, 2006), and there is some correlational evidence for such a link between affect regulation and memory specificity: When induced into a frustrated mood, individuals who experienced the greatest amount of frustration (i.e., poorer affect regulation) were also those who recalled the greatest percentage of specific events on an autobiographical memory task (Raes, Hermans, de Decker, Eelen, & Williams, 2003).

Despite this evidence for a positive correlation between affect regulation and specificity, research in which autobiographical memory specificity is experimentally manipulated has demonstrated just the opposite effect. Priming individuals to recall specific (vs. general) autobiographical memories leads to a decrease in self-reported emotional intensity when subsequently recalling emotional events or watching emotional film clips (Philippot, Schaefer, & Herbette, 2003). Similarly, adapting a general information-processing mode during the recall of a stressful social situation (e.g., thinking about the elements of that situation that were common to similar situations) led to greater emotional distress in socially anxious individuals than focusing on specific details from only that event (Vrielynck & Philippot, 2009). Philippot and colleagues (2003) suggest that recalling specific events, which is more cognitively taxing than recalling general events, may act to inhibit the reexperiencing of emotional intensity. Therefore, elaborating on the details of events might be the more effective means by which to achieve affect regulation (Philippot, Baeyens, Douilliez, & Francart, 2004), with the caveat that the details being elaborated upon must concern features that were unique to a given event rather than shared across multiple events (Neumann & Philippot, 2007).

As one way to reconcile these seemingly contradictory findings, Philippot and colleagues (2003) suggest that overgeneral memory results not from increased attempts at affect regulation, but rather from deficits in the executive resources needed to regulate affect in order to recall specific events. This explanation dovetails nicely with findings from the overgeneral memory literature that adopting a more specific retrieval mode is correlated with better treatment outcomes in depressed populations (Williams, Teasdale, Segal & Soulsby, 2000), and may also provide further support for the reduced executive control explanation of overgeneral memory (Dalgleish et al., 2007).

A deficit in the ability to recall particular memories in the service of emotion regulation goals may contribute to the development and maintenance of affective disorders, providing further support for the role of memory in affect regulation (see Gotlib & Joormann, 2010, for a review). For example, healthy individuals with higher levels of subclinical depression are less likely to exhibit mood-incongruent memory following a negative mood induction (Josephson et al., 1996; see also Joorman & Siemer, 2004). Formerly depressed patients do not report enhanced mood upon recalling positive memories, and currently depressed patients actually exhibit *decreases* in mood during such mood-incongruent recall (Joormann, Siemer, & Gotlib, 2007). Similar to the overgeneral memory effect, the ineffective use of mood-incongruent recall for mood repair may be attributed to reduced executive control functioning and increased rumination on negative information in dysphoric and depressed individuals (Joormann & Siemer, 2011).

In addition to event selection or accessibility, the working self can influence the types of details recalled about a particular event, as well as the appraisals we make about those details, so as to influence our current emotional states. Our memories for past emotional states are subject to the same reconstructive processes as our memories for other types of event details (for reviews, see Levine & Pizarro, 2004; Robinson & Clore, 2002). Our emotional states or goals at the time of memory retrieval can bias this constructive process, leaving open the possibility that specific events can be constructed in such a way as to make ourselves feel more positive or negative (Pasupathi, 2003).

The ability to reconstruct the emotions we remember experiencing during a particular event can be quite functional in hedonic affect regulation and may have important implications for well-being. For example, individuals may reconstrue their romantic partners' negative actions or faults into positive traits (e.g., "integrity" rather than "stubbornness"), an action that may help quell doubt or uncertainty about a partner (Murray & Holmes, 1993). In addition to helping maintain relationships, individuals may reconstrue their experienced emotions to maintain a stable sense of self. Levine, Safer, and Lench (2006) demonstrated that extraverted individuals, who often strive to achieve and maintain higher levels of positive affect (Tamir, 2009), are more likely to remember experiencing less anxiety prior to an exam than they had reported. This bias in recall may help extraverted individuals maintain their goal of increased positive affect and self-identity as extraverts.

Older adults may use a similar process to achieve their emotion regulation goals. One line of work hypothesizes that positive emotions and hedonic emotion regulation goals are particularly salient for older adults (e.g., Carstensen & Turk-Charles, 1998; Mather, 2006). In keeping with this hypothesis, older (vs. younger) adults are more likely to reframe their past negative events in a positive manner (Comblain, D'Argembeau, & Van der Linden, 2005) and to forget the negative emotions associated with events (Levine & Bluck, 1997). One longitudinal study asked a large sample of nuns to rate their present and past emotional states at several time points. The results revealed that the older participants were more likely to recall the past as more positive than they had rated it at the time (Kennedy, Mather, & Carstensen, 2004).

Emotion regulation via memory recall can also occur by reframing past events in a more negative light, so as to perceive improvement in the present (Ross, 1989). This type of reframing is also relevant in romantic relationships. In one study, wives were asked to rate their current and past levels of marital satisfaction over the course of 20 years (Karney & Coombs, 2000). Those who showed the greatest amount of negative biasing when recalling their past levels of satisfaction (i.e., more likely to remember the past as being more negative than it was) were also the ones who had the highest current perceptions of marital satisfaction.

The studies reviewed above suggest that individuals can recall the past in such a way as to change how they are feeling and thereby meet their affect regulation goals, and that a failure to recruit memories in such a way is associated with affective disorders. However, this line of research has yet to shed light on how the details of a particular memory can be recalled differently at two different time points depending on one's emotion regulation goals. In one study in our laboratory (Holland, Tamir, & Kensinger, 2010), we attempted to manipulate participants' regulation goals by telling them that they would be meeting with an experimenter who was either very happy or very sad, with the idea being that social situations are powerful motivators for regulating one's emotions (Huntsinger, Lun, Sinclair, & Clore, 2009). Following this goal manipulation, participants recalled three autobiographical events (e.g., high school graduation). When the recall following the manipulation was compared to a baseline recall of the same events 2 weeks prior, it was revealed that those individuals who thought they would be meeting with a sad experimenter increased the proportion of negative emotion words written in their narrative recalls. Individuals expecting to meet with a happy experimenter demonstrated the opposite trend. This experiment provided preliminary evidence that the construction of details at recall can be modulated by emotional goals.

Taken together, the research reviewed in this section suggests that recalling emotional information can influence or regulate individuals' current affective states. It seems that affect regulation goals can influence either which events or which details about a particular event are most likely to be recalled. Much of the work in this domain is in its infancy, however; it will be critical for future work to examine the efficacy of using memory recall as an affect regulation strategy, as well as how different emotional goals might modulate event and detail selection, in both healthy and clinical populations.

The Role of Individual Differences

As these sections have highlighted, there is a delicate interplay between the emotion elicited by an event, the affective state of the individual at the time, and the likelihood that an event—or particular details of an event—will be remembered. It is perhaps not surprising, therefore, that there can be systematic individual differences in this interplay. Some of these differences are likely to stem from how the event was initially experienced. For instance, those who view an event as highly self-relevant may be more likely to focus on event-related details than those who view the event from the perspective of an outside observer (Muscatell, Addis, & Kensinger, 2010; Pezdek, 2003).

Other differences may stem from trait or personality differences: People higher in anxiety or neuroticism may focus attention, and elaborative resources, on negative event details, causing them to remember those details better (e.g., MacLeod & Matthews, 2004), but at the expense of less negative contextual information (e.g., Chan, Goodwin, & Harmer, 2007; Waring, Payne, Schacter, & Kensinger, 2010). Still other differences are likely to reflect a person's goal state while an event unfolded (see Levine & Edelstein, 2009, for a review); as just one example, those who are attempting to regulate their emotions are likely to remember different details of an experience than those who experience the event without the attempts for reappraisal (Richards & Gross, 2000; Steinberger, Payne, & Kensinger, 2011). Other factors may come into play when the information is retrieved from memory. Individuals who view their time as limited, such as older adults who feel they are approaching the end of their life, may be more likely to reflect on their past in a positive way, seeing the "silver lining" even in their past struggles (Kennedy et al., 2004). By contrast, those who are depressed may have difficulty remembering the specifics of past experiences (e.g., Williams et al., 2007) and may dwell on the feeling that their past has been filled with unpleasant outcomes and with thwarted goals (Hertel, 2004). Although research to date has primarily focused on what is in common across all individuals as they encode, consolidate, and retrieve emotional experiences, an area still ripe for exploration surrounds the question of how individual differences moderate the way that emotion influences each of these stages of memory.

Acknowledgments

Preparation of this chapter was assisted by funding from the National Institute of Mental Health (Grant No. MH080833), from the National Science Foundation (No. BCS 0963581), and from the U.S. Department of Defense (National Defense Science and Engineering Graduate fellowship to Alisha C. Holland). We thank Jessica Payne for helpful discussion regarding the contents of this chapter.

References

Anderson, A. K. (2005). Affective influences on the attentional dynamics supporting awareness. *Journal of Experimental Psychology: General, 134*(2), 258–281.

Anderson, A. K., & Phelps, E. A. (2001). Lesions of the human amygdala impair enhanced perception of emotionally salient events. *Nature, 411*, 305–309.

Anderson, A. K., Yamaguchi, Y., Grabski, W., & Lacka, D. (2006). Emotional memories are not all created equal: Evidence for selective memory enhancement. *Learning and Memory, 13*, 711–718.

Beck, A. T. (1976). *Cognitive therapy and the emotional disorders*. New York: International Universities Press.

Beck, A. T., & Clark, D. A. (1988). Anxiety and depression: An information-processing perspective. *Anxiety Research, 1*, 23–36.

Blaney, P. H. (1986). Affect and memory: A review. *Psychological Bulletin, 99*, 229–246.

Bluck, S., Alea, N., Habermas, T., & Rubin, D. C. (2005). A tale of three functions: The self-reported uses of autobiographical memory. *Social Cognition, 23*, 91–117.

Bower, G. H. (1981). Mood and memory. *American Psychologist, 36*, 129–148.

Brainerd, C. J., Stein, L. M., Silveira, R. A., Rohenkohl, G., & Reyna, V. F. (2008). How does negative emotion cause false memories? *Psychological Science, 19*, 919–925.

Brewer, D., Doughtie, E. B., & Lubin, B. (1980). Induction of mood and mood shift. *Journal of Clinical Psychology, 36*, 215–226.

Brown, R., & Kulik, J. (1977). Flashbulb memories. *Cognition, 5*, 73–99.

Buchanan, T. W., & Adolphs, R. (2002). The role of the human amygdala in emotional modulation of long-term declarative memory. In S. Moore & M. Oaksford (Eds.), *Emotional cog-*

nition: From brain to behavior (pp. 9—34). London: John Benjamins.

Buchanan, T. W., & Lovallo, W. R. (2001). Enhanced memory for emotional material following stress-level cortisol treatment in humans. *Psychoneuroendocrinology, 26,* 307–317.

Cahill, L., Babinsky, R., Markowitsch, H. J., & McGaugh, J. L. (1995). The amygdala and emotional memory. *Nature, 377,* 295–296.

Cahill, L., Haier, R. J., Fallon, J. M, Alkire, M. T., Tang, C., Keator, D., et al. (1996). Amygdala activity at encoding correlated with long-term, free recall of emotional information. *Proceedings of the National Academy of Sciences of the United States of America, 93,* 8016–8021.

Cahill, L., Haier, R. J., White, N. S., Fallon, J., Kilpatrick, L., Lawrence, C., et al. (2001). Sex-related difference in amygdala activity during emotionally influenced memory storage. *Neurobiology of Learning and Memory, 71,* 1–9.

Canli, T., Zhao, Z., Brewer, J., Gabrieli, J. D., Cahill, L. (2000). Event-related activation in the human amygdala associates with later memory for individual emotional experience. *Journal of Neuroscience, 21,* RC99.

Carstensen, L. L., & Turk-Charles, S. (1998). Emotion in the second half of life. *Current Directions in Psychological Science, 7,* 144–149.

Chan, S. W., Goodwin, G. M., & Harmer, C. J. (2007). Highly neurotic never-depressed students have negative biases in information processing. *Psychological Medicine, 37,* 1281–1291

Christianson, S., & Loftus, E. F. (1991). Remembering emotional events: The fate of detailed information. *Cognition and Emotion, 5,* 81–108.

Clark, M. S., & Isen, A. M. (1982). Toward understanding the relationship between feeling states and social behavior. In A. H. Hastorf & A. M. Isen (Eds.), *Cognitive social psychology* (pp. 73–108). New York: Elsevier.

Comblain, C., D'Argembeau, A., & Van der Linden, M. (2005). Phenomenal characteristics of autobiographical memories for emotional and neutral events in older and younger adults. *Experimental Aging Research, 31,* 173–189.

Conway, M. A. (2005). Memory and the self. *Journal of Memory and Language, 53,* 594–628.

Conway, M. A., & Pleydell-Pearce, C. W. (2000). The construction of autobiographical memories in the self-memory system. *Psychological Review, 107,* 261–288.

Crick, F., & Mitchison, G. (1983). The function of dream sleep. *Nature, 304,* 111–114.

Dalgleish, T., Williams, J. M. G., Golden, A. J., Perkins, N., Feldman Barrett, L., Barnard, P. J., et al. (2007). Reduced specificity of autobiographical memory and depression: The role of executive control. *Journal of Experimental Psychology: General, 136,* 23–42.

Daselaar, S. M., Rice, H. J., Greenberg, D. L., Cabeza, R., LaBar, K. S., & Rubin, D. C. (2008). The spatiotemporal dynamics of autobiographical memory: Neural correlates of recall, emotional intensity, and reliving. *Cerebral Cortex, 18*(1), 217–229.

Dolan, R. J., Lane, R., Chua, P., & Fletcher, P. (2000). Dissociable temporal lobe activations during emotional episodic memory retrieval. *NeuroImage, 11,* 203–209.

Dolcos, F., LaBar, K. S., & Cabeza, R. (2005). Remembering one year later: Role of the amygdala and the medial temporal lobe memory system in retrieving emotional memories. *Proceedings of the National Academy of Sciences of the United States of America, 102,* 2626–2631.

Dudai, Y. (2002). Molecular bases of long-term memories: A question of persistence. *Current Opinion in Neurobiology, 12,* 211–216.

Easterbrook, J. S. (1959). The effect of emotion on cue utilization and the organization of behavior. *Psychological Review, 66,* 183–201.

Ellenbogen, J. M., Payne, J. D., & Stickgold, R. (2006). The role of sleep in declarative memory consolidation: Passive, permissive, active or none? *Current Opinion in Neurobiology, 16,* 716–722.

Forgas, J. P. (1995). Mood and judgment: The affect infusion model (AIM). *Psychological Bulletin, 117,* 39–66.

Forgas, J. P. (2000). Managing moods: Towards a dual-process theory of spontaneous mood regulation. *Psychological Inquiry, 11,* 172–177.

Fredrickson, B. L. (2001). The role of positive emotions in positive psychology: The broaden-and-build theory of positive emotions. *American Psychologist, 56,* 218–226.

Fredrickson, B. L., & Branigan, C. (2005). Positive emotions broaden the scope of attention and thought–action repertoires. *Cognition and Emotion, 19,* 313–332.

Gable, P. A., & Harmon-Jones, E. (2008). Approach-motivated positive affect reduces breadth of attention. *Psychological Science,* *19,* 476–482.

Gais, S., & Born, J. (2004). Declarative memory consolidation: Mechanisms acting during human sleep. *Learning and Memory, 11,* 679–685.

Goodale, M. A., & Milner, A. D. (1992). Separate visual pathways for perception and action. *Trends in Neuroscience, 15,* 20–5.

Gotlib, I. H., & Joormann, J. (2010). Cognition and depression: Current status and future directions. *Annual Review in Clinical Psychology, 6,* 285–312.

Gross, J. J. (1998). The emerging field of emotion regulation: An integrative review. *Review of General Psychology, 2,* 271–299.

Hamann, S. B. (2001). Cognitive and neural mechanisms of emotional memory. *Trends in Cognitive Sciences, 5,* 394–400.

Hamann, S. B., Cahill, L., McGaugh, J. L., & Squire, L. (1997). Intact enhancement of declarative memory by emotional arousal in amnesia. *Learning and Memory, 4,* 301–309.

Hasselmo, M. (1999). Neuromodulation: Acetylcholine and memory consolidation. *Trends in Cognitive Sciences, 3,* 351–359.

Hertel, P. T. (2004). Memory for emotional and nonemotional events in depression: A question of habit? In P. T. Hertel & D. Reisberg (Eds.), *Memory and emotion* (pp. 182–216). New York: Oxford University Press.

Holland, A. C., & Kensinger, E. A. (2010). Emotion and autobiographical memory. *Physics of Life Review, 7,* 88–131.

Holland, A. C., Tamir, M., & Kensinger, E. A. (2010). The effect of regulation goals on emotional event specific knowledge. *Memory, 18,* 504–521.

Hu, P., Stylos-Allan, M., & Walker, M. P. (2006). Sleep facilitates consolidation of emotionally arousing declarative memory. *Psychological Science, 10,* 891–898.

Huntsinger, J. R., Lun, J., Sinclair, S., & Clore, G. L. (2009). Contagion without contact: Anticipatory mood matching in response to affiliative motivation. *Personality and Social Psychology Bulletin, 35,* 910–923.

Isen, A. M. (1985). Asymmetry of happiness and sadness in effects on memory in normal college students: Comment on Hasher, Rose, Zacks, Sanft, and Doren. *Journal of Experimental Psychology: General, 114,* 388–391.

Joormann, J., & Siemer, M. (2004). Memory accessibility, mood regulation, and dysphoria: Difficulties in repairing sad mood with happy memories? *Journal of Abnormal Psychology, 113,* 179–188.

Joormann, J., & Siemer, M. (2011). Affective processing and emotion regulation in dysphoria and depression: Cognitive biases and deficits in cognitive control. *Social and Personality Psychology Compass, 5,* 13–28.

Joormann, J., Siemer, M., & Gotlib, I. H. (2007). Mood regulation in depression: Differential effects of distraction and recall of happy memories on sad mood. *Journal of Abnormal Psychology, 116,* 484–490.

Josephson, B. R., Singer, J. A., & Salovey, P. (1996). Mood regulation and memory: Repairing sad moods with happy memories. *Cognition and Emotion, 10,* 437–444.

Karney, B. R., & Coombs, R. H. (2000). Memory bias in long-term close relationships: Consistency or improvement? *Personality and Social Psychology Bulletin, 26,* 959–970.

Kennedy, Q., Mather, M., & Carstensen, L. L. (2004). The role of motivation in the age-related positivity effect in autobiographical memory. *Psychological Science, 15,* 208–214.

Kensinger, E. A. (2009). Remembering the details: Effects of emotion. *Emotion Review, 1,* 99–113.

Kensinger, E. A., Addis, D. R., & Atapattu, R. K. (2011). Amygdala activity at encoding corresponds with memory vividness and with memory for select episodic details. *Neuropsychologia, 49,* 663–673.

Kensinger, E. A., & Choi, E. S. (2009). Hemispheric processing and the visual specificity of emotional memories. *Journal of Experimental Psychology: Learning, Memory, and Cognition, 35,* 247–253

Kensinger, E. A., & Corkin, S. (2003). Memory enhancement for emotional words: Are emotional words more vividly remembered than neutral words? *Memory and Cognition, 31,* 1169–1180.

Kensinger, E. A., & Corkin, S. (2004). Two routes to emotional memory: Distinct neural processes for valence and arousal. *Proceedings of the National Academy of Sciences of the Unitd States of America, 101,* 3310–3315.

Kleinsmith, L. J., & Kaplan, S. (1963). Paired-associate learning as a function of arousal and interpolated interval. *Journal of Experimental Psychology, 65,* 190–193.

Koole, S. L. (2009). The psychology of emotion regulation: An integrative review. *Cognition and Emotion, 23,* 4–41.

LaBar, K. S., & Cabeza, R. (2006). Cognitive

neuroscience of emotional memory. *Nature Reviews Neuroscience, 7,* 54–56.

LaBar, K. S., & Phelps, E. A. (1998). Arousal-mediated memory consolidation: Role of the medial temporal lobe in humans. *Psychological Science, 9,* 490–493.

Lechner, H. A., Squire, L. R., & Byrne, J. H. (1999). 100 years of consolidation: Remembering Müller and Pilzecker. *Learning and Memory, 6,* 77–87.

Levine, L. J., & Bluck, S. (1997). Experienced and remembered emotional intensity in older adults. *Psychology and Aging, 12,* 514–523.

Levine, L. J., & Edelstein, R. S. (2009). Emotion and memory narrowing: A review and goal relevance approach. *Cognition and Emotion, 23,* 833–875

Levine, L. J., & Pizarro, D. A. (2004). Emotion and memory research: A grumpy overview. *Social Cognition, 22,* 530–554.

Levine, L. J., Safer, M. A., & Lench, H. C. (2006). Remembering and misremembering emotions. In L. J. Sanna & E. C. Chang (Eds.), *Judgments over time: The interplay of thoughts, feelings, and behaviors* (pp. 271–290). New York: Oxford University Press.

Lewis, P. A., Cairney, S., Manning, L., & Critchley, H. D. (2011). The impact of overnight consolidation upon memory for emotional and neutral encoding contexts. *Neuropsychologia, 49,* 2619–2629.

Loftus, E. F. (1979). The malleability of human memory. *American Scientist, 67,* 312–320.

Loftus, E. F., Loftus, G. R., & Messo, J. (1987). Some facts about weapon focus. *Law and Human Behavior, 11,* 55 62.

MacLeod, C., & Matthews, A. (2004). Selective memory effects in anxiety disorders: An overview of research findings and their implications. In D. Reisberg & P. Hertel (Eds.), *Memory and emotion* (pp. 155–185). New York: Oxford University Press.

Mahmood, D., Manier, D., & Hirst, W. (2004). Memory for how one learned of multiple deaths from AIDS: Repeated exposure and distinctiveness. *Memory and Cognition, 32,* 125–134.

Maratos, E. J., Dolan, R. J., Morris, J. S., Henson, R. N., & Rugg, M. D. (2001). Neural activity associated with episodic memory for emotional context. *Neuropsychologia, 39,* 910–920.

Mather, M. (2006). Why memories may become more positive as people age. In B. Uttl, N. Ohta, & A. L. Siegenthaler (Eds.), *Memory and emotion: Interdisciplinary perspectives* (pp. 135–159). Boston: Blackwell.

Mather, M., & Sutherland, M. R. (2011). Arousal-biased competition in perception and memory. *Perspectives on Psychological Science, 6,* 114–133.

Matt, G. E., Vazquez, C., & Campbell, W. K. (1992). Mood-congruent recall of affectively tones stimuli: A meta-analytic review. *Clinical Psychology Review, 12,* 227–255.

McGaugh, J. L. (2000). Memory: A century of consolidation. *Science, 287,* 248–51.

McGaugh, J. L. (2004). The amygdala modulates the consolidation of memories of emotionally arousing experiences. *Annual Review of Neuroscience, 27,* 1–28.

McIntyre, C. K., & Roozendaal, B. (2007). Adrenal stress hormones and enhanced memory for emotionally arousing experiences. In F. Bermúdez-Rattoni (Ed.), *Neural plasticity and memory: From genes to brain imaging* (pp. 265–284). Boca Raton, FL: CRC Press.

Mickley, K. R., & Kensinger, E. A. (2008). Neural processes supporting subsequent recollection and familiarity of emotional items. *Cognitive, Affective, and Behavioral Neuroscience, 8,* 143–152.

Mickley Steinmetz, K. R., Addis, D. R., & Kensinger, E. A. (2010). The effect of arousal on the emotional memory network depends on valence. *NeuroImage, 53,* 318–324.

Mickley Steinmetz, K. R., & Kensinger, E. A. (2009). The effects of valence and arousal on the neural activity leading to subsequent memory. *Psychophysiology, 46,* 1190–1199.

Mickley Steinmetz, K. R., & Kensinger, E. A. (in press). the emotion-induced memory trade-off: More than an effect of overt attention? *Memory and Cognition.*

Mishkin, M., & Ungerleider, L. G. (1982). Contribution of striate inputs to the visuospatial functions of parieto–preoccipital cortex in monkeys. *Behavioral Brain Research, 6,* 57–77.

Müller, G. E., & Pilzecker A. (1900). [Experimental contributions to the science of memory]. *Zeitschrift für Psychologie und Physiologie der Sinnesorgane, 1,* 1–300.

Murray, S. L., & Holmes, J. G. (1993). Seeing virtues in faults: Negativity and the transformation of interpersonal narratives in close relationships. *Journal of Personality and Social Psychology, 65,* 707–722.

Muscatell, K. A., Addis, D. R., & Kensinger, E. A. (2010). Self-involvement modulates the effective connectivity of the autobiographical memory network. *Social, Cognitive, and Affective Neuroscience, 5*, 68–76.

Neumann, A., & Philippot, P. (2007). Specifying what makes a personal memory unique enhances emotion regulation. *Emotion, 7*, 566–578.

Nieuwenhuis, I. L., & Takashima, A. (2011). The role of the ventromedial prefrontal cortex in memory consolidation. *Behavioral Brain Research, 218*, 325–334.

Ochsner, K. N. (2000). Are affective events richly recollected or simply familiar?: The experience and process of recognizing feelings past. *Journal of Experimental Psychology: General, 129*, 242–261.

Öhman, A., Flykt, A., & Esteves, F. (2001). Emotion drives attention: Detecting the snake in the grass. *Journal of Experimental Psychology: General, 130*, 466–478.

Parker, E. S., Cahill, L., & McGaugh, J. L. (2006). A case of unusual autobiographical remembering. *Neurocase, 12*, 35–49.

Parrott, W. G., & Sabini, J. (1990). Mood and memory under natural conditions: Evidence for mood incongruent recall. *Journal of Personality and Social Psychology, 59*, 321–336.

Pasupathi, M. (2003). Social remembering for emotion regulation: Differences between emotions elicited during an event and emotions elicited when talking about it. *Memory, 11*, 151–163,

Payne, J. D., & Kensinger, E. A. (2010). Sleep's role in the consolidation of emotional episodic memories. *Current Directions in Psychological Science, 19*, 290–295.

Payne, J. D., & Kensinger, E. A. (2011). Sleep leads to changes in the emotional memory trace: Evidence from fMRI. *Journal of Cognitive Neuroscience, 23*, 1285–1297.

Payne, J. D., Stickgold, R., Swanberg, K., & Kensinger, E. A. (2008). Sleep preferentially enhances memory for emotional components of scenes. *Psychological Science, 19*, 781–788.

Pessoa, L. (2005). To what extent are emotional visual stimuli processed without attention and awareness? *Current Opinion in Neurobiology, 15*, 188–196.

Pezdek, K. (2003). Event memory and autobiographical memory for the events of September 11, 2001. *Applied Cognitive Psychology, 17*, 1033–1045.

Phelps, E. A., & LeDoux, J. E. (2005). Contributions of the amygdala to emotion processing: From animal models to human behavior. *Neuron, 48*, 175–187.

Philippot, P., Baeyens, C., & Douilliez, C. (2006). Specifying emotional information: Modulation of emotional intensity via executive processes. *Emotion, 6*, 560–571.

Philippot, P., Baeyens, C., Douilliez, C., & Francart, B. (2004). Cognitive regulation of emotion: Application to clinical disorders. In P. Philippot & R. S. Feldman (Eds.), *The regulation of emotion* (pp. 71–98). New York: Erlbaum.

Philippot, P., Schaefer, A., & Herbette, G. (2003). Schematic versus propositional processing of emotional information: Impact of generic versus specific autobiographical memory priming on emotion elicitation. *Emotion, 3*, 270–283.

Pierce, B. H., & Kensinger, E. A. (2011). Effects of emotion on associative recognition: Valence and retention interval matter. *Emotion, 11*, 139–144.

Posner, J., Russell, J. A., & Peterson, B. S. (2005). The circumplex model of affect: An integrative approach to affective neuroscience, cognitive development, and psychopathology. *Developmental Psychopathology, 17*, 715–734

Raes, F., Hermans, D., de Decker, A., Eelen, P., & Williams, J. M. G. (2003). Autobiographical memory specificity and affect regulation: An experimental approach. *Emotion, 3*, 201–206.

Reisberg, D., & Heuer, F. (1992). Flashbulbs and memory for detail from emotional events. In E. Winograd & U. Neisser (Eds.), *Affect and accuracy in recall: The problem of "flashbulb" memories* (pp. 162–190). New York: Cambridge University Press.

Reisberg, D., & Heuer, F. (2004). Remembering emotional events. In D. Reisberg & P. Hertel (Eds.), *Memory and emotion* (pp. 3–41). New York: Oxford University Press.

Ribot, T. (1881). *Les maladies de la mémoire* [Diseases of memory]. Paris: Baillière.

Richards, J. M., & Gross, J. J. (2000). Emotion regulation and memory: The cognitive costs of keeping one's cool. *Journal of Personality and Social Psychology, 79*, 410–424.

Riggs, L., McQuiggan, D. A., Farb, N., Anderson, A. K., & Ryan, J. D. (2011). The role of overt attention in emotion-modulated memory. *Emotion, 11*, 776–785.

Ritchey, M., LaBar, K. S., & Cabeza, R. (2011). Level of processing modulates the neural correlates of emotional memory formation. *Journal of Cognitive Neuroscience, 23*, 757–771.

Robinson, M. D., & Clore, G. L. (2002). Belief and feeling: Evidence for an accessibility model of emotional self-report, *Psychological Bulletin, 128,* 934–960.

Rogers, T. B., Kuiper, N. A., & Kirker, W. S. (1977). Self-reference and the encoding of personal information. *Journal of Personality and Social Psychology, 35,* 677–688.

Ross, M. (1989). Relation of implicit theories to the construction of personal histories. *Psychological Review, 96,* 341–357.

Russell, J. A. (1980). A circumplex model of affect. *Journal of Personality and Social Psychology, 39,* 1161–1178.

Rusting, C. L. (1998). Personality, mood, and cognitive processing of emotional information: Three conceptual frameworks. *Psychological Bulletin, 124,* 165–196.

Sakaki, M., Gorlick, M., & Mather, M. (2011). Differential interference effects of negative emotional states on subsequent semantic and perceptual processing. *Emotion, 11,* 1263–1278.

Saletin, J. M., Goldstein, A. N., & Walker, M. P. (2011). The role of sleep in directed forgetting and remembering of human memories. *Cerebral Cortex, 21,* 2534–2541.

Schacter, D. L., & Addis, D. R. (2007). On the constructive episodic simulation of past and future events. *Behavioral and Brain Sciences, 30,* 299–351.

Schmitz, T. W., De Rosa, E., & Anderson, A. K. (2009). Opposing influences of affective state valence on visual cortical encoding. *Journal of Neuroscience, 29*(22), 7199–7207.

Sharot, T., & Yonelinas, A. P. (2008). Differential time-dependent effects of emotion on recollective experience and memory for contextual information. *Cognition, 106,* 538–547.

Singer, J. A., & Salovey, P. (1988). Mood and memory: Evaluating the network theory of affect. *Clinical Psychology Review, 8,* 211–251.

Smith, A. P., Henson, R. N., Rugg, M. D., & Dolan, R. J. (2005). Modulation of retrieval processing reflects accuracy of emotional source memory. *Learning and Memory, 12,* 472–479.

Steinberger A., Payne J. D., & Kensinger E. A. (2011). The effect of cognitive reappraisal on the emotional memory trade-off. *Cognition and Emotion, 25,* 1237–1245.

Strange, B., & Dolan, R. (2006). Anterior medial temporal lobe in human cognition: Memory for fear and the unexpected. *Cognitive Neuropsychiatry, 11,* 198–218.

Symons, C. S., & Johnson, B. T. (1997). The self-reference effect in memory: A meta-analysis. *Psychological Bulletin, 121,* 371–394.

Talarico, J. M., & Rubin, D. C. (2003). Confidence, not consistency, characterizes flashbulb memories. *Psychological Science, 14,* 455–461.

Talmi, D., & Moscovitch, M. (2004). Can semantic relatedness explain the enhancement of memory for emotional words? *Memory and Cognition, 32,* 742–751.

Tamir, M. (2009). Differential preferences for happiness: Extraversion and trait-consistent emotion regulation. *Journal of Personality, 77,* 447–470.

Tamir, M., Mitchell, C., & Gross, J. J. (2008). Hedonic and instrumental motives in anger regulation. *Psychological Science, 19,* 324–328.

Taylor, S. F., Liberzon, I., Fig, L. M., Decker, L. R., Minoshima, S., & Koeppe, R. A. (1998). The effect of emotional content on visual recognition memory: A PET activation study. *NeuroImage, 8,* 188–197.

Teasdale, J. D. (1983). Negative thinking in depression: Cause, effect, or reciprocal relationship? *Advances in Behaviour Research and Therapy, 5,* 3–25.

Teasdale, J. D. (1988). Cognitive vulnerability to persistent depression. *Cognition and Emotion, 2,* 247–274.

Tulving, E. (1983). *Elements of episodic memory.* Oxford, UK: Oxford University Press.

Vrielynck, N., & Philippot, P. (2009). Regulating emotion during imaginal exposure to social anxiety: Impact of the specificity of information processing. *Journal of Behaviour Therapy and Experimental Psychiatry, 40,* 274–282.

Vuilleumier, P., & Driver, J. (2007). Modulation of visual processing by attention and emotion: Windows on causal interactions between human brain regions. *Philosophical Transactions of the Royal Society of London, B Series, Biological Sciences, 362,* 837–855.

Wagner, U., Gais, S., & Born, J. (2001). Emotional memory formation is enhanced across sleep intervals with high amounts of rapid eye movement sleep. *Learning and Memory, 8,* 112–119.

Wagner, U., Hallschmid, M., Rasch, B., & Born, J. (2006). Brief sleep after learning keeps emotional memories alive for years. *Biological Psychiatry, 60*, 788–790.

Wagner, U., Kashyap, N., Diekelmann, S., & Born, J. (2007). The impact of post-learning sleep vs. wakefulness on recognition memory for faces with different facial expressions. *Neurobiology of Learning and Memory, 97*, 679–697.

Walker, E. L., & Tarte, R. D. (1963). Memory storage as a function of arousal and time with homogeneous and heterogeneous lists. *Journal of Verbal Learning and Verbal Behavior, 2*, 113–119.

Waring, J. D., & Kensinger, E. A. (2009). Effects of emotional valence and arousal upon memory trade-offs with aging. *Psychology and Aging, 24*, 412–422.

Waring, J. D., & Kensinger, E. A. (2011). How emotion leads to selective memory: Neuroimaging evidence. *Neuropsychologia, 49*, 1831–1842.

Waring, J. D., Payne, J. D., Schacter, D. L., & Kensinger, E. A. (2010). Impact of individual differences upon emotion-induced memory trade-offs. *Cognition and Emotion, 24*, 150–167.

Watkins, E., & Teasdale, J. D. (2001). Rumination and overgeneral memory in depression: Effects of self-focus and analytic thinking. *Journal of Abnormal Psychology, 110*, 353–357.

Westermann, R., Kordelia, S., Stahl, G., & Hesse, F. W. (1996). Relative effectiveness and validity of mood induction procedures: A meta-analysis. *European Journal of Social Psychology, 26*, 557–580.

Williams, J. M. G. (1996). Depression and the specificity of autobiographical memory. In D. C. Rubin (Ed.), *Remembering our past: Studies in autobiographical memory* (pp. 244–267). New York: Cambridge University Press.

Williams, J. M. G., Barnhofer, T., Crane, C., Hermans, D., Raes, F., Watkins, E., et al. (2007). Autobiographical memory specificity and emotional disorder. *Psychological Bulletin, 133*, 122–148.

Williams, J. M. G., Teasdale, J. D., Segal, Z. V., & Soulsby, J. (2000). Mindful meditation reduces overgeneral autobiographical memory in depressed patient. *Journal of Abnormal Psychology, 109*, 150–155.

CHAPTER 10

Goals and Emotion

Charles S. Carver and Michael F. Scheier

Not so very long ago, emotions were considered mysterious and irrational, aspects of the human experience that were outside the domain of logic or understanding. Today, emotions are seen instead to serve critical functions in the elaborate enterprise of negotiating a world that is both alluring and dangerous. Without emotions, that world would seem neither dangerous, nor alluring, nor satisfying.

This chapter describes a viewpoint in which emotions are intimately connected to other aspects of a systematic network of influences on behavior. This view of behavior is grounded in the common-sense goal concept, but with a bit of a twist. In this view, goals are seen as embedded in self-regulating systems of a particular kind. The systems act to regulate people's actions with respect to diverse kinds of goals (e.g., values, plans, strategies, intentions, and even whims), so that life's incentives are successfully approached and threats successfully avoided.

The viewpoint we take on self-regulation is one in which behavior reflects the outputs of feedback control processes. We propose that two layers of control manage two different aspects of behavior, jointly situating behavior in time as well as space. We argue that one of these layers is responsible for the existence of affect, the evaluative core

of emotions. We argue further that such an arrangement is useful both for the attainment of a single goal and for the handling of a life space in which multiple tasks compete for attention. More specifically, the system described in this chapter can help transform simultaneous concerns with many different goals into a stream of actions that shifts repeatedly from one goal to another over time.

Behavior as Goal Directed and Feedback Controlled

We begin by briefly describing a feedback-based view of action control, starting with the goal concept. The goal concept is prominent in today's psychology, under a wide variety of names (Austin & Vancouver, 1996; Elliot, 2008; Johnson, Chang, & Lord, 2006). The concept is broad enough to cover both long-term aspirations (e.g., creating and maintaining a good impression among colleagues) and the end points of very short-term acts (e.g., reaching to pick up a water glass without knocking it over). Goals generally can be reached in diverse ways, and a given action often can be done in the service of diverse goals—resulting in, potentially, vast complexity in the organization of action.

The goal concept has acquired a considerable foothold in personality psychology. People who think about goals as an organizing construct tend to assume that understanding a person means understanding that person's goals—indeed, that the substance of the self consists partly of the person's abstract goals and the organization among them (cf. Mischel & Shoda, 1995).

Feedback Loops

Our main point in this section actually is less about goals themselves than about the process of attaining them. Long ago we adopted the view that movement toward a goal reflects the functioning of a discrepancy-reducing feedback loop (MacKay, 1966; Miller, Galanter, & Pribram, 1960; Powers, 1973; Wiener, 1948). Such a loop involves the sensing of some present condition, which is compared to a desired or intended condition (as a reference value). If there is a discrepancy between the two, the discrepancy is countered by subsequent action to change the sensed condition. The overall effect of such an arrangement is to bring the sensed condition into conformity with the intended one (Powers, 1973). If the intended condition is thought of as a goal, the overall effect is to bring behavior into conformity to the goal—thus, goal attainment.

There also exist discrepancy-enlarging loops, which increase deviations from the comparison point rather than decrease them. The value in this case is a threat, an "anti-goal." Effects of discrepancy enlargement in living systems are typically constrained by discrepancy-reducing processes. Thus, for example, people often are able to avoid something aversive by the very act of approaching something else. Such dual influence occurs in instances of what is called *active avoidance:* An organism fleeing a threat spots a relatively safe location and approaches it.

People sometimes infer from descriptions such as the preceding one that feedback loops act only to create and maintain steady states and are therefore irrelevant to behavior. In reality, some reference values (and goals) *are* static, but others are dynamic (e.g., taking a vacation trip across Europe, raising children to be good citizens). In the latter cases, the goal is the process of traversing the changing trajectory of the activity, not just the arrival at the end point. The principle of feedback control applies easily to moving targets (Beer, 1995).

We bring to the conversation about goals (although we are not the first to have done so by any means) the idea that goal-directed action involves feedback control. Why this emphasis on feedback control? Many think of feedback as an engineering concept (engineers do use it), but the concept has older roots in physiology and other fields. Homeostasis, the processes by which the body self-regulates physical parameters such as temperature, blood sugar, and heart rate, is the prototypic feedback process (Cannon, 1932). The concept has been useful enough in many fields that it is sometimes suggested that feedback processes are some of the fundamental building blocks of all complex systems.

We believe there is merit in recognizing functional similarities between the processes that underlie behavior and those underlying other complex systems (cf. Ford, 1987; von Bertalanffy, 1968). Nature appears to be a miser and a recycler. It seems likely that an organizational property that emerges in one complex system will emerge over and over in other complex systems. For the same reason, it seems likely that principles embodied in physical movement control (which also rely, in part, on principles of feedback) have something in common with principles embodied in higher mental functions (Rosenbaum, Carlson, & Gilmore, 2001). For these reasons, we have continued to use the principle of feedback control as a conceptual heuristic over the years.

Levels of Abstraction

A couple more points about goals: The goal concept can seem a bit overwhelming because of the fact that goals exist at many levels of abstraction. You can have the goal of being socially responsible, but you can also have the goal of conserving resources—a more restricted goal that contributes to being socially responsible. One way to conserve resources is the process of recycling. Recycling entails other, more concrete goals: placing newspapers and empty bottles into containers and moving them to a pickup location. All of these are goals, values to be approached, but they exist at varying levels of abstraction.

It is often said that people's goals form a hierarchy (Powers, 1973; Vallacher & Wegner, 1987), in which abstract goals are achieved by attaining the concrete goals that help define them. Lower-level goals are attained by briefer sequences of action (formed from subcomponents of motor control; e.g., Rosenbaum, Meulenbroek, Vaughan, & Jansen, 2001). Some sequences of action have a self-contained quality, in that they run off fairly autonomously once triggered.

Viewed from the other direction, sequences can be organized into programs of action (Powers, 1973). Programs are more planful than sequences and require choices at various points. Programs, in turn, are sometimes (though not always) enacted in the service of principles—more abstract values that provide a basis for making decisions within programs and which suggest that certain programs be undertaken or not. What Powers (1973) called *principles* are roughly equivalent to what social psychologists call *values* (Schwartz & Bilsky, 1990; Schwartz & Rubel, 2005). Even that is not the end of potential complexity, though. Patterns of values can coalesce to form a very abstract sense of desired (and undesired) self or a sense of desired (and undesired) community.

All these classes of goals, from very concrete to very abstract, can in principle serve as reference points for self-regulation. When self-regulation is undertaken regarding a goal at one level, control presumably is simultaneously invoked at all levels of abstraction below that one. Control is not necessarily exerted at higher levels than that one, however. Indeed, it is even possible for a person to knowingly take an action that turns out to conflict with a higher-level goal, which creates problems when the person later thinks about that higher goal. This is an issue that can be very important in certain contexts, but it is outside the focus of this chapter.

Feedback Processes and Affect

Control of action provides a jumping-off point for addressing the focal concern of this chapter, which is affect or emotion. Two

fundamental questions about affect are what it consists of and where it comes from. It is often said that affect pertains to one's desires and whether they are being met (e.g., Clore, 1994; Frijda, 1986, 1988; Ortony, Clore, & Collins, 1988). But what exactly is the internal mechanism by which affect arises?

Some address this question at a neurobiological level, others at a cognitive level. We have proposed an answer that is neither of these, though we believe it to be compatible with both of them. The answer we posed (Carver & Scheier, 1990, 1998, 1999a, 1999b) focuses on some of the functional properties that affect seems to display in the person who experiences it. We used feedback control again as an organizing principle, but applied it somewhat differently than in the foregoing description. We suggested that the feeling properties that represent the core of emotions emerge from a feedback process that runs automatically, simultaneously with the behavior-guiding process, and in parallel to it. The easiest way to convey the sense of this second process is to say that it is checking on how well the first process (the behavior loop) is doing at reducing *its* discrepancies (we focus first on approach loops, then consider avoidance loops). Thus, the input for the second loop is some representation of the *rate of discrepancy reduction in the action system over time*.

An analogy may be useful. An action implies a change between states. Change in state is distance. Thus, behavior is analogous to distance. If the action loop controls distance, and if the affect loop assesses the action loop's progress, then the affect loop is assessing the psychological analogue of velocity, the first derivative of distance over time. To the extent that this analogy is meaningful, the perceptual input to the affect loop should be the first derivative over time of the input used by the action loop.

Input per se does not create affect (a given rate of progress has different affective implications in different circumstances). We believe that, as in any feedback system, this input is compared to a reference value (cf. Frijda, 1986, 1988). In this case, the reference is an acceptable or desired or intended rate of behavioral discrepancy reduction. As in other feedback loops, the comparison checks for deviation from the standard. If there is one, the output function changes.

We propose that the comparison in this loop yields an error signal (a representation of the discrepancy), which is manifested subjectively as affect—positive or negative valence. If the sensed rate of progress is below the criterion, affect is negative. If the rate is high enough to exceed the criterion, affect is positive. If the rate is not distinguishable from the criterion, affect is neutral. In essence, the argument is that feelings with a positive valence mean you are doing better at something than you need to, and feelings with a negative valence mean you are doing worse than you need to (for details, see Carver & Scheier, 1998, Chs. 8 and 9).

One implication of this line of thought is that, for any given goal-directed action, the potential for affective valence should form a bipolar dimension. That is, for any given action, affect can be positive, neutral, or negative, depending on how well or poorly the action is going. This is a point with several implications, to be addressed later.

What determines the criterion for this loop? When the activity is unfamiliar, the criterion is rather arbitrary and tentative. In those cases it is likely to shift easily. If the activity is familiar, the criterion is likely to reflect the person's accumulated experience, in the form of an expected rate (indeed, the more experience you have, the more you know what is reasonable to expect). Sometimes the criterion is a "desired" or "needed" rate of progress. Whether it is an expected rate or a desired rate doubtlessly depends on the context.

The criterion can also change, a phenomenon identified with the term *hedonic treadmill* (Brickman & Campbell, 1971). How fast the criterion changes depends on additional factors. The less experience the person has in a domain, the more fluid the criterion is likely to be; in a familiar domain, change is slower. Still, repeated overshoot of the criterion automatically yields an upward drift of the criterion (e.g., Eidelman & Biernat, 2007); repeated undershoots yield a downward drift. Thus, the system recalibrates over repeated experience in such a way that the criterion stays somewhere within the range of those experiences (Carver & Scheier, 2000). An ironic effect of recalibration would be to keep the balance of a person's affective experience in a given domain (positive to negative) relatively similar across time, even when the rate criterion changes considerably.

Evidence

Evidence of the role of the velocity function in affective reactions to situations comes from several sources (see also Carver & Scheier, 1998). Initial support came from research by Hsee and Abelson (1991), who came to the velocity hypothesis independently. In one study, participants read descriptions of paired hypothetical scenarios and indicated which they would find more satisfying. For example, they chose whether they would be more satisfied if their class standing had gone from the 30th percentile to the 70th over the past 6 weeks, or if it had done so over the past 3 weeks. Given positive outcomes, they preferred improving to a high outcome over a constant high outcome; they preferred a fast velocity over a slow one; and they preferred fast small changes to slower larger changes. When the change was negative (e.g., salaries got worse), they preferred a constant low salary to a salary that started high and fell to the same low level; they preferred slow falls to fast falls; and they preferred large slow falls to small fast falls.

A later study conceptually replicated aspects of these findings, but with an event that was personally experienced rather than hypothetical (Lawrence, Carver, & Scheier, 2002). Success feedback was manipulated on an ambiguous task over an extended period. Subjects in a neutral condition received feedback of 50% correct on the first and last block, and 50% average across all blocks. Others experienced a positive change in performance, starting poorly and gradually improving to 50%. Others experienced a negative change, starting well and gradually worsening to 50%. The patterns of feedback thus converged, such that feedback on block 6 was identical for all subjects at 50% correct. All rated their mood before starting and again after block 6 (which they did not know ended the session). Those whose performances were improving reported mood improvement, those whose performances were deteriorating reported mood deterioration, compared to those with a constant performance.

Another early study that appears to bear on this view of affect, although not having this purpose in mind, was reported by Brunstein (1993). It examined subjective well-being among college students over the course of an academic term, as a function of several perceptions, including perception of progress toward goals. Of greatest interest at present, perceived progress at each measurement point was strongly correlated with concurrent well-being.

More recently, Chang, Johnson, and Lord (2010) reported another pair of studies on this topic. The first was a field study of employees' job satisfaction. Participants rated various aspects of their current jobs with respect to existing and desired job characteristics. They also rated their perceptions of how quickly each job characteristic was changing to more closely approximate the ideal, and they rated the desired velocity of change for each job characteristic. Results indicated that velocity considerations play an important role in participants' job satisfaction. In a second study using a laboratory study, Chang and colleagues found that satisfaction with task performance was similarly affected by perceptions of velocity toward their performance goal.

Convergent Evidence

The plausibility of the general line of reasoning behind this theoretical model is indirectly supported by two other lines of work, one from neuropsychology and one from neurobiology. One of them concerns the existence of timing devices in the nervous system. Our view is predicated on the existence of an ability to assess change over time. Doing so requires some representation of time. Neural structures clearly do exist that represent time in some manner (e.g., Handy, Gazzaniga, & Ivry, 2003; Ivry & Richardson, 2002; Ivry & Spencer, 2004).

A second source of indirect support concerns consequences of the detection of discrepancies between actual and expected events. Our affect model rests on the assumption that discrepancies above and below a velocity criterion are detected. Recent reviews of dopamine function appear to point to an analogous function. Specifically, dopaminergic neurons respond to rewards that are expected; they respond even more intensely to unexpected rewards; and their responses diminish when a reward that

is expected fails to occur (Schultz, 2000, 2006). This pattern of response appears to indicate that dopamine neurons are involved in detecting when things are going better than expected or worse than expected (see also Holroyd & Coles, 2002). Though the evidence regarding dopamine is not directly supportive of our theory (which deals with progress rather than outcome), the pattern has a very strong parallelism to it.

Two Kinds of Behavioral Loops, Two Dimensions of Affect

The preceding discussion focused exclusively on discrepancy-reducing loops. Now consider discrepancy-enlarging loops. The view just outlined rests on the idea that positive feeling results when an action system is making rapid progress in *doing what it is organized to do*. There is no obvious reason why this principle should not also apply to systems that enlarge discrepancies. If that kind of a system is making rapid progress doing what it is organized to do, there should be positive affect. If it is doing poorly, there should be negative affect.

The idea that affects of both valences can potentially occur would seem comparable across both approach and avoidance systems. That is, both approach and avoidance have the potential to induce positive feelings (by doing well), and the potential to induce negative feelings (by doing poorly). But doing well at *approaching an incentive* is not quite the same experience as doing well at moving *away from a threat*. Thus, the two positives may not be quite the same, nor may the two negatives.

Based on this line of thought, and drawing as well on insights from Higgins (e.g., 1987, 1996) and his collaborators, we assume two sets of affects, one relating to approach, the other to avoidance (Carver & Scheier, 1998). The former reflect doing well versus poorly at gaining an incentive; the latter reflect doing well versus poorly at avoiding a threat. Thus, approach can lead to such positive affects as eagerness, excitement, and elation, and to such negative affects as frustration, anger, and sadness (Carver, 2004; Carver & Harmon-Jones, 2009a). Avoidance can lead to such positive affects as relief and contentment (Carver, 2009) and such negative affects as fear, guilt, and anxiety (for application of this view to social relations, see Laurenceau, Troy, & Carver, 2005). The two sets of affects are assumed to have independent origins (see Figure 10.1). Given the fact that approach and avoidance functions can be engaged simultaneously, however, the affects that people subjectively experience are not always purely one or the other.

The view shown in Figure 10.1 is similar to the view proposed for different reasons by Rolls. Rolls's (1999, 2005) theory starts with reinforcement contingencies, identifying emotions in terms of the occurrence of reinforcers and punishers and the omission or termination of reinforcers and punishers. Consistent with our view, Rolls differentiated between the occurrence of a punisher (which yields fear) and the omission of a reinforcer (which yields frustration and anger). Similarly, he distinguished between the occurrence of a reinforcer (which yields elation) and the omission of a punisher (which yields relief).

Merging Affect and Action

The two-layered viewpoint described in the preceding sections implies a natural link between affect and action. If the input function of the affect loop is a sensed rate of progress in action, the output function must involve a change in rate of that action. Thus, the affect loop has a direct influence on what occurs in the action loop.

Some changes in rate output are straightforward. If you are lagging behind, you push harder (Brehm & Self, 1989; Wright, 1996). Sometimes the changes are less straightforward. The rates of many "behaviors" are defined not by pace or intensity of physical action but by choices among actions or entire programs of action. For example, increasing the rate of progress on a work project may mean choosing to spend a weekend working on it rather than camping. Increasing your rate of kindness means choosing to do an action that reflects that value when an opportunity arises. Thus, adjustment in rate must often be translated into other terms, such as concentration or allocation of time and effort.

The idea of two feedback systems functioning in concert with one another is something we more or less stumbled onto. It turns out, however, that such an arrangement is common in control engineering (e.g., Clark, 1996). Engineers have long recognized that having two feedback systems functioning together—one controlling position, one controlling velocity—permits the device in which they are embedded to respond in a way that is both quick and stable, without overshoots and oscillations (Carver & Scheier, 1998, pp. 144–145).

The combination of quickness and stability is valuable in the kinds of devices with which engineers deal, but its value is not limited to such artificial devices. A person

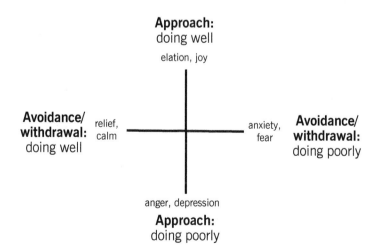

FIGURE 10.1. Carver and Scheier's (1998) view of two orthogonal dimensions of self-regulatory function and examples of the affects that can emerge from them.

who is highly reactive emotionally is prone to overreact to experiences and to oscillate behaviorally. A person who is emotionally unreactive is slow to respond even to urgent events. A person whose reactions are between these two extremes responds quickly but without undue overreaction and consequent oscillation.

For biological entities, being able to respond quickly yet accurately confers a clear adaptive advantage. We believe that the possibility of having the combination of quick and stable responding is a consequence of having both behavior-managing and affect-managing control systems. Affect causes people's responses to be quicker (because this control system is time-sensitive) and, provided that the affective system is not overresponsive, the responses are also stable.

Our focus here is on how affects influence behavior, emphasizing the extent to which they are interwoven. Note, however, that the behavioral responses that are related to the affects also lead to a *reduction of the affects*. Thus, in a very basic sense, the affect system is itself self-regulating (cf. Campos, Frankel, & Camras, 2004). Certainly people also make voluntary efforts to regulate emotions (Gross, 2007), but the affect system does a good deal of that self-regulation on its own. Indeed, if the affect system is optimally responsive, affect will generally not be intense, because the relevant deviations are countered before they become intense (cf. Baumeister, Vohs, DeWall, & Zhang, 2007).

Affect Issues

This theoretical model differs from others in several ways. At least two of the differences appear to have interesting and important implications.

Divergent Views of the Dimensionality Underlying Affect

One difference concerns relationships among various affects. A number of theories conceptualize affects as aligned along dimensions (though certainly not all do so). Our view fits that picture, in a sense. That is, we argue that affects have the potential to be either positive or negative, whether they are related to approach or to avoidance. Thus

we assume a *bipolar dimension of potential affective valence for each core motivational direction.*

Most dimensional models of affect, however, take a very different form. The most widely known dimensional models assume a view in which each core motivational system is responsible for affect of one valence only. This view yields *two unipolar dimensions, each of them linked to the functioning of a motivational system.* This is essentially the position that has been taken by Gray (e.g., 1990, 1994), Lang and colleagues (e.g., Lang, 1995; Lang, Bradley, & Cuthbert, 1990), Cacioppo and colleagues (e.g., Cacioppo & Berntson, 1994; Cacioppo, Gardner, & Berntson, 1999), and Watson and colleagues (Watson, Wiese, Vaidya, & Tellegen, 1999).

What does the evidence say on this issue? There is not a wealth of information from studies targeting it, but there is some. Least studied is "doing well" in threat avoidance. Here are some examples of findings relevant to it. Higgins, Shah, and Friedman (1997, Study 4) found that having an avoidance orientation to a task (instructions to avoid failing) plus a good outcome led to elevations in reports of calmness. Calmness was not affected, however, with an approach orientation (instructions to succeed). Thus, calmness was linked to doing well at avoidance, not doing well at approach. Other studies have asked people to respond to hypothetical scenarios in which a threat was introduced, then removed (Carver, 2009). Reports of relief related principally to individual differences in threat sensitivity.

A larger accumulation of evidence links certain negative affects to "doing poorly" in approaching incentives; just a few are noted here (see Carver & Harmon-Jones, 2009b, for details). In the study by Higgins, Shah, and Friedman (1997) that was just described, people with an approach orientation who experienced failure reported elevated sadness. This did not occur with an avoidance orientation. This pattern suggests a link between sadness and doing poorly at approach.

The broader literature of self-discrepancy theory also makes a similar point. Many studies have found that sadness relates uniquely (controlling for anxiety) to discrepancies between actual selves and ideal selves (see Higgins, 1987, 1996, for reviews). Ideals are qualities the person intrinsically desires: aspirations, hopes, positive images for the self. There is evidence that pursuing an ideal is an approach process (Higgins, 1996). Thus, this literature also suggests that sadness stems from a failure of approach.

Another study bearing on this question examined the situation of frustrative nonreward. Participants were led to believe that they could obtain a reward if they performed well on a task (Carver, 2004). All were told they had done poorly, however, and got no reward. Sadness and discouragement at that point related to sensitivity of the approach system, but not sensitivity of the avoidance system.

There is also a good deal of evidence linking the approach system to anger (for a review, see Carver & Harmon-Jones, 2009b). As one example, Harmon-Jones and Sigelman (2001) induced anger in some persons but not others, then examined cortical activity. They found elevated left anterior activity, which previous research (e.g., Davidson, 1992) had linked to activation of the approach system. In other studies (Carver, 2004), people reported the feelings they experienced in response to hypothetical events (Study 2) and after the destruction of the World Trade Center (Study 3). Reports of anger related to sensitivity of the approach system, whereas reports of fear and anxiety related to sensitivity of the avoidance system.

On the other hand, there is also an accumulation of evidence that contradicts this position, locating all negative affects on one dimension and all positive affects on another dimension. This evidence, briefly summarized by Watson (2009), consists primarily of a large number of studies in which people reported their moods at a particular time or across a particular span of time. As Carver and Harmon-Jones (2009a) pointed out, however, an affective response to a particular event differs in important ways from a mood. Among other things, moods aggregate experiences over multiple events. It seems likely that different influences come into play in the creation or maintenance of moods than underlie focused affective responses to specific events.

We have devoted a good deal of space here to the issue of how affects might be organized. Why? This is an important issue because of its implications with regard to a conceptual mechanism underlying affect. Theories postulating two unipolar dimensions appear to equate greater activation or engagement of a motivational system to more affect of that valence. If the approach system actually relates to feelings of both valences, such a mechanism is not tenable. A conceptual mechanism is needed that addresses both positive and negative feelings within the approach function (and, separately, the avoidance function). The mechanism that was described here does so.

One more word about dimensionality. Our view is dimensional in the sense that it is predicated on a dimension of system functioning (from very well to very poorly). However, the affects that fall on that dimension do not themselves form a dimension, apart from the fact that they represent two valences and a neutral point (Figure 10.1). For example, depression (which arises when things are going extremely poorly) is not simply a more intense state of frustration (which arises when things are going poorly, but less poorly). The affects themselves appear to be nonlinear consequences of linear variation in system functioning. Anger and depression are both potential consequences of approach going poorly; which one emerges appears to depend on whether the goal seems lost or not (see also Rolls, 1999, 2005).

Coasting When Exceeding Criterion

Another potentially important issue also differentiates this model from most other viewpoints on the meaning and consequences of affect (Carver, 2003). Recall the idea that affect reflects the error signal in a feedback loop. Affect thus would be a signal to adjust progress—and that would be true whether rate is above the criterion or below it. This is intuitive for negative feelings: Frustration leads to increase in effort. But what about positive feelings?

Here theory becomes counterintuitive. In this model, positive feelings arise when things are going better than they need to. But the feelings still reflect a discrepancy, and the function of a negative feedback loop is to minimize sensed discrepancies. If so, such a system "wants" to see neither negative nor positive affect. Either one would represent an "error" and lead to changes in output that eventually would reduce it (see also Izard, 1977).

This view argues that exceeding the criterion rate of progress (thus creating positive feelings) automatically results in a tendency to reduce effort in this domain. The person "coasts" a little. This does not mean stopping altogether, but easing back, such that subsequent progress returns to the criterion. The impact on affect would be that the positive feeling is not sustained for very long. It begins to fade.

We should be clear that expending effort to catch up when behind, and coasting when ahead, are both presumed to be specific to the goal to which the affect is linked. Usually (though not always) this is the goal from which the affect arises in the first place. We should also be clear about time frames. This view pertains to the current, ongoing episode. This is *not* an argument that positive affect makes people less likely to do the behavior again later on. That obviously is incorrect. Emotions have important effects on learning, but those effects of emotion are outside the scope of this chapter (see Baumeister et al., 2007).

A system of the sort we are postulating would operate in the same way as a car's cruise control. If progress is too slow, negative affect arises. The person responds by increasing effort, trying to speed up. If progress is better than needed, positive affect arises, leading to coasting. A car's cruise control displays similar properties. A hill slows you down; the cruise control feeds the engine more fuel, speeding back up. If you come across the crest of a hill and roll downward too fast, the system restricts fuel and the speed drags back down.

The analogy is intriguing partly because both sides are asymmetrical in the consequences of deviation from the criterion. In both cases, addressing the problem of going too slowly requires expending further resources. Addressing the problem of going too fast entails only cutting back. A cruise control does not apply the brakes; it only reduces fuel. The car must coast back to the setpoint.

The effect of the cruise control on an excessively high rate of speed thus depends partly on external circumstances. If the downward slope is steep, the car may exceed the setpoint all the way to the valley below. In the same fashion, people generally do not respond to positive affect by trying to dampen the feeling. They only ease back a little on resources that are devoted to the domain in which the affect arose. The feelings may stay for a long time (depending on circumstances), as the person coasts down the subjective hill. Eventually, though, the reduced resources would cause the positive affect to fade. In the long run, then, the system would act to prevent great amounts of pleasure as well as great amounts of pain (Carver, 2003; Carver & Scheier, 1998).

Does positive affect (or making greater than expected progress) lead to coasting? To test this idea, a study must assess coasting with respect to the goal underlying the affect (or the unexpectedly high progress). Many studies have created positive affect in one context and assessed its influence elsewhere (e.g., Isen, 1987, 2000; Schwarz & Bohner, 1996), but that does not test this question.

A few studies satisfy these criteria. Mizruchi (1991) found that professional basketball teams in playoffs tend to lose after winning. It is unclear, however, whether the prior winner slacked off, the loser tried harder, or both. Louro, Pieters, and Zeelenberg (2007) explicitly examined the role of positive feelings from surging ahead in the context of multiple-goal pursuit. In three studies they found that when people were relatively close to a goal, positive feelings prompted decrease in effort toward that goal and a shift of effort to an alternate goal. They also found a boundary on this effect (it occurred only when people were relatively close to their goal).

Another more recent study used an intensive experience sampling procedure across a 2-week period (Fulford, Johnson, Llabre, & Carver, 2010). Participants made a set of judgments three times a day about each of three goals that they were pursuing over that period. The ratings they made included perceptions of progress for each time block, which could be compared to expected progress for that block. The data showed that greater than expected progress toward a goal was followed by reduction in effort toward that goal during the next time period.

Coasting and Multiple Concerns

The idea that positive affect promotes coasting, which eventually results in reduction of the positive affect, strikes some people as improbable at best. Why should a process possibly be built into people that limits positive feelings—indeed, that reduces them? After all, a truism of life is that people are organized to seek pleasure and avoid pain.

There are at least two potential bases for this tendency. One is that it is adaptive for organisms not to spend energy needlessly (Brehm & Self, 1989; Gendolla & Richter, 2010). Coasting is a mechanism that works against that. A second basis stems from the fact that people have multiple simultaneous concerns (Atkinson & Birch, 1970; Carver, 2003; Carver & Scheier, 1998; Frijda, 1994). Given multiple concerns, people do not optimize performance on any one of them, but rather "satisfice" (Simon, 1953)—do a good-enough job on each concern to deal with it satisfactorily. This permits the person to handle many concerns adequately, rather than just one (see also Fitzsimons, Friesen, Orehek, & Kruglanski, 2009; Kumashiro, Rusbult, & Finkel, 2008).

A tendency to coast with respect to a given goal would virtually define *satisficing* regarding that goal. That is, reducing effort would prevent the attainment of the best possible outcome for that goal. A tendency to coast would also promote satisficing regarding a broader array of goals. That is, if progress toward goal attainment in one domain exceeds current needs, a tendency to coast in that particular domain (satisficing) would make it easier to devote energy to another domain. This would help ensure satisfactory goal attainment in the other domain and, ultimately, across multiple domains.

In contrast, continued pursuit of one goal without letup can have adverse effects. Continuing a rapid pace in one arena may sustain positive affect pertaining to that arena, but by diverting resources from other goals it also increases the potential for problems elsewhere. This would be even truer of an effort to *intensify* the positive affect, which would further divert resources from other goals. Indeed, a single-minded pursuit of yet-more-positive feelings in one domain can even be lethal, if it causes the person to disregard threats looming elsewhere.

A pattern in which positive feelings lead to easing back and an openness to shifting the focus of one's energies would minimize such problems. It is important to realize that this view does not require a shift in goals, given positive feelings. It simply holds that

openness to a shift is a consequence—and a potential benefit—of the coasting tendency. This line of thought would, however, begin to account for why people do eventually turn away from pleasurable activities.

Priority Management as a Core Issue in Self-Regulation

This line of argument begins to implicate positive emotion in a broad organizational function within the organism. This function is priority management across time: the shifting from one goal to another as focal in behavior (Dreisbach & Goschke, 2004; Shallice, 1978; Shin & Rosenbaum, 2002). This basic and very important function is often overlooked, but it deserves closer examination. Humans usually pursue many goals simultaneously, but only one can have top priority at a given moment. People attain their many goals by shifting among them. Thus there are changes over time in which goal has the top priority. An important question is how those changes are managed.

What we regard as an extremely insightful view of priority management was proposed many years ago by Simon (1967). He noted that although goals with less than top priority are largely out of awareness, ongoing events still can be relevant to them. Sometimes events that occur during the pursuit of the top-priority goal create problems for a goal with a lower priority. Indeed, the mere passing of time can sometimes create a problem for the goal with the lower priority, because passing of time may make its attainment less likely. If the lower-priority goal is also important, an emerging problem for its attainment needs to be taken into account. If a serious threat to that goal arises, a mechanism is needed for changing priorities, so that the second goal replaces the first one as focal.

Feelings and Reprioritization

Simon (1967) proposed that emotions are calls for reprioritization. He suggested that emotion arising with respect to a goal that is outside awareness eventually induces people to interrupt what they are doing and give that goal a higher priority than it had. The stronger the emotion, the stronger is the claim being made that the unattended goal should have a higher priority than the goal that is currently focal. Simon did not address negative affect that arises with respect to a currently focal goal, but the same principle seems to apply. In that case, negative affect seems to be a call for an even greater investment of resources and effort in that focal goal than is now being made.

Simon's analysis applies easily to negative feelings, cases in which a nonfocal goal demands a higher priority and *intrudes* on awareness. However, another way in which priority ordering can shift is that the currently focal goal can *relinquish its place*. Simon acknowledged this possibility obliquely, noting that goal attainment terminates pursuit of that goal. However, he did not address the possibility that an as-yet-unattained goal might also yield its place in line.

Carver (2003) expanded on that possibility, suggesting that positive feelings represent a cue to *reduce* the priority of the goal to which the feeling pertains. This view appears consistent with the sense of Simon's analysis, but suggests that the prioritizing function of affect pertains to affects of both valences. Positive affect regarding an act of avoidance (relief or tranquility) indicates that a threat has dissipated, that it no longer requires as much attention as it did and can now assume a lower priority. Positive affect regarding approach (happiness, joy) indicates that an incentive is being attained. Even if it is not yet attained, the affect is a signal that you could temporarily withdraw effort from this goal, because you are doing so well.

What follows from a reduction in priority of a currently focal goal? In principle, this situation is less directive than the situation that exists when a nonfocal goal demands higher priority. What happens next in this case depends partly on what else is waiting in line and whether the context has changed in important ways while you were absorbed with the focal goal. Opportunities to attain incentives sometimes appear unexpectedly, and people put aside their plans to take advantage of such unanticipated opportunities (Hayes-Roth & Hayes-Roth, 1979; Payton, 1990). It seems reasonable that people experiencing positive affect should be most prone to shift goals at this point if something else needs fixing or doing (regarding

a next-in-line goal or a newly emergent goal) or if an unanticipated opportunity for gain has appeared.

On the other hand, sometimes neither of these conditions exists. In such a case, no shift in goal would occur. That is, even with the downgrade in priority, the focal goal still has a higher priority than the alternatives. Thus, positive feeling does not *require* that there be a change in direction. It simply sets the stage for such a change to be more likely.

Apart from evidence of coasting per se (discussed earlier), there is also other evidence consistent with the idea that positive affect tends to promote shifting of focus to other areas that need attention (for a broader discussion, see Carver, 2003). As an example, Trope and Neter (1994) induced a positive mood in some people but not others, gave them all a social sensitivity test, then told them that they had performed well on two parts of the test but poorly on a third. The participants then indicated their interest in reading more about their performances on the various parts of the test. Those in a positive mood showed more interest in the part they had failed than did controls, suggesting that they were inclined to shift their focus to an area that needed their attention. This effect was conceptually replicated by Trope and Pomerantz (1998) and Reed and Aspinwall (1998).

Phenomena such as these have contributed to the emergence of the view that positive feelings represent psychological resources (see also Aspinwall, 1998; Fredrickson, 1998; Isen, 2000; Tesser, Crepaz, Collins, Cornell, & Beach, 2000). The idea that positive affect serves as a resource for exploration resembles the idea that positive feelings open people up to noticing and turning to emergent opportunities, to being distracted into enticing alternatives—to opportunistic behavior.

Indeed, there is some evidence that fits this idea more directly (Kahn & Isen, 1993). Kahn and Isen (1993) gave people opportunities to try out choices within a food category. Those who had been put into a state of positive affect beforehand switched among choices more than did controls. Isen (2000, p. 423) interpreted this as showing that positive affect promotes "enjoyment of variety and a wide range of possibilities," which sounds much like opportunistic foraging. In the same vein, Dreisbach and Goschke (2004) found that positive affect decreased perseveration on a task strategy and increased distractibility. Both of these findings are consistent with the reasoning presented in this section.

Priority Management and Dysphoria

One more important aspect of priority management should be addressed here. It concerns the idea that goals sometimes are not attainable and are better abandoned. Sufficient doubt about goal attainment creates an impetus to reduce effort to reach the goal and even to give up the goal itself (Carver & Scheier, 1998, 1999a, 1999b). This sense of doubt is accompanied by sadness or dysphoria. The abandonment of a goal reflects a decrease in its priority. How does this sort of reprioritization fit into the picture just outlined?

At first glance, this outcome seems to contradict Simon's (1967) position that negative affect is a call for higher priority. After all, sadness is a negative affect. However, we think that there is an important difference between two classes of approach-related negative affects, which forces an elaboration of Simon's thinking. As noted earlier, our view on affect rests on a dimension that ranges from doing well to doing poorly (Figure 10.1), though the affects themselves do not form a true continuum (e.g., depression is not more intense anger). We would argue that inadequate movement forward (or no movement, or loss of ground) gives rise initially to frustration, irritation, and anger (Figure 10.2). These feelings (or the mechanism that underlies them) serve to engage effort more completely, so as to overcome obstacles and enhance progress. This case clearly fits the priority management model of Simon.

Sometimes, however, continued effort does not produce adequate movement forward. Indeed, if the situation is one of loss, movement forward is precluded because the goal is gone. When failure is (or seems) assured, the feelings are instead sadness, depression, dejection, despondency, grief, and hopelessness (cf. Finlay-Jones & Brown, 1981). Behaviorally, this is paralleled by disengagement from active effort toward the goal (Klinger, 1975; Lewis, Sullivan, Ram-say, & Allessandri, 1992; Mikulincer, 1988; Wortman & Brehm, 1975).

Despite this reduction of effort, this goal may not immediately have assumed a lower priority, although in adaptive functioning it will eventually do so. People often ruminate about the source of their dysphoria (Nolen-Hoeksema, Wisco, & Lyubomirsky, 2008; Watkins, 2008). The rumination, which keeps that goal in, or at least close to, consciousness, implies that the goal thus far retains a relatively high priority. Ceasing of rumination, which generally (though not inevitably) comes with time, is a sign that the goal's priority has now fallen.

Two additional points about the portion of Figure 10.2 to the right of the vertical criterion line are worth noting. First, this part of the figure has much in common with several other depictions of variations in effort when difficulty in moving toward a goal gives way to loss of the goal (for details, see Carver & Scheier, 1998, Ch. 11). Perhaps best known is Wortman and Brehm's (1975) integration of reactance and helplessness. They described a region of threat to control, in which there is enhanced effort to regain control, and a region of loss of control, in which efforts diminish. Indeed, the figure they used to illustrate those regions greatly resembles the right side of Figure 10.2. Another view with the same character is Brehm and Self's (1989) subsequent refinement of that model.

Another point concerns the fact that the right side of Figure 10.2 is drawn with a rather abrupt shift from anger to sadness (which is also true of the Brehm & Self, 1989, view). The degree of abruptness of the transition in this figure is arbitrary. There likely are cases in which the transition is abrupt and also cases in which it is not. These two sets of cases may be distinguished by the relative importance of the goals involved. Importance as a variable has largely been ignored in this discussion, but it obviously must play a very large role in determining the intensity of affective and motivational experiences (cf. Pomerantz, Saxon, & Oishi, 2000).

We reemphasize that the two kinds of negative feelings we have been discussing here both have adaptive properties for the contexts in which they arise. In the first situation—when the person falls behind, but

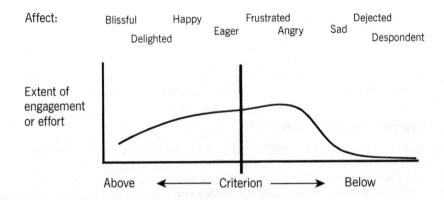

FIGURE 10.2. Hypothesized approach-related affects as a function of doing well versus doing poorly compared to a criterion velocity. The vertical dimension depicts the degree of behavioral engagement posited to be associated with affects at different degrees of departure from neutral. Based on Carver (2004).

the goal is not identified as lost—feelings of frustration and anger accompany an increase in effort, a struggle to gain the goal despite setbacks. This struggle is adaptive (and thus the affect is adaptive) to the extent that the struggle fosters goal attainment. And it often (though not always) does so.

In the second situation—when effort appears futile—feelings of sadness and depression accompany reduction of effort. Sadness, depression, and despondency imply that things cannot be set right, that effort is pointless. Reducing effort in this circumstance is also adaptive (Carver & Scheier, 2003; Wrosch, Scheier, Carver, & Schulz, 2003; Wrosch, Scheier, Miller, Schulz, & Carver, 2003): It conserves energy rather than waste it in pursuit of the unattainable (Nesse, 2000). If reducing effort also helps diminish commitment to the goal (Klinger, 1975), it eventually readies the person to take up other goals in place of this one.

Clinical Implications

The ideas presented in this chapter were intended to focus on the realm of normal experience, but they also have clear relevance for a number of areas of clinical psychology. The clearest relevance is to mood disorders, both depression and mania. In this section we briefly consider how the ideas have been applied to those topics.

Clinical Depression

Although clinical depression involves a great deal more than the affective experience of sadness, sadness is generally part of the picture. The experience of clinical depression is both similar to, and different from, the preceding description of sadness as an affect. One similarity is that the experience of clinical depression is partly a feeling of being unable to move forward to attain desired goals. Along with this comes the sense that even tasks that objectively are easy to accomplish require great effort (Brinkmann & Gendolla, 2008).

One salient difference between the experiences is that normal states of sadness diminish relatively quickly, in part because of diminishing commitment to the goal that seems out of reach. Life entails a good many adjustments of that sort, in which one goal is abandoned and others are taken up. Vulnerability to clinical depression, in contrast, often seems characterized by a relative inability to abandon what seem to be unattainable goals (Carver & Scheier, 1998, Chs. 12–13). It has been suggested that this vulnerability reflects a continuing attempt to demonstrate a condition of self-worth (Rothbaum, Morling, & Rusk, 2009). Whereas it may be easy to reduce one's commitment to goals that are not deeply embedded in the self, it is far harder to give up on the goal of self-worth. Thus, being committed to demonstrating one's self-worth creates problems in the face of failure (Crocker & Park, 2004). As the person tries to hang on to something that is perceived as being out of reach, the result is continuing negative affect (Pyszczynski & Greenberg, 1992).

Mania

Mania is a period of positive or irritable mood, accompanied by symptoms that include increased psychomotor activation, extreme self-confidence, pressured speech, racing thoughts, and pursuit of rewarding activities without attention to risks. Based on a hypothesis suggested by Depue and Iacono (1989), evidence has accumulated that mania is linked to oversensitivity of a general approach system (Alloy & Abramson, 2010; Fowles, 1988; Johnson, 2005; Johnson, Edge, Holmes, & Carver, 2012; Urošević, Abramson, Harmon-Jones, & Alloy, 2008). There is evidence that people vulnerable to mania engage greater effort on difficult tasks than other people (Harmon-Jones et al., 2008). Of particular interest at present, there is also evidence that positive emotions are more persistent among people vulnerable to mania than among other people (Gruber, 2011).

Why are positive emotions more persistent among persons vulnerable to mania? Evidence from one recent study tested the hypothesis that people vulnerable to mania are less likely than other people to coast after having made unexpectedly high progress toward their goals. This study (Fulford et al., 2010) was mentioned earlier in the chapter as providing evidence of coasting—reducing effort—after making better than expected progress toward daily life goals. What was not mentioned earlier is that this study examined both healthy controls and people with bipolar disorder. The pattern of reduced effort emerged for both groups, but it was significantly less pronounced among people with bipolar disorder than among healthy controls. This finding suggests that one problem underlying bipolar disorder may be a failure of this normal homeostatic function.

Summary and Conclusion

In this chapter we have sketched the outlines of a theoretical view of the origin and some of the functions of affect, based on the organizing principle of feedback control processes. This is a functional analysis, in which affect serves the purpose of regulating degree of engagement in goal pursuit across time. The general structure of the model is applicable to any organism that is goal directed and experiences greater or lesser urgency in reaching those goals. Although we have described the model in terms of affective experience—subjective valence—it is not at all clear that consciousness per se is required for the processes we have described to take place. We construe this mechanism as a set of functions that occur simultaneously with the functions that create action, in parallel to them, constantly, automatically, and unbidden. We take no position on the question of whether it is the affects themselves, or the mechanisms that underlie them and create them, that are responsible for the functions that follow.

This is not a biological model. However, it clearly incorporates implicit assumptions about neural processing. It assumes the existence of brain structures that evaluate changes in the relative favorability of situations. This requires both structures that can recognize incentives and threats and also structures that map experience over some range of time. Although these are assumptions, the assumptions appear plausible.

This is not really a cognitive model, either. It does not deal with appraisals, except in the limited sense that perceptions regarding the rate of goal-related progress are appraisals. However, it is relatively easy to integrate this view with the overall sense of appraisal models. Appraisal models all assume that an important property of emotions is that they pertain to events that are valenced. The strength of appraisal models is the nuance they provide *within* the categories "bad" and "good." Our model has no such nuances. But our analysis can be inserted in place of "bad outcome" and "good outcome" in appraisal models, thereby adding to those models the reminder that emotions arise during the flow of experiences, not just at the end.

It is also worth noting that this model ties the creation of information specifying valence to some experience regarding an incentive or a threat. Once information that specifies valence has become attached to other information in memory, it can of course be reevoked by activation of that memory. But in the first cases—those in which affect emerges online—it has to come from somewhere, created via some mechanism. We argue for a particular mechanism. It is a general-purpose mechanism, in the sense that doing poorly with respect to desired goals of great diversity leads to affect of negative valence. Is there modularity within it, with different classes of goals yielding negative affect of slightly different flavor when things are going poorly? We are generally agnostic on that issue.

This view of affect can be brought to bear on one of the most obvious but least examined aspects of human behavior: the fact that people pursue multiple goals over a given period of time, but shift repeatedly from one to another. Affect probably is not the only influence on priority management, but it is an important one. Apart from the role of emotion in learning, its role in priority management may turn out to be its most important function.

Acknowledgments

Preparation of this chapter was facilitated by support from the National Cancer Institute (Grant No. CA64710), the National Science Foundation (Grant No. BCS0544617), and the National Heart, Lung, and Blood Institute (Grant Nos. HL65111, HL65112, HL076852, and HL076858).

References

Alloy, L. B., & Abramson, L. Y. (2010). The role of the behavioral approach system (BAS) in bipolar spectrum disorders. *Current Directions in Psychological Science, 19,* 189–194.

Aspinwall, L. G. (1998). Rethinking the role of positive affect in self-regulation. *Motivation and Emotion, 22,* 1–32.

Atkinson, J. W., & Birch, D. (1970). *The dynamics of action.* New York: Wiley.

Austin, J. T., & Vancouver, J. B. (1996). Goal constructs in psychology: Structure, process, and content. *Psychological Bulletin, 120,* 338–375.

Baumeister, R. F., Vohs, K. D., DeWall, C. N., & Zhang, L. (2007). How emotion shapes behavior: Feedback, anticipation, and reflection, rather than direct causation. *Personality and Social Psychology Review, 11,* 167–203.

Beer, R. D. (1995). A dynamical systems perspective on agent–environment interaction. *Artificial Intelligence, 72,* 173–215.

Brehm, J. W., & Self, E. A. (1989). The intensity of motivation. *Annual Review of Psychology, 40,* 109–131.

Brickman, P., & Campbell, D. T. (1971). Hedonic relativism and planning the good society. In M. H. Appley (Ed.), *Adaptation level theory: A symposium* (pp. 287–302). New York: Academic Press.

Brinkmann, K., & Gendolla, G. H. E. (2008). Does depression interfere with effort mobilization?: Effects of dysphoria and task difficulty on cardiovascular response. *Journal of Personality and Social Psychology, 94,* 146–157.

Brunstein, J. C. (1993). Personal goals and subjective well-being: A longitudinal study. *Journal of Personality and Social Psychology, 65,* 1061–1070.

Cacioppo, J. T., & Berntson, G. G. (1994). Relationship between attitudes and evaluative space: A critical review, with emphasis on the separability of positive and negative substrates. *Psychological Bulletin, 115,* 401–423.

Cacioppo, J. T., Gardner, W. L., & Berntson, G. G. (1999). The affect system has parallel and integrative processing components: Form follows function. *Journal of Personality and Social Psychology, 76,* 839–855.

Campos, J. J., Frankel, C. B., & Camras, L. (2004). On the nature of emotion regulation. *Child Development, 75,* 377–394.

Cannon, W. B. (1932). *The wisdom of the body.* New York: Norton.

Carver, C. S. (2003). Pleasure as a sign you can attend to something else: Placing positive feelings within a general model of affect. *Cognition and Emotion, 17,* 241–261.

Carver, C. S. (2004). Negative affects deriving from the behavioral approach system. *Emotion, 4,* 3–22.

Carver, C. S. (2009). Threat sensitivity, incentive sensitivity, and the experience of relief. *Journal of Personality, 77,* 125–138.

Carver, C. S., & Harmon-Jones, E. (2009a). Anger and approach: Reply to Watson (2009) and Tomarken and Zald (2009). *Psychological Bulletin, 135,* 215–217.

Carver, C. S., & Harmon-Jones, E. (2009b). Anger is an approach-related affect: Evidence and implications. *Psychological Bulletin, 135,* 183–204.

Carver, C. S., & Scheier, M. F. (1990). Origins and functions of positive and negative affect: A control–process view. *Psychological Review, 97,* 19–35.

Carver, C. S., & Scheier, M. F. (1998). *On the self-regulation of behavior.* New York: Cambridge University Press.

Carver, C. S., & Scheier, M. F. (1999a). Several more themes, a lot more issues: Commentary on the commentaries. In R. S. Wyer, Jr. (Ed.), *Advances in social cognition* (Vol. 12, pp. 261–302). Mahwah, NJ: Erlbaum.

Carver, C. S., & Scheier, M. F. (1999b). Themes and issues in the self-regulation of behavior. In R. S. Wyer, Jr. (Ed.), *Advances in social cognition* (Vol. 12, pp. 1–105). Mahwah, NJ: Erlbaum.

Carver, C. S., & Scheier, M. F. (2000). Scaling back goals and recalibration of the affect system are processes in normal adaptive self-regulation: Understanding "response shift" phenomena. *Social Science and Medicine, 50,* 1715–1722.

Carver, C. S., & Scheier, M. F. (2003). Three human strengths. In L. G. Aspinwall & U. M. Staudinger (Eds.), *A psychology of human strengths: Fundamental questions and future directions for a positive psychology* (pp. 87–102). Washington, DC: American Psychological Association.

Chang, C.-H., Johnson, R. E., & Lord, R. G. (2010). Moving beyond discrepancies: The importance of velocity as a predictor of satisfaction and motivation. *Human Performance, 23,* 58–80.

Clark, R. N. (1996). *Control system dynamics.* New York: Cambridge University Press.

Clore, G. L. (1994). Why emotions are felt. In P. Ekman & R. J. Davidson (Eds.), *The nature of emotion: Fundamental questions* (pp. 103–111). New York: Oxford University Press.

Crocker, J., & Park, L. E. (2004). The costly pursuit of self-esteem. *Psychological Bulletin, 130,* 392–414.

Davidson, R. J. (1992). Anterior cerebral asymmetry and the nature of emotion. *Brain and Cognition, 20,* 125–151.

Depue, R. A., & Iacono, W. G. (1989). Neurobehavioral aspects of affective disorders. *Annual Review of Psychology, 40,* 457–492.

Dreisbach, G., & Goschke, T. (2004). How positive affect modulates cognitive control: Reduced perseveration at the cost of increased distractibility. *Journal of Experimental Psychology: Learning, Memory, and Cognition, 30,* 343–353.

Eidelman, S., & Biernat, M. (2007). Getting more from success: Standard raising as esteem maintenance. *Journal of Personality and Social Psychology, 92,* 759–774.

Elliot, A. J. (Ed.). (2008). *Handbook of approach and avoidance motivation.* Mahwah, NJ: Erlbaum.

Finlay-Jones, R., & Brown, G. W. (1981). Types of stressful life event and the onset of anxiety and depressive disorders. *Psychological Medicine, 11,* 803–815.

Fitzsimons, G. M., Friesen, J., Orehek, E., & Kruglanski, A. W. (2009). Progress-induced goal shifting as a self-regulatory strategy. In J. P. Forgas, R. F. Baumeister, & D. M. Tice (Eds.), *Psychology of self-regulation: Cognitive, affective, and motivational processes* (pp. 183–197). New York: Psychology Press.

Ford, D. H. (1987). *Humans as self-constructing living systems: A developmental perspective on behavior and personality.* Hillsdale, NJ: Erlbaum.

Fowles, D. C. (1988). Psychophysiology and psychopathology: A motivational approach. *Psychophysiology, 25,* 373–391.

Fredrickson, B. L. (1998). What good are positive emotions? *Review of General Psychology, 2,* 300–319.

Frijda, N. H. (1986). *The emotions.* Cambridge, UK: Cambridge University Press.

Frijda, N. H. (1988). The laws of emotion. *American Psychologist, 43,* 349–358.

Frijda, N. H. (1994). Emotions are functional, most of the time. In P. Ekman & R. J. Davidson (Eds.), *The nature of emotion: Fundamental questions* (pp. 112–126). New York: Oxford University Press.

Fulford, D., Johnson, S. L., Llabre, M. M., & Carver, C. S. (2010). Pushing and coasting in dynamic goal pursuit: Coasting is attenuated in bipolar disorder. *Psychological Science, 21,* 1021–1027.

Gendolla, G. H. E., & Richter, M. (2010). Effort mobilization when the self is involved: Some lessons from the cardiovascular system. *Review of General Psychology, 14,* 212–226.

Gray, J. A. (1990). Brain systems that mediate both emotion and cognition. *Cognition and Emotion, 4,* 269–288.

Gray, J. A. (1994). Three fundamental emotion systems. In P. Ekman & R. J. Davidson (Eds.), *The nature of emotion: Fundamental ques-*

tions (pp. 243–247). New York: Oxford University Press.

Gross, J. J. (Ed.). (2007). Handbook of emotion regulation. New York: Guilford Press.

Gruber, J. (2011). Can feeling too good be bad?: Positive emotion persistence (PEP) in bipolar disorder. Current Directions in Psychological Science, 20, 217–221.

Handy, T., Gazzaniga, M., & Ivry, R. B. (2003). Cortical and subcortical contributions to the representation of temporal information. Neuropsychologia, 41, 1461–1473.

Harmon-Jones, E., Abramson, L. Y., Nusslock, R., Sigelman, J. D., Urošević, S., Turonie, L. D., et al. (2008). Effect of bipolar disorder on left frontal cortical responses to goals differing in valence and task difficulty. Biological Psychiatry, 63, 693–698.

Harmon-Jones, E., & Sigelman, J. D. (2001). State anger and prefrontal brain activity: Evidence that insult-related relative left-prefrontal activation is associated with experienced anger and aggression. Journal of Personality and Social Psychology, 80, 797–803.

Hayes-Roth, B., & Hayes-Roth, F. (1979). A cognitive model of planning. Cognitive Science, 3, 275–310.

Higgins, E. T. (1987). Self-discrepancy: A theory relating self and affect. Psychological Review, 94, 319–340.

Higgins, E. T. (1996). Ideals, oughts, and regulatory focus: Relating affect and motivation to distinct pains and pleasures. In P. M. Gollwitzer & J. A. Bargh (Eds.), The psychology of action: Linking cognition and motivation to behavior (pp. 91–114). New York: Guilford Press.

Higgins, E. T., Shah, J., & Friedman, R. (1997). Emotional responses to goal attainment: Strength of regulatory focus as moderator. Journal of Personality and Social Psychology, 72, 515–525.

Holroyd, C. B., & Coles, M. G. H. (2002). The neural basis of human error processing: Reinforcement learning, dopamine, and the error-related negativity. Psychological Review, 109, 679–709.

Hsee, C. K., & Abelson, R. P. (1991). Velocity relation: Satisfaction as a function of the first derivative of outcome over time. Journal of Personality and Social Psychology, 60, 343–347.

Isen, A. M. (1987). Positive affect, cognitive processes, and social behavior. In L. Berkowitz (Ed.), Advances in experimental social psychology (Vol. 20, pp. 203–252). San Diego, CA: Academic Press.

Isen, A. M. (2000). Positive affect and decision making. In M. Lewis & J. M. Haviland-Jones (Eds.), Handbook of emotions (2nd ed., pp. 417–435). New York: Guilford Press.

Ivry, R. B., & Richardson, T. (2002). Temporal control and coordination: The multiple timer model. Brain and Cognition, 48, 117–132.

Ivry, R. B., & Spencer, R. (2004). The neural representation of time. Current Opinion in Neurobiology, 14, 225–232.

Izard, C. E. (1977). Human emotions. New York: Plenum Press.

Johnson, R. E., Chang, C.-H., & Lord, R. G. (2006). Moving from cognitive to behavior: What the research says. Psychological Bulletin, 132, 381–415.

Johnson, S. L. (2005). Mania and dysregulation in goal pursuit. Clinical Psychology Review, 25, 241–262.

Johnson, S. L., Edge, M. D., Holmes, M. K., & Carver, C. S. (2012). The behavioral activation system and mania. Annual Review of Clinical Psychology, 8, 243–267.

Kahn, B. E., & Isen, A. M. (1993). The influence of positive affect on variety-seeking among safe, enjoyable products. Journal of Consumer Research, 20, 257–270.

Klinger, E. (1975). Consequences of commitment to and disengagement from incentives. Psychological Review, 82, 1–25.

Kumashiro, M., Rusbult, C. E., & Finkel, E. J. (2008). Navigating personal and relational concerns: The quest for equilibrium. Journal of Personality and Social Psychology, 95, 94–110.

Lang, P. J. (1995). The emotion probe: Studies of motivation and attention. American Psychologist, 50, 372–385.

Lang, P. J., Bradley, M. M., & Cuthbert, B. N. (1990). Emotion, attention, and the startle reflex. Psychological Review, 97, 377–395.

Laurenceau, J.-P., Troy, A. B., & Carver, C. S. (2005). Two distinct emotional experiences in romantic relationships: Effects of perceptions regarding approach of intimacy and avoidance of conflict. Personality and Social Psychology Bulletin, 31, 1123–1133.

Lawrence, J. W., Carver, C. S., & Scheier, M. F. (2002). Velocity toward goal attainment in immediate experience as a determinant of affect. Journal of Applied Social Psychology, 32, 788–802.

Lewis, M., Sullivan, M. W., Ramsay, D. S., &

Allessandri, S. M. (1992). Individual differences in anger and sad expressions during extinction: Antecedents and consequences. *Infant Behavior and Development, 15,* 443–452.

Louro, M. J., Pieters, R., & Zeelenberg, M. (2007). Dynamics of multiple-goal pursuit. *Journal of Personality and Social Psychology, 93,* 174–193.

MacKay, D. M. (1966). Cerebral organization and the conscious control of action. In J. C. Eccles (Ed.), *Brain and conscious experience* (pp. 422–445). Berlin: Springer-Verlag.

Mikulincer, M. (1988). Reactance and helplessness following exposure to learned helplessness following exposure to unsolvable problems: The effects of attributional style. *Journal of Personality and Social Psychology, 54,* 679–686.

Miller, G. A., Galanter, E., & Pribram, K. H. (1960). *Plans and the structure of behavior.* New York: Holt, Rinehart & Winston.

Mischel, W., & Shoda, Y. (1995). A cognitive–affective system theory of personality: Reconceptualizing the invariances in personality and the role of situations. *Psychological Review, 102,* 246–268.

Mizruchi, M. S. (1991). Urgency, motivation, and group performance: The effect of prior success on current success among professional basketball teams. *Social Psychology Quarterly, 54,* 181–189.

Nesse, R. M. (2000). Is depression an adaptation? *Archives of General Psychiatry, 57,* 14–20.

Nolen-Hoeksema, S., Wisco, B. E., & Lyubomirsky, S. (2008). Rethinking rumination. *Perspectives on Psychological Science, 3,* 400–424.

Ortony, A., Clore, G. L., & Collins, A. (1988). *The cognitive structure of emotions.* New York: Cambridge University Press.

Payton, D. W. (1990). Internalized plans: A representation for action resources. In P. Maes (Ed.), *Designing autonomous agents: Theory and practice from biology to engineering and back* (pp. 89–103). Cambridge, MA: MIT Press.

Pomerantz, E. M., Saxon, J. L., & Oishi, S. (2000). The psychological trade-offs of goal investment. *Journal of Personality and Social Psychology, 79,* 617–630.

Powers, W. T. (1973). *Behavior: The control of perception.* Chicago: Aldine.

Pyszczynski, T., & Greenberg, J. (1992). *Hanging on and letting go: Understanding the onset, progression, and remission of depression.* New York: Springer-Verlag.

Reed, M. B., & Aspinwall, L. G. (1998). Self-affirmation reduces biased processing of health-risk information. *Motivation and Emotion, 22,* 99–132.

Rolls, E. T. (1999). *The brain and emotion.* Oxford, UK: Oxford University Press.

Rolls, E. T. (2005). *Emotion explained.* Oxford, UK: Oxford University Press.

Rosenbaum, D. A., Carlson, R. A., & Gilmore, R. O. (2001). Acquisition of intellectual and perceptual–motor skills. *Annual Review of Psychology, 52,* 453–470.

Rosenbaum, D. A., Meulenbroek, R. G. J., Vaughan, J., & Jansen, C. (2001). Posture-based motion planning: Applications to grasping. *Psychological Review, 108,* 709–734.

Rothbaum, F., Morling, B., & Rusk, N. (2009). How goals and beliefs lead people into and out of depression. *Review of General Psychology, 13,* 302–314.

Schultz, W. (2000). Multiple reward signals in the brain. *Nature Reviews, 1,* 199–207.

Schultz, W. (2006). Behavioral theories and the neurophysiology of reward. *Annual Reviews of Psychology, 57,* 87–115.

Schwartz, S. H., & Bilsky, W. (1990). Toward a theory of the universal content and structure of values: Extensions and cross-cultural replications. *Journal of Personality and Social Psychology, 58,* 878–891.

Schwartz, S. H., & Rubel, T. (2005). Sex differences in value priorities: Cross-cultural and multimethod studies. *Journal of Personality and Social Psychology, 89,* 1010–1028.

Schwarz, N., & Bohner, G. (1996). Feelings and their motivational implications: Moods and the action sequence. In P. M. Gollwitzer & J. A. Bargh (Eds.), *The psychology of action: Linking cognition and motivation to behavior* (pp. 119–145). New York: Guilford Press.

Shallice, T. (1978). The dominant action system: An information-processing approach to consciousness. In K. S. Pope & J. L. Singer (Eds.), *The stream of consciousness: Scientific investigations into the flow of human experience* (pp. 117–157). New York: Wiley.

Shin, J. C., & Rosenbaum, D. A. (2002). Reaching while calculating: Scheduling of cognitive and perceptual–motor processes. *Journal of Experimental Psychology: General, 131,* 206–219.

Simon, H. A. (1953). *Models of man.* New York: Wiley.

Simon, H. A. (1967). Motivational and emotional controls of cognition. *Psychology Review, 74,* 29–39.

Tesser, A., Crepaz, N., Collins, J. C., Cornell, D., & Beach, S. R. H. (2000). Confluence of self-esteem regulation mechanisms: On integrating the self-zoo. *Personality and Social Psychology Bulletin, 26,* 1476–1489.

Trope, Y., & Neter, E. (1994). Reconciling competing motives in self-evaluation: The role of self-control in feedback seeking. *Journal of Personality and Social Psychology, 66,* 646–657.

Trope, Y., & Pomerantz, E. M. (1998). Resolving conflicts among self-evaluative motives: Positive experiences as a resource for overcoming defensiveness. *Motivation and Emotion, 22,* 53–72.

Urošević, S., Abramson, L. Y., Harmon-Jones, E., & Alloy, L. B. (2008). Dysregulation of the behavioral approach system (BAS) in bipolar spectrum disorders: Review of theory and evidence. *Clinical Psychology Review, 28,* 1188–1205.

Vallacher, R. R., & Wegner, D. M. (1987). What do people think they're doing?: Action identification and human behavior. *Psychological Review, 94,* 3–15.

von Bertalanffy, L. (1968). *General systems theory.* New York: Braziller.

Watkins, E. (2008). Constructive and unconstructive repetitive thought. *Psychological Bulletin, 134,* 163–206.

Watson, D. (2009). Locating anger in the hierarchical structure of affect: Comment on Carver and Harmon-Jones (2009). *Psychological Bulletin, 135,* 205–208.

Watson, D., Wiese, D., Vaidya, J., & Tellegen, A. (1999). The two general activation systems of affect: Structural findings, evolutionary considerations, and psychobiological evidence. *Journal of Personality and Social Psychology, 76,* 820–838.

Wiener, N. (1948). *Cybernetics: Control and communication in the animal and the machine.* Cambridge, MA: MIT Press.

Wortman, C. B., & Brehm, J. W. (1975). Responses to uncontrollable outcomes: An integration of reactance theory and the learned helplessness model. In L. Berkowitz (Ed.), *Advances in experimental social psychology* (Vol. 8, pp. 277–336). New York: Academic Press.

Wright, R. A. (1996). Brehm's theory of motivation as a model of effort and cardiovascular response. In P. M. Gollwitzer & J. A. Bargh (Eds.), *The psychology of action: Linking cognition and motivation to behavior* (pp. 424–453). New York: Guilford Press.

Wrosch, C., Scheier, M. F., Carver, C. S., & Schulz, R. (2003). The importance of goal disengagement in adaptive self-regulation: When giving up is beneficial. *Self and Identity, 2,* 1–20.

Wrosch, C., Scheier, M. F., Miller, G. E., Schulz, R., & Carver, C. S. (2003). Adaptive self-regulation of unattainable goals: Goal disengagement, goal re-engagement, and subjective well-being. *Personality and Social Psychology Bulletin, 29,* 1494–1508.

CHAPTER 11

Emotion Regulation and Cognition

Gaurav Suri, Gal Sheppes, and James J. Gross

Imagine two job candidates waiting for an important interview. They are both terribly nervous and can't stop their hands from trembling. Each feels sick to his stomach, and each worries that his fear will interfere with his interview performance. If only they could calm down and regain their confidence! The first candidate decides to direct his attention away from his fearful thoughts and think instead about calming things. The second candidate decides to attend to the interview but to reinterpret it as an opportunity to find whether the company is good enough for *him*, to see whether *he* would enjoy working there. Both of these options lessen the anxiety of the candidates, and they feel more confident as the receptionist buzzes them in.

This vignette begins with an emotion—fear—whose alleviation consists of two types of regulating cognitive processes. In this chapter our goal is to provide an introduction to the research and theories on how people regulate their emotions, with a particular emphasis on how cognitive processes enable important types of emotion regulation. In the first section we provide an overview of emotion and emotion regulation and present a framework that has proved useful for organizing the many different types of emotion regulation strategies. We then discuss the role cognition plays in

this framework. In the second section we analyze the neural systems that give rise to our abilities to cognitively regulate emotion. We specifically examine two different types of cognitive control—attention based and meaning based—that are useful in regulating emotional responses. In the third section we outline individual differences in emotion regulation. In particular, we describe adaptive and maladaptive variations in attention-based and meaning-based strategies. We conclude by outlining future directions in the field of emotion regulation, emphasizing the areas where a consideration of cognitive approaches is likely to continue to yield exciting new results.

Emotion and Emotion Regulation

Emotions have been said to represent the "wisdom of the ages" (Lazarus, 1991, p. 820), providing time-tested responses to recurrent adaptive problems. This idea has been developed by functionalist perspectives that highlight the crucial benefits of emotion: Emotions prepare time-tested behavioral responses (Cosmides & Tooby, 2000), improve decision making for events that are personally relevant (Damasio, 1999), enhance memory for events that are important to remember (Phelps, 2006), and facilitate interpersonal interactions (Keltner & Kring, 1998). That said, emotions are not always helpful—sometimes they can work against us (Parrott, 1993). This can happen when an emotion is of the wrong type, or if it occurs at the wrong time, or with an intensity that may be out of place. In such situations, we may be motivated to regulate our emotions. But to understand the mechanisms of emotion regulation, we must first consider its target—namely, emotion itself.

What Is Emotion?

The word *emotion* came to psychology from everyday usage and it does not have a well-defined boundary. This means that many different phenomena fall under this heading. Emotions vary in their intensity, ranging from mild to overwhelming, panic-like responses; they also vary in their duration and in the speed of their onset and decline. Some emotions, such as sadness, rise and fall slowly, whereas other emotions, such as disgust, quickly rise to their peak and return to baseline just as quickly (Davidson, 1998). Therefore, to provide a single, tidy definition of emotion that spans all its instances has proven to be a challenging task. Nevertheless, progress is possible if we consider prototypical features that tend to be common across most instances of emotion. Here we consider three such features.

First, emotions arise when an individual attends to a situation that he or she deems meaningful to his or her goals (Lazarus, 1991). The goals may be enduring (writing a novel) or ephemeral (having another slice of pizza), biologically based (hunting for food) or culturally derived (respecting one's elders), peripheral (finding the shortest grocery checkout lane) or central to one's self concept (being a good father), widely shared and accepted (wanting to be good at one's profession), or personal and idiosyncratic (staging beetle fights). But whatever the end goal, it is the meaning attached to the goal-relevant situation that generates emotion. It is of note that the meaning may be generated by a cognitive or an emotional process, or some combination of both. In our opening example, the interview (the situation) was cognitively meaningful to the candidate's goal of gainful employment and it therefore generated an emotion: fear.

Second, emotions can be conceptualized as multifaceted, embodied phenomena that involve loosely coupled changes in subjective experience, behavior, and peripheral physiology (Mauss, Evers, Wilhem, & Gross, 2006). The subjective experience part of emotion—typically called *feeling*—is an internal representation of the changes invoked by the unfolding emotion (Damasio, 1999). The behavioral part of emotion can include changes in activity of the muscles of the face (e.g., being happy can make us smile) and body (e.g., fear can make us freeze), and in what one says, as well as more general changes in basic motivational states such as the likelihood of approach or withdrawal from a relevant stimulus in the environment (Frijda, 1986). The peripheral physiological part of emotion includes the autonomic and neuroendocrine responses that provide metabolic support for anticipated and actual behavioral responses (Levenson, 1999).

Third, emotions are often malleable. Yes, they can interrupt what we're doing and force themselves on our awareness (Frijda, 1986). However, in doing so, they must compete with other cognitions and other emotions that may well take precedence. In our opening example the interview situation produced anxiety, but it was partially overruled by a new construal. This essential malleability of emotions was first emphasized by William James (1884), who viewed emotions as response tendencies that could be modulated in a large number of ways. Cognitive control is surely an important path to modulating emotion; in other words, cognition is central to emotion regulation.

The Modal Model of Emotion

These three core features of emotion—its generation from meaningful situations; its experiential, behavioral, and physiological aspects; and its core malleability—constitute what we refer to as the *modal model* of emotion. This model underlies intuitions about emotion (Feldman Barrett, Ochsner, & Gross, 2007; Gross 1998b) and represents several points of agreement among emotion researchers and theorists. According to this model, emotion arises in the context of a person–situation transaction that compels attention, has a particular meaning to an individual, and gives rise to a coordinated yet malleable multisystem response to the ongoing person–situation transaction. Importantly, situations may be attended to and appraised with conscious awareness, or the attention–appraisal process steps may occur unconsciously. The attention–appraisal process steps, occurring within the brain, connect the emotion-generating situation to the emotional response.

To illustrate the modal model, let's say one is cut off in traffic (or, alternatively, recall a time when one was cut off in traffic). Regardless of whether the situation is external or internal, directed attention and appraisal constitute one's assessment of, among other things, the situation's familiarity and value relevance (Ellsworth & Scherer, 2003). In our example, an emotional response is the result of first attending to this incident and then appraising that the traffic injustice was particularly flagrant. It is the combined effect of attention to emotional features and a particular appraisal that lead to an emotional response.

As noted previously, the emotional responses generated by attention and appraisals are thought to involve changes in experiential, behavioral, and physiological response systems. In this example, one may respond with a feeling of rage, a rude hand gesture, and amygdala activation, respectively. However, if a response does occur, it could change the situation that generated the response. Thus, an angry gesture could lead to an apologetic gesture from the driver of the offending car, which in turn could lead to one being forgiving rather than angry.

What Is Emotion Regulation?

Like emotion, the concept of *emotion regulation* has many possible meanings—in part because the concept inherits all of the complexities that are inherent in the term *emotion*. However, we can again make progress by postulating a general definition and by outlining dimensions along which prototypical instances of emotion regulation occur. These dimensions, and their endpoints, sketch the boundary conditions within which episodes of emotion regulation are most likely to reside.

We begin with a high-level definition. In general, *emotion regulation* refers to processes that influence which emotions we have, when we feel them, and how we experience or express them (Gross, 1998b). Emotion regulation is defined by the activation of a goal to modify the emotion-generating process and involves the motivated recruitment of one or more processes to influence emotion generation (Gross, Sheppes, & Urry, in press).

The first dimension of variation across emotion regulation episodes is whether the emotion-regulating goal is activated in the individual who is having (or is likely to have) an emotion episode, or in someone else. The former—which we refer to as *intrinsic regulation*—involves the activation of a regulation goal in the person who is having the emotion. As we have already seen by way of example, intrinsic emotion regulation can be rooted in cognition. The latter—which we refer to as *extrinsic regulation*—involves the activation of a regulation goal in a person other than the one who is having the emotion in question. In extrinsic regulation, social communication is involved and is thus partly cognitive.

A second dimension of variation across emotion regulation episodes is whether the motivation to engage in emotion regulation is short-term hedonic (to feel less negative or more positive in the near term) or instrumental (to achieve one's long-term goals) (Tamir, 2009). Both types of emotion regulation often arise from cognitive processes.

A third dimension of variation across emotion regulation episodes is whether the emotion-regulating goal is explicit or implicit (Bargh, Gollwitzer, Lee-Chai, Barndollar, & Trotschel, 2001). Implicit goals are activated outside of an individual's awareness, such as when an individual unconsciously stands next to the exit sign and feels calm while standing there. Explicit goals are activated with some measure of awareness, such as when an individual realizes that he or she is feeling grumpy and makes a conscious effort to look cheerful. Both implicit and explicit goals can be governed by cognitive processes.

The Process Model of Emotion Regulation

One of the challenges in thinking about emotion regulation is finding a conceptual framework that can help to organize the numerous forms of emotion regulation. The modal model suggests one approach, in that it specifies a sequence of processes involved in emotion generation, each of which is a potential target for emotion regulation. In Figure 11.1, we present the process model of emotion regulation, which highlights the five points in the modal model where individuals can regulate their emotions. These points correspond to five families of emotion regulation processes: situation selection, situation modification, attentional deployment, cognitive change, and response modulation. Below we elaborate on each of these families, particularly focusing on two regulation families that are most unambiguously cognitive in nature: attentional deployment and cognitive change.

Situation selection refers to efforts an individual makes to influence the situation he or she will encounter, with a view to increasing (or decreasing) the likelihood that certain emotions will arise. Situation selection may best be captured in the classic conceptualization of choosing between approaching and avoiding a situation. Our job candidates from the opening paragraph of this chapter may, for example, choose to reduce their anxiety by deciding to go back home and eschewing the interview entirely. Avoidance functions as a very strong regulatory option that intersects the emotion generative process at the earliest point. Nevertheless, it can be clearly maladaptive if overused (Campbell-Sills & Barlow, 2007).

Situation modification consists of efforts to modify the situation directly so as to alter its emotional impact. For example, when a conservative family member visits, situation modification may consist of removing controversial politically themed artwork.

Attentional deployment refers to the direction of attention in a way that alters the emotion response trajectory. This takes place after an emotional situation has been encountered. An important feature of attentional deployment is that, unlike situation selection and situation modification, the emotion regulation is primarily cognitive. There are several attention regulation options:

1. *Distraction* involves a shift in attention either away from the emotional aspects of the situation or away from the situation altogether. If one of our job candidates decided to think about the exploits of the 2010 San Francisco Giants instead of dwelling on the upcoming interview, he would be using distraction to lessen his fear. Distraction as a regulatory strategy involves loading working memory with independent neutral contents (Van Dillen & Koole, 2007). The strategy involves replacing current emotional information with independent neutral information. Distraction also filters incoming emotional information, which competes with emotion-regulating processes at an early processing stage, before stimuli are represented in working memory for further semantic evaluative processing. That is, dis-

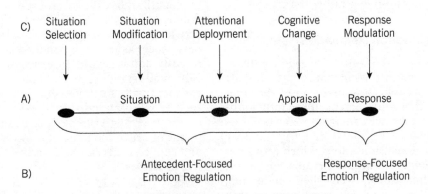

FIGURE 11.1. The process model of emotion regulation. (A) Components of emotion generation. (B) Antecedent-focused versus response-focused emotion regulation strategies. (C) Five emotion regulation families. Adapted from Sheppes and Gross (in press). Copyright by Sage Publications. Adapted by permission.

traction prevents the affective meaning of a stimulus from being processed by blocking it via an early attentional filter. Studies have indicated that distraction is equally effective in attenuating negative affect under low and high levels of emotional intensity (Sheppes & Meiran, 2007).

2. *Rumination* is an emotion regulation strategy that involves directing attention inward, focusing on negative aspects of the self in an abstract, passive, and repetitive way (Nolen-Hoeksema, Wisco, & Lyubomirsky, 2008; Watkins, 2008). Rumination could be viewed as asking big "why" questions (e.g., "Why am I sad?" "Why do these bad things happen to me?") about the causes of negative events, without a translation into a concrete way to deal with things.

3. In recent years, influential accounts from Eastern philosophy and Buddhism have introduced *mindfulness* as an additional form of attentional regulation. Mindfulness involves attending to emotional experiences by focusing on immediate here-and-now aspects with an orientation of curiosity, openness, and acceptance (Bishop et al., 2004). Mindfulness has proven to be an adaptive way to regulate negative emotions and has been incorporated into cognitive treatments of anxiety and depression (Goldin, McRae, Ramel, & Gross, 2008).

Cognitive change refers to changing one's appraisal(s) in a way that alters the situation's emotional significance, by changing how one thinks about the situation itself or about one's capacity to manage its demands. One form of cognitive change that has been extensively studied is *reappraisal*, which involves changing the situation's meaning in such a way that there is a change in the person's emotional response to that situation. For example, one of the job candidates from the opening paragraph reappraised the interview's meaning from a situation in which he was being judged to one where he was doing the judging! Studies of reappraisal have provided evidence that it leads to decreased negative emotion experience and expressive behavior (Dandoy & Goldstein, 1990; Gross, 1998b), decreased startle responses (Dillon & LaBar, 2005; Jackson, Malmstadt, Larson, & Davidson, 2000), decreased neuroendocrine responses (Abel-son, Liberzon, Young, & Khan, 2005), and decreased autonomic responses (Stemmler, 1997; but see Gross, 1998b). Comparable effects have been observed when research participants use reappraisal in the lab (Egloff, Schmukle, Burns, & Schwerdfeger, 2006) or in everyday life (Gross & John, 2003). Consistent with these behavioral and physiological findings, reappraisal is associated with decreased activation in subcortical emotion-generating regions such as the insula and the amygdala. We discuss the neural architecture of emotion regulation in detail in the next major section.

Response modulation refers to attempting to change one or more of the experiential, behavioral, or physiological components of an activated emotion response. In this final stage of the emotion-generating process (shown on the right side of Figure 11.1), experiential, behavioral, and physiological emotional response tendencies have been launched. Regulation targets one of these response systems. For example, exercise can be used to decrease physiological and experiential effects of certain emotions. Another modulation strategy that targets the behavioral response tendency is *expressive suppression*, which involves inhibiting emotion-expressive facial behavior (Richards & Gross, 1999, 2000).

Cognitive Consequences of Emotion Regulation

Each of the above regulation strategies may result in different cognitive consequences. For example, Richards and Gross (2000) contrasted the impact of reappraisal and suppression on memory. Participants watched a series of slides that either elicited high or low levels of negative emotion. Some participants were randomly assigned to view the slides while inhibiting their ongoing emotion-expressive behavior (expressive suppression), whereas others were assigned to view the slides with the detached interest of a medical professional (cognitive reappraisal). A third group was asked to simply view the slides (control). As slides were presented, participants were informed that the study was designed to understand how people use visual and biographical information when "forming impressions of people who have been injured." Specifically, participants were told that they would see several slides of people who had all been severely injured, either recently (high negative emotion) or in the distant past (low negative emotion), and that they would hear each person's name, occupation, and type of accident. The suppression participants fared worse than the control participants in a test where subjects were asked to write down details associated with each slide as it was presented a second time. The drop in performance occurred for both low- and high-intensity slides. By contrast, reappraisal did not impact performance on the memory test.

More recently, Hayes and colleagues (2010) used functional imaging to investigate the neural processes of memory formation during emotion regulation. Participants viewed negative pictures while alternately engaging in cognitive reappraisal, expressive suppression, or passive viewing. They were asked to return 2 weeks later for a surprise memory test. Behavioral results showed a reduction in negative affect and a retention advantage for reappraised stimuli relative to expressive suppression. Imaging results showed that successful encoding during reappraisal was uniquely linked with increased coactivation of the left inferior frontal gyrus, amygdala, and hippocampus.

The Neural Bases of Emotion and Emotion Regulation

To better understand attention-based strategies (e.g., distraction) and meaning-based strategies (e.g., reappraisal), it is useful to consider underlying neural mechanisms. Historically, there have been two approaches to understanding the neural bases of emotional processes. One is a bottom-up approach that emphasizes the affective properties of stimuli. The second is a top-down approach that analyzes the higher-level cognitive processes that interpret the meaning of the stimuli in the context of an individual's current goals, wants, and needs (Scherer, Schorr, & Johnstone, 2001). Distraction and reappraisal are primarily top-down processes that act upon generative processes that could themselves be top down or bottom up. To understand interactions between various types of processes, we must rely upon methods that are integrative across both approaches.

The Bottom-Up Approach

The bottom-up approach characterizes emotions as a response to stimuli with intrinsic or learned reinforcing properties (e.g., Rolls, 1999). As such, emotions are seen as inevitable consequences of perceiving certain kinds of stimuli. Early animal research supported this approach. Experiments suggested that direct electrical stimulation could trigger either aggressive or prosocial behavior, depending on the specific site of the stimulation. This research focused on subcortical structures such as the hypothalamus and the amygdala as well as on the cortical systems with which these regions were connected (Cannon, 1915; Panksepp, 1998).

Modern recording and lesion studies have built on these findings by elaborating complementary roles for subcortical and cortical systems in emotional learning. For example, it has been shown that the amygdala is implicated in aversive learning, and the medial and orbital frontal cortex supports extinctions and alteration of the stimulus–reinforcer associations (LeDoux, 2000). The main thrust of the bottom-up approach is that emotion is a response to stimulus properties that could be perceived and encoded directly. Participants were simply asked to passively perceive purportedly affective stimuli as their responses were recorded in a scanner.

Although the emotion-as-stimulus property yielded stable results among nonhuman animals, imaging studies on humans have led to more variable results. For example, amygdala activation in response to emotional stimuli was only found inconsistently (Phan, Wager, Taylor, & Liberzon, 2002; Wager et al., 2008). Other studies (for a review, see Ochsner & Gross, 2005) showed that prefrontal systems—not important in animal work—are reliably activated in studies of human emotion generation. It seemed that studying emotion generation in humans involves something more than mapping the neural signals resulting from the bottom-up processing of affective stimuli.

Top-Down Approaches

Top-down approaches have helped to fill in our understanding of the neural bases of emotion generation and regulation. They describe emotion as the product of cognitive appraisal processes that evaluate the meaning of stimuli in relation to an individual's current context—his or her goals, wants, and needs (Scherer et al., 2001). Although some of these appraisals arise in subcortical structures, others seem to require engagement of prefrontal cortical systems. For example, a delayed order in a restaurant could be appraised as incompetence and lead to anger, or it could be seen as the result of an overburdened staff and lead to patient understanding. As such, cognitive reappraisals could be involved in emotion regulation. Similarly, top-down attentional distraction could direct regulatory processes.

A key foundational principle underlying top-down approaches is that unlike other mammals, humans possess a large capacity to make conscious and deliberative choices about the way they construe, respond to, and regulate emotionally evocative situations. Regulatory processes, in particular, rely on cognitive systems such as selective attention, working memory, language, inhibitory control, and long-term memory.

These higher cognitive processes have been associated with regions of the lateral and medial prefrontal cortex (PFC) thought to implement processes important for regulatory control, and regions of the dorsal anterior cingulate cortex (ACC) thought to monitor the extent to which control processes are achieving their goals (e.g., Botvinick, Braver, Barch, Carter, & Cohen, 2001). The use of top-down approaches may help explain some of the apparent inconsistencies of the early (bottom-up) emotion imaging literature. It is possible that individuals in these studies spontaneously used cognitive regulatory strategies—a phenomenon quite common in behavioral research (Drabant, McRae, Manuck, Hariri, & Gross, 2009; Erber, 1996). Additionally, the participants may have controlled their attention to, and appraisal of, emotionally evocative stimuli. This could help to explain some instances of PFC activity and also explain failures to observe amygdala activity.

Despite its promise, the top-down approach does not directly address the fact that humans are not immune from brain electrical and chemical manipulations from subcortical regions (Panksepp, 2003). It seems likely that there is some conservation of subcortical emotional processes in humans. Everyday experience suggests that top-down generative and regulatory processes often interact with bottom-up processes. In the next section, we consider how bottom-up and top-down approaches might be integrated.

Integrating Bottom-Up and Top-Down Approaches

It is likely that the distinction between bottom-up and top-down processing is relative rather than absolute and that there is a continuum along which processes can be arrayed, with the two approaches at each end point. Nonetheless, the distinction is a useful heuristic for guiding thinking about the way in which the two types of processes interact with each other and how they may be usefully integrated.

Ochsner and Gross (2007) suggested an initial integrative working framework of the cognitive control of emotions. According to this framework, emotion generation and regulation involve the interaction of fast appraisal systems (e.g., the amygdala) that encode the affective properties of stimuli in a bottom-up fashion, with control systems implemented in the prefrontal and cingulate cortex that support controlled top-down stimulus appraisals (Ochsner, Bunge, Gross, & Gabrieli, 2002; Ochsner & Gross, 2005; McRae, Ochsner, & Gross, 2011).

The framework posits that emotions can be generated and modulated either by bottom-up or top-down processes. For instance, top-down processes can focus attention on particular stimuli, and in so doing have the capacity to regulate emotions by selectively determining the information that has access to generative, bottom-up processes. Once the bottom-up generation begins, top-down processes can regulate or alter the way in which triggering stimuli are appraised. To illustrate how this model might be applied to specific types of emotion regulation processes, we next detail two cognitive forms of emotion regulation that have, to date, received a great deal of empirical attention: attentional distraction and cognitive reappraisal.

Attentional Distraction

Attention is a basic cognitive process that acts as a gatekeeper by allowing passage of goal-relevant information for further processing. Processes that are not affected by attentional manipulation can be defined as automatic; other processes generate altered responses—behavioral and neural—when attention is directed toward them.

According to the integrative framework, attentional deployment in the context of emotion should work much the same way as it does in nonemotional cognitive contexts. For example, looking at photographs of faces activates the fusiform face area, whereas directing attention to other stimuli decreases its activation (Kanwisher, Stanley, & Harris, 1999). We could therefore expect that, in the case of emotion, if attention is directed, automatically or willfully, toward emotionally evocative stimuli, there should be increased activity in regions such as the amygdala that participate in appraising these stimuli. Conversely, directing attention away from such stimuli should decrease, for example, amygdala activity. In attentional distraction, a secondary task is engaged to divert attention from processing a primary target stimulus. As such, incoming emotional information competes with the secondary task at an early processing stage, before stimuli are represented in working memory for further semantic evaluative processing (Sheppes & Gross, in press).

Most studies on distraction have focused on examining the impact of performing a cognitive task on responses to (often aversive) affective stimuli. For example, one study used fear faces as stimuli and found that amygdala responses diminished when participants performed a line orientation judgment task (Pessoa, McKenna, Gutierrez, & Ungerleider, 2002; see also Pessoa & Pereira, Chapter 4, this volume). Other studies have shown that performing a verbal fluency task (Frankenstein, Richter, McIntyre, & Remy, 2001), the Stroop task (Bantick et al., 2002; Valet et al., 2004), or simply being asked to think about "something else" (Tracey et al., 2002) diminishes the aversiveness of pain and may reduce activity in cortical and subcortical pain-related regions, including the mid-cingulate cortex, insula, thalamus, and periaqueductal gray. Tracey and colleagues (2002) applied heat stimulation to the hands of subjects who were asked to either focus on or distract themselves from the painful stimuli, which were cued using colored lights. Functional imaging revealed that activation in the periaqueduc-

tal gray was significantly decreased during the distraction condition.

Additionally, as predicted by the model above, regions such as the orbitofrontal cortex (OFC), medial PFC, ACC, and dorsolateral PFC may be more active during distraction (Frankenstein et al., 2001; Tracey et al., 2002; Valet et al., 2004). More recently, it has become possible to specifically distinguish the neural bases of distraction from those of cognitive reappraisal. We detail these differences below, after first surveying the neural correlates of cognitive reappraisal.

Cognitive Reappraisal

Appraisal theorists have described the cognitive steps needed to transform a percept into something that elicits emotion. *Cognitive change* refers to changing how we appraise the situation we are in to alter its emotional significance, either by changing how we think about the situation or about our capacity to manage the demands it poses. As discussed above, cognitive reappraisal entails attending to an emotional stimulus and reinterpreting its meaning in a way that alters its emotional impact (e.g., Gross, 1998b).

As would be predicted by the integrative working model above, several studies (for a review, see Ochsner & Gross, 2008) published to date indicate that reappraisal depends on interactions between prefrontal and cingulate regions implicated in cognitive control and frequently (subcortical) regions such as the amygdala and insula that have been implicated in emotional responding. Neuroimaging studies also show that reappraisal is cognitively complex and requires processes for generating, implementing, and maintaining an alternative cognitive construal of a situation (Ochsner & Gross, 2008). During reappraisal, activated regions include dorsal portions of the PFC implicated in working memory and selective attention, ventral portions of the PFC that have been implicated in language or response inhibition, dorsal portions of the ACC implicated in monitoring control processes, and portions of the medial PFC implicated in reflecting upon one's own or someone else's affective states. It further appears that reappraisal may modulate systems involved in bottom-up appraisal—including the amygdala, which has been implicated in the detection and encoding of affectively arousing stimuli, and the insula, which receives visceral–sensory inputs and may play a general role in affective experience.

Although top-down systems such as the PFC and ACC are consistently activated during reappraisal, the specific regions of activity vary across studies. This variation may well occur because cognitive reappraisal may include a variety of different operationalizations that include (1) reinterpreting the situational aspects of the stimuli (e.g., the sick child in the picture will soon get better) or (2) distancing of oneself by adopting a detached third-person perspective (e.g., viewing the sick child in the picture as an unfamiliar person whom the participant does not know). Oschsner and colleagues (2004) showed that the latter type of regulation recruited medial prefrontal regions implicated in internally focused processing, whereas situation-focused regulation recruited lateral prefrontal regions implicated in externally focused processing. This finding suggests that both common and distinct neural systems support different forms of reappraisal and that which particular prefrontal systems modulate the amygdala in different ways depends on the regulatory goal and strategy employed.

Comparing Neural Correlates of Distraction and Reappraisal

As we have seen, attentional distraction and cognitive reappraisal recruit partially overlapping brain regions: each one depends on interactions between the PFC, interpreted as implementing cognitive control, and subcortical regions, interpreted as mediating emotional responses. However, the process model would suggest that the two strategies have fundamental differences: They may draw upon different neural mechanisms and drive different emotional consequences. For example, we would expect that distraction and reappraisal vary in (1) when they act upon the emotion-generating process and (2) the neural bases that support both strategies. Specifically, we would predict that attentional distraction should reduce emotional salience early on, before emotional information is represented in working memory. By contrast, reappraisal should allow for elaborated emotional processing prior to its mod-

ulation. In terms of neural bases, this would lead to the prediction that distraction should engage an attentional control network, and reappraisal would be supported by a neural network that transmits affective meaning.

In a recent event-related potential (ERP) study, we have shown that distraction modulated an electrocortical component that denotes enhanced emotional processing (the late positive potential) at its earliest point, and reappraisal modulated this component only at a late point (Thiruchselvam, Blechert, Sheppes, Rydstrom, & Gross, 2011). The early modulation in distraction represents a time point when emotional processing is being represented in working memory. By contrast, the late modulation in reappraisal denotes a time point when the meaning of received emotional information has already been elaborated.

Two additional recent studies provide support for partially dissociable neural bases of distraction and reappraisal (McRae et al., 2010). Relative to distraction, reappraisal led to greater decreases in self-reported negative affect and to greater increases in the activation of regions associated with processing affective meaning (medial prefrontal and anterior temporal cortices). Relative to reappraisal, distraction led to greater decreases in amygdala activation and to greater increases in activation in prefrontal and parietal regions. Taken together, these data suggest that distraction and reappraisal differentially engage neural systems involved in attentional deployment and cognitive reframing and have different emotional consequences.

As we have seen in this section, recently developed methods in neuroscience have enabled a better understanding of the mechanisms underlying two types of emotion regulation. This is an instance of a broader trend: As emotion regulation further captures the attention of neuroscientists and cognitive psychologists, a more extensive and sophisticated array of tools, techniques, and empirical methods has become available to the field. Cognitive-experimental methods allow emotion regulation researchers to assess the role of cognitive processes, such as selective attention, without relying upon self-reported measures (Joormann & Gotlib, 2010). Similarly, in addition to the results discussed in this section, neuroscience has proven extremely helpful in studying the brain bases of emotion regulation (Berkman & Lieberman, 2009).

Individual Differences in Emotion Regulation

We have now examined the neural process involved in attentional distraction and cognitive reappraisal. Next, we examine how people vary in implementing these cognitive regulation strategies. We consider both adaptive and maladaptive variations in attentional deployment and cognitive change.

Individual Differences in Attentional Deployment

When attentional strategies are used adaptively, pleasant or neutral distractions could be used to alter an emotional response. Then, if necessary, one can commence problem solving (Nolen-Hoeksema, 1991). As we have noted above, distracting responses are thoughts and behaviors that help divert one's attention away from one's undesirable emotional state and its consequences and turn it to pleasant or benign thoughts and activities that are absorbing, engaging, and capable of providing positive reinforcement (Csikszentmihalyi, 1990; Nolen-Hoeksema, 1991). For example, concentrating on a project at work may help take one's mind off a disturbing argument until more resources are available to tackle the underlying issue. However, just as some individuals are instrumental in their attentional deployment strategies, others are burdened by them. We specifically examine one such response style—rumination.

Rumination is a mode of responding to distress that involves repetitively and passively focusing one's attention on symptoms of distress and on the possible causes and consequences of these symptoms. Contrary to distraction, habitual rumination has been shown to maintain and exacerbate depression by enhancing negative thinking, impairing problem solving, interfering with instrumental behavior, and eroding social support (Nolen-Hoeksema et al., 2008). Specifically, longitudinal studies have shown that people who engage in rumination when distressed have more prolonged periods of depression and are more likely to develop depressive

disorders (Just & Alloy, 1997; Kuehner & Weber, 1999; Nolan, Roberts, & Gotlib, 1998); similar results were found in samples of adolescents or children (Abela, Brozina, & Haigh, 2002). Other measures of rumination—in particular, those assessing a perseverative focus on the self and one's problems—have demonstrated similar links to depression (Luminet, 2004).

In addition, chronic ruminators appear to behave in ways that are counterproductive to their support relationships. In a study of bereaved adults, ruminators were more likely to reach out for social support after their loss, but they reported more social friction and less emotional support from others (Nolen-Hoeksema & Davis, 1999).

Lastly, it is important to mention that chronic use of distraction without subsequently engaging in reappraisal or problem solving may morph into avoidance of negative emotions through maladaptive avoidance behaviors. Wenzlaff and Luxton (2003) suggest that avoidance can, in turn, fuel rumination. Similarly, engaging in behavioral avoidance can also contribute to rumination when these behaviors create more problems in individuals' lives. This is supported by the findings that adolescent girls who engage in binge eating (a common avoidance behavior) display increases in rumination over time (Nolen-Hoeksema, Stice, Wade, & Bohon, 2007).

Individual Differences in Cognitive Change

As we have noted above, cognitive reappraisal is a form of cognitive change that involves construing a potentially emotion-eliciting situation in a way that changes its emotional impact. In this literature, the adaptive profile of reappraisal is contrasted with the maladaptive profile of expressive suppression, which is a form of response modulation that involves inhibiting ongoing emotion-expressive behavior. According to the process model of emotion regulation discussed above (Gross, 1998a), reappraisal—which occurs relatively early in the emotion-generating process—changes the entire emotional sequence, with minor physiological, cognitive, or interpersonal costs. By contrast, suppression—which occurs later in the emotion-generating process—comes with substantial emotional, cognitive, and social costs (see Gross, 2002, for a review).

Individual differences in the habitual use of reappraisal and suppression revealed several differential associations with emotion experience, cognition, relationships, and well-being. For example, habitual use of reappraisal correlated negatively with depression, and use of suppression correlated positively with depression (Gross & John, 2003; John & Gross, 2004). In addition, habitual use of reappraisal correlated positively with positive emotion and negatively with negative emotion.

Thus, adaptive, habitual use of cognitive reappraisals can provide several benefits. But habitual use of certain regulatory strategies may not reflect fixed or immutable traits— rather this habitualization may be socially acquired and be sensitive to individual development. Specifically, Dweck (e.g., 1999) and her colleagues have suggested that the beliefs people hold about the malleability of personal attributes impact the amount of control they have on their emotions: Individuals who hold entity beliefs view attribution as relatively fixed (e.g., "The truth is, people have very little control over their emotions") and therefore difficult to control, whereas individuals who hold incremental beliefs view emotions as malleable (e.g., "If they want to, people can change their emotions") and controllable.

These general beliefs should influence the individual's emotion regulation efforts. For example, people who believe that emotions are fixed and cannot be changed will likely apply those beliefs to their own emotions as well. If they have no reason to think regulatory strategies would be successful, they are unlikely to expend energy implementing them. In contrast, individuals who believe emotions are not fixed but can be controlled should have high levels of emotion regulation efficacy. This prediction should certainly apply to cognitive reappraisal.

The effect of an individual's beliefs about emotions and emotion regulation on their emotion regulation strategies has been examined. Researchers have used the Emotion Regulation Questionnaire Cognitive Reappraisal Scale to show that implicit theories of emotion are indeed related to individuals' sense of efficacy in emotion regulation (Tamir, John, Srivastava, & Gross, 2007).

Individuals who viewed emotion as more malleable were indeed more likely to report actively modifying their emotions by using reappraisals.

Directions for Future Research

Using our process model of emotion regulation, we have considered the neural correlates of two cognitive regulation strategies and individual differences in the operationalization of these two strategies. In this last section, we consider three growth points that we consider particularly exciting: (1) developing more detailed process models of emotion regulation, (2) finding neural correlates to support such models, and (3) exploring the sources of individual differences in emotion regulation choice and efficacy.

As a conceptual model, the process model (Figure 11.1) has proved to be remarkably enduring. However, as the field of emotion regulation has expanded, there is a need for more detailed understanding of the processes postulated by the process model. One important contribution has been work establishing the importance of the emotional intensity that one faces when regulating emotions, strategies underlying cognitive operations, and whether the goal of a particular strategy is to provide short-term relief or long-term adaptation (Sheppes & Gross, in press). As the field continues to mature, our understanding will become increasingly nuanced as we develop better descriptions of underlying regulatory operations due to a better understanding of their temporal dynamics and neural bases, as well as other factors such as individual differences, the nature of the stimuli one is facing, and availability of cognitive resources, to name a few areas of improvement.

As our understanding of the neural bases of emotion and emotion regulation has expanded, it has become clear how important it will be to employ new and more sophisticated methods. For example, electroencephalographic (EEG) studies are now being used to evaluate more clearly the temporal dynamics and unfolding of different emotion regulation strategies (e.g., Hajcak, MacNamara, & Olvet, 2010), and neuroimaging studies are being designed that can better probe the neural bases of different strategies (see Ochsner & Gross, 2005, 2008; Wager et al., 2008, for reviews). A new generation of studies may be possible that involve coregistration of ERPs and functional magnetic resonance imaging (fMRI), which may help the field to make better inferences regarding the tight links between rapid temporal dynamics captured best by ERPs and the fine spatial dynamics enabled by fMRIs. Furthermore, sophisticated connectivity analysis may reveal antecedent and projecting networks involved in emotion regulation.

We have noted that people differ in their regulation choice and efficacy. One intriguing puzzle is how these differences arise. There are diverse possibilities, and it is likely that all of them play a role. However, disassociating the circumstances that could isolate the influence of each has not been yet been comprehensively attempted. Genetics, for example, may play a part in shaping individual differences in regulation strategies as well as explanatory styles. It is known, for example, that the explanatory styles of monozygotic twins are more highly correlated than the explanatory style of dizygotic twins (Schulman, Keith, & Seligman, 1993). This finding does not necessarily imply that there is a gene related to explanatory style. Genes may influence other factors, such as intelligence, which could then in turn lead to certain types of beliefs. How genes might influence habitual regulation choice and efficacy is unknown.

Another possibility is that teachers could also help to create individual differences. Teachers' comments about children's performance may affect children's attribution about their successes and failures in the classroom. But positive comments do not always drive helpful attributions. Mueller and Dweck (1998) found that teachers praising children for their intelligence led to greater helplessness characteristics in the face of difficulty, compared to situations in which children were praised for their effort.

Researchers have also analyzed the relationships between how a particular explanatory style of parents might impact their offspring (e.g., Seligman et al., 1984). The broad conclusion appears to be that explanatory style is transmitted to children by parents, but not universally so. Future studies must explore moderators of this potential link; plausible candidates include the time spent by the parents and children and the type of their interaction. It is known that children from happy and supportive homes are more likely as adults to have an optimistic explanatory style for bad events (Franz, McClelland, Weinberger, & Peterson, 1994). Trauma, media, and social networks may also play a part in shaping regulatory differences. However, a comprehensive view across all these influences has yet to emerge.

References

Abela, J. R. Z., Brozina, K., & Haigh, E. P. (2002). An examination of the response styles theory of depression in third- and seventh-grade children: A short-term longitudinal study. *Journal of Abnormal Child Psychology, 30*, 515–527.

Abelson, J. L., Liberzon, I., Young, E. A., & Khan, S. (2005). Cognitive modulation of the endocrine stress response to a pharmacological challenge in normal and panic disorder subjects. *Archives of General Psychiatry, 62*, 668–675.

Bantick, S. J., Wise, R. G., Ploghaus, A., Clare, S., Smith, S. M., & Tracey, I. (2002). Imaging how attention modulates pain in humans using functional MRI. *Brain, 125*(Pt. 2), 310–319.

Bargh, J. A., Gollwitzer, P. M., Lee-Chai, A., Barndollar, K., & Trotschel, R. (2001). The automated will: Nonconscious activation and pursuit of behavioral goals. *Journal of Personality and Social Psychology, 81*, 1014–1027.

Berkman, E. T., & Lieberman, M. D. (2009). Using neuroscience to broaden emotion regulation: Theoretical and methodological considerations. *Social and Personality Psychology Compass, 3*, 475–493.

Bishop, S. R., Lau, M., Shapiro, S., Carlson, L., Anderson, N. D., Carmody, J., et al. (2004). Mindfulness: A proposed operational definition. *Clinical Psychology: Science and Practice, 11*, 230–241.

Botvinick, M. M., Braver, T. S., Barch, D. M., Carter, C. S., & Cohen, J. D. (2001). Conflict monitoring and cognitive control. *Psychological Review, 108*, 624–652.

Campbell-Sills, L., & Barlow, D. H. (2007). Incorporating emotion regulation into conceptualizations and treatments of anxiety and mood disorders. In J. J. Gross (Ed.), *Hand-*

book of emotion regulation (pp. 542–559). New York: Guilford Press.

Cannon, W. B. (1915). *Bodily changes in pain, hunger, fear and rage: An account of recent researches into the function of emotional excitement*. New York: Appleton.

Cosmides, L., & Tooby, J. (2000). Evolutionary psychology and the emotions. In M. Lewis & J. M. Haviland-Jones (Eds.), *Handbook of emotions* (2nd ed., pp. 41–115). New York: Guilford Press.

Csikszentmihalyi, M. (1990). *Flow: The psychology of optimal experience*. New York: Harper & Row.

Damasio, A. R. (1999). *The feeling of what happens: Body and emotion in the making of consciousness*. New York: Harcourt, Brace.

Dandoy, A. C., & Goldstein, A. G., (1990). The use of cognitive appraisal to reduce stress reaction: A replication. *Journal of Social Behavior and Personality, 5*, 275–285.

Davidson, R. J. (1998). Affective style and affective disorders: Perspectives from affective neuroscience. In *Neuropsychological perspectives on affective and anxiety disorders* (p. 307). Hove, UK: Psychology Press.

Dillon, D. G., & LaBar, K. S. (2005). Startle modulation during conscious emotion regulation is arousal dependent. *Behavioral Neuroscience, 119*, 1118–1124.

Drabant, E. M., McRae, K., Manuck, S. B., Hariri, A. R., & Gross, J. J. (2009). Individual differences in typical reappraisal use predict amygdala and prefrontal responses. *Biological Psychiatry, 65*, 367–373.

Dweck, C. S. (1999). *Self-theories: Their role in motivation, personality, and development*. New York: Psychology Press.

Egloff, B., Schmukle, S. C., Burns, L. R., & Schwerdfeger, A. (2006). Spontaneous emotion regulation during evaluated speech tasks: Associations with negative affect, anxiety expression, memory, and physiological responding. *Emotion, 6*, 356–366.

Ellsworth, P. C., & Scherer, K. R. (2003). Appraisal processes in emotion. In R. J. Davidson, K. R. Scherer, & H. H. Goldsmith (Eds.), *Handbook of affective sciences* (pp. 572–595). New York: Oxford University Press.

Erber, R. (1996). The self regulation of moods. In L. L. Martin & A. Tesser (Eds.), *Striving and feeling: Interactions among goals, affect, and self-regulation* (pp. 251–275). Mahwah, NJ: Erlbaum.

Feldman Barrett, L., Ochsner, K. N., & Gross, J. (2007). On the automacity of emotion. In J. Bargh (Ed.), *Social psychology and the unconscious: The automacity of higher mental processes* (pp 173–217). New York: Psychology Press.

Frankenstein, U. N., Richter, W., McIntyre, M. C., & Remy, F. (2001). Distraction modulates anterior cingulate gyrus activations during the cold pressor test. *NeuroImage, 14*, 827–836.

Franz, C. E., McClelland, D. C., Weinberger, J., & Peterson, C. (1994). Parenting antecedents of adult adjustment: A longitudinal study. In C. Perris, W. A. Arrindell, & M. Eismann (Eds.), *Parenting and psychopathology* (pp. 127–144). San Diego, CA: Academic Press.

Frijda, N. H. (1986). The current status of emotion theory. *Bulletin of the British Psychological Society, 39*, A75–A75.

Goldin, P. R., McRae, K., Ramel, W., & Gross, J. J. (2008). The neural bases of emotion regulation: Reappraisal and suppression of negative emotion. *Biological Psychiatry, 63*, 577–586.

Gross, J. J. (1998a). Antecedent and response focused emotion regulation: Divergent consequences for experience, expression, and physiology. *Journal of Personality and Social Psychology, 74*, 224–237.

Gross, J. J. (1998b). The emerging field of emotion regulation: An integrative review. *Review of General Psychology, 2*, 271–299.

Gross, J. J. (2002). Emotion regulation: Affective, cognitive, and social consequences. *Psychophysiology, 39*, 281–291.

Gross, J. J., & John, O. P. (2003). Individual differences in two emotion regulation processes: Implications for affect, relationships, and well-being. *Journal of Personality and Social Psychology, 85*, 348–362.

Gross, J. J., Sheppes, G., & Urry, H. L. (in press). Emotion generation and emotion regulation: A distinction we should make (carefully). *Cognition and Emotion*.

Hajcak, G., MacNamara, A., & Olvet, D. M. (2010). Event-related potentials, emotion, and emotion regulation: An integrative review. *Developmental Neuropsychology, 35*, 129–155.

Hayes, J. P., Morey, R. A., Petty, C. M., Seth, S., Smoski, M. J., McCarthy, G., et al. (2010). Staying cool when things get hot: Emotion regulation modulates neural mechanisms of memory encoding. *Frontiers in Human Neuroscience, 4*, 230.

Jackson, D. C., Malmstadt, J. R., Larson, C. L., & Davidson, R. J. (2000). Suppression and enhancement of emotional responses to unpleasant pictures. *Psychophysiology, 37,* 515–522.

James, W. (1884). What is an emotion? *Mind, 9,* 188–205.

John, O. P., & Gross, J. J. (2004). Healthy and unhealthy emotion regulation strategies: Personality processes, individual differences, and life-span development. *Journal of Personality, 72,* 1301–1333.

Joormann, J., & Gotlib, I. H. (2010). Emotion regulation in depression: Relation to cognitive inhibition. *Cognition and Emotion, 24,* 281–298.

Just, N., & Alloy, L. B. (1997). The response styles theory of depression: Tests and an extension of the theory. *Journal of Abnormal Psychology, 106,* 221–229.

Kanwisher, N., Stanley, D., & Harris, A. (1999). The fusiform face area is selective for faces not animals. *NeuroReport, 10,* 183–187.

Keltner, D., & Kring, A. (1998). Emotion, social function, and psychopathology. *Review of General Psychology, 2,* 320–342.

Kuehner, C., & Weber, I. (1999). Responses to depression in unipolar depressed patients: An investigation of Nolen-Hoeksema's response styles theory. *Psychological Medicine, 29,* 1323–1333.

Lazarus, R. S. (1991). Progress on a cognitive–motivational–relational theory of emotion. *American Psychologist, 46,* 819–834.

LeDoux, J. E. (2000). Emotion circuits in the brain. *Annual Review of Neuroscience, 23,* 155–184.

Levenson, R. W. (1999). The intrapersonal functions of emotion. *Cognition and Emotion, 13,* 481–504.

Luminet, O. (2004). Measurement of depressive rumination and associated constructs. In C. Papageorgiou & A. Wells (Eds.), *Depressive rumination: Nature, theory, and treatment* (pp. 187–215) New York: Wiley.

Mauss, I. B., Evers, C., Wilhelm, F. H., & Gross, J. J. (2006). How to bite your tongue without blowing your top: Implicit evaluation of emotion regulation predicts affective responding to anger provocation. *Personality and Social Psychology Bulletin, 32,* 589–602.

McRae, K., Hughes, B., Chopra, S., Gabrieli, J. D., Gross, J. J., & Ochsner, K. N. (2010). The neural correlates of cognitive reappraisal and distraction: An fMRI study of emotion regulation. *Journal of Cognitive Neuroscience, 22,* 248–262.

McRae, K., Ochsner, K. N., & Gross, J. J. (2011). The reason in passion: A social cognitive neuroscience approach to emotion regulation. In K. D. Vohs & R. F. Baumeister (Eds.), *Handbook of self-regulation: Research, theory, and applications* (2nd ed., pp. 186–203). New York: Guilford Press.

Mueller, C. M., & Dweck, C. S. (1998). Praise for intelligence can undermine children's motivation and performance. *Journal of Personality and Social Psychology, 99,* 156–165.

Nolan, S. A., Roberts, J. E., & Gotlib, I. H. (1998). Neuroticism and ruminative response style as predictors of change in depressive symptomatology. *Cognitive Therapy and Research, 22,* 445–455.

Nolen-Hoeksema, S. (1991). Responses to depression and their effects on the duration of depressive episodes. *Journal of Abnormal Psychology, 100,* 569–582.

Nolen-Hoeksema, S., & Davis, C. G. (1999). "Thanks for sharing that": Ruminators and their social support networks. *Journal of Personality and Social Psychology, 77,* 801–814.

Nolen-Hoeksema, S., Stice, E., Wade, E., & Bohon, C. (2007). Reciprocal relations between rumination and bulimic, substance abuse, and depressive symptoms in female adolescents. *Journal of Abnormal Psychology, 116,* 198–207.

Nolen-Hoeksema, S., Wisco, B. E., & Lyubomirsky, S. (2008). Rethinking rumination. *Perspectives on Psychological Science, 3,* 400.

Ochsner, K. N., Bunge, S. A., Gross, J. J., & Gabrieli, J. D. (2002). Rethinking feelings: An fMRI study of the cognitive regulation of emotion. *Journal of Cognitive Neuroscience, 14,* 1215–1229.

Ochsner, K. N., & Gross, J. J. (2005). The cognitive control of emotion. *Trends in Cognitive Sciences, 9,* 242–249.

Ochsner, K. N., & Gross, J. J. (2007). The neural architecture of emotion regulation. In J. J. Gross (Ed.), *Handbook of emotion regulation* (pp. 87–109). New York: Guilford Press.

Ochsner, K. N., & Gross, J. J. (2008). Cognitive emotion regulation: Insights from social cognitive and affective neuroscience. *Current Directions in Psychological Science, 17,* 153–158.

Ochsner, K. N., Ray, R. D., Cooper, J. C., Robertson, E. R., Chopra, S., Gabrieli, J. D., et al. (2004). For better or for worse: Neural systems supporting the cognitive down- and up-regulation of negative emotion. *NeuroImage, 23,* 483–499.

Panksepp, J. (1998). *Affective neuroscience.* New York: Oxford University Press.

Panksepp, J. (2003). At the interface of the affective, behavioral, and cognitive neurosciences: Decoding the emotional feelings of the brain. *Brain and Cognition, 52,* 4–14.

Parrott, W. G. (1993). Beyond hedonism: Motives for inhibiting good moods and maintaining bad moods. In D. M. Wegner & J. W. Pennebaker (Eds.), *Handbook of mental control* (pp. 278–305). Englewood Cliffs, NJ: Prentice-Hall.

Pessoa, L., McKenna, M., Gutierrez, E., & Ungerleider, L. G. (2002). Neural processing of emotional faces requires attention. *Proceedings of the National Academy of Sciences of the United States of America, 99,* 11458–11463.

Phan, K. L., Wager, T., Taylor, S. F., & Liberzon, I. (2002). Functional neuroanatomy of emotion: A meta-analysis of emotion activation studies in PET and fMRI. *NeuroImage, 16,* 331–348.

Phelps, E. A. (2006). Emotion and cognition: Insights from studies of the human amygdala. *Annual Review of Psychology, 57,* 27–53.

Richards, J. M., & Gross, J. J. (1999). Composure at any cost?: The cognitive consequences of emotion suppression. *Personality and Social Psychology Bulletin, 25,* 1033–1044.

Richards, J. M., & Gross, J. J. (2000). Emotion regulation and memory: The cognitive costs of keeping one's cool. *Journal of Personality and Social Psychology, 79,* 410–424.

Rolls, E. T. (1999). *The brain and emotion.* Oxford, UK: Oxford University Press.

Scherer, K. R., Schorr, A., & Johnstone, T. (2001). *Appraisal processes in emotion: Theory, methods, research.* New York: Oxford University Press.

Schulman, P., Keith, D., & Seligman, M. E. P. (1993). Is optimism heritable?: A study of twins. *Behavior Research and Therapy, 31,* 569–574.

Seligman, M. E. P., Peterson, C., Kaslow, N. J., Tannenbaum, R. L., Alloy, L. B., & Abramson, L. Y. (1984). Attributional style and depressive symptoms among children. *Journal of Abnormal Psychology, 93,* 235–238.

Sheppes, G., & Gross, J. J. (in press). Is timing everything?: Temporal considerations in emotion regulation. *Personality and Social Psychology Review.*

Sheppes, G., & Meiran, N. (2007). Better late than never?: On the dynamics of on-line regulation of sadness using distraction and cognitive reappraisal. *Personality and Social Psychology Bulletin, 33,* 1518–1532.

Stemmler, G. (1997). Selective activation of traits: Boundary conditions for the activation of anger. *Personality and Individual Difference, 22,* 213–233.

Tamir, M. (2009). What do people want to feel and why?: Pleasure and utility in emotion regulation. *Current Directions in Psychological Science, 18,* 101–105.

Tamir, M., John, O. P., Srivastava, S., & Gross, J. J. (2007). Implicit theories of emotion: Affective and social outcomes across a major life transition. *Journal of Personality and Social Psychology, 92,* 731–744.

Thiruchselvam, R., Blechert, J., Sheppes, G., Rydstrom, A., & Gross, J. J. (2011). The temporal dynamics of emotion regulation: An EEG study of distraction and reappraisal. *Biological Psychology, 87,* 84–92.

Tracey, I., Ploghaus, A., Gati, J. S., Clare, S., Smith, S., Menon, R. S., et al. (2002). Imaging attentional modulation of pain in the periaqueductal gray in humans. *Journal of Neuroscience, 22,* 2748–2752.

Valet, M., Sprenger, T., Boecker, H., Willoch, F., Rummeny, E., Conrad, B., et al. (2004). Distraction modulates connectivity of the cingulo-frontal cortex and the midbrain during pain: An fMRI analysis. *Pain, 109,* 399–408.

Van Dillen, L. F., & Koole, S. L. (2007). Clearing the mind: A working memory model of distraction from negative mood. *Emotion, 7,* 715–723.

Wager, T. D., Feldman Barrett, L., Bliss-Moreau, E., Lindquist, K., Duncan, S., Kober, H., et al. (2008). The neuroimaging of emotion. In M. Lewis, J. M. Haviland-Jones, & L. Feldman Barrett (Eds.), *Handbook of emotions* (3rd ed., pp. 249–271). New York: Guilford Press.

Watkins, E. R. (2008). Constructive and unconstructive repetitive thought. *Psychological Bulletin, 134,* 163–206.

Wenzlaff, R. M., & Luxton, D. D. (2003). The role of thought suppression in depressive rumination. *Cognitive Therapy and Research, 22,* 293–308.

SOCIAL COGNITION

CHAPTER 12

The Embodied Perspective
on Cognition–Emotion Interactions

Piotr Winkielman and Liam C. Kavanagh

The sleuths of experimental psychology have now established, beyond a reasonable doubt, that cognition and emotion are entwined in many intimate interactions (see this entire volume). In this chapter, we flesh out the mechanistic details of these interactions from the perspective of embodiment theories. As we develop later in the chapter, the fundamental idea of embodiment theories is that higher-level processing is grounded in the organism's sensory and motor experiences—hence, embodiment theories are often called *grounded cognition* theories (Barsalou, 2008; Wilson, 2002). According to such theories (elaborated on shortly), information processing for a number of items and domains—for example, tools, flavors, driving directions, emotional words and faces, and even processing of abstract emotional and mental state concepts, along with many other kinds of information—is influenced, informed, associated with, and sometimes dependent on perceptual, somatosensory, and motor resources. As we illustrate in the chapter, this perspective sheds new light on many empirical phenomena and forces rethinking of some fundamental theoretical questions about emotion–cognition interactions.

As an organizational preview, we begin this chapter by contrasting embodiment theories with their main competitors—theories that emphasize the amodal, propositional nature of mental representations. We then briefly review some evidence for embodied processing in nonemotional domains, showing that embodiment occurs across a variety of situations. Next, we describe in more detail research on embodied processing in emotional perception and emotional language comprehension, the role of embodied metaphor in understanding interpersonal relations and morality, as well as the role of mimicry in social judgment. Finally, we discuss applications of embodiment theory for understanding, and perhaps helping, individuals with autism.

To preview our bottom line, we conclude that a fully fleshed-out embodied account of emotion–cognition interactions is still a work in progress. In fact, we personally believe that it is unlikely that all emotional cognition is embodied (challenges and limitations are highlighted throughout). However, we strongly believe that an embodiment perspective is remarkably generative in terms of both producing new findings and explaining major phenomena. As such, a comprehensive and accurate picture of emotion–cognition interactions is now impossible without taking embodiment into account.

The "Traditional" View: Amodal Processing

Until recently, the mechanisms underlying emotion–cognition interactions were understood using primarily the framework of semantic networks theories—a standard approach for understanding mental processes (e.g., Bower, 1981). On a most general level, such semantic networks represent knowledge as a set of abstract language-like propositions—sentences in the language of thought (Fodor, 1975). Critically, these propositions are *amodal*. This means that they discard much of the perceptual and motor input that gave rise to them. For example, a person's experience with an instance of the number *4* becomes distilled (transduced) into an abstract concept of "four," regardless of whether it was encountered as *IV, IIII, 4*, Spanish *cuatro*, German *vier*, or Polish *cztery*. Similarly, an actual physical experience when handling a searing hot, neon green, and yucky-greasy cup might get conceptually distilled into a propositional concept of "a cup with properties hot + green + slippery." Psychologists have long endorsed this form of knowledge representation because it allows for *generalizability* (e.g., one can easily think of many different kinds of cups) and *compositionality* (one can think of cups with all sorts of properties and easily combine different concepts). Cognitive scientists also like propositional representations for easy and flexible implementability—they can be realized by pretty much any information-processing system and have indeed been used to model knowledge and reasoning in computers.

More specifically, in terms of emotion knowledge representation, the framework of semantic networks theories assumes that a particular emotional state is represented as a node (e.g., *happiness*), which is linked to antecedents *(kittens, sunsets)*, beliefs ("The best things in life are free," "Stop and smell the roses"), and correlations ("Happy people are friendlier"). When happiness is experienced, the happiness node is activated, and it then diffuses activation to these associated concepts. These associated concepts then become more accessible to consciousness and thus more relevant for interpreting and generating behavior. Conversely, activation can spread from semantic nodes associated with happiness to the happiness node, associatively generating the experience of emotion itself. Of course, the emotion nodes can be linked to perceptual, physiological, and bodily patterns associated with them (e.g., for happiness, relaxed posture, warm feeling, smiling face). However, these patterns do not do any cognitive "work." They are just associations, passive by-products of "real" information processing that occur via transforming amodal propositions (see Barsalou, Niedenthal, Barbey, & Ruppert, 2003; Niedenthal, 2007).

The Embodied Perspective

Embodied accounts break with the idea that information processing is best understood as transformation of amodal, abstract, language-like propositions that can be realized in any arbitrary physical system (Fodor, 1975). Instead, embodied theories propose that information processing is "somehow" shaped by the specific form of the human body and nervous system, along with its interactions with the actual, physical world (Wilson, 2002). A recurring theme emerging from accounts motivated by this perspective is that thinking (offline processing) involves partial reproduction or "simulation" of experiential and motor states presented when the perceiver actually encountered the object (Barsalou, 1999, 2008). For example, when trying to describe our most disliked high school teacher to a friend, we recall traces of direct perceptual experiences of that teacher, perhaps using them to mimic the "funny" movements he or she made or the "irritating" sound of his or her voice. In a more future-oriented example, when thinking about making a new kind of soup (e.g., ginger-cumin-bisque with freshly ground pepper), we might generate visual, olfactory, gustatory, and motor images. Critically, these simulations (grounded in our past experiences) will act as integral resources in our current project (e.g., help us determine proportions of various ingredients, time and effort to grind the pepper).

Similarly, emotional experiences are tied to bodily states, as recognized long ago by James (1896/1994). So, the embodied perspective should apply particularly well to thinking about emotion (Niedenthal, Barsalou, Winkielman, Krauth-Gruber, & Ric, 2005; Winkielman, Niedenthal, & Oberman, 2008). For example, when we retell the story of our most embarrassing personal moment, we also reproduce a trace of the state of embarrassment. Critically, we also simulate such states when thinking abstractly about the definition of embarrassment. For example, the reader may find it hard to describe the difference between embarrassment and shame without resorting to at least a partial simulation of each emotion. In essence, embodiment theories hold that, far from being incidental, this kind of reproduction is sometimes crucial to thinking about emotional concepts, emotional perception, and interpreting emotional language.

It is worth noting that the experience-based simulations posited by the embodiment account do not have to be conscious, full-blown emotional episodes. Instead, simulation may only involve reinstantiating enough of the original experience to be useful in conceptual processing. Importantly, as we develop later, such simulations do not simply result from associative connections of emotion concepts to somatic states. Instead, they are constructive reinstantiations done when it is necessary to represent this form of content in information processing.

Evidence for Embodied Models from Nonemotional Domains

Convergent evidence from various experimental paradigms has helped embodiment theories to be taken seriously as an alternative to the amodal view of cognition. In this section, we briefly review some important experiments and paradigms from cognitive psychology and cognitive neuroscience.

Perhaps the most researched area to date is the involvement of sensory modalities in the comprehension and production of conceptual information. One paradigm for testing the role of sensory modalities in conceptualization is the property verification task. In this task, participants are asked to verify or deny that a certain object has a certain property (i.e., answer a question such as "Do cats have WINGS?"). Results here showed that speed of property verification—a conceptual

task—is related to the perceptual salience of the feature in questions (Solomon & Barsalou, 2004). For example, properties that were larger were verified more rapidly, presumably because they were easier to "see" on a recalled or "simulated" visual representation. Another paradigm, the feature generation task, asks participants to produce lists of features for a particular object. Here, research has shown that the likelihood that participants will generate specific features of a particular object (i.e., the visual or auditory features) varies as a function of presumably irrelevant perceptual variables (Wu & Barsalou, 2009). For example, when participants had to list the features of the concept, HALF WATERMELON, they were more likely to spontaneously produce the features *seeds* and *red* compared to when they had to list the features of the concept, WATERMELON. Presumably, the interior visual features of the watermelon were "revealed" in simulating the former concept and not the latter. These findings also extended to novel concepts such as GLASS CAR (as opposed to CAR). This is important, as it shows that the patterns of performance could not be due purely to stored associations between amodal propositions and thus cannot be explained fully via simple associative priming.

Several classic embodiment studies focused on the phenomenon of modal "switching costs"—decreased performance when changing the modality in which conceptual information is presented, mirroring previous findings in perception. Perception researchers have shown that when attention shifts from one modality to another (e.g., switching from audition to vision), the second stimulus is processed more slowly than it would have been had the two stimuli both used the same modality. This implies a time cost to switching modalities (e.g., Spence, Nicholls, & Driver, 2001). Diane Pecher and colleagues reasoned that, if conceptual processing also takes place in sensory modalities, then a switching cost should also be found for conceptual processing (Pecher, Zeelenberg, & Barsalou, 2004). This was demonstrated in a series of experiments that showed that participants verified features of a concept in one modality more slowly if they had just verified a feature from another (vs. the same) modality—for example, BOMB-loud followed by LEMON-tart (vs. LEAVES-rustle). The reasoning is that, if a just-used modality is appropriate for the processing of the next concept, then it should already be "online" or activated when the next concept is processed, so one might expect the next concept to be processed more quickly. Importantly, the results in these studies cannot be interpreted as due to simple priming, because stimuli were selected such that there were no prestored strong associative connections between concepts within a modality (e.g., BOMB and LEAVES).

Another well-known set of findings from the grounded cognition literature focused on the interaction of high-order sentence processing with perception and action. These experiments showed that the speed of object recognition increases when the images are consistent with the particular visualization implied by a sentence that participants have just read. In one study (Stanfield & Zwaan 2001), investigators constructed sentences that were identical except for one critical word or phrase that would influence the spatial orientation of a particular object. For example, the sentence "The carpenter hammered the nail into the {floor/wall}" would cue participants to simulate the viewing of a nail in either a vertical or horizontal orientation, depending on which of the two possible final words are used. After reading such sentences, participants would see images and would be asked to verify that they had appeared in the sentence. Critical trials were those in which the object shown in the image actually was in the sentence (a nail). There were two images for all such objects, each one corresponding to a simulation of one version of the sentence (e.g., pictures of horizontally or vertically oriented nails). Results showed that participants responded faster to targets that had perceptual properties that were consistent with a visualization of the just-presented sentence. A very similar study used sentence pairs that would cause the same item to be differently shaped during simulations. For example, on critical trials, after reading a sentence such as "The Ranger saw an eagle in {the sky/its nest}," participants would have to verify that an image of either a perched eagle or a flying eagle on a critical trial matched with the content of the sentence (Zwaan, Stanfield, & Yaxley, 2002). The results again showed

that images that were consistent with a contextualized visual representation of a sentence (i.e., perched eagles were verified more quickly after participants read about eagles in nests) were recognized more quickly.

Perhaps one could argue that sentences in these studies were parsed via regular semantic networks, but that the networks end states would effectively prime some images more than others during subsequent verification tasks. One could have several images of an eagle in memory, and perhaps images of eagles in flight were primed more by the processing of the words *eagle* and *sky*. This argument, however, would have a hard time explaining additional studies, such as Horton and Rapp's (2003) demonstration that objects described as being occluded from view in a sentence were recognized more slowly than those described as seen. Just as difficult to explain is Yaxley and Zwaan's result (2007), which showed that when participants read sentences describing objects as hazy or viewed through blurry goggles, low resolution (blurry) images of those objects were recognized more quickly than when the same objects were described as being seen clearly. As predicted, the reverse was true for objects described as clearly seen. These results are exactly what one would expect if participants were visually simulating the content of sentences.

The above-mentioned studies are representative of cognitive psychology findings supporting embodiment in a nonemotional domain. However, there are now many others, and the reader is invited to consult some classic papers and reviews (Barsalou, 2008; Gallese & Metzinger, 2003; Glenberg & Kaschak, 2002; Pecher, Zeelenberg, & Barsalou, 2003; for a review of the embodiment of linguistic meaning, see also Gibbs, 2003).

Evidence for embodiment is also found in the literature on cognitive neuroscience. Embodiment theory predicts that modality-specific areas of the brain, such as the auditory and visual cortices, should be involved when verifying or generating properties that pertain to the given modality. This idea has been investigated via experiments that wed neuroimaging to standard cognitive psychology paradigms. Kan, Barsalou, Solomon, Minor, and Thompson-Schill (2003) found that brain areas involved in a certain perceptual modality (i.e., visual cortex, gustatory cortex, or auditory cortex) were activated during verification of conceptual properties that refer to the same modality (e.g., verifying BOMB-loud activated the auditory cortex). Patterns of brain activation during feature generation yielded similar results (Simmons, Hamann, Harenski, Hu, & Barsalou, 2008). These results are nicely consistent with research suggesting some somatotopic specificity in the processing of abstract language (for a review, see Pulvermueller & Fadiga 2010).

An intriguing line of recent evidence for embodiment of conceptual processing comes from brain-imaging studies comparing right-handed and left-handed individuals. Participants showed increased activation in the brain hemisphere contralateral to their dominant hand when imagining actions such as grasping or cutting (actions usually done with the dominant hand), but not when imagining action verbs whose actual performance does not involve the hands, such as *kneel* (Willems, Toni, Hagoort, & Casasanto, 2009). One possible explanation for these patterns of activation is that these brain areas were engaging in simple action planning, rather than processing conceptual meaning. In order to rule out the idea that action planning alone explained these activation patterns, a later experiment showed that these activation patterns hold when participants are asked simply to read words representing actions performed with the dominant hand, without being asked to imagine the action (Willems, Toni, Hagoort, & Casasanto, 2010).

Is There Any Amodal Processing at All?

Significant differences in opinion exist between embodiment theorists on the relative prevalence and importance of embodied processing in our cognitive life. Some authors believe that much of our mental life is modality-based (e.g., Gibbs, 2003). However, in the view of others (including us), the traditional description of cognition is accurate for some cases. Certainly, our conceptual skills allow us to construct representations that are not slaves to their perceptual instantiations (Camarazza & Mahon, 2006). Returning to an earlier example, we can understand the essential, functional features

of the number *four* regardless of whether we encountered it as *IV, IIII, 4, cuatro, vier*, or *cztery*. Similarly, we can think about how to solve a storage problem using an abstract idea of a container, without having to commit to its particular size, color, and shape. Of course, there might always be a concrete, perceptual component to these representations, but the point is that often, we can easily abstract from it in our thought process (e.g., 2 + IV = six). In another more social example, most legal concepts—such as *copyright, eminent domain, liability, invention*, and *negligence*—are essentially nonperceptual. Also, the features of many abstract concepts have such strong semantic links to that concept itself that accessing a perceptual trace memory, or constructing a perceptual simulation, is unnecessary in order to verify a feature. For example, we don't need to construct perceptual number representations when doing basic mental arithmetic. Nor do we need to retrieve perceptual trace memories of a bull to verify that it can be "grabbed by its horns." Finally, as we will see, even in the emotion domain, we can sometimes answer questions about emotions without necessarily simulating their concrete, perceptual instances (e.g., we can determine conceptually that one way in which anger differs from guilt is that anger involves another person's fault and guilt involves my fault).

One provocative hypothesis offered by Jean Mandler (2008) is that embodied simulation may be very prevalent in early stages of development (while abstract reasoning is underdeveloped) and that embodied processing may be progressively replaced by more abstract general reasoning representations. It may also be that if, say, an embodied metaphor is reused often enough and the results of its use can be represented well by a semantic network, then semantic processing will be an efficient shortcut, eliminating the need for simulation.

Perceptual simulation is most useful, and therefore most likely to take place, when there are either no preexisting semantic associations (e.g., to the novel concept of GLASS CAR) or when those associations are relatively weak or ambiguous. This is not unlike mental imagery, which is most useful if there is no easy way of reasoning to the answer (e.g., when you, dear reader, enter your office, is the door handle on the left or right?). The use of a particular embodied simulation also depends on the specific situated conceptualization or the context in which the concept is being processed (Barsalou, 2003). For example, if the task does not require the generation of internal properties, then they are not simulated (Wu & Barsalou, 2009). We return to these questions when we talk about conditionality of embodiment in emotion processing.

Embodiment in Emotional Processing

Most of the research on embodied emotional cognition can be divided roughly into two main areas. The largest area has established that the somatosensory–motor elements of emotional experience, such as the physical sensations of emotional expressions (e.g., the bodily feeling of smiling), contribute to higher-order emotional processing. The other area of research has established that when we use emotional metaphors, such as those relating physical distance to emotional engagement, or those relating temperature to emotional engagement, we

make use of our capacities for sensing heat and appreciating physical distance. We cover some core research in these two areas below. After that, we discuss potential relations of embodiment research to human mimicry and the application of embodiment research in autism.

Emotional Processing and Embodied Simulation

William James (1896/1994) was famously one of the predecessors of modern embodiment theories, and his canonical example of coming upon a bear in the woods is still a fine place to begin discussing modern embodied emotion theories. James said, roughly, this: You see a scary stimulus, then your autonomic nervous system is automatically activated (i.e., your heart rate and blood pressure elevate, your stomach churns, your face freezes, and your legs want to carry you backward). Upon noticing your changed bodily state, you recognize that you are afraid, and you conceptualize the object in world as *scary* (see Figure 12.1). Mod-

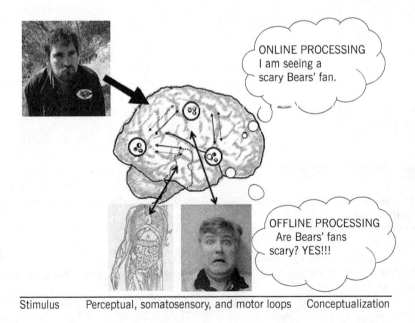

Stimulus   Perceptual, somatosensory, and motor loops   Conceptualization

FIGURE 12.1. Embodied account of online and offline processing of emotion-related information. In online processing, the stimulus (an angry fan of Chicago Bears) triggers a set of bodily responses (visceral feedback, motor reactions in the face and limbs, etc.). These response are centrally represented via somatosensory areas (large circles, with small circles representing specific features). In offline processing, the perceiver partially reinstates somatosensory states to process emotional language.

ern emotion theories, of course, see emotional causation as a much more complex event. Furthermore, they do not take actual changes in bodily states to be necessary to experience an emotion, instead focusing on brain representations of somatosensory and motor processes (e.g., Damasio, 1998). In fact, modern embodiment theories emphasize that a partial reactivation of the brain somatic representation of experience might be sufficient for much of online, as well as offline, emotional processing (again, see Figure 12.1). However, the essential Jamesian point remains: Mentally represented bodily states are an integral part of emotional experience. Furthermore, they are an integral component of conceptualizing not only one's own state (e.g., our fear) but also our understanding of the external world (e.g., that something is scary).

Somatic Involvement in Processing of Approach and Avoidance Information

There are now a number of experimental results showing that the processing of emotional information is affected by the simultaneous performance of bodily actions that are, themselves, affect-laden. In an early demonstration, Chen and Bargh (1999) had participants indicate the valence of presented words (e.g., *love, hate*) using a lever that could either be pushed or pulled. The experiment was motivated by the observation that we use the motor action of pushing (either as a practical action or as a communicative gesture) to avoid things we don't like, but pull objects that we like toward us or indicate our liking of objects to others via a pulling-type gesture. Combined with the notion that specific motor actions are tied to abstract valence representations, this led the investigators to hypothesize that reactions to the task would be facilitated when the valence of the physical action was congruent with that of the concept being evaluated. This reasoning was born out by the data, which showed that response times for correct responses were lower when pushes indicated words with negative valence and pulls indicated positive valence. Others have reported similar findings (Cacioppo, Priester, & Berntson, 1993; Förster & Strack, 1997, 1998; Neumann & Strack, 2000), though follow-up studies have also warned against simplis-

tic interpretations of the valence–action link (Eder & Rothermund, 2008; Markman & Brendl, 2005; Rotteveel & Phaf, 2004). In this context, it is worth mentioning some recent evidence that adopting approach-type postures (e.g., leaning forward) leads to physiological changes characteristic of approach situations (Harmon-Jones, Gable, & Price, 2011; Price, Dieckman & Harmon-Jones, 2012).

Affect as a Type of Modality

As discussed earlier, one way to examine whether abstract knowledge is tied to modalities, rather than being amodal, is via the switching cost paradigm (as used by the Pecher et al. study discussed above). Interestingly, some studies on emotional knowledge suggest that both positive and negative affect can be considered modalities unto themselves, just like vision, audition, or taste (Vermeulen, Niedenthal, & Luminet, 2007). In these experiments, participants had to verify (TRUE/FALSE) features of nouns that were auditory (KEYS-jingling) and visual (TREASURE-bright). The experimenters selected features so that they were either neutral or strongly affective (either positive or negative). Each concept–feature target pair was preceded by a priming pair (e.g., TRIUMPH-exhilarating) followed by a target pair (e.g., COUPLE-happy). The structure of these pairs was experimentally manipulated so that participants had to consecutively verify properties either of the same or different modalities (visual, taste, auditory, affective) with either similar or different valences (positive or negative). For example, a same-modality same-valence pair might be (SPIDER-black, WOUND-open), whereas a different-modality same-valence pair might be (SPIDER-black, SOB-moaning), and a different-valence different-modality could be (SPIDER-black, VICTORY-sung). The findings showed that verifying features of concepts from different sensory modalities produced costs of longer reaction times and higher error rates than concepts from the same modality. Critically, there was also a cost of switching between the verification of features with positive affective value to the verification of those with negative value, and vice versa, even when controlling for associative links between the concepts. There was also a cost to switching between either of these valences and neutral modalities. These results follow naturally from an embodied perspective on which modality activation is an intrinsic part of accessing knowledge. In other words, it appears that we simulate the perceptual aspects of conceptual knowledge, including its valence. These results are harder to account for within an amodal, purely propositional model of concept representation, which views modalities as irrelevant to abstract knowledge processing and affect, in particular, as just another node in the semantic networks.

Recent experiments pushed further the idea that conceptual processes rely on perceptual resources, even when dealing with abstract knowledge about emotion. One set of studies focused on the role of "perceptual perspective" in understanding concepts referring to mental states (Oosterwijk et al., 2012). These states can be affective (e.g., anger, happiness) or cognitive (e.g., thinking, remembering). The idea here was that the understanding of mental state concepts can vary depending on what perceptual perspective is activated, and thus what specific aspects of the mental state are simulated. Specifically, many mental states have a clear internal component—people "feel" a certain way when they are in these states (e.g., anger feels hot, memory retrieval feels effortful). These internal experiences may be simulated when people understand conceptual references to mental states. However, mental states can also be described from an "external" perspective. In those cases, simulation of visible outside features may be more relevant for understanding (e.g., anger makes the face red, memory retrieval involves head scratching). In a switching-costs paradigm, participants saw semantically unrelated sentences describing emotional and nonemotional mental states while manipulating their "internal" or "external" focus. For example, an internally focused emotional sentence might be "Being at the party filled her with happiness," whereas an externally focused emotional sentence would be "His nose wrinkled with disgust." Results showed that switching costs were incurred when participants shifted between sentences with an internal and external focus, regardless of whether both sentences were emotional or nonemotional. These results suggest that

different forms of simulation underlie our understanding of mental states from different points of view. This conclusion is important because it shows that even very abstract concepts are perceptually grounded and subject to "perspective effects," in which different properties of abstract mental states are revealed. Again, these effects are hard to predict from the perspective of a purely abstract, amodal knowledge representation where such perceptual perspective effects should not matter.

Embodiment of Facial Emotions

Many examples of how bodily experiences can augment emotion processing come from research on the recognition of emotional facial expressions. Until recently, expression recognition was thought to be mostly a matter of detecting features (e.g., curves at the corners of the mouth, lines in the corners of the eyes, etc) that are probabilistically associated with an expression (e.g., smile). In other words, the recognition of a smile was assumed to be very much like the recognition of any other stimuli (e.g., recognizing that an analogue clock is showing 2:45). In contrast, embodied accounts of expression detection emphasize the role that somatosensory representations of our own faces play in the process (Barsalou, 1999; Damasio, 1999; Niedenthal et al., 2005). From the embodied perspective, one can think of the act of smiling, for example, as a partial simulation of the state of happiness, which can verify (via facial feedback) a match between one's own state and the mood of the person whom we are imitating.

There is much evidence for the correlational links between expression recognition and both activation of spontaneous facial motor movements (e.g., Dimberg, 1982) and greater activity in the somatosensory areas of the brain (e.g., Carr, Iacoboni, Dubeau, Mazziotta, & Lenzi, 2003). Critically, research on the recognition of facial expressions also provides some evidence for the causal, constitutive role of embodied simulation in emotion recognition. For example, preventing participants from engaging expression-relevant facial muscles impairs their ability to detect briefly presented or relatively ambiguous facial expressions that involve those muscles (Niedenthal, Brauer,

Halberstadt, & Innes-Ker, 2001; Oberman, Winkielman, & Ramachandran, 2007; Stel & Van Kippenberg, 2008). Lesion studies that examined the effects of (1) damage to the sensory–motor areas and (2) temporary inactivation of the face area with repetitive transcranial magnetic stimulation (TMS) further support the idea that motor representations causally contribute to the recognition of facial emotion (Adolphs, Damasio, Tranel, Cooper, & Damasio, 2000; Pitcher, Garrido, Walsh, & Duchaine, 2008). Of course, this does not mean that embodiment is always involved in the processing of facial expressions or that it is always causally necessary. For example, patients with facial paralysis (Moebius syndrome) can learn to recognize expression using nonembodied routes (Bogart & Matsumoto, 2010). Furthermore, participants with autism can also develop alternative routes to recognition (see below). The critical point here is that typical perceivers will activate the somatosensory networks in the course of everyday processing, especially when the recognition cannot be achieved via simple or highly automated pattern recognition strategies.

Facing Language

Recent evidence highlights interesting links between the facial feedback process and the processing of emotional language. In one provocative study, authors first used subcutaneous injections of Botox to temporarily paralyze the facial muscle used in frowning, and then had participants read emotional sentences (Havas, Glenberg, Gutowski, Lucarelli, & Davidson, 2010). Data suggested that participants were slower to understand sentences whose emotional meaning involved the use of the paralyzed muscle. Another study explored the links between embodied processing of emotion words and embodied processing of faces (Halberstadt, Winkielman, Niedenthal, & Dalle, 2009). The idea was that people's actual facial reactions to other individuals' faces interact with conceptual information about those faces communicated via language, and that these motor–conceptual interactions might serve to support and hold as well as distort memories of other people's facial expressions. In studies of Halberstadt and colleagues (2009), participants were

first asked to look at faces of several different individuals with ambiguous facial expressions and think about why each of these individuals might possibly feel "happy" or "angry" (concept label was randomly paired with the face). Later, participants were asked to recall which exact expression was presented for each individual. The data showed that participants' memory of facial expression was biased in the direction of the earlier language concept (e.g., remembering a face as happier when it was earlier associated with a happy label). Critically, this memory distortion was related to the degree to which the conceptual label assigned to the expression (happy or angry) elicited a corresponding facial electromyographic (EMG) response during the initial perception of the face. Presumably, this concept-driven motor representation got tied with the actual perceptual representation of the face and later served as a retrieval cue. As Zajonc (1980) pointed out, the body is often where perception and conceptions meet.

The Conditional Use of Somatic Simulation to Understand Abstract Concepts

As described above, many recent studies report involvement of somatic processes, such as facial action, when people process abstract emotional stimuli. These studies nicely complement earlier observations that emotional imagery (offline cognition) triggers bodily signs of the corresponding emotion. For instance, Grossberg and Wilson (1968) found systematic changes in heart rate and skin conductance during imagery of fearful situations versus neutral situations. Similarly, Schwartz and his colleagues found that when individuals engaged in positive imagery, there was greater spontaneous activity over the zygomaticus major muscle (the smiling muscle), but when individuals engaged in negative imagery, there was greater activity over the corrugator supercilii (the frowning muscle) (Brown & Schwarz, 1980; Schwartz, Fair, Salt, Mandel, & Klerman, 1976).

Note, however, that all such studies could be interpreted as evidence of emotional *stimulation* (physically expressed emotional response to an abstract object), rather than *simulation* (attempt to build a physically grounded representation of the abstract concept). Interestingly, recent studies suggest that people engage in such bodily movements more, or only, when this is necessary in order to grasp the meaning of an abstract emotion concept (Niedenthal, Winkielman, Mondillon, & Vermeulen, 2009). In one experiment, participants viewed both emotional and nonemotional nouns (e.g., SUN, SLUG, FIGHT, CUBE). Some participants were simply asked whether the word was capitalized (a perceptual task), whereas others were asked whether or not the word was associated with a particular emotion (conceptual task). During the task, the activation of participants' facial muscles was measured via EMG. Consistent with the idea of the context-dependent, strategic use of modal processing, the results showed that facial muscles were subtly activated in emotion-specific patterns when participants were evaluating the meaning of the words but not when they made judgments of letter case.

A second experiment was similar to the first, except that abstract adjectives, rather than concrete nouns, were used (e.g., FURIOUS, FOUL, JOYFUL). Results were similar, with participants generating emotion-specific EMG responses when processing the stimuli in an emotion-relevant way. This finding shows that the processing of emotional adjectives—a more abstract word type—is also associated with embodiment. Critically, both experiments argue against a pure "stimulation" account of these results, in which embodiments are just reflexive reactions to reading the word.

A third experiment repeated the methodology of the first two, but focused more directly on the critical question of whether embodiments are simply by-products of emotional processing or causally contribute to emotional understanding (Niedenthal et al., 2009). In this experiment, half of the participants received instructions to hold a pen in their mouth—a manipulation shown in earlier studies to interfere with production of expressions of happiness and disgust (e.g., Oberman et al., 2007). Thus, this manipulation should also interfere with the processing of abstract emotion concepts if motor expressions are indeed important. Consistent with this hypothesis, participants were less accurate in classifying words related to the specific emotions of happiness and disgust when the pen blocked the facial movements specific to these emotions.

In a fourth and final experiment, Niedenthal and colleagues asked participants to generate features related to 32 concepts that were evenly divided among the following categories: neutral, anger-related, disgust-related, and happiness-related. Participants were told that the features were being produced for an audience that was described (depending on condition) either as being interested in "hot" emotional features of the concepts or in "cold" features of the emotion concepts. EMG measurements were taken during the performance of these tasks. Interestingly, participants were able to come up with normatively appropriate emotion features in both the "hot" and "cold" conditions. However, the physiological results showed that there was greater activation of the expected sets of facial muscles when participants were asked for features of emotion words in the "hot" condition than there was in the "cold" condition. This shows, again, that embodied simulations are selectively recruited in concept understanding, but only if they are relevant for solving the task (cf. Wu & Barsalou, 2009). Presumably in this (but not the other) condition, participants try to mentally generate features of, say, FRUSTRATION, by first recreating a relevant experience and then "reading off" its features from associated embodiments. This point is important because it argues against the idea that embodiments are simply passive by-products of conceptual processing (sensory–motor reflexes that are just there "for the ride"). On the other hand, the study somewhat qualifies a very strong embodiment position on which all understanding of emotion requires somatosensory simulation. After all, participants in the "cold" condition were able to successfully generate features of emotional states, albeit in a more dictionary-like way. Of course, future studies are needed to determine whether such generation was purely "cold" or whether it was still "perceptual" but involved an alternative modality (e.g., visual). Studies should also explore to what extent the turning-on and -off of embodied simulation is a function of a particular perspective taken on the event, a topic to which we return shortly.

Embodied Emotional Metaphor

In addition to relying on emotion-specific modalities to abstractly reason about emotion, we can also use nonemotional perceptual input to think about emotions. This is enabled by our use of metaphor—conceptual mappings between an abstract target domain and a usually more concrete source domain (Lakoff & Johnson, 1999). Consider a restaurant where you feel most at home. It may have a "warm" waiter who talks to you in a familiar way. In contrast, the places you least like to go (e.g., government offices) may be described as being "cold." Our high school friend can be described as being "close" to us, or perhaps we have gone different directions since and have actually gotten quite "distant" from one another. When happy, we are feeling "up," "tall," and see a bright future. When sad, we are feeling "down," "small," and see dark days ahead.

There is now much evidence that concepts of valence are related to a variety of perceptual and spatial metaphors. Thus, good things are brighter, whiter, higher, taller, etc. (for a review, see Landau, Meier, & Keefer, 2010). Perhaps more surprisingly, several lines of research suggest that emotional cognition is metaphorically tied to sheer physical distance. One set of studies found that manipulations of physical distance could increase feelings of emotional distance (Williams & Bargh, 2008b). In these studies, participants were primed with a manipulation that asked them to plot two points on a two-dimensional space, with some participants plotting points that were very close together and others plotting points quite far apart. Subsequently, participants who plotted two points very far apart perceived themselves as having weaker emotional attachment to their hometowns and family members. In two other studies, participants plotting more distant points enjoyed a story about embarrassment more and were less affected by a story relating a harrowing and violent experience than were participants plotting close points (presumably because they felt more distance from the situations presented).

There are potentially interesting links between the just discussed work on distance and research looking at how emotional reactions are influenced by the level and type of construal. Such construal may differ on the dimensions of abstractness versus concreteness, as described by the action identification theory (Vallacher & Wegner, 1987). Construal may also depend on different forms of psychological distance (temporal, physical, and social), as described by the construal theory (Trope & Liberman, 2003). However, the links between construal and emotion reactivity appear complex. For example, there is clinical evidence that more abstract processing *enhances* emotional reactivity, presumably because it highlights the deeper meaning of the episode (Watkins, Moberly, & Moulds, 2008). On the other hand, enhancing psychological distance to an event via self-distancing (or "a fly-on-the-wall perspective") may decrease reactivity (Kross & Ayduk, 2008). And, in the reverse direction, increasing emotion intensity decreases perceived psychological distance (Van Boven, Kane, McGraw, & Dale, 2010). Finally, as mentioned earlier, thinking about emotional concepts from the perspective of a "technical" audience reduces relevant physiological activation (Study 4 in Niedenthal et al., 2009). Clearly, the processes of construal level, distance, and perspective interact in complex ways when determining an emotional response.

Returning to emotional metaphors, several lines of research suggest that emotion is linked to the notion of temperature. One set of provocative studies primed participants with physical sensations that bear on the embodied metaphor for warmth (Williams & Bargh, 2008a). These studies showed that participants found an interaction partner to be a "warmer" person when, in an unrelated task, they were holding a warm cup of coffee rather than a cold one. In a related line of research, Zhong and Leonardelli (2008) asked some participants to recall an experience of social rejection while others were instructed to recall an experience of inclusion. Afterward, both groups were asked to estimate the temperature in the room. Those who recalled a feeling of exclusion guessed significantly lower than did those who recalled inclusion (21.44 degrees Celsius vs. 24 degrees Celsius). A second experiment in the same study involved the "cyberball" manipulation in which participants played

language and fundamentally "alinguistic," perhaps so much so that transduction would be either counterproductive or impossible. It is perhaps worth noting here that much of nonverbal communication functions like this, making exploration of this process of even more general interest.

The theory and evidence summarized above seems to suggest that mimicking another's gestures and postures may help us to better understand his or her emotional states, allowing us to think in the same way. Pushing one's arms forward in the same way as another does, or even merely simulating the act, will induce in oneself a similar modal state. The previously cited research on the importance of modal thinking also points out how important the attainment of a similar modal state can be. The modal states that seem most likely to be captured by mimicry are emotional and somatic. The impulse to put oneself in the same somatic and emotional states as another would seem to reveal a desire to understand the other. Because such changes in expressions and posture are inherently visible, the act of putting oneself in a similar somatic and emotional state can, by its nature, be simultaneously a communication of this intention. This communication may explain why mimicry seems to play a causal role in affecting the feelings of the model toward the mimic.

Embodiment as a Tool for Improved Social Behavior

Understanding embodiment may even shed light on certain developmental disorders with a large social component, such as autism. For example, in contrast to typical participants, individuals with autism do not spontaneously reproduce (mimic) facial expressions when they "just watch" them—that is, without any prompts to recognize the expressions or to react to them (McIntosh, Reichmann-Decker, Winkielman, & Wilbarger, 2006). Even when those individuals are explicitly asked to focus on recognizing them, their mimicry is delayed (Oberman et al., 2007). Because numerous other studies have shown that spontaneous mimicry aids emotion recognition, there is reason to suppose that such deficits may hinder understanding of nonverbal cues by individuals with autism (see Winkielman,

McIntosh, & Oberman, 2009, for a fuller review of theory and evidence in this area). People affected by autism have also been shown to have impairments in nonemotional empathy and understanding of "other minds" (i.e., mentalizing). As discussed, these skills are partially supported by the ability to construct an embodied simulation of the other.

Interestingly, if it is indeed true that embodiment is part of the autistic deficit, it should be possible to improve these individuals' real-life emotional communication skills by training embodiment. Success in such a program would also provide a powerful example of how theories of social cognition can inform and facilitate actual interpersonal behavior. One domain where this can be easily achieved is facial mimicry, where quick motor reactions to faces can be developed by frequently pairing a stimulus and motor response (smile to smile, frown to frown). We are currently testing this idea in our lab by using a training paradigm in which typical participants and those with autism spectrum disorder (ASD) produce facial expressions in response to schematic facial stimuli in a video game, which previously was used to train face recognition (Tanaka et al., 2010). We are also planning an intervention program with a humanoid robot that makes realistic facial expressions (Wu, Butko, Ruvolo, Bartlett, & Movellan, 2009). An interested reader can find several videos of this robot via a simple Internet search with the words "*Einstein robot ucsd.*" We hypothesize that these perception–action pairings will enhance the ability of participants with ASD to quickly mirror facial expressions, which will not only facilitate their recognition of faces but will also make others judge these participants' own expressions (produced in everyday life) as more socially appropriate.

Conclusion

The current chapter presented an embodiment perspective on emotion–cognition interactions. We agree with most psychologists that, when and if science arrives at a satisfactory account of the human mind, this account will include components that are similar to traditional amodal models of cognition, such as networks of semantic propositions. However, explanations of many types of behavior (particularly emotional matters) will be inadequate without considering modal, analogical representations and processing mechanisms that actively utilize the perceptual, somatosensory, and motor resources. As we have illustrated in the chapter, such embodied resources are routinely activated in higher-order conceptual tasks, can play a causal and necessary role in understanding, and can be flexibly deployed by perceivers in order to facilitate mental processing. As such, the heuristic and explanatory value of an embodied perspective on emotion–cognition interactions is likely to grow.

Acknowledgments

We appreciate generous feedback from the editors, comments from Evan Carr and Mark Rotteveel, and many years of discussion about these issues with Paula Niedenthal.

References

Adolphs, R., Damasio, H., Tranel, D., Cooper, G., & Damasio, A. R. (2000). A role for somatosensory cortices in the visual recognition of emotion as revealed by three dimensional lesion mapping. *Journal of Neuroscience, 20,* 2683–2690.

Barsalou, L. W. (1999). Perceptual symbol system. *Behavioral and Brain Sciences, 22,* 577–660.

Barsalou, L. W. (2003). Situated simulation in the human conceptual system. *Language and Cognitive Processes, 18,* 513–562.

Barsalou, L. W. (2008). Grounded cognition. *Annual Review of Psychology, 59,* 617–645.

Barsalou, L. W., Niedenthal, P. M., Barbey, A., & Ruppert, J. (2003). Social embodiment. In B. Ross (Ed.), *The psychology of learning and motivation* (Vol. 43, pp. 43–92). San Diego, CA: Academic Press.

Bernieri, F. (1988). Coordinated movement and rapport in teacher–student interactions. *Journal of Nonverbal Behavior, 12,* 120–138.

Bogart, K. R., & Matsumoto, D. (2010). Facial expression recognition by people with Moebius syndrome. *Social Neuroscience, 5,* 241–251.

Bower, G. H. (1981). Emotional mood and memory. *American Psychologist, 36,* 129–148.

Brown, S. L., & Schwartz, G. E. (1980). Relationships between facial electromyography and subjective experience during affective imagery. *Biological Psychology, 11,* 49–62.

Cacioppo, J. T., Priester, J. R., & Berntson, G. G. (1993). Rudimentary determination of attitudes: II. Arm flexion and extension have differential effects on attitudes. *Journal of Personality and Social Psychology, 65,* 5–17.

Camarazza, A., & Mahon, B. (2006). The organization of conceptual knowledge in the brain: The future's past and some future directions. *Cognitive Neuropsychology, 23,* 13–38.

Carr, L., Iacoboni, M., Dubeau, M. C., Mazziotta, J. C., & Lenzi, G. L. (2003). Neural mechanisms of empathy in humans: A relay from neural systems for imitation to limbic areas. *Proceedings of the National Academy of Science of the United States of America, 100,* 5497–5502.

Chartrand, T. L., & Bargh, J. A., (1999). The chameleon effect: The perception–behavior link and social interaction. *Journal of Personality and Social Psychology, 76,* 893–910.

Chartrand, T. L., & van Baaren, R. (2009). Human mimicry. *Advances in Experimental Social Psychology, 41,* 219–274

Chen, M., & Bargh, J. A. (1999). Consequences of automatic evaluation: Immediate behavioral predispositions to approach or avoid the stimulus. *Personality and Social Psychology Bulletin, 25,* 215–224.

Damasio, A. R. (1999). *The feeling of what happens: Body and emotion in the making of consciousness.* New York: Harcourt, Brace.

Dimberg, U. (1982). Facial reactions to facial expressions. *Psychophysiology, 19,* 643–647.

Eder, A., & Rothermund, K. (2008). When do motor behaviors (mis)match affective stimuli?: An evaluative coding view of approach and avoidance reactions. *Journal of Experimental Psychology: General, 137,* 262–281.

Fodor, J. (1975). *The language of thought.* Cambridge, MA: Harvard University Press.

Förster, J., & Strack, F. (1997). Motor actions in retrieval of valenced information: A motor congruence effect. *Perceptual and Motor Skills, 85,* 1419–1427.

Förster, J., & Strack, F. (1998). Motor actions in retrieval of valenced information: II. Boundary conditions for motor congruence effects. *Perceptual and Motor Skills, 86,* 1423–1426.

Gallese V., & Metzinger T. (2003). Motor ontology: The representational reality of goals, actions, and selves. *Philosophical Psychology, 13*(3), 365–388.

Gibbs, R. W. (2003). Embodied experience and linguistic meaning. *Brain and Language, 84,* 1–15.

Glenberg, A. M., & Kaschak, M. P. (2002). Grounding language in action. *Psychonomic Bulletin and Review, 9, 558–565.*

Grossberg, J. M., & Wilson, H. K. (1968). Physiological changes accompanying the visualization of fearful and neutral situations. *Journal of Personality and Social Psychology, 10,* 124–133.

Halberstadt, J., Winkielman, P., Niedenthal, P. M., & Dalle, N. (2009). Emotional conception: How embodied emotion concepts guide perception and facial action. *Psychological Science, 20,* 1254–1261.

Harmon-Jones, E., Gable, P. A., & Price, T. F. (2011). Leaning embodies desire: Evidence that leaning forward increases relative left frontal cortical activation to appetitive stimuli. *Biological Psychology, 87,* 311–313.

Havas, D. A., Glenberg, A. M., Gutowski, K. A., Lucarelli, M. J., & Davidson, R. J. (2010). Cosmetic use of botulinum toxin-A affects processing of emotional language. *Psychological Science, 21,* 895–900.

Horton, W. S., & Rapp, D. N. (2003). Occlusion and the accessibility of information in narrative comprehension. *Psychonomic Bulletin and Review, 10,* 104–109.

James, W. (1994). The physical basis of emotion. *Psychological Review, 101,* 205–210. (Original work published 1896)

Kan, I. P., Barsalou, L. W., Solomon, K. O., Minor, J. K., & Thompson-Schill, S. L. (2003). Role of mental imagery in a property verification task: fMRI evidence for perceptual representations of conceptual knowledge. *Cognitive Neuropsychology, 20,* 525–540.

Kavanagh, L., Suhler, C., Churchland, P., & Winkielman, P. (2011). When it's an error to mirror: The surprising reputational costs of mimicry. *Psychological Science, 22,* 1274–1276.

Kross, E., & Ayduk, Ö. (2008). Facilitating adaptive emotional analysis: Distinguishing distanced-analysis of depressive experiences from immersed-analysis and distraction. *Personality and Social Psychology Bulletin, 34,* 924–938.

Lakin, J. L., Jefferis, V. E., Cheng, C. M., & Chartrand, T. L. (2003), The chameleon effect as social glue: Evidence for the evolutionary significance of nonconscious mimicry. *Journal of Nonverbal Behavior, 27,* 145–162.

Lakoff, G., & Johnson, M. (1999). *Philosophy in the flesh: The embodied mind and its challenges to Western thought.* New York: Basic Books.

Landau, M. J., Meier, B. P., & Keefer, L. A. (2010). A metaphor-enriched social cognition. *Psychological Bulletin, 136,* 1045–1067.

Lee, S. W. S., & Schwarz, N. (2010). Of dirty hands and dirty mouths: Embodiment of the moral purity metaphor is specific to the motor modality involved in moral transgression. *Psychological Science, 21,* 1423–1425.

Mandler, J. M. (2008). On the birth and growth of concepts. *Philosophical Psychology, 21,* 207–230.

Markman, A. B., & Brendl, C. M. (2005). Constraining theories of embodied cognition. *Psychological Science, 16,* 6–10.

McIntosh, D. N., Reichmann-Decker, A., Winkielman, P., & Wilbarger, J. L. (2006). When the social mirror breaks: Deficits in automatic, but not voluntary mimicry of emotional facial expressions in autism. *Developmental Science, 9,* 295–302.

Neumann, R., & Strack, F. (2000). "Mood contagion": The automatic transfer of mood between persons. *Journal of Personality and Social Psychology, 79,* 211–223.

Niedenthal, P. M. (2007). Embodying emotion. *Science, 316,* 1002–1005.

Niedenthal, P. M., Barsalou, L., Winkielman, P., Krauth-Gruber, S., & Ric, F. (2005). Embodiment in attitudes, social perception, and emotion. *Personality and Social Psychology Review, 9,* 184–211.

Niedenthal, P. M., Brauer, M., Halberstadt, J. B., & Innes-Ker, Å. (2001). When did her smile drop?: Facial mimicry and the influences of emotional state on the detection of change in emotional expression. *Cognition and Emotion, 15,* 853–864.

Niedenthal, P. M., Winkielman, P., Mondillon, L., & Vermeulen, N. (2009). Embodiment of emotional concepts: Evidence from EMG measures. *Journal of Personality and Social Psychology, 96,* 1120–1136.

Oberman, L. M., Winkielman, P., & Ramachandran, V. S. (2007). Face to face: Blocking expression-specific muscles can selectively impair recognition of emotional faces. *Social Neuroscience, 2,* 167–178.

Oosterwijk, S., Winkielman, P., Pecher, D.,

Zeelenberg, R., Rotteveel, M., & Fischer, A. H. (2012). Mental states inside out: Processing sentences that differ in internal and external focus produces switching costs. *Memory and Cognition, 40*, 93–100.

Pecher, D., Zeelenberg, R., & Barsalou, L. W. (2003). Verifying different-modality properties for concepts produces switching costs. *Psychological Science, 14*, 119–124.

Pecher, D., Zeelenberg, R., & Barsalou, L. W. (2004). Sensorimotor simulations underlie conceptual representations: Modality-specific effects of prior activation. *Psychonomic Bulletin and Review, 11*, 164–167.

Pitcher, D., Garrido, L., Walsh, V., & Duchaine, B. (2008). TMS disrupts the perception and embodiment of facial expressions. *Journal of Neuroscience, 28*, 8929–8933.

Price, T. F., Dieckman, L., & Harmon-Jones, E. (2012). Embodying approach motivation: Body posture influences startle eyeblink and event-related potential responses to appetitive stimuli. *Biological Psychology, 90*, 211–217.

Pulvermueller, F., & Fadiga, L. (2010). Active perception: Sensorimotor circuits as a cortical basis for language. *Nature Reviews Neuroscience, 11*, 351–360.

Rotteveel, M., & Phaf, R. II. (2004). Automatic affective evaluation does not automatically predispose for arm flexion and extension. *Emotion, 4*, 156–172

Schnall, S., Benton, J., & Harvey, S. (2008). With a clean conscience: Cleanliness reduces the severity of moral judgments. *Psychological Science, 19*, 1219–1222.

Schwartz, G. E., Fair, P. L., Salt, P., Mandel, M. R., & Klerman, G. L. (1976). Facial muscle patterning to affective imagery in depressed and nondepressed subjects. *Science, 192*, 489–491.

Simmons, W. K., Hamann, S. B., Harenski, C. N., Hu, X. P., & Barsalou, L. W. (2008). fMRI evidence for word association and situated simulation in conceptual processing. *Journal of Physiology—Paris, 102*, 106–119.

Solomon, K. O., & Barsalou, L. W. (2004). Perceptual simulation in property verification. *Memory and Cognition, 32*, 244–259.

Spence, C., Nicholls, M. E. R., & Driver, J. (2001). The cost of expecting events in the wrong sensory modality. *Perception and Psychophysics, 63*, 330–336.

Stanfield, R. A., & Zwann, R. A. (2001). The effect of implied orientation derived from verbal context on picture recognition. *Psychological Science, 12*, 153–156.

Stel, M., & Van Knippenberg, A. (2008). The role of facial mimicry in the recognition of affect. *Psychological Science, 19*, 984–985.

Tanaka, J. W., Wolf, J. M., Klaiman, C., Koenig, K., Cockburn, J., Herlihy, L., et al. (2010). Using computerized games to teach face recognition skills to children with autism spectrum disorder: The Let's Face It! program. *Journal of Child Psychology and Psychiatry, 51*, 944–995.

Trope, Y., & Liberman, N. (2003). Temporal construal. *Psychological Review, 110*, 403–421.

Vallacher, R. R., & Wegner, D. M. (1987). What do people think they're doing?: Action identification and human behavior. *Psychological Review, 94*, 3–15.

Van Boven, L., Kane, J., McGraw, A. P., & Dale, J. (2010). Feeling close: Emotional intensity reduces perceived psychological distance. *Journal of Personality and Social Psychology, 98*, 872–885.

Vermeulen, N., Niedenthal, P. M., & Luminet, O. (2007). Switching between sensory and affective systems incurs processing costs. *Cognitive Science, 31*, 183–192.

Watkins, E., Moberly, N. J., Moulds, M. L. (2008). Processing mode causally influences emotional reactivity: Distinct effects of abstract versus concrete construal on emotional response. *Emotion, 8*, 364–378.

Willems, R. M., Toni, I., Hagoort, P., & Casasanto, D. (2009). Body specific motor imagery of hand actions: Neural evidence from right and left-handers. *Frontiers in Human Neuroscience, 3*, 1–9.

Willems, R. M., Toni, I., Hagoort, P., & Casasanto, D. (2010). Neural dissociations between action verb understanding and motor imagery. *Journal of Cognitive Neuroscience, 22*, 2387–2400.

Williams, L. E., & Bargh, J. A. (2008a). Experiencing physical warmth promotes interpersonal warmth. *Science, 322*, 606–607.

Williams, L. E., & Bargh, J. A. (2008b). Keeping one's distance: The influence of spatial distance cues on affect and evaluation. *Psychological Science, 19*, 302–308.

Wilson, M. (2002). Six views of embodied cognition. *Psychonomic Bulletin and Review, 9*, 625–636.

Winkielman, P., McIntosh, D. N., & Oberman, L. (2009). Embodied and disembodied emotion processing: Learning from and about typical and autistic individuals. *Emotion Review, 2*, 178–190.

Winkielman, P., Niedenthal, P., & Oberman, L. (2008). The embodied emotional mind. In G. R. Semin & E. R. Smith (Eds.), *Embodied grounding: Social, cognitive, affective, and neuroscientific approaches* (pp. 263–288). New York: Cambridge University Press.

Wu, L. L., & Barsalou, L. W. (2009). Perceptual simulation in conceptual combination: Evidence from property generation. *Acta Psychologica, 132*, 173–189.

Wu, T., Butko, N. J., Ruvolo, P., Bartlett, M. S., & Movellan, J. (2009, June). *Learning to make facial expressions.* Proceedings of the 8th International Conference on Development and Learning, Shanghai, China.

Yaxley, R. H., & Zwaan, R. A. (2007). Simulating visibility during language comprehension. *Cognition, 150*, 229–236.

Zajonc, R. B. (1980). Feeling and thinking: Preferences need no inferences. *American Psychologist, 35*, 151–175.

Zhong, C. B., & Leonardelli, G. J. (2008). Cold and lonely: Does social exclusion feel literally cold? *Psychological Science, 19*, 838–842.

Zhong, C. B., & Liljenquist, K. (2006). Washing away your sins: Threatened morality and physical cleansing. *Science, 313*, 1451–1452.

Zhong, C. B., Strejcek, B., & Sivanathan, N. (2010). A clean self can render harsh moral judgment. *Journal of Experimental Social Psychology, 46*, 859–862.

Zwaan, R. A., Stanfield, R. A., & Yaxley, R. H. (2002). Language comprehenders mentally represent the shapes of objects. *Psychological Science, 13*, 168–171.

CHAPTER 13

Mood Effects on Cognition

Joseph P. Forgas and Alex S. Koch

Humans are a moody species. Fluctuating positive and negative affective states accompany, underlie, and color everything we think and do, and our thoughts and behaviors are often determined by prior affective reactions. It is all the more surprising that empirical research on how moods influence the way people think, remember, and deal with information is a relatively recent phenomenon. Yet understanding the delicate interplay between feeling and thinking or affect and cognition has been one of the greatest puzzles about human nature since time immemorial. This chapter reviews recent research documenting the multiple roles that moods play in influencing both the *content* and the *process* of cognition.

After a brief introduction reviewing early work and theories exploring the links between mood and cognition, the chapter is divided into two main parts. First, research documenting the way moods influence the *content and valence* of cognition is reviewed, focusing on mood congruence in cognition and behavior. The second part of the chapter presents evidence for the *processing effects* of moods, showing that mood states influence the quality of information processing as well. The chapter concludes with a discussion of the theoretical and applied implications of this work, and future prospects for these lines of inquiry are considered.

We define moods as "relatively low-intensity, diffuse, subconscious, and enduring affective states that have no salient antecedent cause and therefore little cognitive content" (Forgas, 2006, pp. 6–7). Distinct emotions, in contrast, are more intense, conscious, and short-lived experiences (e.g., fear, anger, or disgust). Moods tend to have relatively more robust, reliable, and enduring cognitive consequences, and the research reported here largely focused on the effects of mild, nonspecific positive and negative moods on thinking and behavior, although more specific states such as anger have also been studied (e.g., Unkelbach, Forgas, & Denson, 2008).

Historical Background

Since the dawn of Western civilization, a long list of writers and philosophers have explored the role of moods in the way we think, remember, and form judgments. Apart from some early exceptions (e.g., Rapaport, 1942/1961; Razran, 1940), concentrated empirical research on this phenomenon in psychology is but a few decades old, perhaps because the affective nature of human beings has long been considered secondary and inferior to the study of rational thinking (Adolphs & Damasio, 2001; Hilgard, 1980). Neither of the two paradigms that dominated the brief history of our discipline (behaviorism and cognitivism) assigned much importance to the study of affective states or moods. Radical behaviorists considered all mental events such as moods beyond the scope of scientific psychology. The emerging cognitive paradigm in the 1960s was largely directed at the study of cold, affectless mental processes, and initially had little interest in the study of affect and moods. In contrast, research since the 1980s has shown that moods play a central role in how information about the world is represented, and affect determines the cognitive representation of many of our social experiences (Forgas, 1979).

Early Evidence Linking Mood and Cognition

Although radical behaviorists generally showed little interest in exploring the nature of mood effects, Watson's research with Little Albert may be viewed as an early demonstration of affect congruence in judgments (Watson, 1929; Watson & Rayner, 1920). These studies showed that evaluations of a neutral stimulus, such as a live rabbit, became more negative after being associated with threatening stimuli such as a loud noise. Watson thought that most complex affective reactions are acquired in a similar manner throughout life due to cumulative stimulus associations. In another early mood study, Razran (1940) showed that people evaluated sociopolitical messages more favorably when in a good rather than in a bad mood, induced either by a free lunch (!) or aversive smells, respectively. This work also provides an early demonstration of mood congruence (see also Bousfield, 1950). In another pioneering study, Feshbach and Singer (1957) induced negative affect in subjects through electric shocks and then instructed some of them to suppress their fear. Fearful subjects' evaluations of another person were more negative, and ironically, this effect was even greater when subjects were trying to suppress their fear (Wegner, 1994). Fesh-

bach and Singer explained this response in terms of the psychodynamic mechanism of projection, suggesting that "suppression of fear facilitates the tendency to project fear onto another social object" (p. 286). Mood-congruent effects on evaluative judgments were also found by Byrne and Clore (1970; Clore & Byrne, 1974) using a classical conditioning approach. They used pleasant or unpleasant environments (the unconditioned stimuli) to elicit good or bad moods (the unconditioned response), and then assessed evaluations of a person encountered in this environment (the conditioned stimulus; Gouaux, 1971; Gouaux & Summers, 1973; Griffitt, 1970). These early studies paved the way for the emergence of more focused research on mood congruence in thinking and judgments in the 1980s.

Informational Effects of Moods

Early studies focused on informational effects—that is, ways that positive and negative moods may influence the *content and valence* of cognition. This research tradition is considered first here. Three main theories accounting for mood congruence are reviewed: (1) *associative network* theories emphasizing memory processes (Bower, 1981; Bower & Forgas, 2000), (2) *affect-as-information* theory relying on inferential processes (Clore, Gasper, & Garvin, 2001; Clore & Storbeck, 2006; Schwarz & Clore, 1983), and (3) an integrative *affect infusion model* (AIM; Forgas, 1995, 2002).

Associative Network Model

Bower (1981) assumes that moods are linked to an associative network of memory representations. A mood state may thus automatically prime or activate representations linked to that mood, which in turn are more likely to be used in subsequent constructive cognitive tasks. Several experiments found support for such *affective priming*. For example, happy or sad people were more likely to recall mood-congruent details from their childhood and also remembered more mood-congruent events that occurred in the past few weeks (Bower, 1981). Mood congruence was also observed in how people interpreted ongoing social behaviors (Forgas, Bower, & Krantz, 1984) and formed impressions of others (Forgas & Bower, 1987). Further research found that mood congruence is subject to several boundary conditions (see Blaney, 1986; Bower, 1987; Singer & Salovey, 1988). Mood congruence in memory and judgments is most reliable (1) when moods are intense (Bower & Mayer, 1985) and (2) meaningful (Bower, 1991), (3) when the subsequent task is self-referential (Blaney, 1986), and (4) when open, elaborate thinking (or constructive processing) is used. In particular, tasks requiring constructive processing such as associations, inferences, impression formation, and interpersonal behaviors are most likely to show mood-congruent effects (e.g., Bower & Forgas, 2000; Fiedler, 1990; Mayer, Gaschke, Braverman, & Evans, 1992), because open, elaborate processing amplifies the opportunities for affectively primed incidental memories and information to become incorporated into a newly constructed response. Tasks that require little or no constructive processing, such as recognition or the simple reproduction of existing reactions, are unlikely to show mood congruence (Forgas, 1995, 2002, 2006), because narrow and targeted thinking offers little opportunity for affectively primed information to be incorporated into a response.

Affect-as-Information Theory

This alternative approach seeks to explain mood congruence by suggesting that "rather than computing a judgment on the basis of recalled features of a target, individuals may . . . ask themselves: 'how do I feel about it?' [and] in doing so, they may mistake feelings due to a pre-existing state as a reaction to the target" (Schwarz, 1990, p. 529; see also Clore & Storbeck, 2006; Schwarz & Clore, 1983). Thus, people misattribute a preexisting mood state as indicative of their reaction to an unrelated target. The model is closely derived from research on misattribution and judgmental heuristics. However, its predictions are often empirically indistinguishable from those derived from earlier conditioning models that assumed blind associative learning processes (e.g., Clore & Byrne, 1974). Evidence shows that people mainly rely on their mood as a simple and convenient heuristic cue to infer their

evaluative reactions when "the task is of little personal relevance, when little other information is available, when problems are too complex to be solved systematically, and when time or attentional resources are limited" (Fiedler, 2001, p. 175). If the task is of high personal relevance and there are cognitive resources available, then affective priming is the most likely strategy resulting in mood congruence.

For example, mood induced by good or bad weather was found to influence judgments on a variety of unexpected and unfamiliar questions in a telephone interview (Schwarz & Clore, 1983). In another study, Forgas and Moylan (1987) found mood congruence in survey responses of almost 1,000 subjects who completed a questionnaire after they had seen funny or sad films at the cinema. As in the study by Schwarz and Clore (1983), respondents presumably had little time, interest, motivation, or capacity to engage in elaborate constructive processing, and so relied on their mood as a simple and convenient heuristic shortcut to infer their reactions. Because the informational value of a mood state is not fixed but rather depends on the situational context (Martin, 2000), such mood effects may also be highly context-specific. Furthermore, the affect-as-information model mostly applies to evaluative judgments and may have difficulty accounting for mood congruence in attention, learning, and memory. In one sense misattributing mood to an unrelated target is probably the exception rather than the norm in real-life mood effects on cognition.

Affect Infusion Model (AIM)

The AIM (Forgas, 1995, 2002) suggests that mood effects on cognition depend on the kind of information-processing strategy used and identifies four processing strategies that vary in terms of (1) their *constructiveness* and (2) the degree of *effort* exerted in seeking a solution. The first, *direct access* strategy involves the simple and direct retrieval of a preexisting response. This response is most likely when the task is highly familiar and there is no reason to engage in more elaborate thinking (e.g., retrieving a friend's mobile number). As this is a low-effort, low-constructive processing strategy, affect infusion should not occur. The second, *motivated process-*

ing strategy refers to effortful, yet highly selective and targeted thinking that is dominated by a particular motivational objective (e.g., drafting a message about how to get to your place). This strategy again involves little open, constructive processing and therefore should be impervious to affect infusion and may even produce mood-incongruent effects (Clark & Isen, 1982; Sedikides, 1994). *Heuristic processing* refers to constructive but truncated, low-effort processing, which might be adopted when time and personal resources such as motivation, interest, attention, and working memory capacity are scarce (e.g., evaluating your friend's new company car). Heuristic processing may result in mood congruence when affect is used as a heuristic cue, as predicted by the AIM (Schwarz & Clore, 1983; see also Clore et al., 2001; Clore & Storbeck, 2006). Finally, *substantive processing* involves both high effort and open, constructive thinking, and is used whenever the task is demanding and there are no ready-made direct-access responses or motivational goals available to guide the response. Substantive processing is most likely to produce affect infusion into cognition as mood may selectively prime or enhance the accessibility of mood-congruent thoughts, memories, and interpretations (Forgas, 1994, 1999a, 1999b). Furthermore, the AIM identifies a range of contextual variables related to the task, the person, and the situation that jointly determine processing choices (Forgas, 2002; Smith & Petty, 1995), and recognizes that affect itself can influence processing choices (Bless & Fiedler, 2006).

The key prediction of the AIM is the absence of affect infusion when direct access or motivated processing is used, and the presence of affect infusion during heuristic and substantive processing. Affect infusion is most likely in the course of constructive processing that involves the substantial transformation, rather than the mere reproduction, of existing information. Such processing requires a relatively open information search strategy and a significant degree of generative elaboration of the available stimulus details. Thus, affect "will influence cognitive processes to the extent that the cognitive task involves the active generation of new information as opposed to the passive conservation of information given" (Fiedler,

1990, pp. 2–3). The implications of this model have now been supported in a number of the experiments, considered below. In particular, mood congruence in cognition turns out to be *greater* when *more extensive* and *elaborate* processing is required to deal with a more complex, demanding task (Forgas, 2002; Sedikides, 1995).

Mood Congruence in Memory and Attention

Several studies found that people are better at retrieving both early and recent autobiographical memories that match their prevailing mood (Bower, 1981; Miranda & Kihlstrom, 2005), and depressed patients preferentially remember aversive experiences and negative information (Direnfeld & Roberts, 2006). Implicit tests of memory provide evidence of mood congruence as well. For example, depressed people completed more word stems (e.g., *can-*) with negative rather than positive words they had studied earlier (e.g., *cancer* vs. *candy*; Ruiz-Caballero & Gonzalez, 1994), and happy and sad people selectively remembered more positive and negative details, respectively, about people they had read about (Forgas & Bower, 1987).

These mood-congruent memory effects occur because of the selective activation of an affect-related associative base, resulting in mood-congruent information receiving greater attention and more extensive processing and encoding (Bower, 1981). That is, people spend longer reading mood-congruent material, integrating it into a richer network of primed associations, and as a result, they are better able to remember such information (see Bower & Forgas, 2000). There is growing evidence for mood congruence at the attention stage: In a recent inattentional blindness study (Becker & Leinenger, 2011), mood selectively influenced participants' attentional filter, increasing the chance to notice unexpected faces that carried a mood-congruent emotional expression. Other research demonstrated that positive mood led to attentional bias toward rewarding words (Tamir & Robinson, 2007) and broadened attention to positive images (Wadlinger & Isaacowitz, 2006). Depressed patients also paid greater attention to negative information (Koster, De Raedt, Goeleven, Franck, & Crombez, 2005) and showed better learning and memory for depressive words (Watkins, Mathews, Williamson, & Fuller, 1992) and negative facial expressions (Gilboa-Schechtman, Erhard-Weiss, & Jecemien, 2002).

It should be noted that sad people eventually may escape the vicious circle of focusing on and remembering negative information by means of deliberately employing *mood-incongruent* attention and memory. Consistent with the hypothesis of such motivational *mood repair* (Isen, 1985), Josephson, Singer, and Salovey (1996) showed that after initially retrieving negative memories, nondepressed participants in a negative mood deliberately shifted to retrieving positive memories in order to lift their mood (see also Detweiler-Bedell & Salovey, 2003; Heimpel, Wood, Marshall & Brown, 2002).

Mood-Dependent Memory

Mood has another significant influence on memory by selectively facilitating the retrieval of information that has been learned in a matching rather than a nonmatching mood. Such *mood-dependent memory* may play a role in the memory deficits found in patients with alcoholic blackout, chronic depression, dissociative identity, and other psychiatric disorders (Goodwin, 1974; Reus, Weingartner, & Post, 1979; Schacter & Kihlstrom, 1989). However, these effects are rather subtle (Bower & Mayer, 1989; Kihlstrom, 1989; Leight & Ellis, 1981), and there are several moderating factors that influence their occurrence. Constructive tasks such as free recall are more sensitive to mood-dependent memory than are reproductive tasks such as recognition (Bower, 1992; Eich, 1995; Fiedler, 1990; Kenealy, 1997). The effects are most reliable when people generate their own events to be remembered and their own retrieval cues rather than when they are confronted with fixed materials and predetermined retrieval cues (Beck & McBee, 1995; Eich & Metcalfe, 1989). It seems that the more a person needs to rely on self-constructed information, the more likely that memory for corresponding events will be mood-dependent. Eich, Macaulay, and Ryan (1994) confirmed this, reporting that mood dependence effects were markedly greater when the recalled events were self-generated. Recall was consistently better when encoding mood and retrieval mood were matched rather than different, and this effect pattern was obtained with different mood induction methods (Eich, 1995; Eich et al., 1994). Similar mood dependence in memory was demonstrated in patients with bipolar disorder (Eich, Macaulay, & Lam, 1997).

Mood-dependent memory is also enhanced when the intensity, authenticity, or distinctiveness of encoding and retrieval moods is high rather than low (Eich, 1995; Eich & Macauley, 2000; Eich & Metcalf, 1989; Ucros, 1989). Given that individual differences in personality play an important part in mood-congruent memory (Bower & Forgas, 2000; Smith & Petty, 1995), such factors may also moderate mood-dependent memory. Thus, mood-dependent memory is less likely to occur in experiments that employ simple, irrelevant tasks such as list-learning experiments, and when the mood induction is weak and not particularly distinctive to be effective as a retrieval cue. In terms of the AIM (Forgas, 1995, 2002), the higher the level of constructive processing and affect infusion that occurs, both at the encoding and at the retrieval stages, the more likely that mood dependence can be demonstrated.

Mood Congruence in Inferences and Associations

The selective priming of mood-consistent materials in memory can have a marked influence on how complex or ambiguous information is interpreted (Bower & Forgas, 2000; Clark & Waddell, 1983). For example, people generated more mood-congruent ideas when daydreaming or free associating to Thematic Apperception Test (TAT) pictures, and happy subjects generated more positive than negative associations to words such as *life* (e.g., *love* and *freedom* vs. *struggle* and *death*) than did sad subjects (Bower, 1981). The selective priming of mood-congruent constructs can also influence social judgments, such as perceptions of faces (Forgas & East, 2008a; Gilboa-Schechtman et al., 2002; Schiffenbauer, 1974), impressions of people (Forgas & Bower, 1987), and self-perceptions (Sedikides, 1995). These associative effects are diminished when the targets to be judged are simpler and more clear-cut (e.g., Forgas, 1994, 1995), confirming that open, constructive processing is crucial for mood congruence to occur.

Mood Congruence in Judgments

Consistent with the AIM, several studies have found that the more people need to think in order to compute a judgment, the greater the likelihood that affectively primed ideas will influence the outcome. For example, mood had a greater influence on judgments about unusual, complex characters that require more constructive and elaborate processing than on judgments of simple, typical targets (Forgas, 1992). Mood also had a greater influence on judgments about unusual, badly matched couples than on typical, well-matched couples (e.g., Forgas, 1993).

Judgments about one's real-life partners showed similar mood congruence (Forgas, 1994). Mood significantly influenced the evaluation of one's partner and relationship conflicts, and paradoxically, these effects were stronger for judgments about complex, difficult conflicts that required more constructive processing, confirming that affect infusion into social judgments depends on the processing strategy recruited by the task at hand. Some personality characteristics, such as trait anxiety, may moderate such mood congruence effects on judgments, as highly anxious people are less likely to process information in an open, constructive manner (Ciarrochi & Forgas, 1999). Affect intensity may be another important trait moderator of mood congruence effects, as people who scored high on measures assessing openness to feelings showed greater mood congruence (Ciarrochi & Forgas, 2000).

Moods also exert an important influence on self-related judgments (Sedikides, 1995). Students in a positive mood were more likely to claim credit for success in a recent exam, and made more internal and stable attributions for their high test scores, but were less willing to assume personal responsibility for failure. Those in a negative mood blamed themselves more for failure and took less credit for success (Forgas, Bower, & Moylan, 1990). These findings were replicated in a study by Detweiler-Bedell and Detweiler-Bedell (2006), who concluded that consistent with the AIM, "constructive processing accompanying most self-judgments is critical in producing mood-congruent perceptions of personal success" (p. 196).

Sedikides (1995) also found support for the AIM, reporting that well-rehearsed "central" conceptions of the self were processed more automatically and less constructively and thus were less influenced by mood than were "peripheral" self-conceptions that required more substantive processing and showed stronger mood congruence. Individual differences in self-esteem may also influence affect infusion into self-judgments, as mood-congruent effects on self-related memories were stronger for low rather than high self-esteem people (Smith & Petty, 1995), in line with the assumption that the former have a less clearly defined and less stable self-concept (Brown & Mankowski, 1993). Consistent with the AIM, these results show that low self-esteem is linked to the more open and constructive processing of information about the self, increasing the scope for mood-related associations to influence the outcome. Other work suggests that mood congruence may be spontaneously corrected as a result of shifting to the motivated processing strategy, as initially mood-congruent thoughts were spontaneously reversed over time (Sedikides, 1994). Further research by Forgas and Ciarrochi (2002) replicated these results and found that the spontaneous reversal of negative self-judgments was strongest in people with high self-esteem, consistent with the operation of a homeostatic process of mood management.

Mood-Congruent Effects on Social Behaviors

Because planning strategic social behaviors necessarily requires some degree of constructive, open information processing (Heider, 1958), moods may also produce behavioral effects. Positive mood, by priming positive evaluations and inferences, should elicit more optimistic, positive, confident, and cooperative behaviors, whereas negative mood may produce more avoidant, defensive, and unfriendly behaviors. In one experiment, happy or sad mood was induced in people before they engaged in a strategic negotiation task (Forgas, 1998c). Those in a happy mood employed more trusting, optimistic, and cooperative negotiating strategies, and achieved better outcomes, whereas those in a negative mood were more pessimistic and competitive in their negotiating moves. Other experiments examined the effects of induced mood on the way people formulate and use verbal requests (Forgas, 1999a). These studies found that due to more optimistic inferences about the receptiveness/willingness of the persons receiving the request, positive mood resulted in more confident and less polite request formulations. In contrast, negative affect triggered a more cautious, polite, and elaborate requesting strategy as a result of rather pessimistic inferences regarding the request's chance of success.

Another unobtrusive field experiment showed that moods also influence how people *respond* to an impromptu request (Forgas, 1998a). Mood was induced by leaving folders containing mood-inducing materials (pictures as well as text) on empty library desks. After occupying the desks and examining the mood induction materials, students received an unexpected polite or impolite request from a confederate asking for paper needed to complete an essay. Results revealed a clear mood-congruent response

pattern: Negative mood resulted in less compliance and more critical, negative evaluations of the request and requester, whereas positive mood yielded the opposite results. Again, the effects were stronger when the request was formulated in an unusual and impolite way and therefore recruited more substantive processing.

Some strategic interpersonal behaviors, such as *self-disclosure*, are critical for the development and maintenance of intimate relationships, for mental health, and for social adjustment. It seems that by facilitating mood-congruent associations and inferences about a conversational partner, affective states can directly influence people's preferred self-disclosure strategies (Forgas, 2011a). Several recent experiments found that, consistent with the predicted mood congruence effects, those in a positive mood preferred to disclose information that was more intimate, more varied, more abstract, and more positive than was the case for people in a neutral mood. Negative affect had exactly the opposite effect (Figure 13.1), and this pattern was even stronger when the conversational partner reciprocated with a high degree of disclosure. Thus, these experiments provide convergent evidence that temporary fluctuations in mood can produce marked changes in the quality, valence, and reciprocity of self-disclosure, suggesting

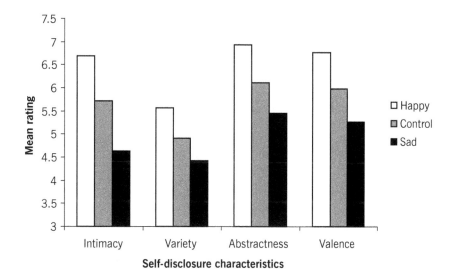

FIGURE 13.1. The effects of positive, neutral, and negative mood on the intimacy, variety, abstractness, and valence of self-disclosing messages.

that mood congruence is likely to occur in the context of many other unscripted and unpredictable strategic interpersonal behaviors.

When considered jointly, the evidence shows that transient moods play an important informative function, influencing the content and valence of memory, attention, associations, inferences, judgments, and social behaviors in a predominantly mood-congruent way. However, these effects are dependent on the information-processing strategy adopted, with open, constructive processing being more likely to be influenced by moods than other kinds of processing strategies (Forgas, 1995, 2002). When such substantive processing is used, affective priming appears to be the most likely mechanism responsible for mood congruence effects (Bower, 1981), and some evaluative judgments made under suboptimal processing conditions may be also become mood congruent as a result of the heuristic affect-as-information mechanism. The overall pattern of results seems consistent with the AIM, suggesting that mood congruence is unlikely when a task can be performed using simple, well-rehearsed direct access or motivated processing, as there is little opportunity for moods to influence cognition. According to the AIM, mood congruence is most likely when individuals engage in substantive, constructive processing.

Mood Effects on Processing Strategies

The evidence surveyed so far clearly shows that mood states can have a significant *informational* influence on the content and valence of cognition, producing mood-congruent effects on memory, attention, associations, judgments, and social behaviors. In addition to influencing cognitive content (i.e., *what* people think), moods may also influence the process of cognition (i.e., *how* people think). This section reviews evidence for the information-processing consequences of moods.

Since the 1980s, a growing number of studies suggests that people experiencing a positive mood rely on a more superficial and less effortful information-processing strategy. Those in a good mood were consistently found to reach decisions more

quickly, use less information, avoid systematic and demanding thinking, and, ironically, they appeared more confident about their decisions. In contrast, negative mood apparently triggered a more effortful, systematic, analytic, and vigilant processing style (Clark & Isen, 1982; Isen, 1984, 1987; Schwarz, 1990). Nevertheless, more recent studies show that positive mood sometimes produces distinct processing advantages. For instance, happy people tend to adopt a more creative, open, and inclusive thinking style, use broader cognitive categories, show greater mental flexibility, and perform better on secondary tasks (Bless & Fiedler, 2006; Fiedler, 2001; Isen & Daubman, 1984; Hertel & Fiedler, 1994). How can we explain these processing differences?

Initially, explanations emphasized the *motivational* consequences of good and bad moods. According to the *mood maintenance–mood repair* hypothesis, those in a positive mood may be motivated to maintain this rewarding state by avoiding effortful activity such as elaborate information processing. In contrast, a negative mood should motivate people to engage in more vigilant, effortful information processing as an adaptive strategy to relieve their aversive state (Clark & Isen, 1982; Isen, 1984, 1987). More recently, several studies also showed that the cognitive consequences of affective states may depend on whether the mood state is high or low in approach motivation intensity. For example, low-approach positive affect seems to broaden cognitive categorization and attention, but high-approach positive affect tends to narrow cognitive categorization (Gable & Harmon-Jones, 2008; Price & Harmon-Jones, 2010).

An alternative *cognitive-tuning* account (Schwarz, 1990) argues that positive and negative moods have a fundamental signaling/tuning function, informing the person whether a relaxed, effort-minimizing (positive mood) or a vigilant, effortful (negative mood) processing style is required. Both these models rely on a functionalist/evolutionary view of moods as fulfilling adaptive functions (Forgas, Haselton & von Hippel, 2007). Yet another theory focuses on the impact of moods on *information-processing capacity*, suggesting that mood states may influence processing style because they take up scarce processing capacity. Curiously, both positive mood (Isen, 1984) and negative mood (Ellis & Ashbrook, 1988) are hypothesized to reduce processing capacity.

Assimilation–Accommodation Model

The various explanations all assume that moods influence processing style by altering the degree of motivation, vigilance, and effort exerted. However, this view has been challenged by some experiments demonstrating that positive mood does not necessarily impair processing effort, as performance on simultaneously presented secondary tasks was not impaired (e.g., Fiedler, 2001; Hertel & Fiedler, 1994). An alternative theory, Bless and Fiedler's (2006) assimilation–accommodation model, suggests that the fundamental, evolutionary significance of moods is not to regulate processing effort, but rather to trigger equally effortful but qualitatively different *processing styles*. The model identifies

> two complementary adaptive functions, *assimilation* and *accommodation* (cf. Piaget, 1954). Assimilation means to impose internalized structures onto the external world, whereas accommodation means to modify internal structures in accordance with external constraints. With respect to affective influences the role of positive mood is to facilitate assimilation, whereas the role of negative mood is to strengthen accommodation functions. (Bless & Fiedler, 2006, p. 66)

Several lines of evidence now support the assimilative–accommodative processing dichotomy. For example, those in a positive mood used broader, more assimilative cognitive categories (Isen, 1984), sorted stimuli into fewer and more inclusive groups (Isen & Daubman, 1984), and classified behavioral descriptions into fewer and more inclusive types (Bless, Hamilton, & Mackie, 1992). Positive affect also recruited more assimilative and abstract representations in language choices, as happy people produced more abstract event descriptions than sad participants (Beukeboom, 2003), and were more likely to retrieve a generic rather than specific representation of a persuasive message (Bless, Mackie, & Schwarz, 1992). Similar mood-induced effects on processing style were found with nonverbal tasks. For example, happy mood resulted in greater focus on the global rather than the local features of geometric patterns (Gasper & Clore, 2002; Sinclair, 1988).

What is the reason for these mood-induced differences in processing style? Bless and Fiedler (2006) suggest that moods perform an adaptive function essentially preparing us to respond to different environmental challenges. Positive mood indicates that the situation is safe and familiar, and that existing knowledge can be relied upon. In contrast, negative mood functions like a mild alarm signal, indicating that the situation is novel and unfamiliar, and that the careful monitoring of new, external information is required. There is supporting evidence suggesting that positive affect increases, and negative affect decreases, the tendency to rely on internal knowledge rather than external information in cognitive tasks, resulting in a selective memory bias for self-generated information (Bless, Bohner, Schwarz, & Strack, 1992; Fiedler, Nickel, Asbeck, & Pagel, 2003).

The theory thus predicts that *both* positive and negative mood can produce processing advantages, albeit in response to different situations requiring different processing styles. Given the almost exclusive emphasis on the benefits of positive affect in our culture, this is an important message with some intriguing real-life implications. Numerous studies now suggest that negative mood can produce definite processing advantages in situations when the careful and detailed monitoring of new, external information is required, as we shall see below.

Memory Performance

One key area where the processing consequences of good or bad moods have been explored is memory performance. If negative mood indeed recruits a more accommodative, externally focused processing style, then it should result in improved memory for incidentally encountered information. In one experiment happy or sad subjects read a variety of essays advocating alternative positions on public policy issues. Later, their cued recall memory of the essays was assessed (Forgas, 1998b, Exp. 3). Results showed that those in a negative mood remembered the details of the essays significantly better than those in a happy mood, consistent with negative mood promoting more externally focused, accommodative thinking.

This effect was further explored in a recent field experiment, when happy or sad shoppers (on sunny or rainy days, respectively) saw a variety of small objects displayed on the checkout counter of a local news agency (Forgas, Goldenberg, & Unkelbach, 2009). After leaving the store, they were asked to recall and recognize the objects they had seen on the counter. It turned out that mood, induced by the weather, had a significant effect. Those in a negative mood (on rainy days) had significantly better memory for what they had seen in the shop than did happy people (on sunny days), confirming that mood states have a subtle but reliable memory effect, and negative mood actually improves memory for incidentally encountered information (see Figure 13.2).

A series of further experiments explored mood effects on eyewitness memory, predicting that, due to promoting more assimilative thinking (Isen, 1987), positive affect should increase, and negative affect should decrease, the tendency of eyewitnesses to incorporate false details into their memories (Forgas, Vargas, & Laham, 2005). In one study (Forgas et al., 2005, Exp. 1), participants viewed pictures of a car crash (negative event) and a wedding party (positive event). One hour later, they received a mood induction (recalling happy or sad events from their past) and answered questions about the initially viewed scenes that either contained or did not contain misleading, false information. After a further 45-minute interval the accuracy of their eyewitness memory for the two scenes was tested. As predicted, positive mood increased, and negative mood decreased the amount of false, misleading information incorporated (assimilated) into their eyewitness memories. In contrast, negative mood almost completely eliminated this "misinformation effect," as confirmed by a signal detection analysis.

In a second, more realistic experiment students witnessed a staged 5-minute aggressive encounter between a lecturer and a female intruder (Forgas et al., 2005, Exp. 2). One week later, while in a happy or sad mood, they received a questionnaire that either did or did not contain planted, misleading information. After a further interval, their eyewitness memory was assessed. Those in a happy mood when exposed to misleading information were more likely to assimilate false details into their memory. In contrast, negative mood eliminated this source of error in eyewitness memory, consistent with negative mood recruiting more accommodative processing and thus improving subject's the ability to discriminate between correct and misleading details (Figure 13.3).

In a further experiment, participants saw videotapes showing a robbery and a wedding scene. After a 45-minute interval they received an audiovisual mood induction and completed a short questionnaire that either contained or did not contain mislead-

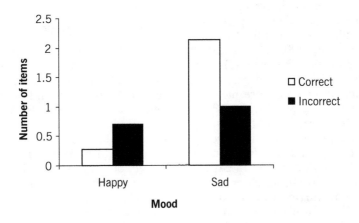

FIGURE 13.2. Mean number of target items seen in a shop recalled as a function of the mood (happy vs. sad) induced by the weather.

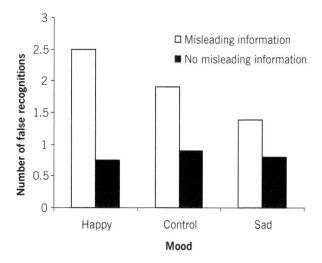

FIGURE 13.3. The interaction between mood and the presence or absence of misleading information on eyewitness memory: Positive mood increased and negative mood decreased the tendency to incorporate false, misleading details (false alarms) into eyewitness reports.

ing information about the events. Additionally, some were instructed to "disregard and control their affective states." Exposure to misleading information reduced eyewitness accuracy most when people were in a happy rather than a sad mood. However, direct instructions to control one's affect proved ineffective to reduce this mood effect.

Conceptually similar results were reported by Storbeck and Clore (2005), who found that "individuals in a negative mood were significantly less likely to show false memory effects than those in positive moods" (p. 785). These authors explain their findings in terms of the affect-as-information mechanism. These experiments offer convergent evidence that negative moods recruit more accommodative thinking and therefore can improve memory performance by means of reducing susceptibility to misleading information. Paradoxically, happy mood *reduced* eyewitness accuracy yet *increased* subjective confidence, suggesting that judges were unaware of the processing consequences of their mood states.

Mood Effects on Judgmental Accuracy

Is it possible that mood states, through their influence on processing style, may also improve or impair the accuracy of our social judgments? For example, can good or

bad mood influence the common tendency for people to form evaluative judgments based on their first impressions? One recent experiment examined mood effects on this "primacy effect," which occurs because people pay disproportionate attention to early rather than later information when forming impressions (Forgas, 2011b). After an autobiographical mood induction (recalling happy or sad past events), participants formed impressions about a character (Jim) described either in an introvert–extravert or an extravert–introvert sequence. As primacy effects occur because of the assimilative processing of later information, the subsequent impression formation judgments revealed that positive mood significantly increased the primacy effect by recruiting more top-down, assimilative processing. In contrast, negative mood, by recruiting a stimulus-based, accommodative processing style, almost eliminated the primacy effect.

Many common judgmental errors in everyday life occur because people are imperfect and often inattentive information processors. For example, the *fundamental attribution error* (FAE) or *correspondence bias* refers to the pervasive tendency by people to infer intentionality and internal causation and underestimate the impact of situational constraints and forces when making judgments about the behavior of others (Gilbert

& Malone, 1995). This error occurs because people focus on central and salient information, that is, the actor, whereas they ignore equally relevant but less salient information about external influences on the actor (Gilbert & Malone, 1995). Because negative mood promotes vigilant, detail-oriented processing, it should reduce the incidence of the FAE by directing greater attention to external influences on actors.

This prediction was tested in one experiment (Forgas, 1998b) in which happy or sad subjects read an essay and made attributions about its writer advocating a popular or unpopular position (for or against nuclear testing). The writer's position was described as either assigned (implies external causation) or freely chosen (implies internal causation). Results showed that happy persons were more likely and sad people were less likely than controls to commit the FAE by incorrectly inferring an internally caused attitude based on a coerced essay.

Such mood-induced differences in judgmental accuracy do occur in real life. In a field study (Forgas, 1998b) happy or sad participants (after watching happy or sad movies) read essays and made attributions about writers advocating popular positions (pro recycling) or unpopular positions (contra recycling). Again, positive affect increased and negative affect decreased the tendency to mistakenly infer internally caused attitudes based on coerced essays. In a further study, recall of the essays was additionally assessed as an index of processing style (Forgas, 1998b, Exp. 3). Negative mood again reduced and positive mood increased the incidence of the FAE. Recall memory data confirmed that those in a negative mood remembered more details, indicating enhanced accommodative processing. Furthermore, a mediation analysis showed that this mood-induced difference in processing style significantly mediated the observed mood effects on the incidence of the FAE. We should note, however, that negative mood only improves judgmental accuracy when relevant stimulus information is actually available. Ambady and Gray (2002) found that in the absence of diagnostic details, "sadness impairs [judgmental] accuracy precisely by promoting a more deliberative information processing style" (p. 947).

Mood Effects on Skepticism and the Detection of Deception

Most of our knowledge about the world is based on second-hand information we receive from others. Many messages, such as most interpersonal communications, are by their very nature ambiguous and not open to objective validation. Other claims (e.g., "urban myths") can potentially be evaluated against objective evidence, although such testing is usually not practicable. One of the most important cognitive tasks people face in everyday life is to decide whether to trust and accept, or distrust and reject, social information. Rejecting valid information (excessive skepticism) is just as dangerous as accepting invalid information (gullibility). What determines whether the information we come across in everyday life is judged true or false?

There is some recent evidence that by recruiting assimilative or accommodative processing, mood states may significantly influence skepticism and gullibility (Forgas & East, 2008a; 2008b). For example, one study asked happy or sad participants to judge the probable truth of a number of urban legends and rumors (Forgas, 2011c). Positive mood promoted greater gullibility for novel and unfamiliar claims, whereas negative mood promoted skepticism, which is consistent with the more externally focused, attentive, and detail-oriented accommodative thinking style. In another experiment, participants' recognition memory was tested 2 weeks after initial exposure to true and false statements taken from a trivia game. Only sad participants were able to correctly distinguish between the true and false claims they had seen previously. In contrast, happy participants tended to rate all previously seen and thus familiar statements as true (in essence, a fluency effect). This pattern suggests that happy mood produced reliance on the "what is familiar is true" heuristic, whereas negative mood conferred a clear cognitive advantage of improving judges' ability to accurately remember the truth or untruth of the statements.

Unlike many urban myths, interpersonal communications are often intrinsically ambiguous and have no objective truth value (Heider, 1958). Accepting or rejecting such messages is particularly problematic, yet critically important for effective social interaction. It turns out that mood effects on processing style may also influence people's tendency to accept or reject interpersonal communications as genuine. People in a negative mood were significantly less likely and those in a positive mood were more likely to accept various facial expressions communicating feelings as authentic (Forgas & East, 2008a).

Taking this line of reasoning one step further, does mood, through its effect on processing styles, influence people's ability to detect deception? In one study, happy or sad participants watched videotaped interrogations of suspects accused of theft who were either guilty or not guilty of this offense (Forgas & East, 2008b). Surprisingly, those in a positive mood were more gullible, as they accepted more denials as true. In contrast, sad mood resulted in more guilty judgments and actually improved the participants' ability to correctly identify targets as deceptive (guilty) or honest, consistent with a more accommodative processing style. These experiments offer convergent evidence that negative mood increases skepticism and may significantly improve people's ability to accurately detect deception.

Mood Effects on Stereotyping

Assimilative processing in happy mood should promote, and accommodative processing in negative mood should reduce, the use of preexisting knowledge structures, such as stereotypes. In two studies, Bodenhausen (1993; Bodenhausen, Kramer, & Süsser, 1994) found that happy participants relied more on ethnic stereotypes when evaluating a student accused of misconduct, whereas negative mood reduced this tendency. Generally speaking, sad individuals tend to pay greater attention to specific, individuating information when forming impressions of other people (Bless, Schwarz, & Wieland, 1996).

Similar effects were demonstrated in a recent experiment where happy or sad subjects had to form impressions about the quality and other aspects of a brief philosophical essay allegedly written by a middle-age male academic (stereotypical author) or by a young, alternative-looking female writer (atypical author). Results showed that

happy mood increased the judges' tendency to be influenced by irrelevant stereotypical information about the age and gender of the author. In contrast, negative mood eliminated this effect (Forgas, 2011d). Again, this pattern is entirely consistent with the predicted assimilative versus accommodative processing style recruited by good or bad moods, respectively.

Could mood-induced differences in processing style also influence reliance on stereotypes in actual social behaviors? We tested this prediction by asking happy or sad people to generate rapid responses to targets that appeared or did not appear to be Muslims, using the "shooter's bias" paradigm to assess subliminal aggressive tendencies (Correll, Park, Judd, & Wittenbrink, 2002). In this task, people are instructed to rapidly shoot at targets only when they carry a gun. Prior work with this paradigm showed that U.S. citizens display a strong implicit bias to shoot more at black than white targets (Correll et al., 2002, 2007).

We expected a "turban effect," that is, Muslim targets may elicit a similar bias. We used morphing software to create targets who did, or did not, appear Muslim (wearing or not wearing a turban or the *hijab*) and who either held a gun or held a similar object (e.g., a coffee mug). Participants indeed shot more at Muslims than at non-Muslims, but the most intriguing finding was that negative mood actually *reduced* this selective response tendency fueled by negative stereotypes (Unkelbach et al., 2008). Positive mood in turn increased shooters' bias against Muslims, consistent with a more top-down, heuristic assimilative processing style (Bless & Fiedler, 2006; Forgas, 2007). Thus, mood effects on information processing styles may extend to influencing actual aggressive behaviors based on stereotypes as well.

Mood Effects on Interpersonal Strategies

Effective interpersonal behavior may be improved by processing external information in a more attentive and accommodative fashion. For instance, moods may optimize the way people process, produce, and respond to persuasive messages. In a number of studies, participants in sad moods showed greater attentiveness to message quality and were more persuaded by strong rather than weak arguments. In contrast, those in a happy mood were not influenced by message quality and were equally persuaded by strong and weak arguments (e.g., Bless et al., 1990; Bless, Mackie, & Schwarz, 1992; Bohner, Crow, Erb, & Schwarz, 1992; Sinclair, Mark, & Clore, 1994; Wegener & Petty, 1997).

Furthermore, mood states may also influence the *production* of persuasive messages. In one experiment, participants received an audiovisual mood induction and were then asked to produce effective persuasive arguments for or against (1) an increase in student fees and (2) Aboriginal land rights (Forgas, 2007). As expected, results showed that participants in a sad mood produced higher quality, more effective persuasive arguments on both issues than did happy participants. A mediation analysis revealed that it was mood-induced variations in argument concreteness that mediated the observed differences in argument quality, consistent with the prediction that negative mood should recruit a more externally oriented, concrete and accommodative processing style (Bless, 2001; Bless & Fiedler, 2006; Fiedler, 2001; Forgas, 2002). Similar effects were found when happy and sad people produced per-

suasive arguments for a "partner" to volunteer for a boring experiment using e-mail exchanges (Forgas, 2007). Once again, negative affect produced a processing benefit, resulting in more concrete and more effective persuasive messages (see Figure 13.4).

Induced moods may also influence the degree of *selfishness* versus *fairness* people display when allocating resources among themselves and others in strategic games, such as the dictator game (Tan & Forgas, 2010). Positive mood, by increasing internally focused, assimilative processing, resulted in more selfish allocations, and this effect was even greater when the other person was a stranger rather than an ingroup member (see Figure 13.5). Negative mood, in contrast, focusing greater attention on external information such as the norm of fairness, resulted in significantly more generous and fair allocations to both ingroup members and strangers.

Summary and Conclusions

Understanding the relationship between feeling and thinking, affect and cognition has been one of the more enduring puzzles about human nature. From Plato to Pascal and Kant, a long line of Western phi-

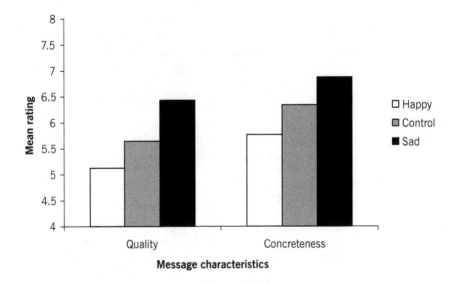

FIGURE 13.4. Mood effects on the quality and concreteness of the persuasive messages produced: Negative affect increased the degree of concreteness of the arguments produced, and arguments produced in negative mood were also rated as more persuasive.

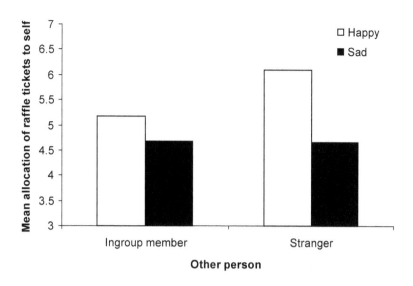

FIGURE 13.5. Mood effects on the degree of selfishness versus fairness on allocations made to ingroup members versus strangers: Positive mood recruited more assimilative, internally focused processing resulting in greater selfishness, and negative mood produced greater attention to fairness norm and fairer allocations.

losophers has tried to analyze the ways that affect can influence our thinking, memory, judgments, and behaviors. Despite a number of promising early studies, psychologists were relatively late to apply empirical methods to study mood effects on cognition. This chapter reviewed the current status of this important research area and suggested that the effects of mood on cognition can be classified into two major kinds of influences: *informational effects* impacting on the content and valence of thinking, usually resulting in mood congruence, and mood effects on *processing strategies*, influencing how people deal with information.

Practical Implications

Contemporary culture places an almost exclusive emphasis on the beneficial effects of positive mood, and the achievement of positive affect seems to be the objective of most applied psychological interventions. In contrast with this view, the results reviewed here highlight the potentially adaptive and beneficial processing consequences of both positive and negative moods, demonstrating that positive affect is not universally desirable. For instance, people in a negative

mood are less prone to judgmental errors (Forgas, 1998b), are more resistant to eyewitness distortions (Forgas et al., 2005), are less likely to rely on stereotypes (Unkelbach et al., 2008), and are better at producing high-quality, effective persuasive messages (Forgas, 2007). Given the consistency of findings across a number of different domains, tasks, and affect inductions, these effects appear reliable. Furthermore, they are broadly consistent with the notion that over evolutionary time, affective states came to operate as adaptive, functional triggers to elicit information-processing patterns that are appropriate in a given situation. In a broader sense, the results presented here suggest that the persistent contemporary cultural emphasis on positivity and happiness may be misplaced, given growing evidence for the important, adaptive benefits of both positive and negative mood states.

It is important to note that the processing advantages of negative affect reported here apply only to mild, temporary negative moods and do not generalize to more intense and enduring negative affective states such as depression, because depression does not necessarily produce more accommodative thinking. In a recent review article on the

cognitive manifestation of depression, Gotlib and Joormann (2010) concluded that
"depression is characterized by increased
elaboration of negative information, by difficulties disengaging from negative material,
and by deficits in cognitive control when
processing negative information" (p. 285).
According to this view, the cognitive dysfunction inherent in depression can rather
be described as of prolonged, gridlocked
mood-congruent information processing,
rather than better accommodation to situational requirements. We should also note
that according to recent evidence, the cognitive consequences of affective states may
also depend on whether the affective state
is low or high in approach motivation. In
several studies, low-approach positive affect
was found to broaden cognitive categorization and attention, but high-approach positive affect had the opposite effect, narrowing categorization (Gable & Harmon-Jones,
2008; Price & Harmon-Jones, 2010).

In conclusion, there is now strong evidence showing that mood states have a powerful, yet often subconscious, influence on
what people think (content effects) as well as
how people think (processing effects). As we
have seen, research shows that these effects
are often subtle and subject to a variety of
boundary conditions and contextual influences. A better understanding of the complex interplay between mood and cognition
remains one of the most important tasks for
psychology as a science. A great deal has
been achieved in the last few decades by
applying empirical methods to exploring this
issue, but in a sense, the enterprise has barely
begun. Hopefully this chapter, and the col-
lection of papers in this volume in general,
will stimulate further research exploring the
fascinating relationship between mood and
cognition.

References

Adolphs, R., & Damasio, A. R. (2001). The
interaction of affect and cognition: A neurobiological perspective. In J. P. Forgas (Ed.),
Handbook of affect and social cognition
(pp. 27–49). Mahwah, NJ: Erlbaum.

Ambady, N., & Gray, H. (2002). On being sad
and mistaken: Mood effects on the accuracy

of thin-slice judgments. *Journal of Personality
and Social Psychology, 83,* 947–961.

Beck, R. C., & McBee, W. (1995). Mood-
dependent memory for generated and repeated
words: Replication and extension. *Cognition
and Emotion, 9,* 289–307.

Becker, M. W., & Leineger, M. (2011). Attentional selection is biased toward mood-
congruent stimuli. *Emotion, 11,* 1248–1254.

Beukeboom, C. (2003). *How mood turns on
language.* Unpublished doctoral dissertation,
Free University of Amsterdam, The Netherlands.

Blaney, P. H. (1986). Affect and memory: A
review. *Psychological Bulletin, 99,* 229–246.

Bless, H. (2001). Mood and the use of general
knowledge structures. In L. L. Martin (Ed.),
*Theories of mood and cognition: A user's
guidebook* (pp. 9–26). Mahwah, NJ: Erlbaum.

Bless, H., Bohner, G., Schwarz, N., & Strack,
F. (1990). Mood and persuasion: A cognitive
response analysis. *Personality and Social Psychology Bulletin, 16,* 331–345.

Bless, H., & Fiedler, K. (2006). Mood and the
regulation of information processing and
behavior. In J. P. Forgas (Ed.), *Hearts and
minds: Affective influences on social cognition and behaviour* (pp. 65–84). New York:
Psychology Press.

Bless, H., Hamilton, D. L., & Mackie, D. M.
(1992). Mood effects on the organization of
person information. *European Journal of
Social Psychology, 22,* 497–509.

Bless, H., Mackie, D. M., & Schwarz, N. (1992).
Mood effects on encoding and judgmental
processes in persuasion. *Journal of Personality and Social Psychology, 63,* 585–595.

Bless, H., Schwarz, N., & Wieland, R. (1996).
Mood and the impact of category member-
ship and individuating information. *European
Journal of Social Psychology, 26,* 935–959.

Bodenhausen, G. V. (1993). Emotions, arousal,
and stereotypic judgments: A heuristic model
of affect and stereotyping. In D. M. Mackie &
D. L. Hamilton (Eds.), *Affect, cognition, and
stereotyping* (pp. 13–37). San Diego, CA: Academic Press.

Bodenhausen, G. V., Kramer, G. P., & Süsser, K.
(1994). Happiness and stereotypic thinking in
social judgment. *Journal of Personality and
Social Psychology, 66,* 621–632.

Bohner, G., Crow, K., Erb, H. P., & Schwarz, N.
(1992). Affect and persuasion: Mood effects
on the processing of message content and con-

text cues. *European Journal of Social Psychology, 22,* 511–530.

Bousfield, W. A. (1950). The relationship between mood and the production of affectively toned associates. *Journal of General Psychology, 42,* 67–85.

Bower, G. H. (1981). Mood and memory. *American Psychologist, 36,* 129–148.

Bower, G. H. (1987). Commentary on mood and memory. *Behaviour Research and Therapy, 25,* 443–455.

Bower, G. H. (1991). Mood congruity of social judgments. In J. P. Forgas (Ed.), *Emotion and social judgments* (pp. 31–53). Oxford, UK: Pergamon.

Bower, G. H. (1992). How might emotions affect learning? In S. A. Christianson (Ed.), *Handbook of emotion and memory* (pp. 3–31). Hillsdale, NJ: Erlbaum.

Bower, G. H., & Forgas, J. P. (2000). Affect, memory, and social cognition. In E. Eich, J. F. Kihlstrom, G. H. Bower, J. P. Forgas, & P. M. Niedenthal (Eds.), *Cognition and emotion* (pp. 87–168). New York: Oxford University Press.

Bower, G. H., & Mayer, J. D. (1985). Failure to replicate mood-dependent retrieval. *Bulletin of the Psychonomic Society, 23,* 39–42.

Bower, G. H., & Mayer, J. D. (1989). In search of mood-dependent retrieval. *Journal of Social Behavior and Personality, 4,* 121–156.

Brown, J. D., & Mankowski, T. A. (1993). Self-esteem, mood, and self-evaluation: Changes in mood and the way you see you. *Journal of Personality and Social Psychology, 64,* 421–430.

Byrne, D., & Clore, G. L. (1970). A reinforcement model of evaluation responses. *Personality, 1,* 103–128.

Ciarrochi, J. V., & Forgas, J. P. (1999). On being tense yet tolerant: The paradoxical effects of trait anxiety and aversive mood on intergroup judgments. *Group Dynamics: Theory, Research, and Practice, 3,* 227–238.

Ciarrochi, J. V., & Forgas, J. P. (2000). The pleasure of possessions: Affect and consumer judgments. *European Journal of Social Psychology, 30,* 631–649.

Clark, M. S., & Isen, A. M. (1982). Towards understanding the relationship between feeling states and social behavior. In A. H. Hastorf & A. M. Isen (Eds.), *Cognitive social psychology* (pp. 73–108). New York: Elsevier.

Clark, M. S., & Waddell, B. A. (1983). Effects of moods on thoughts about helping, attraction and information acquisition. *Social Psychology Quarterly, 46,* 31–35.

Clore, G. L., & Byrne, D. (1974). The reinforcement affect model of attraction. In T. L. Huston (Ed.), *Foundations of interpersonal attraction* (pp. 143–170). New York: Academic Press.

Clore, G. L., Gasper, K., & Garvin, E. (2001). Affect as information. In J. P. Forgas (Ed.). *Handbook of affect and social cognition* (pp. 121–144). Mahwah, NJ: Erlbaum.

Clore, G. L., & Storbeck, J. (2006). Affect as information about liking, efficacy, and importance. In J. P. Forgas (Ed.), *Affect in social thinking and behavior* (pp. 123–142). New York: Psychology Press.

Correll, J., Park, B., Judd, C. M., & Wittenbrink, B. (2002). The police officer's dilemma: Using ethnicity to disambiguate potentially threatening individuals. *Journal of Personality and Social Psychology, 83,* 1314–1329.

Correll, J., Park, B., Judd, C. M., Wittenbrink, B., Sadler, M. S., & Keesee, T. (2007). Across the thin blue line: Police officers and racial bias in the decision to shoot. *Journal of Personality and Social Psychology, 92,* 1006–1023.

Detweiler-Bedell, B., & Detweiler-Bedell, J. B. (2006). Mood-congruent perceptions of success depend on self–other framing. *Cognition and Emotion, 20,* 196–216.

Detweiler-Bedell, J. B., & Salovey, P. (2003). Striving for happiness or fleeing from sadness?: Motivating mood repair using differentially framed messages. *Journal of Social and Clinical Psychology, 22,* 627–664.

Direnfeld, D. M., & Roberts, J. E. (2006). Mood-congruent memory in dysphoria: The roles of state affect and cognitive style. *Behavior Research and Therapy, 44,* 1275–1285.

Eich, E. (1995). Searching for mood dependent memory. *Psychological Science, 6,* 67–75.

Eich, E., & Macaulay, D. (2000). Are real moods required to reveal mood-congruent and mood-dependent memory? *Psychological Science, 11,* 244–248.

Eich, E., Macaulay, D., & Lam, R. (1997). Mania, depression, and mood-dependent memory. *Cognition and Emotion, 11,* 607–618.

Eich, E., Macaulay, D., & Ryan, L. (1994). Mood-dependent memory for events of the personal past. *Journal of Experimental Psychology: General, 123,* 201–215.

Eich, E., & Metcalfe, J. (1989). Mood-dependent

memory for internal versus external events. *Journal of Experimental Psychology: Learning, Memory, and Cognition, 15,* 443–455.

Ellis, H. C., & Ashbrook, P. W. (1988). Resource allocation model of the effects of depressed mood states on memory. In K. Fiedler & J. P. Forgas (Eds.), *Affect, cognition and social behavior* (pp. 25–43). Toronto: Hogrefe.

Feshbach, S., & Singer, R. D. (1957). The effects of fear arousal and suppression of fear upon social perception. *Journal of Abnormal and Social Psychology, 55,* 283–288.

Fiedler, K. (1990). Mood-dependent selectivity in social cognition. In W. Stroebe & M. Hewstone (Eds.), *European review of social psychology* (Vol. 1, pp. 1–32). New York: Wiley.

Fiedler, K. (2001). Affective influences on social information processing. In J. P. Forgas (Ed.), *Handbook of affect and social cognition* (pp. 163–185). Mahwah, NJ: Erlbaum.

Fiedler, K., Nickel, S., Asbeck, J., & Pagel, U. (2003). Mood and the generation effect. *Cognition and Emotion, 17,* 585–608.

Forgas, J. P. (1979). *Social episodes: The study of interaction routines.* New York: Academic Press.

Forgas, J. P. (1992). On bad mood and peculiar people: Affect and person typicality in impression formation. *Journal of Personality and Social Psychology, 62,* 863–875.

Forgas, J. P. (1993). On making sense of odd couples: Mood effects on the perception of mismatched relationships. *Personality and Social Psychology Bulletin, 19,* 59–71.

Forgas, J. P. (1994). Sad and guilty?: Affective influences on the explanation of conflict episodes. *Journal of Personality and Social Psychology, 66,* 56–68.

Forgas, J. P. (1995). Mood and judgment: The affect infusion model (AIM). *Psychological Bulletin, 117,* 39–66.

Forgas, J. P. (1998a). Asking nicely?: Mood effects on responding to more or less polite requests. *Personality and Social Psychology Bulletin, 24,* 173–185.

Forgas, J. P. (1998b). On being happy but mistaken: Mood effects on the fundamental attribution error. *Journal of Personality and Social Psychology, 75,* 318–331.

Forgas, J. P. (1998c). On feeling good and getting your way: Mood effects on negotiating strategies and outcomes. *Journal of Personality and Social Psychology. 74,* 565–577.

Forgas, J. P. (1999a). On feeling good and being rude: Affective influences on language use and requests. *Journal of Personality and Social Psychology, 76,* 928–939.

Forgas, J. P. (1999b). Feeling and speaking: Mood effects on verbal communication strategies. *Personality and Social Psychology Bulletin, 25,* 850–863.

Forgas, J. P. (2002). Feeling and doing: Affective influences on interpersonal behavior. *Psychological Inquiry, 13,* 1–28.

Forgas, J. P. (Ed.). (2006). *Affect in social thinking and behavior.* New York: Psychology Press.

Forgas, J. P. (2007). When sad is better than happy: Mood effects on the effectiveness of persuasive messages. *Journal of Experimental Social Psychology, 43,* 513–128.

Forgas, J. P. (2011a). Affective influences on self-disclosure strategies. *Journal of Personality and Social Psychology. 100*(3), 449–461.

Forgas, J. P. (2011b). Can negative affect eliminate the power of first impressions?: Affective influences on primacy and recency effects in impression formation. *Journal of Experimental Social Psychology, 47,* 425–429.

Forgas, J. P. (2011c). *Mood effects on skepticism and gullibility.* Unpublished manuscript, University of New South Wales, Sydney, Australia.

Forgas, J. P. (2011d). *She just doesn't look like a philosopher . . . ?: Affective influences on the halo effect in impression formation.* Manuscript submitted for publication.

Forgas, J. P., & Bower, G. H. (1987). Mood effects on person perception judgments. *Journal of Personality and Social Psychology, 53,* 53–60.

Forgas, J. P., Bower, G. H., & Krantz, S. (1984). The influence of mood on perceptions of social interactions. *Journal of Experimental Social Psychology, 20,* 497–513.

Forgas, J. P., Bower, G. H., & Moylan, S. J. (1990). Praise or blame?: Affective influences on attributions. *Journal of Personality and Social Psychology, 59,* 809–818.

Forgas, J. P., & Ciarrochi, J. V. (2002). On managing moods: Evidence for the role of homeostatic cognitive strategies in affect regulation. *Personality and Social Psychology Bulletin, 28,* 336–345.

Forgas, J. P., & East, R. (2008a). How real is that smile?: Mood effects on accepting or rejecting the veracity of emotional facial expressions. *Journal of Nonverbal Behavior, 32,* 157–170.

Forgas, J. P., & East, R. (2008b). On being happy

and gullible: Mood effects on skepticism and the detection of deception. *Journal of Experimental Social Psychology, 44,* 1362–1367.

Forgas, J. P., Goldenberg, L., & Unkelbach, C. (2009). Can bad weather improve your memory?: A field study of mood effects on memory in a real-life setting. *Journal of Experimental Social Psychology, 54,* 254–257.

Forgas, J. P., Haselton, M. G., & von Hippel, W. (Eds.). (2007). *Evolution and the social mind.* New York: Psychology Press.

Forgas, J. P., & Moylan, S. J. (1987). After the movies: the effects of transient mood states on social judgments. *Personality and Social Psychology Bulletin, 13,* 478–489.

Forgas, J. P., Vargas, P., & Laham, S. (2005). Mood effects on eyewitness memory: Affective influences on susceptibility to misinformation. *Journal of Experimental Social Psychology, 41,* 574–588.

Gable, P. A., & Harmon-Jones, E. (2008). Approach-motivated positive affect reduces breadth of attention. *Psychological Science, 19,* 476–482.

Gasper, K., & Clore, G. L. (2002). Attending to the big picture: Mood and global versus local processing of visual information. *Psychological Science, 13,* 34–40.

Gilbert, D. T., & Malone, P. S. (1995). The correspondence bias. *Psychological Bulletin, 117,* 21–38.

Gilboa-Schechtman, E., Erhard-Weiss, D., & Jeccmien, P. (2002). Interpersonal deficits meet cognitive biases: Memory for facial expressions in depressed and anxious men and women. *Psychiatry Research, 113,* 279–293.

Goodwin, D. W. (1974). Alcoholic blackout and state-dependent learning. *Federation Proceedings, 33,* 1833–1835.

Gotlib, I. H., & Joormann, J. (2010). Cognition and depression: Current status and future directions. *Annual Review of Clinical Psychology, 6,* 285–312.

Gouaux, C. (1971). Induced affective states and interpersonal attraction. *Journal of Personality and Social Psychology, 20,* 37–43.

Gouaux, C., & Summers, K. (1973). Interpersonal attraction as a function of affective states and affective change. *Journal of Research in Personality, 7,* 254–260.

Griffitt, W. (1970). Environmental effects on interpersonal behavior: Temperature and attraction. *Journal of Personality and Social Psychology, 15,* 240–244.

Heider, F. (1958). *The psychology of interpersonal relations.* New York: Wiley.

Heimpel, S. A., Wood, J. V., Marshall, M., & Brown, J. (2002). Do people with low self-esteem really want to feel better?: Self-esteem differences in motivation to repair negative moods. *Journal of Personality and Social Psychology, 82,* 128–147.

Hertel, G., & Fiedler, K. (1994). Affective and cognitive influences in a social dilemma game. *European Journal of Social Psychology, 24,* 131–145.

Hilgard, E. R. (1980), The trilogy of the mind: Cognition, affect, and conation. *Journal of the History of the Behavioral Sciences, 16,* 107–117.

Isen, A. M. (1984). Towards understanding the role of affect in cognition. In R. S. Wyer, Jr. & T. K. Srull (Eds.), *Handbook of social cognition* (Vol. 3, pp. 179–236). Mahwah, NJ: Erlbaum.

Isen, A. M. (1985). Asymmetry of happiness and sadness in effects on memory in normal college students: Comment on Hasher, Rose, Zacks, Sanft, and Doren. *Journal of Experimental Psychology: General, 114,* 388–391.

Isen, A. M. (1987). Positive affect, cognitive processes, and social behaviour. In L. Berkowitz (Ed.), *Advances in experimental social psychology* (Vol. 20, pp. 203–253). New York: Academic Press.

Isen, A. M., & Daubman, K. A. (1984). The influence of affect on categorization. *Journal of Personality and Social Psychology, 47,* 1206–1217.

Josephson, B. R., Singer, J. A., & Salovey, P. (1996). Mood regulation and memory: Repairing sad moods with happy memories. *Cognition and Emotion, 10,* 437–444.

Kenealy, P. M. (1997). Mood-state-dependent retrieval: The effects of induced mood on memory reconsidered. *Quarterly Journal of Experimental Psychology, 50A,* 290–317.

Kihlstrom, J. F. (1989). On what does mood-dependent memory depend? *Journal of Social Behavior and Personality, 4,* 23–32.

Koster, E. H. W., De Raedt, R., Goeleven, E., Franck, E., & Crombez, G. (2005). Mood-congruent attentional bias in dysphoria: Maintained attention to and impaired disengagement from negative information. *Emotion, 5,* 446–455.

Leight, K. A., & Ellis, H. C. (1981). Emotional mood states, strategies, and state-dependency in memory. *Journal of Verbal Learning and Verbal Behavior, 20*, 251–266.

Martin, L. (2000). Moods don't convey information: Moods in context do. In J. P. Forgas (Ed.), *Feeling and thinking: The role of affect in social cognition* (pp. 153–177). New York: Cambridge University Press.

Mayer, J. D., Gaschke, Y. N., Braverman, D. L., & Evans, T. W. (1992). Mood-congruent judgment is a general effect. *Journal of Personality and Social Psychology, 63*, 119–132.

Miranda, R., & Kihlstrom, J. (2005). Mood congruence in childhood and recent autobiographical memory. *Cognition and Emotion, 19*, 981–998.

Piaget, J. (1954). *The construction of reality in the child.* New York: Free Press.

Price, T. F., & Harmon-Jones, E. (2010). The effect of embodied emotive states on cognitive categorization. *Emotion, 10*, 934–938.

Rapaport, D. (1961). *Emotions and memory.* New York: Science Editions. (Original work published 1942)

Razran, G. H. (1940). Conditioned response changes in rating and appraising sociopolitical slogans. *Psychological Bulletin, 37*, 481–493.

Reus, V. I., Weingartner, H., & Post, R. M. (1979). Clinical implications of state-dependent learning. *American Journal of Psychiatry, 136*, 927–931.

Ruiz-Caballero, J. A., & Gonzalez, P. (1994). Implicit and explicit memory bias in depressed and non-depressed subjects. *Cognition and Emotion, 8*, 555–570.

Schacter, D. L., & Kihlstrom, J. F. (1989). Functional amnesia. In F. Boller & J. Grafman (Eds.), *Handbook of neuropsychology* (Vol. 3, pp. 209–230). New York: Elsevier.

Schiffenbauer, A. I. (1974). Effect of observer's emotional state on judgments of the emotional state of others. *Journal of Personality and Social Psychology, 30*, 31–35.

Schwarz, N. (1990). Feelings as information: Informational and motivational functions of affective states. In E. T. Higgins & R. M. Sorrentino (Eds.), *Handbook of motivation and cognition: Vol. 2. Foundations of social behavior* (pp. 527–561). New York: Guilford Press.

Schwarz, N., & Clore, G. L. (1983). Mood, misattribution and judgments of well-being: Informative and directive functions of affective states. *Journal of Personality and Social Psychology, 45*, 513–523.

Sedikides, C. (1994). Incongruent effects of sad mood on self-conception valence: It's a matter of time. *European Journal of Social Psychology, 24*, 161–172.

Sedikides, C. (1995). Central and peripheral self-conceptions are differentially influenced by mood: Tests of the differential sensitivity hypothesis. *Journal of Personality and Social Psychology, 69*, 759–777.

Sinclair, R. C. (1988). Mood, categorization breadth, and performance appraisal: The effects of order of information acquisition and affective state on halo, accuracy, and evaluations. *Organizational Behavior and Human Decision Processes, 42*, 22–46.

Sinclair, R. C., Mark, M. M., & Clore, G. L. (1994). Mood-related persuasion depends on misattributions. *Social Cognition, 12*, 309–326.

Singer, J. A., & Salovey, P. (1988). Mood and memory: Evaluating the network theory of affect. *Clinical Psychology Review, 8*, 211–251.

Smith, S. M., & Petty, R. E. (1995). Personality moderators of mood congruency effects on cognition: The role of self-esteem and negative mood regulation. *Journal of Personality and Social Psychology, 68*, 1092–1107.

Storbeck, J., & Clore, G. L. (2005). With sadness comes accuracy; with happiness, false memory: Mood and the false memory effect. *Psychological Science, 16*, 785–791.

Tamir, M., & Robinson, M. D. (2007). The happy spotlight: Positive mood and selective attention to rewarding information. *Personality and Social Psychology Bulletin, 33*, 1124–1136.

Tan, H. B., & Forgas, J. P. (2010). When happiness makes us selfish, but sadness makes us fair: Affective influences on interpersonal strategies in the dictator game. *Journal of Experimental Social Psychology, 46*, 571–576.

Ucros, C. G. (1989). Mood state-dependent memory: A meta-analysis. *Cognition and Emotion, 3*, 139–167.

Unkelbach, C., Forgas, J. P., & Denson, T. F. (2008). The turban effect: The influence of Muslim headgear and induced affect on aggressive responses in the shooter bias paradigm. *Journal of Experimental Social Psychology, 44*, 1409–1413.

Wadlinger, H., & Isaacowitz, D. M. (2006). Positive affect broadens visual attention to positive stimuli. *Motivation and Emotion, 30,* 89–101.

Watkins, T., Mathews, A. M., Williamson, D. A., & Fuller, R. (1992). Mood congruent memory in depression: Emotional priming or elaboration. *Journal of Abnormal Psychology, 101,* 581–586.

Watson, J. B. (1929). *Behaviorism.* New York: Norton.

Watson, J. B., & Rayner, R. (1920). Conditioned emotional reactions. *Journal of Experimental Psychology, 3,* 1–14.

Wegener, D. T., & Petty, R. E. (1997). The flexible correction model: The role of naïve theories of bias in bias correction. In M. P. Zanna (Ed.), *Advances in experimental social psychology* (Vol. 29, pp. 141–208). New York: Academic Press.

Wegner, D. M. (1994). Ironic processes of mental control. *Psychological Review, 101,* 34–52.

CHAPTER 14

Cognition and Emotion in Judgment and Decision Making

Daniel Västfjäll and Paul Slovic

Judgment and decision making (JDM) research has shown a dramatic increase in interest in the interplay of emotional and cognitive processes during the last 15 years (Schwarz, 2000; Slovic & Västfjäll, 2010). In a 2001 review, "Problems for Judgment and Decision Making," emotions and decisions were highlighted as an important, but still largely unexplored, research area (Hastie, 2001). A focus on cognitive processes was still prevailing. In a more recent *Annual Review of Psychology* article titled "Mindful Judgment and Decision Making," Weber and Johnson (2009) write that "the emotions revolution of the past decade or so has tried to correct this overemphasis (on cognitive processes) by documenting the prevalence of affective processes, depicting them as automatic and essentially effort-free inputs that orient and motivate adaptive behavior" (p. 65). Weber and Johnson even conclude, "the emotions revolution has put affective processes on a footing equal to cognitive ones" (p. 53). Indeed, emotion is today seen as an integral part of the decision process. More importantly, it is considered a phenomenon that can be quantified and studied in a JDM context. The goal of this chapter is to review research on affect and decision making to highlight how cognition and emotion jointly influence JDM.

We begin by situating emotion in what have been cognitive theories of JDM. Next, we examine dual-process accounts of JDM where cognition–emotion interactions are central. Finally, we present a framework to classify different "decision emotions."

The Emergence of Emotion in Cognitive JDM Theories

Traditional decision research has mainly examined behavioral violations of rational choice models (Mellers, Schwartz, & Cooke, 1998; Weber & Johnson, 2009). Rational choice is often expressed as a single "correct" choice on the basis of a cognitive evaluation of the outcomes (Elster, 1999; Loewenstein, 1996). The desirability of an alternative or set of alternatives may then be described by the utility derived from each alternative (Read & Loewenstein, 1999). Alternative X is chosen over Y because the utility of X exceeds the utility of Y. In this research tradition, utility is inferred from the choices people make. Moreover, the probability or belief of the occurrence of an outcome is, in these theories, an important determinant of the overall utility for each alternative (i.e., subjective expected utility theory: Savage, 1954). Normative choice as subjective expected utility theory, have dominated JDM research (Mellers, 2000). Nevertheless, the utility of a certain alternative can be described in many different fashions. A reexamination of the concept of utility in decision making research has led to a renewed interest in the role of emotion, in particular, through the introduction of the concept of *experienced utility*; that is, the utility a decision maker experiences from the outcome of a chosen alternative (Kahneman, 2011; Kahneman & Snell, 1990). Kahneman, Wakker, and Sarin (1997) returned to Benthams's (1789/1984) original proposition that *utility* refers to the pleasure and pain that we derive from outcomes. In this sense, utility is about emotional experiences themselves. More specifically, *utility* refers to the pleasure–displeasure or comfort–discomfort that is derived from each outcome. Emotional experience guides choice in that one seeks to maximize pleasure and avoid pain (Higgins, 1997). Experienced utility is, however, only one of several variants of utility that may influence choice. Kahneman and colleagues further distinguish between (1) *instantaneous utility*, which is the continuous experienced utility from sensory input; (2) *remembered utility*, which influences postdecision evaluations (e.g., regret and disappointment with a decision outcome); (3) *predicted utility*, the decision maker's anticipation or prediction of experienced utility; and (4) *decision utility*, the utility influencing the actual decision.

Utility has both an affective and cognitive component (e.g., Kahneman, 2011; Kahneman & Snell, 1990; Kahneman et al., 1997; Rottenstreich & Hsee, 2001). For instance, the monetary value of an outcome of a gamble is presumably the most important aspect attended to either before gambling or when the outcome is later experienced. Yet, the gambler may also react with emotion to varying degrees, depending on the person and situation. Contrast this to a choice of listening to music. In this case, anticipating an affective reaction or subsequently reacting affectively is probably the most important aspect (Juslin & Västfjäll, 2008). Everyday decisions can be characterized as having both utilitarian and emotional components (Böhm & Pfister, 1996; Dhar & Wertenbroch, 2000).

The Importance of Specific Emotions and Affect

Affect, in all its various forms, serves different functions in motivating behavior. For example, strong visceral emotions such as fear and anger sometimes play a role in risk assessment. These two emotions appear to have opposite effects: Fear amplifies risk estimates, and anger attenuates them (Lerner, Gonzalez, Small, & Fischhoff, 2003; Lerner & Keltner, 2000). Lerner and colleagues have explained these differences by proposing that fear arises from appraisals of uncertainty and situational control, whereas anger arises from appraisals of certainty and individual control.

Fortunately, most of the time people are in a calmer state, being guided by much subtler feelings. We use the term *affect* to mean the specific quality of "goodness" or "badness" (1) experienced as a feeling state (with or without consciousness) and (2) demarcating a positive or negative quality of a stimulus (including variations in arousal, thus making it similar to what Russell [2003] termed *core affect*). A characteristic of core affect is that it is always present in one form or another. This form of affect is therefore likely to be used in judgments and decisions. We have used the term *affect heuristic* to characterize reliance on such feelings (Slovic, Finucane, Peters, & MacGregor, 2002). The idea is that the experienced feelings are used as information to guide judgment and decision making (Schwarz & Clore, 1983). Importantly, both integral affect (positive and negative feelings about a stimulus that are experienced while considering the stimulus) and incidental affect (positive and negative feelings, such as mood states, that are independent of a stimulus, but can be misattributed to it) are used in judgments and decisions.

A large body of research documents the importance of affect in conveying meaning and motivating behavior. Without affect, information lacks meaning and will not be used in judgment and decision making (Peters, 2006). However, affect serves other functions as well. For instance, many theorists have given affect a direct and primary role in motivating behavior. Pleasant feelings motivate actions that people anticipate will intensify those feelings. Unpleasant feelings motivate actions that people anticipate will diminish those feelings (Västfjäll & Gärling, 2006).

Affect can also serve as a spotlight, guiding information processing (Peters, 2006), and as a "common currency," so to speak, allowing decision makers to compare apples to oranges (Cabanac, 1992). Montague and Berns (2002) link this notion to "neural responses in the orbitofrontal–striatal circuit which may support the conversion of disparate types of future rewards into a kind of internal currency, that is, a common scale used to compare the valuation of future behavioral acts or stimuli" (p. 265). By translating more complex thoughts into simpler affective evaluations, decision makers can compare and integrate good and bad feelings rather than attempting to make sense out of a multitude of conflicting logical considerations (Peters, Västfjäll, Gärling, & Slovic, 2006).

Two Modes of Thinking

Affect thus appears to play a central role in what are known as dual-process theories of thinking (Sloman, 1996; Stanovich & West, 2000). According to these theories, people apprehend reality in two fundamentally different ways: one intuitive, automatic, natural, nonverbal, narrative, and experiential (system 1 or fast thinking), and the other analytical, deliberative, and verbal (system 2 or slow thinking) (see Epstein, 1994; Kahneman, 2011; see also Table 14.1). One of the

main characteristics of the intuitive, experiential system is its affective basis. Although analysis is certainly important in some decision-making circumstances, reliance on affect is generally a quicker, easier, and more efficient way to navigate in a complex, uncertain, and sometimes dangerous world.

It is important to note that there are strong elements of rationality in both systems of thinking (Pham, 2007). The experiential system enabled human beings to survive as they evolved. Intuition, instinct, and gut feeling were relied upon to determine whether an animal was safe to approach or water was safe to drink. As life became more complex and humans gained more control over their environment, analytic tools such as probability theory, risk assessment, and decision analysis were invented to "boost" the rationality of experiential thinking.

Evidence for Cognition–Emotion Interactions in JDM

Ample evidence shows that people use both "fast" (lower-order route) and "slow" (higher-order route) thinking to arrive at judgments and decisions (Kahneman, 2011). An illustrative example is given in Shiv and Fedorikin (2002). In their research paradigm, Shiv and Fedorikin let participants choose between a chocolate cake (more positive affect, less favorable cognitions) and a fruit salad (less positive affect, more favorable cognitions) while exposed to different experimental manipulations (in specific,

TABLE 14.1. Two Modes of Thinking: Comparison of the Experiential and Analytic Systems

Experiential system (system 1)	Analytic system (system 2)
1. Holistic	1. Deliberative
2. Affective: Pleasure–pain oriented	2. Logical: Reason oriented (what is sensible)
3. Associative connections	3. Logical connections
4. Behavior mediated by "vibes" from past experiences	4. Behavior mediated by conscious appraisal of events
5. Encodes reality in concrete images, metaphors, and narratives	5. Encodes reality in abstract symbols, words, and numbers
6. *Faster* processing: Oriented toward immediate action	6. *Slower* processing: Oriented toward delayed action
7. Self-evidently valid: "experiencing is believing"	7. Requires justification via logic and evidence

Note. Based on Epstein (1994) and Kahneman (2011).

time pressure, and cognitive load). When participants had little processing capabilities and time, the low-order route controlled choices, but when participants had time and resources to deliberate on the alternatives, the high-order route influenced decisions.

In his Nobel Prize address, Kahneman notes that the operating characteristics of system 1 are similar to those of human perceptual processes (Kahneman, 2003). He points out that one of the functions of system 2 is to monitor the quality of the intuitive impressions formed by system 1. Kahneman and Frederick (2002) suggest that this monitoring is typically rather lax and allows many intuitive judgments to be expressed in behavior, including some that are erroneous. Kahneman (2011, p. 282) argues that judgments of value and probability are, to a large extent, driven by system 1 thinking. System 1 thinking is often correct but breaks down in some contexts, such as when dealing with large numbers (Slovic & Västfjäll, 2010).

The Affect Heuristic and Responses to Probability

Evidence of risk as feelings was present in early studies of risk perception (Lichtenstein, Slovic, Fischhoff, Layman, & Combs, 1978). Those studies showed that feelings of dread were the major determiner of public perception and acceptance of risk for a wide range of hazards. This explains, for example, why many people judge radiation exposure from nuclear power plants (highly dreaded) as far riskier than radiation from medical X-rays—an assessment not shared by risk experts. In today's world, terrorism has replaced nuclear power at the top of the list of widely dreaded risks.

Research has found that, whereas risk and benefit tend to be positively correlated across hazardous activities in the world (i.e., high-risk activities tend to have greater benefits than do low-risk activities), they are negatively correlated in people's minds and judgments (i.e., high risk is associated with low benefit, and vice versa). The significance of this phenomenon was not realized until a study by Alhakami and Slovic (1994), who found that the inverse relationship between perceived risk and perceived benefit of an activity (e.g., using pesticides) was linked to the strength of positive or negative affect associated with that activity as measured by rating the activity on bipolar scales such as good–bad, nice–awful, and so forth. This finding implies that people judge a risk not only by what they think about it, but also by how they feel about it. If their feelings toward an activity are favorable, they tend to judge the risks as low and the benefits as high; if their feelings toward the activity are unfavorable, they tend to make the opposite judgment—high risk and low benefit (i.e., the affect heuristic: Finucane, Alhakami, Slovic, & Johnson, 2000; Slovic et al., 2002).

If affect guides perceptions of risk and benefit, then providing information about benefit should change people's perception of risk, and vice versa (see Figure 14.1). For example, information stating that the benefit is high for a technology such as nuclear power should lead to more positive overall affect, which should, in turn, decrease perceived risk (Figure 14.1A).

Finucane and colleagues (2000) tested this hypothesis for various technologies, providing information designed to manipulate affect by increasing or decreasing perceived benefit for the technology or by increasing or decreasing its perceived risk. Their predictions were confirmed. Further support for the affect heuristic came from a second experiment by Finucane et al., showing that the inverse relationship between perceived risks and benefits increased greatly under time pressure, when opportunity for analytic deliberation was reduced. Coupled with the findings of Alhakami and Slovic (1994), these experiments indicate that affect influences judgment directly and is not simply a response to analytic considerations.

Rottenstreich and Hsee (2001) demonstrated that decision makers react strongly to a small probability of a strongly affective event (they value it highly), but that they are insensitive to increases in that probability (i.e., its evaluation is not much higher despite its greater likelihood). The evaluation of a weak affective event, on the other hand, grows more linearly with its probability. In their studies, decision makers were willing to pay almost as much for a 1% chance as a 99% or 100% chance to receive an affect-rich outcome (e.g., meet and kiss their favorite movie star). At the same time, they would pay substantially less for the small possibility versus the large probability

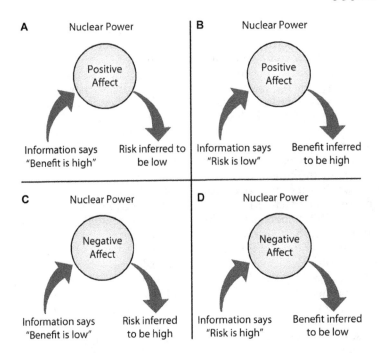

FIGURE 14.1. A model based on the affect heuristic. Support for this model was found by Finucane, Alhakami, Slovic, and Johnson (2000).

of a relatively affect-poor outcome (e.g., $50 in cash). This finding suggests that the shape of the probability weighting function should be different when information is evaluated predominantly by system 1 (as with affect-poor outcomes) than when it is evaluated predominantly by system 2 (affect-rich outcomes; see Figure 14.2). Specifically, the curve for affect-rich options should be quite steep near probabilities of 0.0 and 1.0 and should be flat for intermediate probabilities.

These findings are also very consistent with other research on affect as information. For instance, Damasio (1994) argued that a lifetime of learning leads decision options and attributes to become "marked" by positive and negative feelings linked directly or indirectly to somatic or bodily states. When a negative somatic marker is linked to an outcome, it acts as information by sounding an alarm that warns us away from that choice. When a positive marker is associated with the outcome, it becomes a beacon of incentive drawing us toward that option. Similarly, more recent neuropsychological research suggests that the human brain quickly assesses affect associated with various decision option (Knutson, Wimmer,

Kuhnen, & Winkielman, 2008). It is also suggested that relying on affect is often a beneficial strategy that helps us quickly and efficiently navigate in an uncertain world (Slovic et al., 2002).

As a key element of experiential thinking, the affect heuristic was essential to risk assessment and survival during the evolution of the human species. But, just as overusing deliberation can be detrimental to decision making, affect can also mislead people.

The Affect Heuristic and Responses to Magnitude

Interestingly, the similarity between affect (system 1) and perception has resulted in some limitations of the experiential system in dealing with quantities. The experiential system tends to be an on–off system driven by images. It is relatively insensitive to scope or *different magnitudes* (Hsee & Rottenstreich, 2004; Rottenstreich & Hsee, 2001). Hsee and Rottenstreich (2004) also demonstrated that the value function is different for strongly versus weakly affective decision options (see Figure 14.2). In an ingenious set of studies, they showed that younger-adult

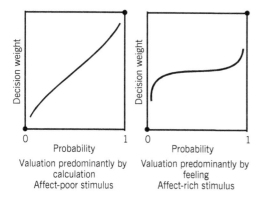

Valuation predominantly by
calculation
Affect-poor stimulus

Valuation predominantly by
feeling
Affect-rich stimulus

FIGURE 14.2. Probability functions for affect-poor and affect-rich decision options. Based on Rottenstreich and Hsee (2001) and Peters et al. (2007).

decision makers value different quantities of an affect-poor stimulus quite differently, whereas they are relatively insensitive to different quantities of an affect-rich stimulus. For example, they asked participants how much they would be willing to pay to save either one or four pandas. When the pandas were represented as affect-poor dots (a single dot vs. four dots), participants were willing to pay almost twice as much for four pandas as they were for one. However, when illustrated with affect-rich pictures of pandas, participants were willing to pay about the same for one versus four pandas. Hsee and Rottenstreich demonstrate that when decision makers rely more on feelings versus calculation, they are sensitive to the existence of a stimulus (vs. its absence), but are relatively insensitive to greater quantities of that stimulus.

The modification of value functions by affect is pertinent to the saving of human lives (Slovic, 2007). The psychophysical model to the right in Figure 14.2 implies that the value of a life diminishes against the backdrop of a larger tragedy. Fetherstonhaugh, Slovic, Johnson, and Friedrich (1997) documented this potential for diminished sensitivity to the value of life—an effect they named *psychophysical numbing*—by evaluating people's willingness to fund various lifesaving medical treatments. In a study involving a hypothetical grant funding agency, nearly two-thirds of the respondents raised their minimum benefit requirements to warrant funding when there was a larger at-risk population, with a median value of 9,000 lives needing to be saved when 15,000 were at risk, compared to a median of 100,000 lives to be saved out of 290,000 at risk. By implication, respondents saw saving 9,000 lives in the "smaller" population as more valuable than saving 10 times as many lives in the larger. Several other studies in the domain of lifesaving interventions (Bartels, 2006; Fetherstonhaugh et al., 1997) have documented similar psychophysical numbing phenomena.

Figure 14.2 may not completely describe the way people respond to increases in the magnitude of the threat. For example, Desvousges and colleagues (1992/2010) carefully elicited people's willingness to pay (WTP) to provide nets that would save 2,000, 20,000, or 200,000 migrating birds from drowning in uncovered oil ponds that the birds mistake for bodies of water. The mean WTP was flat, about $80, although the number of lives saved varied by a range of 100-fold. This "insensitivity to scope" has been explained by Kahneman, Ritov, and Schkade (1999) as possibly resulting from a process whereby a prototype individual (e.g., the image of an oil-covered bird) serves as a proxy for the larger number at risk. Attitudes and emotions toward this mental image create feelings that cue the valuation (a type of affect heuristic: Slovic et al., 2002). Note that this implies a value function that is essentially flat rather than monotonically increasing as the rightward psychophysical function in Figure 14.2 predicts.

Even more dramatic are the implications of research on the so called *singularity effect*. Kogut and Ritov (2005) hypothesized that the processing of information related to a single victim might be fundamentally different from the processing of information concerning a group of victims. They predicted, and subsequently found, that people will tend to feel more distress and compassion when considering an identified single victim than when considering a group of victims, even if identified, resulting in a greater willingness to help the identified individual victim.

Our own research suggests that the decline in response may begin to appear in groups as small as two individuals. Västfjäll, Peters, and Slovic (2011) gave one group of potential donors the opportunity to contribute part of their earnings from an unrelated study to a 7-year-old girl from Mali facing the threat of starvation. Her picture and name were given. A second group was offered the opportunity to donate to a named and pictured 7-year-old boy from Mali, also facing starvation. A third group was shown pictures of both children side by side and asked to give a donation that would go to both the girl and the boy. Feelings of compassion and donation amounts were about identical for the individual children but were lower for the two together, mirroring what Kogut and Ritov (2005) had found for donations to one child versus a group of eight children, both needing the same stated amount of money for cancer therapy. The single child received far greater aid than the group of eight.

This research suggests that our capacity to feel is limited. To the extent that valuation of lifesaving depends on feelings (the affect heuristic), it might follow the function shown in Figure 14.3, where the emotion or affective feeling is greatest at $N = 1$ but begins to decrease at $N = 2$ and collapses at some higher value of N that becomes simply "a statistic."

Decision makers may put lower value on saving more lives when they evaluate each option separately (separate evaluation; SE). In joint evaluation (JE, where helping one vs. two, e.g., is evaluated simultaneously), decision makers typically display a preference for more individuals saved (Kogut & Ritov, 2005). JE and SE can be mapped to dual processes. In SE, people typically use system 1 thinking (affective feelings), wheras for JE, system 2 thinking (reason) tends to dominate. Following this line of thinking, reliance on system 2 may be a way to overcome underreaction to the needs of many.

Different Types of Emotion Have Different Influences on JDM

The research reviewed thus far suggests that emotion plays an important role in JDM: It can both improve and distort decisions. The role of emotion may critically depend on the eliciting conditions. In this section, we review how different types of emotion influence JDM. Figure 14.4 shows the different forms of "decision emotions" that we consider in our subsequent discussion. A first distinction is made between pre- and postdecisional affect (see Mellers, Schwartz, & Ritov, 1999). *Predecisonal* affect is emotion that influences the decision before the decision actually is made. Current mood, anticipatory, and anticipated emotions are such influences. Anticipatory emotions are emotional reactions experienced in the present, brought about by thinking of the future. Anticipated emotions, on the other hand, are primarily cognitive expectations about future emotions without actually experiencing them in the present (Loewenstein, Weber, Hsee, & Welch, 2001).

Postdecisional affect concerns the experienced affect when the outcome of the decision is known. A second distinction, mentioned in the introduction, is that between incidental and integral affect (Lerner & Keltner, 2000; Loewenstein & Lerner, 2003). *Incidental affect* consists of affective influences that are unrelated to the decision task (e.g., a good mood because it is a sunny day), whereas *integral affect* is related to the decision task (e.g., the anticipated unhappiness with the outcome of a gamble or the experienced joy of a win). A third distinction is made between *immediate affect* (affect experienced in the present due to sunny weather or winning $50) and *expected affect* (expectations about affective reactions to future outcomes, such as thinking of possible regret if one receives outcome A and the unobtained outcome B turns out to be better).

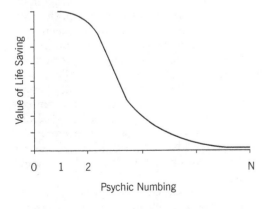

FIGURE 14.3. A collapse value function where $N = 1$ is valued most highly (Slovic, 2007).

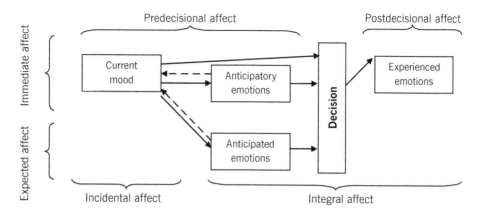

FIGURE 14.4. Different forms of emotion influencing JDM.

These three dimensions represent different foci concerning the interplay of affect and decision making, but they may be complementary, as suggested in Figure 14.4. For instance, current mood may be thought of as incidental, immediate, predecisional affect, whereas experienced affect is integral, immediate, postdecisional affect. In a similar manner, anticipated emotions can be thought of as integral, expected, predecisional affect, whereas anticipatory emotions are integral, immediate, predecisional affect. Thinking about the differential influence of mood and experienced, anticipated, and anticipatory emotions on decision making along the three dimensions of *time of decision* (pre–post decisional), *time of affect* (immediate–expected) and *affect–decision relationship* (incidental–integral) may help us understand the eliciting conditions and effects of each of these components.

Experienced Emotions and Decision Making

Currently experienced emotions may influence decision making in several ways. In general, a division can be made between influences of (1) emotions or mood at the time of decision making, and (2) experienced emotions in relation to the actual outcome or in relation to the decision situation. In the first case, for instance, a decision maker's current mood (positive because of the sunny weather) may result in optimistic thoughts of future success on the stock market and consequently a risky choice to buy high-risk

stocks. The second entity, experienced emotions, may be feelings of regret, self-blame, and disappointment when the high-risk investment fails. Both types of emotions are experienced in the present and are apt to influence decisions, but they have some contrasting features. Most importantly, current mood is unrelated, or *incidental*, to the decision (Loewenstein & Lerner, 2003). Emotions experienced in response to outcomes, on the other hand, are a consequence of the decision and thus related or *integral* to the decision (Lerner & Keltner, 2000). Second, mood states influence while decisions are being made and before the outcome is known (*predecisional affect*), whereas experienced emotions are experienced after the choice and when the outcome is known (*postdecisional affect*) (Zeelenberg et al., 1998).

Incidental Mood

Mood and other affective processes may influence decision making in three different ways (Raghunatan & Pham, 1999): (1) The current mood may influence the content of people's thoughts. For instance, participants in a positive mood may more easily come to think positive thoughts and recall positive memories (Forgas, 1995). This effect has been known as *mood congruence* (Bower, 1981; Wright & Bower, 1992). (2) Other research has shown that positive and negative mood may influence processing capabilities (Luce, Bettman, & Payne, 1997). For instance, happy individuals often tend to process information in a less elaborated and systematic manner than do people in a negative mood (Isen, 2000). (3) People's current mood may influence motives to undertake actions (Andrade, 2005; Raghunatan & Pham, 1999). For example, happy individuals may avoid negative events and outcomes in order to maintain their positive mood state.

Together, these three main effects of mood may influence how outcomes are evaluated. The influence of current mood on risk perception and preference is one of the most studied interplays of cognition and affect in the decision making field. For instance, substantial evidence from Isen and coworkers suggests that positive affect often leads to risk aversion when the decision task is realistic (Arkes, Herren, & Isen, 1988; Isen, 2000). Mood maintenance may be an explanation for the finding that participants in a positive mood are more risk aversive. Participants who are in a positive mood risk "losing" their good feelings if the outcome is negative. Participants in a positive mood may therefore be said to have more to lose than neutral or participants in a negative mood (Isen, 2000). In support of this, Isen showed that positive participants weighed losses more heavily than did neutral participants. At the same time participants in a positive mood state have been shown to give higher estimates of probabilities of success in risky situations (DeSteno, Petty, Rucker, & Wegener, 2000; Johnson & Tversky, 1983; Nygren, Isen, Taylor, & Dulin, 1996). Isen (2000) proposed that probability and utility are influenced in opposite ways by positive affect. Positive affect increases the perceived risk associated with a loss, but also increases the subjective value of gains.

Participants in whom negative affect has been induced have been shown to engage in more careful and deliberate information processing (cognitive tuning; Schwarz & Clore, 1983) and to use less successful decision strategies and repeat themselves more often (Forgas, 1995; Mano, 1992). It has also been shown that participants in a negative mood are willing to take more risks than neutral or happy participants (Mano, 1992). Similarly, negative affective states such as anxiety, depression, and fatigue have been shown to lead to increased risk taking (DeSteno et al., 2000; Raghunathan & Pham, 1999). Mood repair is a possible explanation for this find-

ing. Participants in a negative mood state are motivated to change, or repair, their current mood (Larsen, 2000). One way to improve one's current affect is to win in a gamble and thus to experience positive feelings. In support of the mood repair explanation, studies have shown that positive emotions speed physiological recovery from negative emotions (Fredrickson & Levenson, 1998).

Taken together, current mood has been shown to influence decision making in that it (1) evokes mood-congruent thoughts and memories, (2) influences processing strategies and capabilities, and (3) influences people's motivation for engaging in activities or pursuing alternatives. Common to all these effects is the idea that a primary function of mood and emotional reactions is to inform individuals about the current state of affairs, their well-being, status relative to the environment, and progress toward desired goals (Frijda, 1988). In other words, positive affective states inform people that the world is safe and that personal goals are not threatened. Negative states signal that something is wrong, problematic, or unsafe.

Mood as Information

In the mood-as-information view, it is assumed that individuals utilize mood as information to interpret situations (Schwarz, 2001). Schwarz and Clore (1983) showed that a common heuristic, when asked to make a global evaluation of objects, is to rely on current feelings rather then processing all relevant information. This heuristic has been named the "How do I feel about it?" heuristic (note that this is heuristic is similar to the affect heuristic, but is primarily focused on incidental affect, whereas the affect heuristic was developed to account for integral affect). This view holds that current mood provides relevant information about the current situation. For example, current mood may be used to make judgments about objects and the self. Schwarz (2001) showed that minor mood-influencing events such as finding a coin in a copying machine or the favorite soccer team winning a game influenced ratings of global subjective well-being (Schwarz & Clore, 1983).

However, people only use their current feelings as a basis of judgment when they are perceived to contain valuable information or when they are misattributed as a reaction to the target (Schwarz, 2001). Schwarz and Clore (1983) showed that when participants were made aware that their mood was brought about by something unrelated to the judgmental target, the mood-congruent effect disappeared. Similarly, Pham (1998) showed that when participants believed that their feelings were not relevant to the decision, mood effects diminished. Thus, when mood is representative or relevant to the judgment task, it is more likely to enter into the judgmental process. In addition, Schwarz (2001) and Siemer and Reisenzein (1998) showed that the salience of moods is an important determinant of mood effects on evaluative judgments. More specifically, the more salient moods are, the more weight they will have in the judgmental process. In summary, mood-congruent effects are thus likely to occur when individuals are not able to attribute or explain the cause of their current mood, but are likely to be eliminated when the cause of the current mood is known (Schwarz & Clore, 1983) .

Forgas (1995) proposed an affect infusion model to explain the influence of affect on judgment processes (see Forgas & Koch, Chapter 13, this volume). In this model, the different explanations for mood effects (priming and mood as information) are not exclusive, but complementary. Heuristic processing is used when the judgmental target is simple, and substantive processing is used when the judgmental situation requires learning and processing of information. In the former, but not the latter case, affect has a direct influence on evaluation, judgment, and processing.

Experienced Emotion (Affect Experienced after the Decision)

Affective reactions to stimuli or outcomes have been a focal point in emotion research for a long time. A prominent example is Zajonc's (1980) proposition that "preferences need no inferences." Zajonc argued that affective judgments are often independent of cognitive judgments. Moreover, affective reactions often precede cognitive processes and consequently are fundamental to the evaluation of outcomes (Zajonc, 1980; Zajonc & Markus, 1982; for an opposing

view, see Lazarus, 1991). Ample neuropsychological evidence supports the primacy-of-affect notion (LeDoux, 1996; Panksepp, 1998). An example would be the initial startle response when hearing a sudden noise (Loewenstein et al., 2001). A primary function of such emotional responses is to prepare the individual and mobilize flight–fight tendencies or approach–avoid evaluations (Zajonc, 1998). Cognitions, on the other hand, help the individual to identify the stimulus (Zajonc, 1998). In the example with a sudden noise, the individual may at first experience a sense of mobilization or rapid response to the sound. It is possible that the individual will be frightened. However, after a short time span, the individual will localize the noise-producing source and confirm or disconfirm whether the initial experienced fear was warranted. If the noise-producing source is a tiger, the individual will realize that the initial fear was a correct response. If the noise-producing source turns out to be a loudspeaker, the individual will reevaluate the initial response.

Similar to the affect heuristic work reviewed above (Slovic et al., 2002), Damasio and colleagues argue that affective encoding of different courses of action, *somatic markers*, are essential to efficient decision making (Bechara, Damasio, Tranel, & Damasio, 1997; Damasio, 1994). Drawing on studies of individuals with brain damage, Damasio argues that the prefrontal cortex plays a key role in the interplay of cognitive evaluations and affective reactions (Damasio, 1994). Bechara and colleagues (1997) compared normal participants to participants with prefrontal cortex damage in a gambling experiment. A main result was that participants with prefrontal cortex damage should more risk taking and, after experiencing a loss, returned to high-stakes bets earlier than did normal participants. Bechara and colleagues argued that this finding reflects an inability among the participants with prefrontal cortex damage to experience the fear associated with risky high-stakes gambling. The notion of somatic markers not only applies to experienced emotions, but is essential to anticipated emotions (an issue to which we return later). In the Bechara and colleagues study, it was found that normal participants experienced high arousal or activation (as measured by skin conductance recorded during the experiment) just before the outcome of each gamble was known, whereas no such reaction was observable in participants with damage to the prefrontal cortex. However, both normal participants and participants with prefrontal cortex damage reacted in the same way to actual experienced losses and gains. Bechara at al. thus conclude that anticipated (or rather *anticipatory*; see below) emotions or somatic markers are essential to decision making and to encoding of possible future consequences of a decision.

Counterfactual (Cognitive) Emotions

Emotional reactions to a decision outcome depend strongly on whether the outcome is compared with alternative outcomes or other states of the world (Boninger, Gleicher, & Stratham, 1994; Gleicher et al., 1990; Kahneman & Miller, 1986). *Conterfactual thinking* refers to the mental simulation of comparing the present state with other possible, but not obtained, states (Kahneman & Miller, 1986). Counterfactual thoughts are common in everyday experience and may exert a substantial influence (McMullen, 1997). Research on outcome evaluation has shown that participants feel more strongly about an alternative (either in a positive or negative direction) if counterfactual alternatives are salient (Gleicher et al., 1990). A further distinction is made between *upward* counterfactuals that improve reality (thinking how things could have been better) and *downward* counterfactuals that worsen reality (thinking about how things could have been worse) (Landman, 1993; Sanna, 1998). Upward counterfactuals result in negative affect, whereas downward counterfactuals result in positive affect (McMullen, 1997). This empirical finding has been termed the *affective contrast effect* (McMullen, 1997). It is important to point out that current mood may influence the magnitude and direction of experienced emotions in relation to a decision outcome (cf. mood as information). For instance, Sanna (1998) showed that participants in a negative mood generated more upward counterfactual comparisons, whereas a positive mood was followed by more downward counterfactuals.

The two single most studied experienced and anticipated emotions in decision research are postdecisional *regret* and *disappointment* (Connolly, Ordóñez, & Coughlan, 1997; Landman, 1993; van Dijk & van der Pligt, 1997; Zeelenberg, 1999; Zeelenberg et al., 1998). Regret and disappointment are seen as separate emotions with different effects on decision making (Zeelenberg et al., 1998; Zeelenberg, van Dijk, Manstead, & van der Pligt, 2000). Both are experienced in relation to an unfavorable or undesirable outcome. Regret is experienced when a chosen option turns out to be worse compared to a nonchosen option, whereas disappointment arises when the outcome is worse compared to the expected outcome (Zeelenberg et al., 2000). The experience of regret leads to risk aversion and unwillingness to act (Zeelenberg, 1999). The experience of disappointment results in making choices that match initial expectations or in lowering expectations prior to knowing the outcome (Zeelenberg et al., 2000).

But not only negative experienced emotions such as regret and disappointment are important in decision making. For instance, Mellers and colleagues (1999; Mellers, Schwartz, Ho, & Ritov, 1997) investigated the experience of *elation*. In decision affect theory (Mellers et al., 1999), it is assumed that people become elated or rejoice when receiving a positive outcome (winning a monetary gamble) and disappointed or regretful when facing a negative outcome (losing a monetary gamble). Moreover, the experience of affect is amplified when outcomes are unexpected or surprising (Kahneman & Miller, 1986). In this view, *surprise* is an amplifier of the elation associated with a positive outcome. In decision affect theory, it is assumed that unexpected outcomes intensify either positive or negative emotions, depending on the valence of the outcome.

Moreover, Mellers and colleagues (1997, 1999; Mellers, 2000) found that people's emotional reactions to monetary outcomes depend on both the absolute value (a win of $100) as well as the relative value of the outcome compared to counterfactual outcomes (" . . . but I could have won $1,000"). To account for these findings, Mellers and colleagues formalized the so-called *decision affect theory*, which states that

$$R_u = J[u_a + g(u_a - u_b)(1 - s_u)]$$

where the emotional reaction, R_u, to a gamble with outcomes a and b are dependent on the utilities associated with each gamble (u_a and u_b) and the subjective probability, s_u, of outcome a. The disappointment function, g, takes into account the comparison of obtained and nonobtained outcomes and weighs it by the likelihood of the obtained outcome. The mathematical formulation of decision affect theory has been validated for both chosen and preferred monetary gambles (Mellers, 2000; Mellers et al., 1997, 1999).

Future Emotions and JDM

Since decisions made now have consequences for the future, it is important to know if people will know what they will like and how they will feel in the future. Recent research has raised the question of whether people can accurately anticipate emotional reactions to future outcomes.

Anticipatory Emotions and Affect Imagery

Anticipatory emotions may serve as input to decision making. As already noted, Damasio (1994) showed that *somatic markers* were important to make accurate decisions for the future. Similarly, Loewenstein and colleagues (2001) suggest in their risk-as-feelings hypothesis that immediately experienced emotions are important to risk assessment and choice. Since anticipatory emotions are experienced in the present, findings reviewed in the subsection on experienced emotions are applicable. However, Loewenstein and colleagues argue that emotional reactions (anticipatory or experienced) may deviate from cognitive evaluations, and thus also from expected emotions. In partial support of this idea, several empirical studies have demonstrated a strong relationship between imagery, affect, and decision making (Slovic et al., 2002).

Mental imagery appears to be an important aspect of the presence of anticipatory emotions. Research on emotional imagery has investigated relaxing versus arousing imagery (Carroll, Marzillier, & Merian, 1982), positive versus negative imagery (Haney & Euse, 1976), and imagery of specific emotions (Lang, Kozak, Miller, Levin, & McLean, 1980). Overall, these studies

show that participants use different strategies to imagine different emotions, that some emotions (sadness) are more easily imagined than others (joy), that emotional imagery is accompanied by eletrodermal and visceral responses, and that individual differences in emotional imagery exist (Gollnisch & Averill, 1993). People's abilities to form mental images of objects or situations have been shown to correlate with visceral or bodily responses (Miller et al., 1987). For instance, participants with high self-reported ability for mental imagery can more easily increase or decrease their heart rate as compared to low-ability participants (Carroll, Baker, & Preston, 1979). In an experiment on shock anticipation, Katkin, Wiens, and Öhman (2001) showed that research participants who could utilize visceral cues (introception) and detect heartbeats developed "gut feelings." The overriding function of anticipatory emotions over cognitive processes has been demonstrated with people who have phobias, who, on a cognitive level, know that their object of fear is not harmful but are prevented by their own fear from acting according to this knowledge (Epstein, 1994). Other research has shown that when participants are forced to mentally simulate future emotions, preferences may reverse as compared to when no mental simulation is used (Shiv & Huber, 2000). Thus, the vividness and imaginability of an outcome appear to be important both for the elicitation of anticipatory emotions and their influence on decisions (Loewenstein, 1996).

The vividness of an outcome has been seen as altering the subjective probability of the outcome and activating anticipatory emotions (Loewenstein, 1996). Johnson, Hershey, Meszaros, and Kunreuther (1993) showed that outcome vividness (or mental imagery potential) could affect decisions. Participants were willing to pay more for insurance against "death due to terrorist acts" (the more vivid description) than for insurance against "death due to all possible causes" (a more general and pallid description). Johnson and colleagues and Loewenstein and colleagues (2001) argue that this finding reflects the effect of vivid mental imagery and thus the influence of negative anticipatory emotions.

In summary, anticipatory emotions are emotions experienced in the present when thinking about future states or outcomes. An important determinant of anticipatory emotions is emotional imagery (i.e., vividly thinking about or describing future states). Emotional imagery may also serve as an adaptive tool, in that thinking about a happy memory can make one feel better if one is in a bad mood (Josephson, Singer, & Salovey, 1996). In this sense anticipatory emotions may stem from both anticipated future states as well as memories of past events. In line with this reasoning, Kahneman and colleagues (1997) argued that remembered utility may influence both experienced and predicted utility in that the prediction of future utility or the anticipation of affect is guided by memories of previous experiences. Moreover, Loewenstein and colleagues (2001) argued that anticipatory emotions may be dissociated at times from cognitive evaluations. However, following the definition of Loewenstein et al., *anticipated* or *expected emotions* (primarily thought of as cognitive expectations) may be partially dissociated from both anticipatory emotions and cognitive evaluations.

Affective Forecasting

Anticipated or *expected* emotions concern predictions about the emotional consequences of outcomes without actually experiencing them. In decision making, it is assumed that people predict the emotional outcomes of different alternatives and act in order to maximize positive emotions and minimize negative emotions (Loewenstein & Lerner, 2003). Affective forecasting can be defined as "people's predictions about how they will feel in a particular situation or toward a specific stimulus" (Wilson & Klaaren, 1992, p. 3). The anticipation of future happiness or sorrow is assumed to be a motivator for efficient decision making. In agreement with this view, March (1978) pointed out that all decisions concern predictions about future affect. In counterfactual thinking (what might have been . . .), for example, prediction of future emotions relies on mental simulation of possible future outcomes (what will be . . .).

Anticipation of future emotions may lead to both worsened and improved decision making. A large number of studies has investigated how people make predictions of future states and emotions (*affective forecasting*: Wilson & Gilbert, 2005). In their pioneering work, Kahneman and Snell (1990) showed that people make errors when predicting their future liking for various situations or objects. For instance, they asked participants to make predictions of their liking of yogurt before and after having eaten it 8 days in a row. After having eaten the yogurt eight times, participants indicated that their liking increased, whereas they had predicted that their liking would decrease. Misprediction is serious because the quality of the decision dependens on the accuracy of the prediction. Put differently, if people do not know what they will like in the future, or if they have incorrect intuitive theories about what they will like, they will end up with a bad decision. Gilbert, Wilson, Pinel, Blumberg, and Wheatley (1998) studied assistant professors' predictions of how they would feel before and after a tenure decision, and compared those predictions with professors who already experienced a tenure decision some time ago. It was found that assistant professors predicted themselves to be much happier the first 5 years after a positive outcome, and much more miserable in case of a negative outcome. Actually, those getting the tenure were in general happy, but not as happy as predicted. Those not getting the tenure were, in contrast to their own predictions, not unhappy. In other experiments, Wilson, Gilbert, and colleagues (Gilbert et al., 1998; Gilbert & Wilson, 2000; Wilson & Gilbert, 2005) have shown that people overpredict for how long a new romance or a broken relationship would affect their feelings, and that people overpredict the emotional impact of personal criticism and bad performance.

Other research suggests that people overestimate the intensity and duration of their feelings caused by a single event or outcome. In a classic study, Brickman, Coates, and Janoff-Bulman (1978) compared the self-reported happiness of lottery winners with matched controls. In contrast to lay conception, no significant difference was obtained between the two groups. Schkade and Kahneman (1998) found no differences in self-reported well-being between students living in California and students living in the Midwest region of the United States. However, when the students were asked to rate the well-being of other students living in different parts of the country, large differences were obtained. Students in California believed that they would be less happy in the Midwest, and Midwest students predicted that they would be happier living in California. A possible explanation for these findings is that people focus on a single focal event, failing to take into account other factors or nonfocal events that will contribute to, and meliorate, their general well-being and feelings (Loewenstein & Schkade, 1999; Wilson, Wheatley, Meyers, Gilbert, & Axsom, 2000).

Loewenstein and Schkade (1999) offered three explanations for why people mispredict their future feelings: (1) *People may have "wrong" intuitive theories about hedonics:* For instance, failure to predict adaptation to negative events may stem from people's lack of awareness of their "psychological immune system" (Gilbert & Wilson, 2000). (2) *Differential salience:* People weigh events to which their attention is directed more highly than peripheral events. For instance, participants in Schkade and Kahneman's (1998) study may have exaggerated the impact of climate (California vs. Midwest) on well-being. (3) *The hot–cold empathy gap:* Loewenstein (1996) argued that when people are in a "cold" state, they will have difficulties imagining or predicting how it would be to be in a "hot" state. For instance, hungry people have difficulties predicting what and how much they will eat when they are not hungry (Loewenstein, 1996). Similarly, people in a good mood mispredict how it feels to be in a bad mood.

The research on affective forecasting suggests a complex relationship between cognitive evaluations, expected emotions, and experienced emotions. This complexity may partly be due to the variety of future events previous research has examined. Research restricting the choice set to simpler outcomes (e.g., monetary gambles) finds that people quite accurately can predict their feelings (Mellers, 2000).

Anticipated/Expected Emotions to Future Decision Outcomes

Anticipated emotions to future outcomes are conceived of as primarily cognitive expectations about how one would feel in the future.

As for experienced emotions to decision outcomes, regret and disappointment are the two single most studied anticipated emotions, as noted. In regret and disappointment theories, it is assumed that the actual outcome is compared to counterfactual outcomes and that feelings of regret or disappointment are the result of such comparisons (Bell, 1982; Loomes & Sugden, 1986). Moreover, it is assumed that the emotional consequence of a decision is anticipated and taken into account when making the decision (Zeelenberg et al., 2000). It seems plausible that anticipated emotions thus have a different effect than anticipatory emotions on decision making and choice. The original regret and disappointment theories received only partial support in experimental tests. As Loewenstein and Lerner (2003) propose, this may be due to the fact that people do not anticipate emotions and/or believe that it is irrational to think about the emotional consequences of comparing an actual to a factual outcome (see also Pham, 2007). Another possibility that Loewenstein and Lerner propose is that the original theories were misspecified in that they assumed that the intensity of experienced regret depends only on the comparison of the actual outcome with an outcome that could have been if one had acted differently. Loewenstein and Lerner suggested that the experienced affect may rather stem from feelings of "I should have known better" (recrimination). A number of additional boundary conditions for the anticipation of regret and disappointment have been identified, such as the nature of the decision task, perceived control, omission–commission, and action–inaction (Landman, 1993; van Dijk & van der Pligt, 1997; Zeelenberg, 1999; Zeelenberg et al., 1998, 2000).

In two studies, Mellers and coworkers (1999; Mellers, 2000) extended their decision affect theory to account for anticipated emotional reactions to decision outcomes. As for experienced emotions, anticipated emotions were assumed to depend on the actual outcome, counterfactual outcome, and the probabilities of the outcomes. Similar to regret and disappointment theory, Mellers (2000) formalized the *subjective expected pleasure* (SEP) theory. SEP is related to choice and the relative pleasure of outcomes. For instance, a person making the choice between two options with the possible outcomes A and B (option 1) or the outcomes C and D (option 2) first assesses the overall anticipated pleasure of option 1 as follows:

$$s_A R_A + s_B R_B$$

where s_A and s_B are subjective probabilities of outcomes A and B, and R_A and R_B are predictions of anticipated pleasure of outcomes A and B, respectively. The outcomes C and D are decomposed in the same manner. The simple prediction of the theory is that the decision maker selects the option (A and B or C and D) with the greater average pleasure (Mellers, 2000). Morover, Mellers showed that actual and anticipated pleasure are highly correlated. In studies of monetary outcomes, course grades, pregnancy tests, and dieting, people were asked to rate their anticipated pleasure with future outcomes (winning–losing money, getting an A on the course, finding out that you are pregnant, or finding that you lost or gained weight). When the outcome was experienced (after some time), Mellers and coworkers asked participants to indicate their actual (experienced) pleasure with the outcome. In contrast to many studies in affective forecasting, Mellers reports a very high correspondence between experienced and anticipated emotional reactions. Outside the domain of decision making, Robinson and Clore (2001) found that anticipation of emotional reactions as well as beliefs about appraisal determinants of emotional reactions to pictures were highly similar to actual emotional experiences.

Conclusion

This review shows that emotion has become an important part of decision making theory and research. In the past 15 years, a large set of studies has shown that affect and deliberation jointly influence judgments and choices. Importantly, emotion is now seen as a prerequisite for good decision making in many situations. The notion of "affective rationality" is an important step to acknowledge that emotions can play a role in both normative and descriptive theo-

ries of JDM. In this chapter we reviewed evidence that different forms of emotions may have different influences on JDM. For instance, incidental emotions can be seen as normatively unrelated to decisions and can therefore sometimes distort decision making (Vohs, Baumeister, & Loewenstein, 2007). Integral emotions, on the other hand, are often quite helpful because they are relevant to the decisions to be made (Pham, 2007). Moreover, decision based on currently experienced emotions sometimes differs from decision based on predictions about future emotions. Clarifying the boundary conditions for these effects is an important future research question. In the present review, we have restricted our focus to different types of emotion and cognition–emotion interactions. Understanding the conditions under which people are more or less prone to rely on the different type of system 1 and system 2 processing discussed here is needed (see Pham, 2007).

Even if great progress has been made in understanding how emotions influence JDM, many questions remain unanswered. For instance, we still know relatively little about how emotion influences basic valuation processes such as how we value human life. Future research on cognition–emotion interactions in such domains might help to overcome failure to act when the need is large.

Acknowledgments

This research was supported by the National Science Foundation and Hewlett Foundation.

References

Alhakami, A. S., & Slovic, P. (1994). A psychological study of the inverse relationship between perceived risk and perceived benefit. *Risk Analysis, 14*, 1085–1096.

Andrade, E. B. (2005). Behavioral consequences of affect: Combining evaluative and regulatory mechanisms. *Journal of Consumer Research, 32*, 355–362.

Arkes, H. R., Herren, L. T., & Isen, A. M. (1988). The role of potential loss in the influence of affect on decision making. *Organizational*

Behavior and Human Decision Processes, 47, 181–193.

Bartels, D. M. (2006). Proportion dominance: The generality and variability of favoring relative savings over absolute savings. *Organizational Behavior and Human Decision Processes, 100,* 76–95.

Bechara, A., Damasio, H., Tranel, H., & Damasio, A. R. (1997). Deciding advantageously before knowing the advantageous strategy. *Science, 275,* 1293–1295.

Bell, D. E. (1982). Regret in decision making under uncertainty. *Operations Research, 30,* 961–981.

Bentham, J. (1948). *An introduction to the principles of morals and legislation.* Oxford, UK: Blackwell. (Original work published 1789)

Böhm, G., & Pfister, H.-R. (1996). Instrumental or emotional evaluations: What determines preferences? *Acta Psychologica, 93,* 135–148.

Boninger, D. S., Gleicher, F., & Stratham, A. (1994). Counterfactual thinking: From what might have been to what might be. *Journal of Personality and Social Psychology, 67,* 297–307.

Bower, G. H. (1981). Mood and memory. *American Psychologist, 36,* 129–148.

Brickman, P., Coates, D., & Janoff-Bulman, R. (1978). Lottery winners and accident victims: Is happiness relative? *Journal of Personality and Social Psychology, 36,* 917–927.

Cabanac, M. (1992). Pleasure: The common currency. *Journal of Theoretical Biology, 155,* 173–200.

Carroll, D., Baker, J., & Preston, M. (1979). Individual differences in visual imagery and the voluntary control of heart rate. *British Journal of Psychology, 70,* 39–49.

Carroll, D., Marzillier, J. S., & Merian, S. (1982). Psychophysiological changes accompanying different types of arousing and relaxing imagery. *Psychophysiology, 19,* 75–82.

Connolly, T., Ordóñez, L., & Coughlan, R. D. (1997). Regret and responsibility in the evaluation of decision outcomes. *Organizational Behavior and Human Decision Processes, 70,* 73–85.

Damasio, A. R. (1994). *Descartes' error: Emotion, reason, and the human brain.* New York: Avon.

DeSteno, D., Petty R. E., Rucker, D. D., & Wegener, D. T. (2000). Beyond valence in the perception of likelihood: The role of emotion

specificity. *Journal of Personality and Social Psychology, 78,* 397–419.

Desvousges, W. H., Johnson, F. R., Dunford, R. W., Boyle, K. J., Hudson, S. P., & Wilson, K. N. (2010). Measuring nonuse damages using contingent valuation: An experimental evaluation of accuracy (2nd ed.). Research Triangle Park, NC: RTI International. Retrieved from *www.rti.org/rtipress.* (Original work published 1992)

Dhar, R., & Wertenbroch, K. (2000). Consumer choice between hedonic and utilitarian goods. *Journal of Marketing Research, 37,* 60–71.

Elster, J. (1999). *Alchemies of the mind: Rationality and the emotions.* Cambridge, UK: Cambridge University Press.

Epstein, S. (1994). Integration of the cognitive and the psychodynamic unconscious. *American Psychologist, 49,* 709–724.

Fetherstonhaugh, D., Slovic, P., Johnson, S. M., & Friedrich, J. (1997). Insensitivity to the value of human life: A study of psychophysical numbing. *Journal of Risk and Uncertainty, 14,* 283.

Finucane, M. L., Alhakami, A., Slovic, P., & Johnson, S. M. (2000). The affect heuristic in judgments of risks and benefits. *Journal of Behavioral Decision Making, 13,* 1–17.

Forgas, J. P. (1995). Mood and judgment: The affect infusion model (AIM). *Psychological Bulletin, 117,* 39–66.

Fredrickson, B. L., & Levenson, R. W. (1998). Positive emotions speed recovery from the cardiovascular sequelae of negative emotions. *Cognition and Emotion, 12,* 191–220.

Frijda, N. H. (1988). The laws of emotion. *American Psychologist, 43,* 349–358.

Gilbert, D. T., & Wilson, T. D. (2000). Miswanting: Some problems in the forecasting of future affective states. In J. Forgas (Ed.), *Thinking and feeling: The role of affect in social cognition* (pp. 178–197). Cambridge, UK: Cambridge University Press.

Gilbert, D. T., Wilson, T. D., Pinel, E. C., Blumberg, S. J., & Wheatley, T. P. (1998). Immune neglect: A source of durability in affective forecasting. *Journal of Personality and Social Psychology, 75,* 617–638.

Gleicher, F., Kost, K. A., Baker, S. M., Stratham, A. J., Richman, S. A., & Sherman, S. J. (1990). The role of counterfactual thinking in judgments of affect. *Personality and Social Psychology Bulletin, 16,* 284–295.

Gollnisch, G., & Averill, J. R. (1993). Emotional

imagery: Strategies and correlates. *Cognition and Emotion, 7*, 407–429.

Haney, J. N., & Euse, F. J. (1976). Skin conductance and heart rate responses to neutral, positive, and negative imagery: Implications for covert behavior therapy procedures. *Behavior Therapy, 7*, 494–503.

Hastie, R. (2001). Problems for judgment and decision making. *Annual Review of Psychology, 52*, 653–683.

Higgins, E. T. (1997). Beyond pleasure and pain. *American Psychologist, 52*, 1280–1300.

Hsee, C. K., & Rottenstreich, Y. (2004). Music, pandas, and muggers: On the affective psychology of value. *Journal of Experimental Psychology: General, 133*, 23–30.

Isen, A. M. (2000). Positive affect and decision making. In M. Lewis & J. M. Havieland (Eds.), *Handbook of emotions* (2nd ed., pp. 417–435). London: Guilford Press.

Johnson, E. J., Hershey, J., Meszaros, J., & Kunreuther, H. (1993). Framing, probability, distortions, and insurance decisions. *Journal of Risk and Uncertainty, 7*, 35–51.

Johnson, E. J., & Tversky, A. (1983). Affect, generalization, and the perception of risk. *Journal of Personality and Social Psychology, 45*, 20–31.

Josephson, B. R., Singer, J. A., & Salovey, P. (1996). Mood regulation and memory: Repairing sad moods with happy memories. *Cognition and Emotion, 10*, 437–444.

Juslin, P. N., & Västfjäll, D. (2008). Emotional responses to music: The need to consider underlying mechanisms. *Behavioral and Brain Sciences, 31*, 559–575.

Kahneman, D. (2003). A perspective on judgment and choice: Mapping bounded rationality. *American Psychologist, 58*, 697–720.

Kahneman, D. (2011). *Thinking, fast and slow*. New York: Farrar, Straus & Giroux.

Kahneman, D., & Frederick, S. (2002). Representativeness revisited: Attribute substitution in intuitive judgment. In T. Gilovich, D. W. Griffin, & D. Kahneman (Eds.), *Heuristics and biases: The psychology of intuitive judgment* (pp. 49–81). New York: Cambridge University Press.

Kahneman, D., & Miller, D. T. (1986). Norm theory: Comparing reality to its alternatives. *Psychological Review, 93*, 136–153.

Kahneman, D., Ritov, I., & Schkade, D. (1999). Economic preferences or attitude expressions?: An analysis of dollar responses to pub-

lic issues. *Journal of Risk and Uncertainty, 19*, 203–235.

Kahneman, D., & Snell, J. (1990). Predicting utility. In R. M. Hogarth (Ed.), *Insights in decision making* (pp. 295–310). Chicago: University of Chicago Press.

Kahneman, D., & Tversky, A. (1979). Prospect theory: An analysis of decision under risk. *Econometrica, 47*, 263–291.

Kahneman, D., Wakker, P., & Sarin, R. (1997). Back to Bentham?: Explorations of experienced utility. *Quarterly Journal of Economics, 112*, 375–406.

Katkin, E. S., Wiens, S., & Öhman, A. (2001). Nonconscious fear conditioning, visceral perception, and the development of gut feelings. *Psychological Science, 12*, 366–370.

Knutson, B., Wimmer, G. E., Kuhnen, C. M., & Winkielman, P. (2008). Nucleus accumbens activation mediates the influence of reward cues on financial risk taking. *NeuroReport, 19*, 509–513.

Kogut, T., & Ritov, I. (2005). The "identified victim effect": An identified group or just a single individual? *Journal of Behavioral Decision Making, 18*, 157–167.

Landman, J. (1993). *Regret: The persistence of the possible*. New York: Oxford University Press.

Lang, P. J., Kozak, M. J., Miller, G. A., Levin, D. N., & McLean, A. (1980). Emotional imagery: Conceptual structure and pattern of somatovisceral response. *Psychophysiology, 17*, 179–192.

Larsen, R. J. (2000). Towards a science of mood regulation. *Psychological Inquiry, 11*, 129–141.

Lazarus, R. S. (1991). *Emotion and adaptation*. New York: Oxford University Press.

Lazarus, R. S. (2001). Relational meaning and discreet emotions. In K. R. Scherer, A. Schorr, & T. Johnstone (Eds.), *Appraisal processes in emotion: Theory, methods, and research* (pp. 37–67). New York: Oxford University Press.

LeDoux, J. (1996). *The emotional brain: the mysterious underpinnings of emotional life*. London: Simon & Schuster.

Lerner, J. S., Gonzalez, R. M., Small, D. A., & Fischhoff, B. (2003). Effects of fear and anger on perceived risks of terrorism: A national field experiment. *Psychological Science, 14*, 144–150.

Lerner, J. S., & Keltner, D. (2000). Beyond valence: Toward a model of emotion-specific influences on judgment and choice. *Cognition and Emotion, 14*, 473–493.

Lichtenstein, S., Slovic, P., Fischhoff, B., Layman, M., & Combs, B. (1978). Judged frequency of lethal events. *Journal of Experimental Psychology: Human Learning and Memory, 4,* 551–578.

Loewenstein, G. F. (1996). Out of control: Visceral influences on behavior. *Organizational Behavior and Human Decision Processes, 65,* 272–292.

Loewenstein, G. F., & Lerner, J. S. (2003). The role of affect in decision making. In R. J. Davidson, K. R. Scherer, & H. H. Goldsmith (Eds.), *Handbook of affective sciences* (pp. 619–642). New York: Oxford University Press.

Loewenstein, G. F., & Schkade, D. (1999). "Wouldn't it be nice?": Predicting future feelings. In D. Kahneman, E. Diener, & N. Schwarz (Eds.), *Well-being: The foundation of hedonic psychology* (pp. 85–108). New York: Russell Sage Foundation.

Loewenstein, G. F., Weber, E. U., Hsee, C. K., & Welch, E. S. (2001). Risk as feelings. *Psychological Bulletin, 127,* 267–286.

Loomes, G., & Sudgen, R. (1986). Disappointment and dynamic inconsistency in choice under uncertainty. *Review of Economic Studies, 53,* 271–282.

Luce, M., Bettman, J., & Payne, J. W. (1997). Choice processing in emotionally difficult decisions. *Journal of Experimental Psychology: Learning, Memory, and Cognition, 23,* 384–405.

Mano, H. (1992). Judgments under distress: Assessing the role of unpleasantness and arousal in judgment formation. *Organizational Behavior and Human Decision Processes, 52,* 216–245.

March, J. (1978). Bounded rationality, ambiguity, and the engineering of choice. *Bell Journal of Economics, 9,* 587–608.

McMullen, M. N. (1997). Affective contrast and assimilation in counterfactual thinking. *Journal of Experimental Social Psychology, 33,* 77–100.

Mellers, B. A. (2000). Choice and the relative pleasures of consequences. *Psychological Bulletin, 126,* 910–924.

Mellers, B. A., Schwartz, A., & Cooke, A. D. J. (1998). Judgment and decision making. *Annual Review of Psychology, 49,* 447–477.

Mellers, B. A., Schwartz, A., Ho, K., & Ritov, I. (1997). Decision affect theory: Emotional reactions to the outcomes of risky options. *Psychological Science, 8,* 423–429.

Mellers, B. A., Schwartz, A., & Ritov, I. (1999). Emotion-based choice. *Journal of Experimental Psychology: General, 128,* 332–345.

Miller, G. A., Levin, D. N., Kozak, M. J., Cook, E. W., III, McLean, A., Jr., & Lang, P. (1987). Individual differences in imagery and the psychophysiology of emotion. *Cognition and Emotion, 1,* 367–390.

Montague, P. R., & Berns, G. S. (2002). Neural economics and the biological substrates of valuation. *Neuron, 36,* 265–284.

Nygren, T. E., Isen, A. M., Taylor, P. J., & Dulin, J. (1996). The influence of positive affect on the decision rule in risky situations: Focus on outcome (and especially avoidance of loss) rather than probability. *Organizational Behavior and Human Decision Processes, 66,* 59–72.

Panksepp, J. (1998). *Affective neuroscience. The foundations of human and animal emotions.* New York: Oxford University Press.

Peters, E. (2006). The functions of affect in the construction of preferences. In S. Lichtenstein & P. Slovic (Eds.), *The construction of preference* (pp. 454–463). New York: Cambridge University Press.

Peters, E., Hess, T. M., Västfjäll, D., & Auman, C. (2007). Adult age differences in dual information processes: Implications for the role of affective and deliberative processes in older adults' decision making. *Perspectives on Psychological Science, 2,* 1–23.

Peters, E., Västfjäll, D., Gärling, T., & Slovic, P. (2006). Affect and decision making: A "hot" topic. *Journal of Behavioral Decision Making, 19,* 79–85.

Peters, E., Västfjäll, D., Slovic, P., Mertz, C. K., Mazzocco, K., & Dickert, S. (2006). Numeracy and decision making. *Psychological Science, 17,* 407–413.

Pham, M. T. (1998). Representativeness, relevance, and the use of feelings in decision making. *Journal of Consumer Research, 25,* 144–159.

Pham, M. T. (2007). Emotion and rationality: A critical review and interpretation of empirical evidence. *Review of General Psychology, 11,* 155–178.

Raghunatan, R., & Pham, M. T. (1999). All negative moods are not equal: Motivational influence of anxiety and sadness on decision making. *Organizational Behavior and Human Decision Processes, 79,* 56–77.

Read, D., & Loewenstein, G. (1999). Enduring pain for money: Decisions based on the perception and memory of pain. *Journal of Behavioral Decision Making, 12,* 1–17.

Robinson, M. D., & Clore, G. L. (2001). Simulation, scenarios, and emotional appraisal: Testing the convergence of real and imagined reactions to emotional stimuli. *Personality and Social Psychology Bulletin, 27,* 1520–1532.

Rottenstreich, Y., & Hsee, C. K. (2001). Money, kisses, and electric shocks: On the affective psychology of probability weighting. *Psychological Science, 12,* 185–190.

Russell, J. A. (2003). Core affect and the psychological construction of emotion. *Psychological Review, 110*(1), 145–172.

Sanna, L. J. (1998). Defensive pessimism and optimism: The bitter-sweet influence of mood on performance and prefactual and counterfactual thinking. *Cognition and Emotion, 12,* 635–665.

Savage, L. J. (1954). *The foundations of statistics.* New York: Wiley Press.

Schkade, D. A., & Kahneman, D. (1998). Does living in California make people happy?: A focusing illusion in judgments of life satisfaction. *Psychological Science, 9,* 340–346.

Schwarz, N. (2000). Emotion, cognition, and decision making. *Cognition and Emotion, 14,* 433–440.

Schwarz, N. (2001). Feelings as information: Implications for affective influences on information processing. In L. L. Martin & G. L. Clore (Eds.), *Theories of mood and cognition: A user's guidebook* (pp. 159–176). Hillsdale, NJ: Erlbaum.

Schwarz, N., & Clore, G. L. (1983). Mood, misattribution, and judgments of well-being: Informative and directive functions of affective states. *Journal of Personality and Social Psychology, 45,* 513–523.

Shiv, B., & Fedorikin, A. (2002). Spontaneous versus controlled influences of stimulus-based affect on choice behavior. *Organizational Behavior and Human Decision Processes, 87,* 342–370.

Shiv, B., & Huber, J. (2000). The impact of anticipating satisfaction on consumer choice. *Journal of Consumer Psychology, 27,* 202–216.

Siemer, M., & Reisenzein, R. (1998). Effects of mood on evaluative judgments: Influence of reduced processing capacity and mood salience. *Cognition and Emotion, 12,* 783–805.

Sloman, S. A. (1996). The empirical case for two systems of reasoning. *Psychological Bulletin, 119,* 3–22.

Slovic, P. (2007). "If I look to the mass I will never act": Psychic numbing and genocide. *Judgment and Decision Making, 2,* 79–95.

Slovic, P., Finucane, M. L., Peters, E., & MacGregor, D. G. (2002). The affect heuristic. In T. Gilovich, D. Griffin, & D. Kahneman (Eds.), *Heuristics and biases: The psychology of intuitive judgment* (pp. 397–420). New York: Cambridge University Press.

Slovic, P., & Västfjäll, D. (2010). Affect, moral intuition, and risk. *Psychological Inquiry, 21,* 387–398.

Stanovich, K. E., & West, R. f. (2000). Individual differences in reasoning: Implications for the rationality debate? *Behavioral and Brain Sciences, 23*(5), 645–665.

van Dijk, W. W., & van der Pligt, J. (1997). The impact of probability and magnitude of outcome on disappointment and elation. *Organizational Behavior and Human Decision Processes, 69,* 277–284.

Västfjäll, D., & Gärling, T. (2006). Preference for negative emotions. *Emotion, 6,* 326–329.

Västfjäll, D., Peters, E., & Slovic, P. (2011). *Compassion fatigue: Donations and affect are greatest for a single child in need.* Manuscript submitted for publication.

Vohs, K. D., Baumeister, R. F., & Loewenstein, G. F. (Eds.). (2007). *Do emotions help or hurt decision making?: A hedgefoxian perspective.* New York: Russell Sage.

Weber, E. U., & Johnson, E. J. (2009). Mindful judgment and decision making. *Annual Review of Psychology, 60,* 53–86.

Wilson, T. D., & Gilbert, D. T. (2005). Affective forecasting: Knowing what to want. *Current Directions in Psychological Science, 14,* 131–134.

Wilson, T. D., & Klaaren, K. J. (1992). "Expectation whirls me round": The role of affective expectations. In M. S. Clark (Ed.), *Review of personality and social psychology, emotion and social behavior* (Vol. 14, pp. 1–31). Newbury Park, CA: Sage.

Wilson, T. D., Wheatley, T. P., Meyers, J. M., Gilbert, D. T., & Axsom, D. (2000). Focalism: A source of durability bias in affective forecasting. *Journal of Personality and Social Psychology, 78,* 821–836.

Wright, W. F., & Bower, G. H. (1992). Mood

effect on subjective probability assessment. *Organizational Behavior and Human Decision Processes, 22,* 276–291.

Zajonc, R. B. (1980). Feeling and thinking: Preferences need no inferences. *American Psychologist, 35,* 151–175.

Zajonc, R. B. (1998). Emotions. In D. T. Gilbert, S. T. Fiske, & G. Lindzey (Eds.), *Handbook of social psychology* (pp. 591–632). New York: Oxford University Press.

Zajonc, R. B., & Markus, H. (1982). Affective and cognitive factors in preferences. *Journal of Consumer Research, 9,* 123–131.

Zeelenberg, M. (1999). Anticipated regret, expected feedback and behavioral decision making. *Journal of Behavioral Decision Making, 12,* 93–106.

Zeelenberg, M., van Dijk, W. W., Manstead, A. S. R., & van der Pligt, J. (2000). On bad decisions and disconfirmed expectancies: The psychology of regret and disappointment. *Cognition and Emotion, 14,* 521–541.

Zeelenberg, M., van Dijk, W. W., van der Pligt, J., Manstead, A. S. R., van Empelen, P., & Reinderman, D. (1998). Emotional reactions to the outcomes of decision: The role of counterfactual thought in the experience of regret and disappointment. *Organizational Behavior and Human Decision Processes, 75,* 117–141.

CHAPTER 15

Incidental and Integral Effects of Emotions on Self-Control

Brandon J. Schmeichel and Michael Inzlicht

Probably most human behaviors are impulsive. This seems especially likely to be true for infants and children, who are only beginning to develop the capacity to override impulses. But even for healthy adult humans who are presumed to have a fully developed capacity for self-control, impulsive or automatic behaviors seem to predominate. Given that humans continue to exist (thrive, even) in most corners of the globe, a favorable case can be made that the preponderance of impulsive behaviors has served humankind well.

Self-control is nevertheless an important key to success in life. Knowing how and when to regulate impulsive tendencies and then successfully regulating them increase the flexibility of human behavior. This increased flexibility appears to confer substantial benefits for individuals and for society, as suggested by evidence that success at self-control contributes to physical health, psychological well-being, longevity, occupational attainment, relationship satisfaction, and several other desirable outcomes (for an overview, see Vohs & Baumeister, 2011).

The purpose of this chapter is to consider how self-control is influenced by emotions. Emotions are associated with impulsive or automatic response tendencies, and the traditional view is that emotion and self-control are antagonists. We review evidence supporting this view. Another view is that negative emotions, more so than positive emotions, are likely to undermine self-control, and we also review evidence for that contention. A third view is more nuanced still in recognizing that both positive and negative emotions can impair or improve self-control under the right circumstances, and there's growing evidence for that position (reviewed below). We considered but quickly abandoned a fourth possibility—that emotions have little or no influence on self-control—because few theorists have championed this view, and the relevant published findings usually indicate that emotions have a significant impact on self-control.

The first half of the chapter thus examines the evidence for the effects of emotion on self-control. The guiding question is: Do incidental emotional states (i.e., those that are extrinsic to, or happen to coincide with, a self-control attempt) influence the likelihood of success at self-control? To answer this question, we review the results of experiments that have manipulated emotional states and assessed the consequences for self-control. In particular, we review evidence on the moderating influence of both positive and negative emotion inductions on outcomes associated with dieting and delaying gratification, respectively. Then we discuss the leading explanations for the observed effects.

The second half of the chapter takes a different approach by exploring the integral (as opposed to incidental) influence of emotion in self-control. The guiding question there is: What role do emotions play in stimulating self-control? Rather than treating emotions as outsiders that impinge on the process of self-control, as we do in the first half of the chapter, in the second half we locate emotions inside the mechanisms of self-control and outline the basic conceptual foundations of an *affect alarm model* of self-control.

Before diving into the literature review, we offer two caveats to delimit our approach. First, *emotions are complex*. They involve more or less coordinated changes to subjective experience, physiological responding, and physical (e.g., facial) expression. And they have been categorized along a number of dimensions, including arousal level (from low to high), valence (from positive to negative), and motivational direction (approach or avoidance), among others. Other theorists prefer to think of discrete emotions rather than categorical dimensions. Because the bulk of the literature on the influence of emotion on self-control involves the valence dimension (i.e., effects of positive vs. negative emotions on self-control), likewise our review focuses mainly on the valence dimension.

Second, *self-control is complex*. It involves the capacity to override or alter predominant response tendencies, and it reflects the interplay of cognitive and motivational (or reflective and impulsive) mechanisms. Furthermore, it can be applied to diverse behaviors or tendencies and includes inhibiting or suppressing impulses as well as amplifying or expressing them. To focus our review, we homed in on two well-studied and widely practiced forms of self-control: dieting and delay of gratification. If emotions have a particular impact on self-control, then we should find evidence for it whenever people attempt to restrict their food intake or to forego short-term indulgences in the pursuit of long-term rewards.

Incidental Effects of Emotions on Dieting

Numerous studies have assessed the effects of emotions—particularly negative emotions—on eating behavior in humans (for overviews, see Greeno & Wing, 1994;

Macht, 2008). But do emotions influence the self-control of eating? That is, if a person is trying not to eat, do emotional states help him or her to refrain from eating?

Effects of Negative Emotions on Dieting

The first research to explicitly consider the effect of emotion on the self-control of eating was reported by Herman and colleagues (Herman & Mack, 1975; Herman & Polivy, 1975), who shifted attention away from differences between obese and nonobese individuals and toward differences between restrained versus unrestrained eaters. Restrained eaters are people who are actively attempting to restrict their food consumption—that is, people who are trying to exercise self-control over their eating behavior. Several experiments have found that negative emotions cause restrained eaters to eat more food.

In a sample of female college students, Herman and Polivy (1975) found that the threat of electric shock caused unrestrained eaters to eat less ice cream compared to an impending, nonthreatening tingling sensation. Among restrained eaters, however, threat of shock led to a slight increase in ice cream consumption. Thus, anticipating an anxiety-provoking event caused participants to eat less—unless they were trying to regulate their food consumption.

Similar evidence was reported by Ruderman (1985), who found that taking a test of intelligence and receiving (bogus) feedback indicating failure caused a sample of college-age women to eat more crackers than did receiving success feedback, but only if the women scored high on a self-report measure of dietary restraint. Among these women, the feelings of depression, anxiety, and hostility associated with failure nearly doubled cracker consumption compared to feelings of success. Among women who were not actively trying to restrain eating, cracker consumption was slightly (but nonsignificantly) lower after failure versus success feedback. Here again, unpleasant information that induced negative affect caused only restrained eaters—those who were otherwise trying to regulate their food consumption—to eat more food.

One study suggested that only some aversive events are likely to increase eating among restrained (but not unrestrained) eaters. More specifically, Heatherton, Herman, and Polivy (1991) found that an ego threat— information that threatens or disparages a person's self-views, such as failure at an important task—increases ice cream consumption among restrained eaters, whereas the threat of physical harm (i.e., shock) does not. The threat of physical harm reduced eating among nonrestrained eaters, consistent with earlier research by Schachter and colleagues (e.g., Schachter, 1968; Schachter, Goldman, & Gordon, 1968), but threat of physical harm had no significant effect on eating among restrained eaters. Only self-relevant negative emotions disinhibited eating behavior among restrained eaters (also see Heatherton, Striepe, & Wittenberg, 1998; Wallis & Hetherington, 2004). A more recent study found that restrained eaters ate fewer low-fat snacks under ego threat, suggesting that restrained eaters eat more of only certain types of foods (e.g., high-fat foods) under threat (Wallis & Hetherington, 2009).

In summary, research suggests that negative emotions, perhaps especially ego-threatening or self-relevant negative emotions, can undermine the self-control of eating behavior, even for relatively unpalatable foods (Polivy, Herman, & McFarlane, 1994). Among people who are not dieting, however, negative emotions appear to have a different effect. Several studies have found that fear and anxiety reduce food intake among unrestrained eaters.

Effects of Positive Emotions on Dieting

Experimental research on the effects of positive emotions on eating behavior is fairly rare, and research on the influence of positive emotions on the self-control of eating behavior is rarer still. Eating, and perhaps especially the consumption of diet-busting foods such as cake and ice cream, often accompanies joyous celebrations (e.g., weddings, birthdays). This observation suggests that positive emotions may coincide with disinhibited eating. Indeed, the extant evidence suggests that some positive emotions, like some negative emotions, can increase food consumption among restrained eaters.

A study by Cools, Schotte, and McNally (1992) replicated the now familiar find-

ing that negative emotions increase food intake among restrained eaters. They also found that a positive mood induction (i.e., a comedy film) increases food intake among restrained eaters. These patterns led Cools and colleagues to conclude that emotional arousal, rather than negative emotional valence, plays a central role in disinhibited eating among otherwise restrained eaters.

A more recent study by Yeomans and Coughlan (2009) observed a more nuanced pattern. They found that a subset of restrained eaters—those who also had a tendency toward disinhibited eating—ate more popcorn and raisins while watching an anxiety-provoking clip from the movie *The Shining*. This pattern is consistent with evidence reviewed above regarding the effects of negative emotions on restrained eating. Among unrestrained eaters, however, those with a tendency toward disinhibited eating ate more food while viewing pleasant and humorous clips from the television comedy *Friends*. The anxiety-inducing clip and the humorous clip were equally arousing, so arousal does not easily explain the eating patterns. This study suggests that both positive and negative emotions can increase eating, depending on the eater. Negative emotions led to more eating among some individuals who were actively trying to control their eating behavior, whereas positive emotions led to more eating among a subset of individuals who were not actively trying to control their eating behavior.

One other study is relevant, though it did not directly examine restrained eaters or the self-control of eating. Macht, Roth, and Ellgring (2002) compared the effects of different emotion inductions on liking for chocolate and chocolate consumption. They found divergent effects for sadness and joy, such that joy increased appetite in a sample of men but sadness decreased it. The men in the study also found chocolate more pleasant and more stimulating following a joy induction. These are among the few experimental results pertaining to the influence of positive emotion on eating behavior, and they suggest that (compared to sadness), positive emotions may increase desire for chocolate.

To appreciate fully the influence of emotion on the self-control of eating behavior, much more research on positive emotions is needed. One useful approach for future research may be to compare the effects of different positive emotions, as previous research has focused mainly on the effects of amusement elicited by humorous stimuli. Positive emotions elicited by humorous stimuli may be relatively low in motivation intensity or action orientation and thus may have different effects relative to other positive emotions such as excitement, pride, or determination. Experiments that compare the consequences of low-intensity versus high-intensity positive emotions may also help to clarify the role of arousal in the effects of emotions on eating.

Another potentially useful consideration is self-relevance. As we saw, negative emotions elicited by self-relevant threats (e.g., failure, negative feedback) tend to have different effects on eating behavior compared to other threats (e.g., threat of shock). Positive emotions can also vary in self-relevance, and it may be worthwhile to ask whether flattery, task success, or other self-enhancing events have different effects on eating self-control compared to viewing funny videos. Self-relevant positive emotions may be more intense or arousing than other positive emotions.

Conclusion

Having reviewed the evidence that emotions disrupt the self-control of eating behavior, the next question is: Why do emotions have this effect? The short answer is that no single explanation or theory has emerged to explain the relevant evidence. In the next section of the chapter, after considering the impact of emotions on another classic form of self-control, we review the leading explanations for the effects of emotions in more detail.

Incidental Effects of Emotions on Delay of Gratification

Delay of gratification occurs whenever a person forgoes short-term satisfactions in the pursuit of more distal rewards. Dieting can be seen as delay of gratification (e.g., restraint now to fit into a swimsuit next summer), but delay behavior is more general than dieting insofar as virtually any gratification can be delayed. How do emo-

tions influence delay of gratification? Here we focus on evidence from experiments in which emotional states were induced prior to a measurement of delay of gratification.

Effects of Emotions on Delay of Gratification in Children

Seeman and Schwarz (1974) reported one of the first experiments to find evidence that incidental positive (vs. negative) emotions enhance delay of gratification. They asked a group of 9-year-olds to draw a picture, ostensibly to be reviewed for possible inclusion in an art show. By random assignment, children were told that their pictures had been selected or had not been selected for the show. (Pilot testing had verified that this method reliably induces positive and negative emotions, respectively.) After receiving the news about their drawings, participants were asked to choose between receiving one moderately desirable object now (e.g., one pack of gum) versus receiving a more desirable object later (e.g., two packs of gum in a week).

The results were clear: Children who had been led to believe that their drawing was selected for the art show were more likely to opt for the delayed reward compared to children who had been told their drawings would not be included in the art show. Seeman and Schwarz (1974) concluded that the children's emotional state was a key determinant of their decision to delay gratification. Absent a neutral emotion condition as a control, however, the authors could not discern whether negative emotions reduced delay behavior or positive emotions increased it.

Fry (1975) did include a neutral condition and found conceptually similar results in a sample of 7- and 8-year-olds. Children in this study were asked to think of happy events, think of sad events, or read instructions for a puzzle prior to being introduced to two toys. One toy was more desirable than the other, but the experimenter explicitly instructed the children not to play with this toy; the less desirable toy could be played with at any time. The children then were left alone in a room with both toys and were secretly observed by an experimenter. Children played with the forbidden toy sooner and more often after thinking about sad events than after thinking about happy events or solving a puzzle. And children who thought about happy events waited longer and played less with the forbidden toy compared to both other groups of children. This nice linear pattern suggested unique effects of positive and negative emotions, such that negative emotions decrease and positive emotions increase delay behavior.

Moore, Clyburn, and Underwood (1976) tested the impact of emotions on delay behavior in an even younger sample of children: 3- to 5-year-olds. Like Fry (1975), they asked children to think of happy or sad events prior to the assessment of delay behavior; in a neutral condition subjects completed a counting task. Then the children chose between eating a pretzel right then versus waiting for a lollipop. The sad mood induction caused children to favor the immediate pretzel over the delayed lollipop more often compared to the other conditions. In this experiment, however, delay behavior did not differ between the happy versus neutral conditions.

Fry (1977) manipulated emotional states in a sample of 8- and 9-year-olds using success feedback, failure feedback, or no feedback on a series of cognitive challenges. Then the children were left in a room with two toys but expressly forbidden from playing with the more desirable toy. The induction of positive emotions caused children to wait longer before playing with the forbidden toy, compared to children who received no feedback or negative feedback. And negative feedback caused children to delay less compared to no feedback. Here again, then, positive emotions increased delay behavior, and negative emotions reduced it.

Studies that followed this initial flurry of research activity on emotions and delay behavior in children used more complex methods and found more nuanced variations on the now-familiar pattern of results. For example, Schwarz and Pollack (1977, Experiment 1) used a within-subjects manipulation of happy and sad thoughts and measured delay behavior after each emotion induction. They found that happiness increased delay of gratification relative to sadness, but only in the between-groups comparison (i.e., happy first vs. sad first).

Yates, Lippett, and Yates (1981) found that a positive emotion induction (i.e., thinking happy thoughts) prior to the assessment of delay of gratification increased delay behavior among 8-year-olds but not among 4- and 5-year-olds; the positive emotion induction increased delay behavior among the younger group of children only if they were also reminded to think happy thoughts during the delay period. This study provided a conceptual replication of Mischel, Ebessen, and Zeiss (1972), who had found that encouraging children to think happy thoughts during the delay period increased the duration of delay of gratification.

One clever experiment found that the operative norm in a situation helps to determine whether positive emotions increase or decrease self-indulgence in children. Specifically, Perry, Perry, and English (1985) observed that, compared to completing a simple count task, thinking happy thoughts caused children to indulge (i.e., to take more candy from a candy dish) when there was no hint that taking candy was wrong. However, when the experimenter suggested that they not take too many candies "as that would be greedy," children who had been thinking happy thoughts took significantly fewer candies than other children. Thus, positive emotions caused both increased self-indulgence and increased delay of gratification, depending on the presence or absence of a reminder about an undesirable aspect of self-indulgence.

In summary, emotions have a substantial influence on delay of gratification in children. Negative emotion inductions (particularly, thinking sad thoughts or receiving negative feedback) reduce delay of gratification (i.e., increase immediate gratification) relative to positive mood inductions and neutral states. Furthermore, positive emotion inductions (particularly, thinking happy thoughts or receiving positive feedback) tend to increase delay of gratification relative to neutral emotional states, although a few studies observed only nonsignificant trends in this direction.

Effects of Emotions on Delay of Gratification in Adults

The early research on emotions and delay of gratification involved children as research subjects. Do emotions have the same impact on delay behavior in adults? Fewer studies have examined delay of gratification in adults. This is due in part to the fact that delay behavior is more difficult to study in laboratory experiments with adult subjects. Sadly for self-control researchers, most adult humans easily forgo one marshmallow now for two marshmallows later. Nevertheless, meaningful measures of delay have been devised for adults, and the results suggest that emotions influence delay behavior somewhat differently in adults versus children.

Wertheim and Schwarz (1983) reported one of the first studies assessing the link between emotions and delay of gratification in adults. They found that individuals with higher scores on the Beck Depression Inventory (BDI) chose immediate rewards (e.g., a six-pack of soda now) over delayed rewards (e.g., two six-packs in 3 weeks) more often than did individuals scoring lower on the BDI. Although the correlational nature of the study precluded the authors from making strong causal inferences, their findings fit with the evidence from children indicating that negative emotions decrease (or lack of negative emotions increases) delay of gratification.

Gray (1999) conducted an experiment to examine the effects of threat-related negative emotions on "temporally-extended choice," which is closely related to delay of gratification (see also Knapp & Clark, 1991). Participants earned small monetary rewards for viewing pictures; the more pictures they viewed, the more money they earned. Participants controlled, via button press, how quickly the pictures advanced on the display screen, but the picture-viewing task was arranged so that pressing the button quickly to advance pictures carried a long-term cost. More specifically, advancing pictures quickly increased the rate of picture-viewing in the short term but slowed the rate over the long term, thereby reducing the total amount of money to be earned.

Within the context of this temporally extended choice task, Gray (1999) manipulated emotions by varying the content of the pictures. In the neutral condition, participants viewed images of mundane objects and scenes. In the negative emotions condition, participants viewed unpleasant images from the International Affective Picture System (IAPS; Lang, Bradley, & Cuthbert, 2008), including images of a mutilated body,

a dead animal, and a disgusting toilet. The dependent measure was amount of money participants earned during the last third of the task, after having sufficient opportunity to observe the contingency between button press behavior and subsequent picture durations.

Participants viewing negative pictures earned less money than did participants viewing neutral pictures, suggesting that negative emotions reduce delay of gratification. As Gray (1999) put it, "the aversive group repeatedly favored the option that had beneficial immediate effects, despite larger subsequent costs to the goal of doing well on the task" (p. 71). In a second study, individuals reporting higher stress levels earned less money on the picture-viewing task relative to individuals reporting lower stress levels. Together, the results of these two studies mimic the pattern observed in studies of children: Negative emotions reduce delay of gratification. It is worth noting that the temporally extended choice task was likely to involve other processes (e.g., how quickly and how well participants discerned the contingencies underlying task performance) that may have been influenced by negative emotions, which introduces ambiguity as to whether the results reflect changes in delay or changes in some other process.

As with children, then, the research suggests that adults also become more inclined to seek immediate gratification when they feel negative emotions. Do adults and children show similar effects of positive emotions as well? That is, do positive emotions cause adults to become more inclined to delay gratification?

A study by Hirsh, Guindon, Morisano, and Peterson (2010) tested this hypothesis. Participants completed a series of puzzles faster than a confederate, slower than a confederate, or with no confederate present. Participants then completed a measure of delay discounting, which assesses preferences for immediate versus delayed rewards. This measure asked participants to make a series of choices between hypothetical rewards, one a smaller reward to be received sooner, and the other a larger reward to be delayed (e.g., $2 now or $20 in a year?; $900 now or $1,000 in 6 months?; $18 now or $20 in a week?). Altogether, participants' choices yield idiosyncratic discount rates, such that higher discount rates indicate lower delay of gratification (i.e., a preference for smaller, immediate rewards over larger, delayed ones).

Changes in positive emotions from before to after the puzzle task predicted subsequent discount rates, but only among extraverts. Specifically, among more extraverted individuals, greater increases in positive emotions predicted higher discount rates (i.e., lower delay of gratification). Changes in negative emotions did not predict discount rates. Hirsh and colleagues (2010) proposed that positive emotions potentiate the tendency for extraverted individuals to orient toward opportunities for reward, leading to a bias toward immediate gratification.

The findings of Hirsh and colleagues (2010) are notable because they run counter to the findings from studies of children, which had revealed that positive emotions increase delay of gratification. This research is thus among the first to suggest that positive emotions can reduce delay of gratification, and the findings fit with evidence that sexual arousal makes adult males more likely to discount the future (Wilson & Daly, 2004; see also Ariely & Loewenstein, 2006).

Additional evidence has accumulated to support the idea that, in adults at least, positive emotions can reduce delay behavior. One experiment found that both positive and negative emotions reduce delay of gratification, depending on the person. Specifically, Augustine and Larsen (2011) had participants view positive or negative pictures from the IAPS prior to completing a delay discounting task. Individual differences in neuroticism ended up playing a central role in the results. Participants higher in neuroticism had higher discount rates (i.e., lower delay of gratification) after viewing negative pictures, compared to those lower in neuroticism. The patterns were slightly more complicated among those who viewed positive pictures. Here, only more neurotic individuals who reported little or no unpleasant affect exhibited higher discount rates. Thus, the positive emotion induction (like the negative emotion induction) tended to reduce delay of gratification, but only among more neurotic individuals who experienced lower levels of negative emotions in response to viewing positive pictures.

Two other studies are relevant to the question of how positive emotions influence

self-control. These studies differ from the research reviewed above, insofar as these used a one-shot decision as the key dependent measure. Note, however, that the decision was always between a more indulgent versus a less indulgent option, which is highly relevant to delay of gratification.

Fedorikhin and Patrick (2010) found that viewing a film clip that elicited low-arousal positive emotions caused participants to choose grapes over candy, compared to viewing a neutral film clip. Viewing a film clip that elicited high-arousal positive emotions, however, did not cause participants to choose grapes over candy more often than did viewing a neutral clip. Although the one-shot choice of candy versus fruit does not map perfectly onto delay of gratification as it has been operationalized in the studies reviewed thus far, the results do suggest that positive emotions increase resistance to temptation relative to neutral emotional states, but only if the positive emotions are associated with low levels of arousal.

A series of experiments by Wilcox, Kramer, and Sen (2011) found that pride increases self-indulgence, which is consistent with the notion that positive emotions can reduce delay of gratification. Specifically, after writing about a personal accomplishment of which they were proud, participants were more likely to choose a gift card that could be used to buy entertainment supplies (an indulgent choice) versus a gift card that could be used to buy school supplies (a utilitarian choice). Thinking of a happy memory did not have a significant effect on gift card choice compared to thinking of neutral events.

In summary, the research suggests that emotions influence delay of gratification behavior in adults. Negative emotions mostly reduce delay of gratification, as was found in children. Positive emotions have more mercurial effects. The bulk of the evidence suggests that positive emotions render adults less likely to delay gratification, much like negative emotions do. However, inconsistencies in the literature justify caveats to this conclusion. Positive emotions may reduce delay behavior particularly among extraverts (Hirsh et al., 2010), or among neurotics who experience a drop in negative affect prior to the delay measure (Augustine & Larsen, 2011). And high-arousal positive emotions may be more likely than low-arousal positive emotions to reduce delay of gratification (see also Leith & Baumeister, 1996). Low-arousal positive emotions have been observed to improve resistance to temptation (Fedorikhin & Patrick, 2010), as was typical in research with children, but also low-arousal positive emotions have been found to have no significant effect on resistance to temptation (Wilcox et al., 2011).

Why Do Incidental Emotions Influence Dieting and Delay of Gratification?

In reviewing the research on the effects of incidental emotions on self-control, we found consistent evidence that emotions influence success at both dieting and delay of gratification. Why do emotions influence self-control as they do?

The single most prominent explanation for the influence of negative emotions on self-control is hedonic emotion regulation. Virtually all of the authors and articles reviewed thus far endorsed this view to some degree. The idea is simple. When people feel bad, they become more inclined to do something to feel better. Of course, this is not the case all of the time or for all persons (see Tamir, 2009), but it often seems to be the case for most. If the opportunity to eat (for dieters) or to self-gratify happens along when one is in a bad mood, then one is more likely to eat or to self-gratify, presumably because this helps to alleviate the bad mood.

Or, at the least, people believe that immediate gratification will alleviate bad moods. The evidence that eating food or choosing smaller immediate rewards actually improves mood is far from conclusive. In fact, none of the studies we reviewed provided any evidence that immediate gratification makes people feel better (nor has research on the related topic of binge eating; see Haedt-Matt & Keel, 2011; cf. Dingemans, Martijn, Jansen, & von Furth, 2009). Most studies simply did not assess this possibility. Thus, one obvious avenue for future research is to examine the emotional consequences of seeking immediate gratification when in a bad mood.

One investigation that did examine the effects of negative emotions on self-indulgence found little evidence that indulgence improves mood. In a series of experiments, Tice, Bratslavsky, and Baumeister (2001) manipulated emotional states and assessed their effects on eating, a resource dilemma game, and procrastination. The main finding was that individuals self-indulged when experiencing negative emotions because they believed that self-indulgence would improve their moods. When participants had been led to believe that self-indulgence would not improve their moods, negative emotions did not increase self-indulgence.

For present considerations, the key evidence pertains to the emotional consequences of self-indulgence. Did indulgence actually alleviate participants' negative moods? At the end of two of the experiments reported by Tice and colleagues (2001), participants self-reported their emotional states. Indulgence did not clearly produce an increase in positive emotions in either study. The authors suggested that their mood measures may have lacked sensitivity to find subtle changes in mood, or that the benefits of indulgence were too fleeting to be detected at the end of the experiments. However, they argued against these possibilities and concluded that indulgence does not actually improve mood and that people are mistaken in their belief that indulgence will improve moods. More research is needed on this seeming lack of insight into the hedonic benefits of indulgence and on the limits of indulgence as a mood regulation strategy.

Compared to the hedonic emotion regulation explanation for the effects of negative emotions on self-control, much less consensus exists for explaining the effects of positive emotions on self-control. Perhaps this is because positive emotions can both help and hurt self-control. As we saw, positive emotions tended to increase delay of gratification in kids. A handful of explanations was proposed for this effect, but none has been supported. Fry (1975) speculated that positive emotions heighten self-efficacy and expectations for success, thereby enabling kids to pursue delayed reward. Moore and colleagues (1976) thought that positive emotions allow kids to attend to broader, long-term interests, thereby increasing delay behavior. And Fry (1977) suggested that positive emotions serve as a buffer that allows kids to tolerate the more aversive course of action (e.g., not playing with a desired toy) needed to delay gratification.

In adults, unlike in children, positive emotions tend to reduce delay of gratification, so the proposed explanations here are different. Hirsh and colleagues (2010) proposed that positive emotions prime reward-seeking tendencies, especially for extraverts. Augustine and Larsen (2011) thought that mood regulation accounts for reduced delay under positive emotions. That is, because people tend to want to maintain positive emotions, those who are currently feeling good opt for immediate over delayed gratification to sustain their good moods. Wilcox and colleagues (2011) hypothesized that positive emotions such as pride cause individuals to feel as though they are progressing toward their goals, and these feelings help to justify self-gratification. Ironically, the self-licensing of immediate gratification can negate hard-won progress toward long-term goals.

We think that it is likely that emotions, and particularly positive emotions, can influence self-control via several different mechanisms. Much more evidence and theoretical development is needed before definitive conclusions can be drawn. In the subsequent portions of this chapter, we develop an affect alarm model of self-control that casts negative affect, specifically anxiety, as an integral component of success at self-control. After developing our model, we propose ways to integrate research on the effects of incidental emotions on self-control with our view of negative affect as an integral contributor to self-control. Such integrative efforts promise to advance our understanding of why emotions influence self-control.

Integral Effects of Emotions on Self-Control

Up until now, we have examined the evidence for the idea that incidental emotions moderate the effectiveness of self-control. The evidence indicates that emotional states can undermine or enhance self-control depending on the person and his or her circumstances. We now turn in a different direction to consider the idea that emotions are intrinsic to self-control. That is, rather than viewing emotion as an interloper that impinges upon or moderates self-control

from the outside, we now explore whether emotion is, in fact, integral to the process of self-control, central to the way control is signaled and implemented.

We propose an *affect alarm model of control*, whereby emotion alerts organisms to when self-control is needed. In this sense, emotional processes can be seen as mediating mechanisms of self-control, with emotions acting as information (Schwarz & Clore, 1983) that can tell people when self-control is needed. We should note that although the evidence reviewed above for moderation by incidental emotions is abundant, it is less so for mediation by integral emotions. The evidence we marshal is largely theoretical and our thesis, therefore, more speculative.

One of the "laws" of emotion is that it orients organisms to cues in the environment that signal evolutionarily important needs for survival and reproduction, while tuning out less motivationally relevant information (Frijda, 1988). One class of motivationally relevant events involves needs, desires, and goals that are threatened or at risk of going unmet because they conflict with other needs, desires, and goals. This type of event typically yields negative emotions such as anxiety (Gray & McNaughton, 2000) and is precisely the kind of event in which self-control is needed to bias responding and resolve the conflict. Examples of such goal conflicts include the desire to lose weight coming into conflict with the desire to eat fattening french fries, or the goal of writing a chapter coming into conflict with the goal of reading and replying to e-mail. These forms of goal conflict require attention and resolution so that one can decide what to do and how best to meet long-term goals. In our affect alarm model of control, these types of goal conflicts quickly and automatically elicit negative affect, which serves as an alarm to alert us to possible goal failure and the need to remediate behavior.

We would like to clarify and put boundaries on three aspects of our thesis. First, we suggest that negative emotion, and not positive, acts as an alarm for self-control recruitment. Positive and negative events are both motivationally relevant and thus attract attention (Weinberg & Hajcak, 2010), but only negative events prompt change and remediation. This is because positive affect signals that goals are being met or even exceeded, whereas negative affect signals that goals are threatened and falling short (Carver & Scheier, 2011). So it is negative affect that does the signaling. To be even more specific, we suspect that the negative emotion that fosters self-control is anxiety, an aversive state characterized by vigilance, attention, and inhibition (Gray & McNaughton, 2000). Critically, anxiety is evoked by situations high in goal conflict and other forms of uncertainty (Hirsh, Mar, & Peterson, 2012), which are precisely the situations where self-control is required.

Second, we suggest that affect, rather than full-blown emotions, serves as the signal. Emotions are multifaceted, whole-body responses involving changes to conscious experience, behavior, and physiology that are slow to arise and slow to dissipate. Affect, on the other hand, has been conceptualized as a quick twinge or feeling that may not be conscious, arises very rapidly, possibly within fractions of a second, and may dissipate just as quickly (LeDoux, 1989; Winkielman & Berridge, 2004; Zajonc, 1980). Affect is more likely than full-blown emotions to signal the need for control because consciously experienced emotions are too slow and complex to be useful as self-control signals (see Baumeister, Vohs, DeWall, & Zhang, 2007). In fact, as the first half of this chapter observed, emotions can get in the way of good self-control. Affect, by contrast, is simple, rapid, and automatic and thus well suited to guide ongoing behavior.

Third, we suspect that the kind of control that is triggered by negative affect is inhibition. Researchers who study executive control divide this umbrella concept into smaller subcomponents, including maintaining, switching, and inhibiting (Miyake et al., 2000), and even planning and deciding (Zelazo & Cunningham, 2007). Although these subcomponents tend to tap the same central capacity, we suspect that negative affect most likely signals inhibitory processes. Inhibition involves suppressing or overriding prepotent responses and is triggered by the goal conflicts that produce negative affect (Gray & McNaughton, 2000). Thus, prior research has established a link between negative affect and behavioral inhibition. It is unclear, however, if the other components of executive control are similarly set into motion by negative affect.

Theoretical Models Incorporating Emotions in Self-Control

To make the case that emotion is central to the process of the self-control—that it signals the need for control—we first need to dismiss the notion that emotions are separable from, and unrelated to, cognition. For a number of reasons both historical and cultural, emotion has been considered the antithesis of reason (Solomon, 2008). Emotions are often cast as artifacts of an ancient animal past that hijacks otherwise rational, deliberative minds. The philosophical position of dualism represents a strong version of this view, stating that passionate, animalistic, physical bodies are wholly and completely separate from rational, conscious, nonphysical minds (Descartes, 1649/1989). With this view it is difficult to argue that emotions are an integral part of cognition and, by extension, part of self-control. However, most contemporary researchers do not view emotion and cognition as opposable or mutually exclusive constructs, with some suggesting that they are fully integrated and only minimally decomposable (e.g., Pessoa, 2008). Modern theories view emotions and cognition as interrelated (Frijda, 2008) and thus open the door to the idea that emotions may play a central function in cognition, including higher cognitive functions such as executive control. We now turn to theoretical support for the idea that emotions or affects play an integral role in self-control by signaling the need for control.

Cybernetic Models of Control

Cybernetic or feedback loop models have been very successful in modeling control in humans, but also in simple machines like thermostats. These models invariably identify control with three components: (1) goals/standards, (2) comparators/monitors, and (3) effectors/operators. *Goals/standards* are desired setpoints or criteria; *comparators/monitors* scan the current state of the environment to detect and alert for mismatches with goals and standards; and *effectors/operators* are called upon to make corrections to reduce the size of state–goal mismatches. When a goal or standard is set, control involves one process of monitoring when something shifts away from the criterion and a second process of returning this something to criterion. For example, if the goal is to finish writing a chapter, every glance at an e-mail inbox may trigger the monitoring system to sound the alarm that goal pursuit is going off course and to reorient goal pursuit.

Social and personality psychologists have elaborated upon this structure, postulating, for example, test versus operate mechanisms in action control (Carver & Scheier, 1981) or monitoring versus operating processes in thought control (Wegner, 1994). Similarly, neuroscientists have described cognitive control as relying on two separate neural systems. The first, described as a conflict-monitoring or error-detecting system (Botvinick, Braver, Barch, Carter, & Cohen, 2001; Gehring, Goss, Coles, Meyer, & Donchin, 1993; Holroyd & Coles, 2002), monitors ongoing behavior and detects discrepancies between intended and actual responses. When a discrepancy is detected, this information is passed to the second, regulatory or operating system, which implements the desired response while suppressing incompatible ones. Neuroimaging studies have suggested that these systems are implemented by the anterior cingulate cortex (ACC) and the prefrontal cortex (PFC), respectively (e.g., Kerns et al., 2004).

Although all three components (i.e., standards, monitors, and operators) are important, the monitoring process is fundamental to self-control because it alerts organisms to the need for control and remediation. If the function of the monitoring process sounds like the function we have postulated for negative affect, this is not an accident. Some theorists have hypothesized that the detection of state–goal mismatches is not affectively neutral; rather, mismatches can produce negative affect (Carver & Scheier, 1998, 2011). When people act on their goals and reduce the discrepancy between their goals and current states at an acceptable rate, they experience no affect or possibly positive affect. If, however, the rate of discrepancy reduction is stalled or otherwise too slow, people experience negative affect. This negative affect tends to hasten discrepancy reduction. Negative affect, in other words, can instigate control by orienting people to the fact that a discrepancy was detected and that discrepancy reduction is required.

Returning to our example, when one detects inadequate progress toward completing the goal of writing a chapter, a quick twinge of negative affect may arise and lead the author to correct behavior and once again focus on goal completion. The negative affect produced by the detection of goal–state mismatches can hasten self-control and correction and thereby prevent full-blow emotional reactions from occurring later, if and when the goal is not met. A little negative affect now can prevent a larger amount of negative emotion later.

Reinforcement Sensitivity Theory

According to the revised reinforcement sensitivity theory (RST; Corr, 2008; Gray & McNaughton, 2000), control of behavior depends on three underlying motivational systems. First, the behavioral activation system (BAS) is strongly related to approach motivation and actively increases sensitivity to appetitive stimuli that signal reward or nonpunishment (Carver & White, 1994; Gable & Harmon-Jones, 2008). Second is the fight–flight–freeze system (FFFS), which mediates reactions to aversive stimuli and is associated with avoidance and escape behaviors, with high sensitivity to negative cues. Third is the behavioral inhibition system (BIS), which is associated with anxiety, risk assessment, and worry and helps to resolve conflicts that arise within and between the other two systems. When BIS is activated, it inhibits current behavior to allow alternative response options to be reevaluated.

BIS is the most relevant to the current model. BIS can be conceptualized as the control system because the kinds of conflicts that activate BIS are precisely the kinds of conflicts that instigate inhibitory control. For example, the conflict between saving money for the future versus spending it right now would activate BIS, as would the conflict between reading a word or naming its color. In both cases, one response may be inhibited or suppressed, thereby allowing the second response to take precedence. As with cybernetic models, conflict detection and BIS activation are accompanied by negative affect, specifically anxiety (Gray & McNaughton, 2000). In fact, self-report measures of BIS are dominated by words such as *worry*, *fear*, and *nervousness* (Carver

& White, 1994). Goal conflict produces anxiety that then impels attempts to resolve those conflicts, which includes the inhibition of both approach (BAS) and avoidance (FFFS) behaviors, increases in arousal, and increases in vigilance, all of which stop current behaviors so that the organism can calculate the best course of action.

The point here is that according to revised RST, negative affect plays a prominent role in BIS and therefore in stopping ongoing behaviors so that an organism can reorient and establish control. Evidence suggests that high-trait BIS relates to indices of self-control, including brain-implemented performance monitoring (Amodio, Master, Yee, & Taylor, 2008; Boksem, Tops, Wester, Meijman, & Lorist, 2006), behavioral indices of inhibition (Avila & Parcet, 2001), and corrective behavioral adjustments under some conditions (Boksem, Tops, Kostermans, & De Cremer, 2008). We are quick to note, however, that the relationship between BIS and improved self-control may be restricted to sharp upticks in inhibitory states following phasic releases of noradrenaline (Aston-Jones & Cohen, 2005; Bouret & Sara, 2005), rather than more global trait differences in behavioral inhibition, which are related to improved attention control but also to difficulties with attentional disengagement (Poy, del Carmen Eixarch, & Avila, 2004).

Conflict Monitoring and Adaptive Control

Research in cognitive and affective neuroscience has shed light on how self-control is implemented in the brain. As we discussed above, a prominent theory in neuroscience, *conflict-monitoring theory*, posits that self-regulation relies on two separate neural systems (once goals are set): one for the detection of conflict between competing response tendencies and one that operates on these conflicts and implements control (Yeung, Botvinick, & Cohen, 2004). Conflict-monitoring theory suggests that the ACC plays an important role in monitoring moment-to-moment representations of action tendencies for potential conflicts. Upon detection of conflict, other mechanisms may be engaged to inhibit the unwanted tendency and promote effective goal pursuit. The conflict-monitoring function of the ACC, in other words, appears to signal when control is needed.

Then again, the ACC's signaling of control may be produced not only by the cold detection of conflict but also by the hot reaction to it. The ACC is involved in cognition and control as well as negative affect. For example, the ACC is involved in anxiety, depression, and trait-negative affect (Drevets et al., 1997; Hajcak, McDonald, & Simons, 2004), and is associated with the sympathetic modulation of heart rate (Critchley et al., 2003), skin conductance (Hajcak, McDonald, & Simons, 2003), autonomic control of pupil diameter (Critchley, Tang, Glaser, Butterworth, & Dolan, 2005), levels of basal cortisol (Tops & Boksem, 2011), pain (Rainville, Duncan, Price, Carrier, & Bushnell, 1997), and distress (Eisenberger & Lieberman, 2004).

Shackman and colleagues (2011), along with others (Critchley et al., 2003; Luu & Posner, 2003), have proposed that the anterior midcingulate cortex (aMCC) implements cognitive control by integrating negative affect, pain, and other forms of negative feedback with goal-directed behavior. According to their *adaptive control model* (Shackman et al., 2011), the core function common to negative affect, pain, and cognitive control is the need to determine an optimal course of action in the face of uncertainty. The aMCC is assumed to use affective information to select among alternative courses of action and to bias responding in situations characterized by uncertainty or conflict. Consistent with this view, we suggest that negative affect plays a crucial role in signaling the need for control. And we have found evidence that when negative affect is misattributed to other sources, the alarm function of affect is disabled and control becomes unhinged (Inzlicht & Al-Khindi, in press). The implication is that negative affect allows people to establish control by signaling what needs to be controlled and when.

Errors, Posterror Adjustment, and the Orienting Response

One of the hallmarks of good self-control is the minimization of errors during goal pursuit. By *errors* we mean instances when one fails to reach a standard or goal and instead succumbs to a prepotent response.

Self-control as the minimization of errors is easy to imagine on reaction time tasks such as the Stroop task, in which control is demonstrated by minimizing the number of times one mistakenly reads a word instead of naming its color. Good self-control is also evident whenever a person minimizes the number of times he or she reaches for unhealthy foods while wanting and trying to lose weight.

It turns out that one must notice and orient to errors when they occur to learn from and thereby minimize them. On reaction time tasks, people typically slow down and improve the accuracy of their performance after errors, displaying what researchers call *posterror slowing* or *posterror adjustment*, which is thought to reflect a strategic response to errors characterized by more careful and deliberate behavior to reduce the probability of further error commissions (Botvinick et al., 2001; Rabbitt & Rodgers, 1977). Posterror slowing may also reflect an orienting response to an infrequent event, which causes attentional capture and inhibits subsequent responses (Notebaert et al., 2009). In either case, people typically slow down after errors; and the more they do, the fewer errors they tend to make overall (e.g., Hajcak et al., 2003) and the better outcomes they experience more generally, including outcomes that reflect better self-control (e.g., Compton et al., 2008; Hirsh & Inzlicht, 2010; Robinson, 2007).

Errors thus lead people to take notice, change course, and reestablish control. But why do we notice and orient to them? The answer, we think, is that errors produce negative affect. Errors are not neutral events; rather, errors are distressing because of the negative consequences typically associated with them. Hajcak and colleagues (2003), for example, found that errors prompt rapid changes in autonomic arousal, including increased skin conductance and greater heart rate deceleration. Errors prompt more than an orienting response, however; they are also aversive and anxiety-inducing, with larger startle reflexes—an index of defensiveness—after errors than after correct responses (Hajcak & Foti, 2008). The more aroused people become after they make errors, the fewer errors they tend to make overall (Hajcak et al., 2003). In short, noticing errors contributes to adaptive con-

trol, and the reason people notice errors to begin with is because errors are arousing and aversive. So, here is more evidence that negative affect, in this case, affect associated with errors, signals the need for remediation and control.

Somatic Marker Hypothesis

The final theory we discuss shares a number of features with our own affect alarm model of control. According to Damasio (1994), emotional processes guide and bias behavior, specifically decision-making behavior. This hypothesis emerged in response to a number of observations of neurological patients with focal lesions to "emotional" parts of the brain, namely ventral and medial prefrontal regions. These patients exhibited severe deficits in personal and social decision making, but otherwise exhibited largely intact intellectual abilities (Damasio, 1996). Furthermore, these patients had compromised abilities to express emotion and experience feelings in situations in which emotions would normally have been expected. In other words, along with normal intellect and abnormal decision making, there were abnormalities in emotion and feeling. Damasio (1994, 1996) predicted and later confirmed that the deficits in emotions and feelings directly contributed to these patients' deficits in decision making.

The somatic marker hypothesis states that when we make decisions, we assess the reward value of the available options using both cognitive and emotional processes. When facing complex and conflicting choices, we may be unable to decide using only cognitive processes, which may become overloaded and hence ineffective at guiding decision making. In these cases emotions, or somatic markers, can help by directing attention to more advantageous options and simplifying the decision process (Damasio, 1994). In short, this view suggests that emotions help guide decision making by biasing behavior toward one or more of the response options based on past learning and associations.

The notion that emotions adaptively bias decision making is consistent with our own affect alarm model of self-control, especially insofar as decision making also belongs under the umbrella of self-control (Vohs et al., 2008; Zelazo & Cunningham, 2007). Control is important for decision making, and when control is absent, decision making suffers (Masicampo & Baumeister, 2008). So here is more evidence that emotion aids control, albeit control in the service of making effective decisions. Interestingly, others researchers have found that the same kind of lesion patients that inspired Damasio's somatic marker hypothesis also show deficits in inhibiting previously learned associations (e.g., Rolls, Hornak, Wade, & McGrath, 1994). Emotions, then, seem integral not only for making decisions but also for inhibition. It is important to note that our own model deviates from the somatic marker hypothesis by stressing negatively valenced affect—the quick, automatic form of emotion—and the inhibitory form of control.

Summary and Predictions

We are making only one claim: that emotion, possibly the negative emotion of anxiety and possibly only short-lived, preconscious anxious affect, acts as a kind of alarm that orients people to when self-control is needed. Emotions direct people to motivationally relevant information, and there may be nothing quite as motivating as facing uncertainty about what to do and how to do it, precisely the same kinds of situations where self-control is needed to bias responding in favor of one course of action over another. When we face uncertainty about how to act because goals or response tendencies come into conflict with one another, we have an anxious affective response that directs us to resolve these conflicts by inhibiting ongoing behavior until we settle on a course of action (Gray & McNaughton, 2000).

We have already mentioned that the affect alarm model is largely theoretical at this point, and thus somewhat preliminary. Nonetheless, the model makes a number of predictions that allow it to be distinguished from other theories, including predictions that have now been empirically supported. Space constraints prevent us from listing all predictions and empirical support, so we give only a small sample of them here.

Given the importance of affect in alerting us to the need for control, the affect alarm model of control predicts that temporary increases in integral affect should enhance self-control. A recent study by Moser, Most, and Simons (2010) lends support to this view. When participants in this study "upregulated" their negative emotions, they experienced both more negative affect and improvements in control, suggesting that negative affect helps to enhance cognitive control.

Negative affect is not enough, however; the affect alarm model suggests that people need to attribute their affect to the correct source; otherwise, negative affect will be unmoored from the instigating event (e.g., goal conflict) and will not appropriately alert people to the need for self-control. A recent study supports this view (Inzlicht & Al-Khindi, in press): When people incorrectly attributed the natural, albeit mild, anxiety produced by taking an executive control task, the brain signals related to performance monitoring ceased predicting cognitive control. Self-control, in other words, is thrown off course without negative affect acting as a guide.

The affect alarm model of control further predicts that people who are attuned and aware of their own affective states will show enhanced self-control. Conversely, people who are unaware of their emotions or have difficulty identifying and differentiating between them should show marked decrements in self-control. *Alexithymia* refers to deficiencies in identifying and differentiating emotions, and preliminary research suggests that alexithymia is associated with executive function deficits (Henry, Phillips, Crawford, Theodorou, & Summers, 2006).

In addition to emotional awareness, emotional acceptance may also be important for prompting self-control. Those who acknowledge and approve of their feelings—as opposed to those who judge, reject, and suppress them—may be more inclined to "listen" to what their emotions are trying to say and, as a result, be better attuned to when self-control is required. In support of this view, new research indicates that people who practice mindful meditation show enhanced executive control and enhanced brain-implemented performance monitoring (Teper & Inzlicht, in press). Together, these findings indicate that emotional awareness and acceptance play key roles in improving self-control and are consistent with the affect alarm model of control. Future studies will need to move beyond correlational designs to explore if state enhancements in emotional awareness and acceptance improve self-control.

Integrating Research on the Incidental and Integral Effects of Emotions on Self-Control

Before concluding, we would like to issue a call for future research to integrate the literatures on the incidental and integral effects of emotions on self-control. If subtle twinges of negative affect trigger self-control, as we have proposed, then how do full-blown, conscious emotional states influence these twinges? Why, if negative affect triggers self-control, do full-blown negative emotions tend to impair rather than improve dieting and delay of gratification?

One possibility is that full-blown negative emotions (including long-term negative emotional states such as depression) overwhelm the subtler affective signals that cue the need for self-control. When a person experiences fear at the prospect of receiving an electric shock or receives negative feedback challenging his or her most cherished self-views, perhaps the conflict between consuming fatty foods and sticking to a diet recedes in importance or fails to trigger control because the relevant mechanisms are preoccupied with the more pressing, more intense emotional context. This hypothesis is speculative, but experiments testing it promise to elucidate the relationship between emotions and self-control.

And how do positive emotions alter the affect alarm bell for self-control? One possibility is that, under the influence of positive emotional states, response conflicts cause less or weaker negative affect. In this view, self-control is less likely to occur under positive emotional states because the alarm bell rings too softly. As we saw, however, positive emotions sometimes enhance self-control (particularly in children), so this view is not wholly satisfying. Much more research is needed on the relationship between positive emotions and self-control, particularly as this relates to the affect alarm model we have proposed. As a second possibility, per-haps highly arousing emotions of either positive or negative valence can drown out the affect alarm system, making self-control less likely. Insofar as both positive and negative emotions can disrupt delay of gratification, arousal may help to explain the patterns.

In conclusion, we have reviewed evidence that incidental emotional states are powerful determinants of self-control outcomes, and we have proposed that negative affect can be seen as an integral component of the process of self-control. Research and theory on the integral versus incidental effects of emotions on self-control have lived largely separate lives, much like they did in this chapter. It is high time to integrate them, as the integration promises a more complete picture of the role of emotions in shaping self-control.

References

Amodio, D., Master, S., Yee, C., & Taylor, S. (2008). Neurocognitive components of the behavioral inhibition and activation systems: Implications for theories of self-regulation. *Psychophysiology*, 45, 11–19.

Ariely, D., & Loewenstein, G. (2006). The heat of the moment: The effect of sexual arousal on sexual decision making. *Journal of Behavioral Decision Making*, 19, 87–98.

Aston-Jones, G., & Cohen, J. (2005). An integrative theory of locus coeruleus–norepinephrine function: Adaptive gain and optimal performance. *Annual Review of Neuroscience*, 28, 403–450.

Augustine, A. A., & Larsen, R. J. (2011). Affect regulation and temporal discounting: Interactions between primed, state, and trait affect. *Emotion*, 11, 391–402.

Avila, C., Parcet, M. A. (2001). Personality and inhibitory deficits in the stop-signal task: The mediating role of Gray's anxiety and impulsivity. *Personality and Individual Differences*, 31, 975–986.

Baumeister, R. F., & Heatherton, T. F. (1996). Self-regulation failure: An overview. *Psychological Inquiry*, 7, 1–15.

Baumeister, R. F., Vohs, K. D., DeWall, C. N., & Zhang, L. (2007). How emotion shapes behavior: Feedback, anticipation, and reflection, rather than direct causation. *Personality and Social Psychology Review*, 11, 167–203.

Boksem, M. A. S., Tops, M., Kostermans, E., & De Cremer, D. (2008). Sensitivity to punishment and reward omission: Evidence from error-related ERP components. *Biological Psychology, 79,* 185–192.

Boksem, M. A. S., Tops, M., Wester, A. E., Meijman, T. F., & Lorist, M. M. (2006). Error related ERP components and individual differences in punishment and reward sensitivity. *Brain Research, 1101,* 92–101.

Botvinick, M., Braver, T., Barch, D., Carter, C., & Cohen, J. (2001). Conflict monitoring and cognitive control. *Psychological Review, 108,* 624–652.

Bouret, S., & Sara, S. J. (2005). Network reset: A simplified overarching theory of locus coeruleus noradrenaline function. *Trends in Neuroscience, 28,* 574–582.

Carver, C. S., & Scheier, M. F. (1981). *Attention and self-regulation: A control theory approach to human behavior.* New York: Springer-Verlag.

Carver, C. S., & Scheier, M. F. (1998). *On the self-regulation of behavior.* New York: Cambridge University Press.

Carver, C. S., & Scheier, M. F. (2011). Self-regulation of action and affect. In K. D. Vohs & R. F. Baumeister (Eds.), *Handbook of self-regulation: Research, theory, and applications* (2nd ed., pp. 3–21). New York: Guilford Press.

Carver, C. S., & White, T. L. (1994). Behavioral inhibition, behavioral activation, and affective responses to impending reward and punishment: The BIS/BAS scales. *Journal of Personality and Social Psychology, 67,* 319–333.

Compton, R. J., Robinson, M. D., Ode, S., Quandt, L. C., Fineman, S. L., & Carp, J. (2008). Error-monitoring ability predicts daily stress regulation. *Psychological Science, 19,* 702–708.

Cools, J., Schotte, D. E., & McNally, R. J. (1992). Emotional arousal and overeating in restrained eaters. *Journal of Abnormal Psychology, 101,* 348–351.

Corr, P. J. (2008). Reinforcement sensitivity theory (RST): Introduction. In P. J. Corr (Ed.), *The reinforcement sensitivity theory of personality* (pp. 1–43). Cambridge, UK: Cambridge University Press.

Critchley, H. D., Mathias, C. J., Josephs, O., O'Doherty, J., Zanini, S., Dewar, B.-K., et al. (2003). Human cingulate cortex and autonomic control: Converging neuroimaging and clinical evidence. *Brain, 126,* 2139–2152.

Critchley, H. D., Tang, J., Glaser, D., Butterworth, B., & Dolan, R. J. (2005). Anterior cingulate activity during error and autonomic response. *NeuroImage, 27,* 885–895.

Damasio, A. R. (1994). *Descartes' error: Emotion, reason and the human brain.* New York: Grosset/Putnam.

Damasio, A. R. (1996). The somatic marker hypothesis and the possible functions of the prefrontal cortex. *Proceedings of the Royal Society of London, 351,* 1413–1420.

Descartes, R. (1989). *On the passions of the soul* (S. Voss, Trans.). Indianapolis, IN: Hackett. (Original work published 1649)

Dingemans, A. E., Martijn, C., Jansen, A. T., & von Furth, E. F. (2009). The effect of suppressing negative emotions on eating behavior in binge eating disorder. *Appetite, 52,* 51–57.

Drevets, W. C., Price, J. L., Simpson, J. R., Todd, R. D., Reich, T., Vannier, M., et al. (1997). Subgenual prefrontal cortex abnormalities in mood disorders. *Letters to Nature, 386,* 824–827.

Eisenberger, N. I., & Lieberman, M. D. (2004). Why rejection hurts: A common neural alarm system for physical and social pain. *Trends in Cognitive Sciences, 8,* 294–300.

Fedorikhin, A., & Patrick, V. M. (2010). Positive mood and resistance to temptation: The interfering influence of elevated arousal. *Journal of Consumer Research, 37,* 698–711.

Frijda, N. H. (1988). The laws of emotion. *American Psychologist, 43,* 349–358.

Frijda, N. H. (2008). The psychologist's point of view. In M. Lewis, J. M. Havilland-Jones, & L. Feldman Barrett (Eds.), *Handbook of emotions* (3rd ed., pp. 68–87). New York: Guilford Press.

Fry, P. S. (1975). Affect and resistance to temptation. *Developmental Psychology, 11,* 466–427.

Fry, P. S. (1977). Success, failure, and resistance to temptation. *Developmental Psychology, 13,* 519–520.

Gable, P. A., & Harmon-Jones, E. (2008). Relative left frontal activation to appetitive stimuli: Considering the role of individual differences. *Psychophysiology, 45,* 275–278.

Gehring, W. J., Goss, B., Coles, M. G. H., Meyer, D. E., & Donchin, E. (1993). A neural system for error detection and compensation. *Psychological Science, 4,* 385–390.

Gray, J. A., & McNaughton, N. (2000). *The neuropsychology of anxiety: An enquiry into the functions of the septo-hippocampal sys-*

tem (2nd ed.). Oxford, UK: Oxford University Press.

Gray, J. R. (1999). A bias toward short-term thinking in threat-related negative emotional states. *Personality and Social Psychology Bulletin, 25,* 65–75.

Greeno, G. C., & Wing, R. R. (1994). Stress-induced eating. *Psychological Bulletin, 115,* 444–464.

Haedt-Matt, A. A., & Keel, P. K. (2011). Revisiting the affect regulation model of binge eating: A meta-analysis of studies using ecological momentary assessment. *Psychological Bulletin, 137,* 660–681.

Hajcak, G., & Foti, D. (2008). Errors are aversive: Defensive motivation and the error-related negativity. *Psychological Science, 19,* 103–108.

Hajcak, G., McDonald, N., & Simons, R. F. (2003). To err is autonomic: Error-related brain potentials, ANS activity, and post-error compensatory behavior. *Psychophysiology, 40,* 895–903.

Hajcak, G., McDonald, N., & Simons, R. F. (2004). Error-related psychophysiology and negative affect. *Brain and Cognition, 56,* 189–197.

Heatherton, T. F., Herman, C. P., & Polivy, J. (1991). The effects of physical threat and ego threat on eating. *Journal of Personality and Social Psychology, 60,* 138–143.

Heatherton, T. F., Striepe, M., & Wittenberg, L. (1998). Emotional distress and disinhibited eating: The role of self. *Personality and Social Psychology Bulletin, 24,* 301–313.

Henry, J. D., Phillips, L. H., Crawford, J. R., Theodorou, G., & Summers, F. (2006). Cognitive and psychosocial correlates of alexithymia following traumatic brain injury. *Neuropsychologia, 44,* 62–72.

Herman, C. P., & Mack, D. (1975). Restrained and unrestrained eating. *Journal of Personality, 43,* 647–660.

Herman, C. P., & Polivy, J. (1975). Anxiety, restraint, and eating behavior. *Journal of Abnormal Psychology, 84,* 666–672.

Hirsh, J. B., Guindon, A., Morisano, D., & Peterson, J. B. (2010). Positive mood effects on delay discounting. *Emotion, 10,* 717–721.

Hirsh, J. B., & Inzlicht, M. (2010). Error-related negativity predicts academic performance. *Psychophysiology, 47,* 192–196.

Hirsh, J. B., Mar, R., & Peterson, J. B. (2012). Psychological entropy: A framework for understanding uncertainty-related anxiety. *Psychological Review, 119,* 304–320.

Holroyd, C. B., & Coles, M. G. H. (2002). The neural basis of human error processing: Reinforcement learning, dopamine, and the error-related negativity. *Psychological Review, 109,* 679–709.

Inzlicht, M., & Al-Khindi, T. (in press). ERN and the placebo: A misattribution approach to studying the arousal properties of the error-related negativity. *Journal of Experimental Psychology: General.*

Kerns, J. G., Cohen, J. D., MacDonald, A. W., Cho, R. Y., Stenger, V. A., & Carter, C. S. (2004). Anterior cingulate conflict monitoring and adjustments in control. *Science, 303,* 1023–1026.

Knapp, A., & Clark, M. S. (1991). Some detrimental effects of negative mood on individuals' ability to solve resource dilemmas. *Personality and Social Psychology Bulletin, 17,* 678–688.

Lang, P. J., Bradley, M. M., & Cuthbert, B. N. (2008). *International affective picture system (IAPS): Affective ratings of pictures and instruction manual* (Technical Report A-8). Gainesville, FL: University of Florida.

LeDoux, J. E. (1989). Cognitive–emotional interactions in the brain. *Cognition and Emotion, 3,* 267–289.

Leith, K. P., & Baumeister, R. F. (1996). Why do bad moods increase self-defeating behavior?: Emotion, risk taking, and self-regulation. *Journal of Personality and Social Psychology, 71,* 1250–1267.

Luu, P., & Posner, M. I. (2003). Anterior cingulate regulation of sympathetic activity. *Brain, 126,* 2119–2020.

Macht, M. (2008). How emotions affect eating: A five-way model. *Appetite, 50,* 1–11.

Macht, M., Roth, S., & Ellgring, H. (2002). Chocolate eating in healthy men during experimentally induced sadness and joy. *Appetite, 39,* 147–158.

Masicampo, E. J., & Baumeister, R. F. (2008). Toward a physiology of dual-process reasoning and judgment: Lemonade, willpower, and effortful rule-based analysis. *Psychological Science, 19,* 255–260.

Mischel, W., Ebbesen, E. B., & Zeiss, A. R. (1972). Cognitive and attentional mechanisms in delay of gratification. *Journal of Personality and Social Psychology, 21,* 204–218.

Miyake, A., Friedman, N. P., Emerson, M. J.,

Witzki, A. H., & Howerter, A. (2000). The unity and diversity of executive functions and their contributions to complex "frontal lobe" tasks: A latent variable analysis. *Cognitive Psychology, 41,* 49–100.

Moore, B. S., Clyburn, A., & Underwood, B. (1976). The role of affect in delay of gratification. *Child Development, 47,* 273–276.

Moser, J. S., Most, S. B., & Simons, R. F. (2010). Increasing negative emotions by reappraisal enhances subsequent cognitive control: A combined behavioral and electrophysiology study. *Cognitive Affective and Behavioral Neuroscience, 10,* 195–207.

Notebaert, W., Houtman, F., Opstal, F. V., Gevers, W., Fias, W., & Verguts, T. (2009). Post-error slowing: An orienting account. *Cognition, 111,* 275–279.

Perry, L. C., Perry, D. G., & English, D. (1985). Happiness: When does it lead to self-indulgence and when does it lead to self-denial? *Journal of Experimental Child Psychology, 39,* 203–211.

Pessoa, L. (2008). On the relationship between emotion and cognition. *Nature Reviews Neuroscience, 9,* 148–158.

Polivy, J., Herman, C. P., & McFarlane, T. (1994). Effects of anxiety on eating: Does palatability moderate distress-induced overeating in dieters? *Journal of Abnormal Psychology, 103,* 505–510.

Poy, R., del Carmen Eixarch, M., & Avila, C. (2004). On the relationship between attention and personality: Covert visual orienting of attention in anxiety and impulsivity. *Personality and Individual Differences, 36,* 1471–1481.

Rabbitt, P. M. A., & Rodgers, B. (1977). What does a man do after he makes an error?: An analysis of response programming. *Quarterly Journal of Experimental Psychology, 29,* 727–743.

Rainville, P., Duncan, G. H., Price, D. D., Carrier, B., & Bushnell, M. C. (1997). Pain affect encoded in human anterior cingulate but not somatosensory cortex. *Science, 277,* 968–971.

Robinson, M. D. (2007). Gassing, braking, and self-regulation: Error self-regulation, well-being, and goal-related processes. *Journal of Experimental Social Psychology, 43,* 1–16.

Rolls, E. T., Hornak, J., Wade, D., & McGrath, J. (1994). Emotion-related learning in patients with social and emotional changes associated with frontal lobe damage. *Journal of Neurology, Neurosurgery, and Psychiatry, 57,* 1518–1524.

Ruderman, A. J. (1985). Dysphoric mood and overeating: A test of restraint theory's disinhibition hypothesis. *Journal of Abnormal Psychology, 94,* 78–85.

Schachter, S. (1968). Obesity and eating. *Science, 161,* 751–756.

Schachter, S., Goldman, R., & Gordon, A. (1968). Effects of fear, food deprivation, and obesity on eating. *Journal of Personality and Social Psychology, 10,* 91–97.

Schwarz, J. C., & Pollack, P. R. (1977). Affect and delay of gratification. *Journal of Research in Personality, 11,* 147–164.

Schwarz, N., & Clore, G. L. (1983). Mood, misattribution, and judgments of well-being: Informative and directive functions of affective states. *Journal of Personality and Social Psychology, 45,* 513–523.

Seeman, G. J., & Schwarz, C. (1974). Affective state and preference for immediate versus delayed reward. *Journal of Research in Personality, 7,* 384–394.

Shackman, A. J., Salomons, T. V., Slagter, H. A., Fox, A. S., Winter, J. J., & Davidson, R. J. (2011). The integration of negative affect, pain and cognitive control in the cingulate cortex. *Nature Reviews Neuroscience, 12,* 154–167.

Solomon, R. C. (2008). The philosophy of emotions. In M. Lewis, J. M. Havilland-Jones, & L. Feldman Barrett (Eds.), *Handbook of emotions* (3rd ed., pp. 3–16). New York: Guilford Press.

Tamir, M. (2009). What do people want to feel and why?: Pleasure and utility in emotion regulation. *Current Directions in Psychological Science, 18,* 101–105.

Teper, R., & Inzlicht, M. (in press). Meditation, mindfulness, and executive control: The importance of emotional acceptance and brain-based performance monitoring. *Social Cognitive Affective Neuroscience.*

Tice, D. M., Bratslavsky, E., & Baumeister, R. F. (2001). Emotional distress regulation takes precedence over impulse control: If you feel bad, do it! *Journal of Personality and Social Psychology, 80,* 53–67.

Tops, M., & Boksem, M. A. S. (2011). Cortisol involvement in mechanisms of behavioural inhibition. *Psychophysiology, 48,* 723–732.

Vohs, K. D., & Baumeister, R. F. (Eds.). (2011).

Handbook of self-regulation: Research, theory, and applications (2nd ed.). New York: Guilford Press.

Vohs, K. D., Baumeister, R. F., Schmeichel, B. J., Twenge, J. M., Tice, D. M., & Nelson, N. M. (2008). Making choices impairs subsequent self-control: A limited resource account of decision making, self-regulation, and active initiative. *Journal of Personality and Social Psychology, 94,* 883–898.

Wallis, D. J., & Hetherington, M. M. (2004). Stress and eating: The effects of ego-threat and cognitive demand on food intake in restrained and emotional eaters. *Appetite, 43,* 39–46.

Wallis, D. J., & Hetherington, M. M. (2009). Emotions and eating: Self-reported and experimentally induced changes in food intake under stress. *Appetite, 52,* 355–362.

Wegner, D. M. (1994). Ironic processes of mental control. *Psychological Review, 101,* 34–52.

Weinberg, A., & Hajcak, G. (2010). Beyond good and evil: Implications of examining electrocortical activity elicited by specific picture content. *Emotion, 10,* 767–782.

Wertheim, E. H., & Schwarz, J. C. (1983). Depression, guilt, and self-management of pleasant and unpleasant events. *Journal of Personality and Social Psychology, 45,* 884–889.

Wilcox, K., Kramer, T., & Sen, S. (2011). Indulgence or self-control: A dual process model of the effect of incidental pride on indulgent choice. *Journal of Consumer Research, 38,* 151–163.

Wilson, M., & Daly, M. (2004). Do pretty women inspire men to discount the future? *Proceedings of the Royal Society of London, Series B: Biological Sciences, 271,* 177–179.

Winkielman, P., & Berridge, K. C. (2004). Unconscious emotion. *Current Directions in Psychological Science, 13,* 120–123.

Yates, G. C. R., Lippett, R. M. K., & Yates, S. M. (1981). The effects of age, positive affect induction, and instructions on children's delay of gratification. *Journal of Experimental Child Psychology, 32,* 169–180.

Yeomans, M. R., & Coughlan, E. (2009). Mood-induced eating: Interactive effects of restraint and tendency to overeat. *Appetite, 52,* 290–298.

Yeung, N., Botvinick, M. M., & Cohen, J. D. (2004). The neural basis of error-detection: Conflict monitoring and the error-related negativity. *Psychological Review, 111,* 931–959.

Zajonc, R. (1980). Feeling and thinking: Preferences need no inferences. *American Psychologist, 35,* 151–175.

Zelazo, P. D., & Cunningham, W. A. (2007). Executive function: Mechanisms underlying emotion regulation. In J. J. Gross (Ed.), *Handbook of emotion regulation* (pp. 135–158). New York: Guilford Press.

PART V

INDIVIDUAL DIFFERENCES

CHAPTER 16

The Developmental Polyphony
of Cognition and Emotion

Ross A. Thompson and Abby C. Winer

The interaction between cognition and emotion has long had a unique place in emotions research. Although psychologists agree that they are intimately associated, the field becomes easily polarized by debate over their interaction. Like the nature–nurture debate, these disagreements endure because they tap iconic issues in Western culture concerning human nature: the conflict between the affective and cerebral sides of human experience, the need for rational control over irrational impulses, and the dangers of unrestrained feeling (e.g., see Dalgleish & Power, 1999; De Houwer & Hermans, 2010; Eich, Kihlstrom, Bower, Forgas, & Niedenthal, 2000; Power & Dalgleish, 2008).

Another characteristic of the longstanding debate about the interaction of cognition and emotion is that it tends to lack a developmental orientation. Research and theory typically focus on how affective and mental processes function in maturity rather than studying the origins of their interaction, and one cannot find more than one developmentally oriented chapter in recent volumes on cognition and emotion. Fresh attention to the contributions of a developmental analysis may be warranted, however. Because both cognitive processing and emotional responding mature very rapidly in the early years, a developmental perspective is essential to understanding how these dual aspects of human functioning become intertwined as they develop. Research in developmental neuroscience may provide important contributions to this understanding. Furthermore, a developmental orientation puts some classic issues (e.g., does emotion require cognition?) in a new light, raises new questions about the mutual influences of cognition and emotion, and highlights processes that contribute to their developing interaction that might be otherwise overlooked.

This chapter is concerned with the developing polyphony between emotion and cognition. We use a musical term to denote the distinct character and increasingly complex interplay (sometimes harmoniously, sometimes dissonantly) between emotion and cognition that comes with growth. Developmental work on this topic involves much more than studying the growth of emotion understanding and cognitive appraisals related to emotional arousal. It also includes the emotional processes by which early social cognition develops, the emotional signals by which infants and children evaluate new events, the growth of self-conscious emotions and their effects on self-awareness, the influence of emotion on cognitive achievement, and many other topics. Because this developmental perspective is so rich, our coverage is selective. Interested readers can learn more from a recent volume devoted to developmental perspectives on the cognition–emotion interaction (Calkins & Bell, 2010) and from more classic sources (e.g., Izard, Kagan, & Zajonc, 1984).

Our discussion begins with an outline of the developmental–functionalist approach that guides work in this area, emphasizing the value of a developmental orientation within the context of functionalist emotions theory. We then turn to research illustrations of the developing interaction between cognition and emotion, with an emphasis on those that highlight new ways of thinking about the mutual influences of thinking and feeling at various periods of development. The third section concerns the importance of early experience, particularly in caregiving relationships, as an organizer of cognition–emotion interaction, and some of the processes by which relationships have the effects they do. The chapter ends with concluding reflections on this enduring theme.

A Developmental– Functionalist Perspective

Why is a developmental approach important to understanding the interaction of cognition and emotion? A developmental orientation recognizes that both cognition and emotion begin maturing very early, that they are mutually influential as they develop, and that the growth of each is affected by a variety of other developmental influences, including the quality of early experiences. Consequently, the interaction of emotion with cognition is inherent in how these dual aspects of human functioning mature. A developmental approach thus challenges some of the polarities by which cognition and emotion have been characterized— rational versus irrational, organizational versus disorganizational, regulated versus unregulated, reflective versus impulsive— and which have contributed to longstanding debate about their interaction. Instead, by highlighting the mutual influences of emotion and cognition from early in life, a developmental interactionist perspective underscores that "pure" emotion or cognition exist more often in the theorist's mindset than in the nature of human functioning, and that elucidating the developing interaction of cognition and emotion is an essential way of understanding both.

Neuroscience has been an important contributor to this viewpoint. Neuroimaging studies show, for example, that responses to emotion tasks are widely distributed throughout the brain, including activation of areas commonly regarded as central to emotion (e.g., the amygdala and hypothalamus) and to cognition (including areas of the frontal and prefrontal cortex) (Kober et al., 2008). In a meta-analysis of 162 neuroimaging studies of responses to emotion tasks, Kober and colleagues (2008) reported that these limbic and cortical regions are typically *coactive*, suggesting the involvement of basic perceptual, attentional, and mnemonic processes in emotion activation. Other researchers, using functional magnetic resonance imaging (fMRI), have also reported results indicating that multiple cognitive processes are activated simultaneously with emotion systems in response to affective probes (e.g., Ochsner et al., 2009). Cognitive processes are likewise influenced by the coactivity of emotional responses. Neuroimaging studies suggest that affective representations are important, for example, to perceptual sensitivity, object identification, and other cognitive functions (Feldman Barrett & Bar, 2009; Ochsner et al., 2009; Surguladze et al., 2003). Neuroscience research suggests, therefore, that rather than functioning in mutually inhibitory or in antecedent–consequent associations, the brain regions associated with multiple cognitive and emotive processes are coordinative.

Developmental research helps to explain how these interactions emerge and, in particular, the importance of early experiences as organizers of cognition–emotion interactions. Consider, for example, children who have experienced abuse or neglect. Children living in contexts of chronic stress develop hyperreactive neurobiological stress response systems that cause them to overreact to cues of threat or danger, which may develop as an adaptive response to the need to prepare for challenging events before they occur (Gunnar, Fisher, & the Early Experience, Stress, and Prevention Network, 2006; Gunnar & Vasquez, 2006). The cognitive and perceptual appraisals of maltreated children also make them hypersensitive to adult expressions of anger, although not to other adult negative emotional expressions. In one study, for example, when pictures of adult facial expressions of emotion were progressively "morphed" from one prototypical expression (e.g., sadness) to another (e.g., anger), maltreated children were more likely to identify blended expressions as angry than were nonmaltreated children (Pollak, 2002; Pollak & Kistler, 2002). Abused and neglected children exhibit a lower attentional threshold for detecting anger in the vocal expressions of their mothers (but not of an unfamiliar woman) (Shackman & Pollak, 2005) and have more difficulty attentionally disengaging from perceived angry cues (Pollak & Tolley-Schell, 2003). In a study using event-related brain potentials (ERPs), maltreated children showed higher ERP responses to pictures of angry facial expressions compared to nonabused children, but there were no differences in their responses to pictures of happy or fearful expressions (Pollak, Klorman, Thatcher, & Cicchetti, 2001). Taken together, these studies suggest that antecedent experiences of aberrant care contribute to the development of perceptual biases, altered cognitive appraisals and attentional focusing, and poorly regulated emotional responding that are, together, tied to changes in neurobiological functioning associated with chronic adversity (see Pollak, 2008). These sequelae of maltreatment increase risk for the development of affective psychopathology, with developmental changes in appraisals, emotion regulation, and social-cognitive processes moderating risk status (Thompson, 2010, 2011b; Thompson & Goodman, 2010)

This research is one of many examples of the developing organization of cognition–emotion interactions associated with early experiences. These studies suggest that there are many ways that emotional arousal and cognitive processes are mutually influential as they mature throughout the early years. They include (1) the influence of emotion on perceptual and attentional biases and cognitive appraisals, both immediate and enduring; (2) how typical or atypical cognitive appraisals alter thresholds for emotional arousal, both situationally and chronically; and (3) the effects of emotional arousal on cognitive functioning, such as memory retrieval and perceptual reappraisal, including emotion-related cognitive processes associated with emotion regulation. Although current work in developmental neuroscience suggests that some of these bidirectional

interactions between emotional and cognitive development derive from common neurobiological influences, research on brain development is still at an early stage to fully inform developmental study of cognition–emotion interactions. However, because of the rapid pace and scope of early brain development, there is reason to believe that early experiences are important not only because they contribute to the initial organization of cognition–emotion associations, but also because that initial organization may endure over time. This owes both to the early plasticity of the developing brain, and also because of how perceptual biases, attentional fixation, memory retrieval, emotion thresholds, and self-regulatory processes become mutually reinforcing and thus self-perpetuating as they are incorporated into neural networks. Research on maltreated children and other children at risk offers powerful evidence for these influences.

Functionalist Emotions Theory

The intimate connection between emotion and cognition and its developing organization is readily understood in the context of functionalist emotions theory (Frijda, 1987; Saarni, Campos, Camras, & Witherington, 2006). According to the functionalist view, emotions are fundamentally defined by their association with an organism's goals and their attainment. Emotions not only reflect success or failure in goal achievement, but are also related to changing or maintaining relations between the organism and the environment in ways relevant to these goals. The emotion of anger, for example, is associated with one's goals being blocked, and the action tendencies of anger are directed toward removing the obstacle(s) in order to better achieve the goal. Functionalist approaches thus emphasize the motivational qualities of different emotions, the importance of emotional expressions as social signals (not necessarily as direct reflections of underlying feelings), and the association between emotional arousal and how a person appraises the meaning of environmental events in relation to those goals.

Throughout psychological development, the goal structure of behavior changes and in association with developmental changes in emotional experience (Thompson, 2011a).

Early in life, for example, emotional behavior changes with the growth of means–ends understanding, development of self-produced locomotion, and other advances that enhance the infant's goal-directed behavior. As a result, there is an increase in petulance and anger, especially when the infant's intentions are thwarted (Campos et al., 2000; see also Hendrix & Thompson, 2011). With the growth of psychological understanding in the preschool years, young children connect their emotional experience more self-consciously with the satisfaction or frustration of their desires because of their explicit awareness of the connection between emotions, desires, and intentions (Thompson & Goodvin, 2007). With increasing age, the goals associated with emotional arousal become more socially and psychologically complex and increasingly colored by sociocultural values, including moral obligations, emotional rules of the culture, and concerns with social standing and status (Thompson, 2011a). From the perspective of functionalist emotions theory, therefore, cognition–emotion associations change developmentally with changes in the goal orientation of behavior and the appraisals associated with them.

In practical circumstances, of course, multiple goals simultaneously influence behavioral and emotional responding. Classic studies of delay of gratification in young children illustrate the consequences of competing immediate and long-term goals and that growth in self-regulatory capacities changes how children respond (e.g., Mischel, Shoda, & Rodriguez, 1989). Conflicting immediate and long-term goals can also influence emotional behavior, such as the blended and ambivalent reactions of anger, fear, and distress in a child who has been threatened by a peer, and who must balance immediate goals of coping and self-defense with longer-term goals of avoiding future conflict. In such circumstances, competing goals and goal-related appraisals influence a child's emotions and emotion self-regulation, contributing to responses that may not be optimal.

For children in adversity, the emotional consequences of multiple, conflicting goals may be profound. As earlier noted, the hypersensitivity of maltreated children to adult anger and their biological hyperre-sponsiveness to cues of threat and danger pose long-term risks for healthy emotional development. But these appraisals and emotion responses develop to accomplish the immediate objective of preparing for an adult's attack before it occurs, despite their long-term disadvantages. Similar dilemmas can also be observed in children who are exposed to chronic marital conflict (Davies & Woitach, 2008). Young children who are at risk for the development of anxiety disorders also face biological vulnerabilities affecting their goals and appraisals of threat and danger. A high proportion of at-risk children are temperamentally inhibited and show other qualities that reflect a genetic proneness to fear and anxiety, including heightened neuroendocrine reactivity to novel stressors (Fox, Henderson, Marshall, Nichols, & Ghera, 2005; Gunnar & Vasquez, 2006). Consistent with this finding, these children also show hypervigilance in situations associated with fearful events, attentional orienting to anxiety-provoking stimuli, and a tendency to construe benign situations as disproportionately negative or threatening (Fox et al., 2005; Thompson, 2001). These appraisal and preappraisal processes develop to accomplish the immediate goal of avoiding anxiety-provoking events, even though doing so often has dysfunctional long-term consequences. By the time a young child has been clinically referred, biological vulnerability has contributed to self-reinforcing patterns of appraisal and emotion that are calibrated to the immediate goal of fear avoidance but have coalesced to create heightened risk for affective psychopathology.

A developmental–functionalist perspective thus offers many contributions to understanding cognition–emotion interactions. Fundamentally, it elucidates the many complex ways that cognition and emotion are interactive from the beginning of life. Moreover, it situates this interaction within the context of many other developmental processes that influence thinking and feeling, including changing behavioral capabilities, neurobiological growth, changing goal orientations, developing psychological understanding, and temperamental individuality. In addition, a developmental–functionalist perspective highlights the importance of early experiences not only because of the plasticity of early brain and behavioral systems, but also because of how early experiences contribute to developing interactions between cognition and emotion that may become consolidated over time. As we consider later in this chapter, a central feature of early experiences is the quality of adult–child relationships. Finally, a developmental–functionalist perspective underscores that, because of these processes, it is best to consider cognition and emotion as intersecting behavioral and neurobiological systems, not as independent processes that later connect. In doing so, this perspective argues that the more interesting approach is how early this interaction emerges and how it develops over time.

Cognition–Emotion Interactions in Development

With these conceptual foundations, we profile several examples of developing cognition–emotion interactions in this section. Our purpose is to illustrate, through these different profiles, some of the ways that cognition and emotion are mutually influential as children are growing up, the complexities of this interaction, and important questions for future research. In this section, we focus on four areas: growth in psychological understanding (also known as "theory of mind"), developing self-awareness, cognitive achievement, and understanding of emotion and emotion regulation.

Emerging Theory of Mind

In everyday circumstances, adults use the emotional expressions of other people to guide them in their interpretation of uncertain circumstances. At a social gathering when someone makes an awkward joke, for example, we scan the facial expressions of others to see how they are reacting, and then we respond accordingly. Developmental research indicates that even 1-year-olds have this ability, which is called *social referencing* (see Thompson, 2006b). It can be observed in laboratory experiments and also in everyday circumstances, such as when a baby looks attentively at a sociable stranger in the supermarket and then turns to look at the mother. If the mother looks at the stranger and then turns to the baby with a reassuring expression, the stranger might receive a smile from the baby. If the mother looks surprised, startled, or fearful, then the infant is more likely to withdraw and fuss. The baby has used the emotional cues of the mother's face to derive information about how to evaluate the stranger. In this respect, emotion contributed importantly to social-cognitive understanding.

Although observations like these are common, it is easy to overlook the extent of psychological understanding implicit in the baby's response to the unfamiliar adult. First, the 1-year-old reveals a nonegocentric awareness that although he or she is uncertain about how to respond to the stranger, mother might have knowledge that the baby does not have. The implicit awareness that different people (in this case, mother and baby) have different knowledge is a first step in developing theory of mind—that is, developing an understanding of the mental states of people (Wellman, 2002). The awareness that people have different knowledge is a significant achievement in the 1-year-old's psychological understanding, but that is not all. Second, the baby also understands that mother's visual orientation is important to knowing what is in her mind. This understanding is central to interpreting her emotional expression. In this situation, for example, if the mother appeared reassuring or fearful while looking at her watch, most infants would not respond to the stranger accordingly (see Moses, Baldwin, Rosicky, & Tidball, 2001). Instead, they would try to attract her attention to the stranger. In a sense, therefore, infants are aware that what people are looking at influences what is in their minds, and this is important to social referencing. Mother's emotional expressions are interpretable only in relation to what she is looking at in the moment. Finally, the infant is capable of deriving appropriate meaning from the mother's facial and vocal expressions of emotion (Thompson, 2006b). The baby can use mother's reassuring or fearful expression to provide information about whether the stranger is benign or dangerous.

Emotion is central to many of these early achievements in theory of mind. This is because, in many respects, emotion is an early entrée into another person's mental states (Thompson, 2011b). Within the first 6 months, infants can discriminate facial and vocal expressions of emotion in their caregivers, respond affectively to them, and expect these displays to be expressively congruent (see review by Thompson & Lagattuta, 2006). In the second year, emotional expressions become the basis for understanding others' intentions, desires, and goals (Thompson, 2011b). By 18 months, for example, toddlers can deduce what kind of food—broccoli or goldfish crackers—adults prefer to eat from adults' emotional expressions while eating the item (Repacholi & Gopnik, 1997). Emotions and their causes are prominent in young children's talk about their own internal states and those of others, and are the basis for their judgments of motives for good or bad behavior (Bartsch & Wellman, 1999; Wright & Bartsch, 2008). Emotions are an early gateway into psychological understanding.

Emotions provide an entrée into others' mental states because emotions create a bridge between the baby's internal experience and that of another person during everyday social interactions when emotions are exchanged, elicited, and mirrored (Thompson, 2011b). The intersubjectivity that is created during episodes of social play, shared discoveries, and other interactions enable young infants to connect their own internal experience with another's and with the expressions and actions that are associated with it. To the extent that perceiving another person as "like me" constitutes an early-emerging conceptual framework for understanding others (Meltzoff, 2007), therefore, shared emotional experience contributes significantly to this framework. Moreover, because emotions are so reliably associated with others' goals (their achievement or frustration), desires (fulfilled or unfulfilled), and other mental states (including false belief), emotion understanding gives infants a means of understanding other mental states.

If this is so, it means that early social cognition is colored by children's emotional experiences of other people. This is observed most clearly in the security or insecurity that characterizes early parent–child attachment relationships and the "internal working models" that derive from these attachments and subsequently influence other relation-

ships (Thompson, 2006b). The importance of emotion in early social cognition is also observed in young children's initial trait attributions of other children as "mean" or "nice" (Giles & Heyman, 2005; Heyman & Gelman, 1999), the emergence of attributional biases (including hostile attribution biases) concerning the causes of others' behavior and the development of constructive social problem-solving skills (Raikes & Thompson, 2008), and even early judgments about moral violations that cause harm to others (Smetana, 1989; Wright & Bartsch, 2008). In these and other domains of developing social cognition, emotion is central to how young children perceive others (and, as we shall see, themselves) and others' personalities, motivations, and intentions.

With cognitive growth, of course, social cognition develops to incorporate more nuanced apppraisals of others' internal attributes and strategies of social interaction. Children become more proficient in their interpretation of social behavior, their consideration of multiple social responses and the potential consequences, and their understanding of complex social goals. Emotion remains predominant, however, in children's encoding of social cues and their interpretation, their goals in social interactions, and their decisions about how to respond (Lemerise & Arsenio, 2000). In a sense, the continuing interaction of cognitive growth and emotional responding moves to a higher level of integration with the concurrent growth of social cognition and the emotional dimensions of social interaction. Much more remains to be understood about this developmental interaction.

The early development of theory of mind and the growth of social cognition together illustrate the prominence of emotion in early social interaction and the integration of emotion into developing social understanding. It shows also that as cognitive growth ensues, social cognition develops in a manner that continues to incorporate emotion.

Development of Self-Awareness

At the same time that young children are developing an understanding of other people and their mental states, they are also learning about themselves. Self-awareness is an extended developmental process, with children acquiring a cognitive awareness of different features of themselves with increasing age and cognitive growth (Thompson, 2006b). One milestone in the development of self-awareness occurs when toddlers achieve physical self-recognition. This is commonly assessed by observing young children's responses to their mirror images after their noses have been surreptitiously marked with a spot of rouge. After 18 months of age, but not earlier, toddlers typically touch their noses and often show signs of embarrassment (Lewis & Brooks-Gunn, 1979). The emotional concomitants of physical self-recognition are important in this situation, because they indicate that young children of this age have acquired expectations for their normative appearance (i.e., knowing that their nose is not normally red) and respond self-evaluatively when this expectation is violated.

Indeed, once toddlers have become conceptually aware of themselves as physical beings—and have begun to develop a rudimentary "conceptual self" (Howe & Courage, 1997)—emotions become an increasingly important aspect of developing self-awareness. During the second and third years, for example, young children begin to show a variety of self-conscious emotions, including pride, shame, guilt, shyness, along with embarrassment, in circumstances in which they or their behavior is susceptible to social evaluation (Lagattuta & Thompson, 2007; Lewis, 2008). At this time young children begin calling attention to their achievements and showing signs of pride in response to a parent's applause (Stipek, Recchia, & McClintic, 1992), and behaviors reflecting rudimentary guilt or shame appear in response to an adult's evaluation of the child's conduct (Alessandri & Lewis, 1993). Social evaluations are especially important to the earliest appearance of self-conscious emotions because they help to connect the young child's conduct to an external standard before it has become internalized. Social evaluations also contribute to the emotional dimensions of children's spontaneous self-evaluations.

With increasing age and cognitive growth, of course, young children become self-aware in more complex ways involving attributions of ability and competence; explicit awareness of feelings, needs, and other internal states; categorizing the self by gender and in other ways; enhanced sensitivity to evaluative standards; and assertions of ownership (see Thompson, 2006b, for a review). Young children are also developing a dawning awareness of their psychological characteristics at about the same time that they are attributing psychological traits to others. In studies of 4- and 5-year-olds, using carefully designed interviews, young children reveal self-perceptions of characteristics such as timidity, agreeableness, proneness to becoming upset, as well as positive or negative self-concept (see review by Thompson, 2011b). These self-descriptions have been found to be consistent with the descriptions of these children provided by their mothers, fathers, or teachers (e.g., Brown, Mangelsdorf, Agathen, & Ho, 2008), although the modest strength of these cross-informant associations suggests that young children are not merely appropriating the descriptions of themselves provided by their caregivers, but are also reflecting on their own experiences. One study reported that preschoolers' positive self-concept was associated with more secure mother–child relationships. But for the same children, more negative self-concept was predicted by mothers' reports of stress and depression (Goodvin, Meyer, Thompson, & Hayes, 2008).

Developing self-awareness in early childhood is thus a result of growing cognitive capacities as they interact with the young child's emotional experiences. Indeed, as children reach new milestones in self-awareness, each milestone provides opportunities for different emotions and emotional experiences to become incorporated into their conceptual understanding of themselves. The salience and significance of emotion to developing self-awareness is not surprising. Young children who are temperamentally shy take this emotional attribute with them into daily social situations, where their anxious reserve is more salient to them than it is to others, and the same is true of those who are dispositionally more positive or outgoing. Those who are prone to negative outbursts and tantrums are often more perplexed by their sudden emotional upheavals and its consequences, as are the peers and adults around them. The salient dimensions of emergent personality that color self-awareness are primarily emotional in quality. Because of this, cognitive achievements in self-understanding continuously incorporate emotional experience into the development of self-awareness.

Cognitive Achievement

National attention to school readiness has focused scholarly attention on its origins. One question receiving considerable research attention is this: To what extent is early school achievement primarily a function of antecedent cognitive skills, or does it depend also on emotional, social, and self-regulatory characteristics? The answer has immense practical importance for guiding early education efforts, and it is theoretically significant for understanding how much cognitive ability is integrated with emotional capabilities in predicting learning.

As it turns out, the answer to this question is more complex and nuanced than researchers and policymakers may expect. In a widely publicized report on the analysis of six large-scale longitudinal studies, Duncan and his colleagues reported that late preschool measures of cognitive competence were the strongest predictors of academic performance in early grade school, whereas antecedent measures of social–emotional functioning rarely had much predictive value at all (Duncan et al., 2007). However, subsequent analyses indicated that early elementary school measures of academic skill were poorly predictive of high school completion; rather, emotional and behavioral problems—especially those that persisted in the early primary grades—were significantly predictive of graduation (Magnuson, Duncan, Lee, & Metzger, 2009). In understanding the influence of emotion on cognitive achievement, these findings suggest that the nature of the cognitive outcome is important, as well as the child population on which conclusions are based. Emotional functioning may assume a greater role in predicting cognitive achievement for certain populations of children, such as those who experience stress and disadvantage, compared with others (Thompson & Raikes, 2007; Thompson, Thompson, & Winer, 2012).

Test scores are not necessarily an optimal measure of cognitive achievement, of course, nor are the school years necessarily the best

occasion to study cognition–emotion interactions associated with cognitive achievement. In research on infants and young children, developmental psychologists have often pointed to the importance of emotions for stimulating interest and motivating problem-solving efforts in everyday situations. This is sometimes described as "mastery motivation," and highlights how significantly cognitive achievement in the early years depends on the young child's emotional response to cognitive challenges as well as the social support the child receives for engagement and self-confident action (see MacTurk & Morgan, 1995, for a review). Characteristics such as curiosity, persistence, self-regulation, the ability to delay immediate rewards in favor of longer-term gains, and self-esteem illustrate the indirect influences of emotional qualities on the processes that contribute to cognitive achievement. (These characteristics also constitute some of the "noncognitive skills" that economists such as Heckman [2007] argue are important, along with cognitive ability, to school achievement and adult workforce success.) In a related vein, the developmental research on achievement motivation indicates that early-emerging differences in children's mastery-oriented or helpless atttributions regarding the causes of their prior successes or failures significantly influence persistence and effort on subsequent challenges (Dweck, Mangels, & Good, 2004; Smiley & Dweck, 1994). Taken together, these findings point to the multiple ways that emotions influence the processes underlying cognitive achievement from early in life, consistent with the general role of emotion as a motivator of cognition (Izard, 2010).

Enlisting emotions constructively to motivate cognitive achievement is important for all children, but may be an especially significant concern for children who are at risk for academic failure. For these children, emotional problems and self-regulatory difficulties—manifested in disruptive conduct problems, aggression, or depressive symptomatology—may be significant, perhaps primary, reasons for their poor academic achievement (McClelland, Morrison, & Holmes, 2000; Raver, Garner, & Smith-Donald, 2007). There are several reasons why these influences could be so, including the limitations of these children to attend to and thus benefit from classroom instruction, their poor relationships with teachers and peers and the consequent effects on classroom engagement, how behavioral problems impair cognitive performance and the motivation to achieve, and even the effects of stress neurobiology on learning and memory (National Scientific Council on the Developing Child, 2005; Thompson & Raikes, 2007). In one study with a sample of sociodemographically at-risk children, for example, Trentacosta and Izard (2007) found that kindergarten measures of emotion competence directly predicted academic achievement in first grade. Likewise, emotion knowledge in middle childhood directly predicted academic competence in late childhood for a socioeconomically disadvantaged sample, even when potential mediators such as social skills were included in the model (Trentacosta, Mostow, & Izard, 2005). Understanding emotion–cognition interactions in young children who are at risk of academic failure has practical significance for the design of early education interventions to help improve their school readiness.

Indeed, because of the concurrent development of cognitive delays with the emergence of behavioral problems for these children, several early interventions have been designed to address their emotional and self-regulatory difficulties—sometimes in concert with a cognitively oriented curriculum—to promote cognitive achievement in preschoolers (for reviews, see Domitrovich, Moore, Thompson, & the Collaborative for the Advancement of Social, Emotional, and Academic Learning Preschool to Elementary Assessment Workgroup, 2012; Thompson et al., 2012). Evaluation studies of these interventions underscore the complexity of efforts to improve the cognitive achievement of at-risk children. On one hand, a school readiness intervention focused on strengthening self-regulation skills, the Chicago School Readiness Project, improved low-income children's vocabulary, letter-naming, and math skills as well as self-regulation skills during a year of the program (Raver et al., 2011). On the other hand, the Emotion Course, an intervention designed to improve emotion competence in low-income children, was found to strengthen emotional and behavioral functioning but provided no evidence for improved cognitive or academic skills (Izard et al., 2008). It appears that narrowly focused social–emotional interventions are less likely to contribute to improved cognitive achievement compared with broadly designed programs in which a cognitive language curriculum is supported by interventions to strengthen emotion understanding and behavioral functioning tailored to the needs of young, at-risk children (e.g., see Bierman et al., 2008). This is true, for example, of early intervention programs that target economically disadvantaged children, such as the Perry Preschool Program, which have shown the greatest long-term success (Schweinhart et al., 2005).

Taken together, it seems apparent that understanding the origins of cognitive achievement in children requires attention to more than just the growth of attention, memory, and problem-solving skills. In addition, the development of mastery motivation, curiosity, self-confidence, persistence, and other "noncognitive skills" is also associated with cognitive achievement, with different proportions of variance explained by the varying emotional and self-regulatory influences affecting children facing different amounts of sociodemographic risk. Emotional and self-regulatory problems can impair achievement, especially for children in difficult circumstances who may have to cope with many challenges outside of the classroom. Understanding cognition–emotion interactions that are relevant to cognitive achievement is important for practical reasons, as we have noted, and the design of early education programs to improve school readiness is one of the testing fields in which developmental and intervention research find common ground. One of the lessons from this research is that broadly based interventions that integrate attention to cognitive and emotional skills may have the greatest probability of success.

Developmental Understanding of Emotion and Emotion Regulation

When we consider how cognition and emotion interact in development, it is natural to think of growth in children's understanding of emotion. The expansion of theory of mind as children develop more complex and multifaceted representations of their emotions may alter their emotional experiences as well. Moreover, another consequence of enhanced emotion understanding is that children achieve deeper understanding of how emotions may be managed, which contributes to the growth of their emotion regulation skills.

Children's understanding of their emotions changes considerably as they mature, although in different ways than was formerly understood (Harris, 2008). Based on children's responses to open-ended interview questions, developmental researchers had believed that young children have a narrow, event-based understanding of emotions: Events happen (e.g., encountering a scary dog), and feelings result (e.g., fear). Viewed in this light, preschoolers' emotion understanding is script-like, with different situations leading naturally to different emotions. With increasing conceptual maturity and greater comprehension of the internal, invisible influences on behavior, older children were believed to develop a more psychologically oriented understanding of the origins of emotions.

Further research with more carefully refined methods, however, has revealed a more complex picture. Preschool children actually begin with a surprisingly psychologically oriented understanding of emotions (Harris, 2008). Although they are fully aware of the influence of events on feelings, they also appreciate how emotions are associated with other mental states, such as desires, intentions, needs, and goals, as noted earlier. They understand that emotions can be evoked by thoughts, expectations, and beliefs, such as a child's dismay that an expected treat was not provided. Older preschoolers also understand that mental events alone, independent of the situation, can provoke emotion. They realize, for example, that a girl may feel sad instead of happy when seeing a cute puppy because it reminds her of a favorite pet that was lost last week (Lagattuta & Wellman, 2001). With increasing age, older children acquire a more differentiated emotion lexicon with which to interpret their feelings (words like *contentment, anxiety, fury*) and they understand a broader range of mental processes that may contribute to emotional arousal (e.g., self-referential thoughts). Emotion also becomes increasingly enlisted in their efforts to understand social roles, moral values, and relationships.

Developmental changes in emotion understanding are, not surprisingly, associated with changes in children's understanding of emotion regulation (Thompson, 1990; Thompson, Virmani, Waters, Meyer, & Raikes, 2013). Preschoolers typically endorse practical emotion regulation strategies such as problem solving, restricting exposure to emotionally evocative events (e.g., covering their eyes or ears or leaving the situation), or behavioral distraction (Dennis & Kelemen, 2009; Thompson et al., 2013). Although these simple strategies reflect some psychological insight (covering eyes or ears reveals an awareness that a distressing event must be perceived to evoke emotion), by the end of the preschool years children more reliably endorse psychologically sophisticated emotion regulation strategies, such as reinterpreting the situation or changing their thoughts or goals to alleviate negative feelings (Davis, Levine, Lench, & Quas, 2010; Thompson et al., 2013). Preschoolers recognize that ruminating on sad or distressing events is not good for managing negative feelings, nor does merely venting those feelings contribute to their regulation (see also Watkins, Chapter 21, this volume). Young children also exhibit an awareness that different strategies may be more effective for managing different negative emotions, such as fear, anger, or sadness (Dennis & Kelemen, 2009; Thompson et al., 2013).

These conclusions are based on studies in which children respond to hypothetical story scenarios involving a story character experiencing strong feelings, and children are asked to suggest or endorse alternative strategies of emotion management. Sometimes children are asked to imagine themselves in these stories. In none of this research, however, are children's verbalized strategies of emotion regulation related to their actual behavior in managing their own feelings. This lacuna constitutes one of the most important challenges for future research. In our own research, for example, it was striking to observe how frequently preschoolers recognized that venting is an ineffective self-regulatory strategy for managing emotion in response to hypothetical stories, and then subsequently observe them in a laboratory probe venting emotion when frustrated. Nor did young children exhibit evidence of enacting the psychologically more sophisticated self-regulatory strategies that they endorsed, such as reappraising a frustrating situation (Thompson et al., 2013). Understanding the connection between how children *conceptualize* emotion regulation and how they *enact* emotion regulation is central to understanding cognition–emotion interactions. Unfortunately, there is very little research germane to this developmental question of conceptualization versus enactment of emotion regulation strategies (Harris, 2008).

There are several reasons to question how directly relevant children's developing understanding of emotion regulation is to their practical strategies of emotional self-management. One is simply the power of the situation. Consistent with functionalist emotions theory, children's goals in everyday situations that evoke emotion are likely to be multifaceted and guided, in part, by immediate circumstances. Venting may be perceived as a generally ineffective means of emotional self-control by preschoolers, but it may be strategically useful in a supermarket or at home to achieve one's goals. Another reason for a décalage between understanding of emotion regulation and its enactment is that emotional self-control draws on neurobiological systems that are developmentally immature in young children (Thompson & Nelson, 2001). Consequently, preschoolers may be aware that venting makes you feel worse but be unable to inhibit their emotional outbursts in practical circumstances. Finally, in hypothetical stories and personal situations children are being asked to make very different judgments. In this respect, there may be little reason to anticipate that young children's responses to stories about emotion regulation would be relevant to their actual behavior in situations requiring emotional self-control.

These and other reasons to account for the gap between understanding and behavior highlight some of the challenges in studying cognition–emotion interactions in development. They suggest that with respect to developing cognitive understanding of emotion and emotion regulation, new ways of thinking do not necessarily directly change emotional experience, but rather provide a catalyst for potential developmental change and reorganization. As we consider in the next section, another developmental catalyst consists of how children are encouraged to represent their experiences through their interactions with others.

Early Relationships as Organizers of Cognition–Emotion Interactions

A developmental perspective argues that early experiences are important for organizing cognition–emotion interactions. As previously noted, for example, early experiences of stress and adversity alter neurobiological stress systems that shape emotional reactions to challenge, while simultaneously altering cognitive appraisal processes to render children hypersensitive to cues of threat or danger. As a result, perceptual–cognitive biases function interactively with emotional response tendencies to cause children to overreact to adversity, which can create liabilities for healthy psychosocial functioning. Early social experiences also contribute to the emotional qualities incorporated into self-awareness, such as when young children perceive themselves positively in the context of a secure mother–child relationship, and also color children's self-referential beliefs in ways that help to maintain these self-perceptions. Young children who have difficulty focusing attention and thinking in an early childhood education classroom, owing to family problems, can fall behind academically in ways that undermine their performance in elementary school and diminish achievement motivation and self-confidence.

To be sure, it is not that early experiences are, by nature, determinative of future growth. They are influential, rather, because they have the potential of altering plastic early developmental processes in ways that may become consolidated with increasing age into enduring behavioral tendencies. Because cognition–emotion interactions can, as we have seen, yield mutually reinforcing networks of appraisals and reaction tendencies, these early experiences may be important in shaping the nature of cognition–emotion interactions over time.

In the context of early experiences, parent–child relationships are central to emerging cognition–emotion interactions. These primary relationships influence not only the development of cognitive and emotional competencies in young children, but also how these competencies intersect. In the context of parent–child relationships, for example, infants and toddlers have their initial experiences of gaining insight into another's mental and psychological states through shared emotional experiences. In these relationships, young children begin to understand themselves via complementary conceptual and affective dimensions that derive, in part, from parental responses to the child. Parent–child relationships can be sources of stress or stress-buffering that help to define the threats with which the child must learn to cope and, as a consequence, the intersecting perceptual–cognitive appraisals and emotional response tendencies that develop. In these relationships, parents provide emotion coaching that influences children's developing representations of emotion and their emotion self-regulation. Because some of the most important parenting qualities, such as sensitive responsiveness, have complementary effects on the development of cognitive skills and emotional security (Laible & Thompson, 2007), parent–child relationships are a uniquely important feature of early experience that shapes cognition–emotion interactions.

Parent–Child Relationships and Child Temperament

Yet developing children do not come as empty entities to these interactions. They bring with them temperamental predispositions, unfolding emotional capacities, and developing self-awareness that individualize each transaction with the social world. Temperamental dimensions are, by their nature, emotional in quality (see Table 16.1), as well as reflecting aspects of self-regulation and activity.

How does temperament impact children's cognition and emotion and shape their relationships with their parents? Children's temperament is rooted in their biological, physiological, cognitive, and emotional responses to the social world and affects their tendencies for responding to their environment. In contrast to traditional formulations—that temperament emerges early, is highly consistent across situations and over time, and is directly tied to the growth of personality—current research underscores temperament as a biologically based but developmentally evolving feature of behavior (Rothbart, 2011). For this reason, temperamental attributes become increasingly more consistent over time as temperamental individuality is enveloped into a network of cognitive–emotional processes that include self-perceptions, behavioral preferences, and

TABLE 16.1. Temperament Dimensions as Described by Developmental Temperament Researchers

Common Dimensions	Rothbart & Bates	Thomas & Chess	Buss & Plomin	Goldsmith & Campos
Emotion	Negative affectivity Frustration Fear Discomfort Sadness Soothability	Quality of mood	Emotionality	Individual differences in the arousal and expression of the primary emotions
Self-regulation	Effortful control Attentional control Inhibitory control Perceptual sensitivity Low-intensity pleasure	Rhythmicity Approach/withdrawal Adaptability Distractability Persistence—attention span Sensory threshold of responsiveness		
Activity level	Extraversion/surgency Activity Shyness (low) High-intensity pleasure Smiling and laughter Impulsivity Positive anticipation Affiliation	Activity level Intensity of reaction	Activity level Sociability	

social cognitions that, together, shape developing personality (Thompson, Winer, & Goodvin, 2011).

Contemporary research shows that although temperamental qualities may have direct effects on behavior and development, temperament is more influential as it interacts with characteristics of the caregiving environment (Gallagher, 2002). Current researchers are devoting considerable attention to the interactive and mediated influences of temperamental processes on development. For example, studies have found that early temperamental vulnerability interacts with harsh parenting in the development of conduct disorders in young children (see Owens & Shaw, 2003; Shaw, Miles, Ingoldsby, & Nagin, 2003). Conduct disorders are most strongly predicted by harsh parenting in concert with temperamental negative emotionality and fearlessness.

Further evidence of the role of children's temperament in early emotion–cognition interactions within close relationships comes from research on early conscience development. The growth of conscience incorporates young children's conceptual awareness of moral standards, promoted by parental socialization efforts, with the emotional motivation to comply with those standards. Consistent with this view, studies by Kochanska show that early conscience development is an interaction between the emotional dimensions of early temperament and parental socialization efforts (Kochanska, 1991, 1997). Temperamentally fearful preschoolers are more likely to internalize parental standards of conduct when their caregivers provide gentle guidance, whereas temperamentally fearless children show greater internalization not as a result of parents' discipline efforts, but in the context of a secure parent–child attachment relationship (Kochanska, 1997).

Individual differences in children's temperamental dispositions also play important roles in the development of emotion regulation (Thompson et al., 2011). Children's earliest introduction to emotion regulation comes from the efforts of their caregivers to manage their emotions. Parents attempt to do so by directly intervening to soothe or pacify the child, and they also do so in other ways that are in accord with their perceptions of the child's temperamental strengths and vulnerabilities (Garner & Spears, 2000;

Spinrad, Stifter, Donelan-McCall, & Turner, 2004). With increasing age, children begin to initiate emotionally self-regulatory efforts based on their own perceptions of their temperamental qualities, whether they perceive themselves as dispositionally placid or reactive, positive or negative in mood, or timid or outgoing (Thompson et al., 2011). In these ways, temperament is important both as a direct influence on cognition–emotion relations and as a moderator of those relations.

Unpacking Relational Influences

There are at least two other avenues highlighted in developmental research by which early parent–child relationships are important to cognition–emotion interactions. The first is through the representations that derive from the quality of parent–child relationships, an influence emphasized by attachment theory (Bretherton & Munholland, 2008; Dykas & Cassidy, 2011). According to attachment theorists, a secure parent–child relationship is important for the psychological support it provides the child as well as the positive social skills it fosters. A secure attachment is also important because of its influence on the child's developing representations of self, the attachment figure, and other people. These representations—or "internal working models"—begin to emerge with the rudimentary social expectations for the parent's responsiveness in infancy, and develop into broader and more comprehensive representational systems that influence attention, memory, and social information processing as well as social behavior. Research support for this formulation can be found in an extensive research literature linking security of attachment to social problem-solving skills, more positive self-concept, emotion understanding, diminished negative attribution biases, and other social-cognitive processes as well as memory and attentional processes (see Dykas & Cassidy, 2011; Thompson, 2006b, for reviews). Although the concept of internal working models has been criticized for being overinclusive and vaguely defined, its portrayal of the development of early mental representations that are integrative, affectively colored, and relationally based is a uniquely valuable contribution (Thompson, 2010). As such, it reflects another kind of cognition–emotion interaction in which early relational experience contributes to the development of networked understandings of self and others that integrate affective and conceptual features. The internal working models construct also underscores the importance of studying the development of individual differences in these cognitive–emotional representations.

A second avenue highlighted in developmental research by which parent–child relationships influence the organization of cognition–emotion interactions is research on parent–child conversational discourse (Thompson, 2006a; Wareham & Salmon, 2006). Beginning with studies on the growth of autobiographical memory (Nelson & Fivush, 2004), developmental researchers have studied how the content and quality of parental discourse in conversation with the child influences a range of conceptual advances of early childhood, including the growth of theory-of-mind understanding, event representation and episodic memory, anticipatory event representations, self-understanding, as well as social cognition and emotion understanding (see Thompson, 2006a, 2010, for a review). The manner in which this influence occurs is far more interesting than the view that parental instruction educates young children about these phenomena, although the parent's use of language to clarify and articulate mental processes is no doubt important. Equally important, however, is the *quality* of parental discourse. Developmental researchers have discovered that when mothers enlist an elaborative conversational style, using *wh*-questions (i.e., *who, what, when, where,* and *why*) to elicit the child's understanding and making evaluative statements and contributing knowledge to enhance the child's understanding, young children show greater advances in their conceptual growth compared to children whose mothers use a less enriched, more pragmatic discourse style. Children of elaborative mothers exhibit, for example, greater depth and detail in their autobiographical memory accounts (in part because the mother is a model of mnemonic competence), richer event representations, and enhanced emotion understanding (Nelson & Fivush, 2004). Interestingly, the mothers of securely attached children have also been found to have a more elaborative conversational style in their interactions

with their children, suggesting another avenue by which the internal working models associated with attachment security develop (Thompson, 2010).

The research on parent–child conversation and children's conceptual development suggests that it is not only *what* is said but also *how* it is said—and *who* says it—that influence children's understanding. Because young children rely on the claims of the adults they trust on a wide variety of issues that are important to them, particularly on matters that they cannot confirm independently (Harris, 2007), this research illustrates yet another kind of cognition–emotion interaction in the context of the parent–child relationship. When considered together with the research on parent–child attachment security, it suggests that early relational experience is important to how cognition–emotion interactions become organized early in life because parents are both sources of emotional security and cognitive understanding for young children.

Conclusion

Abe and Izard (1999) have argued that emotionally laden transactions stimulate advances in social-cognitive functioning and, in turn, that advances in social-cognitive understanding contribute to emotional development. As developmental researchers, they have described one of several models of cognition–emotion interactions profiled in this chapter. More complex formulations point to the manner in which cognitive achievements and emotional growth arise from common developmental catalysts (e.g., conversation with an adult about a recent experience), how perceptual–cognitive appraisals are affected by emotional arousal (e.g., in the experience of an anxious child), how cognitive advances provide the opportunity for emotional advances (e.g., in children's understanding of emotion regulation strategies), how mental representations are affectively colored as they develop (e.g., in the growth of internal working models arising from secure or insecure attachments), and how emotional experience infuses cognitive understanding (e.g., in young children's developing self-awareness). In most respects, developmental understanding of cognition–emotion interactions begins not from the perspective of independent systems establishing contact, but rather from the perspective of integrated systems becoming further enmeshed in a developmental cascade.

An important contribution to the theory and research on the development of cognition–emotion interactions has been a new view of emotion in development. Traditionally, emotions—often carefree, irrational, disorganizing, or even disturbing—have long characterized public and scientific views of childhood, with these emotional qualities regarded as hallmarks of childish immaturity. In this view, therefore, maturity requires controlling, regulating, and transforming emotions to enlist them into competent functioning, usually through cognitive means. But developmental studies, including much of the research discussed in this chapter, offers a different view: Emotions are important and adaptive aspects of how young children learn about the world, develop psychological understanding, acquire self-awareness, and interact constructively with others (Thompson, 2011b). Although emotions always retain their capacity in children (and adults) to disorganize and debilitate competent functioning, they also provide uniquely valuable forms of understanding in children (as well as adults). This developmental portrayal of emotion reduces, therefore, the perceived dissonance between cognition and emotion, and makes cognition–emotion interactions part of the fabric of behavioral development.

We expect that as developmental perspectives increasingly become incorporated into mainstream thinking about cognition and emotion, they will lead to diminished concern about the primacy of one over the other or the clash of "order" and "disorder." Instead, we will regard the interaction of cognition and emotion like a polyphonic composition, with continuously interweaving harmonic and dissonant themes that together create a complex and interesting composition.

References

Abe, J. A., & Izard, C. E. (1999). The developmental functions of emotions: An analysis in terms of differential emotions theory. *Cognition and Emotion, 13*, 523–549.

Alessandri, S. M., & Lewis, M. (1993). Parental evaluation and its relation to shame and pride in young chlidren. *Sex Roles, 29*, 335–342.

Bartsch, K., & Wellman, H. (1995). *Children talk about the mind.* Oxford, UK: Oxford University Press.

Bierman, K. L., Domitrovich, C. E., Nix, R. L., Gest, S. D., Welsh, J. A., Greenberg, M. T., et al. (2008). Promoting academic and social–emotional school readiness: The Head Start REDI program. *Child Development, 79*, 1802–1817.

Bretherton, I., & Munholland, K. A. (2008). Internal working models in attachment relationships: Elaborating a central construct in attachment theory. In J. Cassidy & P. R. Shaver (Eds.), *Handbook of attachment: Theory, research, and clinical applications* (2nd ed., pp. 102–127). New York: Guilford Press.

Brown, G. L., Mangelsdorf, S. C., Agathen, J. M., & Ho, M.-H. (2008). Young children's psychological selves: Convergence with maternal reports of child personality. *Social Development, 17*, 161–182.

Calkins, S. D., & Bell, M. A. (Eds.). (2010). *Child development at the intersection of emotion and cognition.* Washington, DC: American Psychological Association.

Campos, J. J., Anderson, D. I., Barbu-Roth, M. A., Hubbard, E. M., Hertenstein, M. J., & Witherington, D. (2000). Travel broadens the mind. *Infancy, 1*, 149–219.

Dalgleish, T., & Power, M. J. (Eds.). (1999). *Handbook of cognition and emotion.* New York: Wiley.

Davies, P. T., & Woitach, M. (2008). Children's emotional security in the interparental relationship. *Current Directions in Psychological Science, 17*, 269–274.

Davis, E. L., Levine, L. J., Lench, H. C., & Quas, J. A. (2010). Metacognitive emotion regulation: Children's awareness that changing thoughts and goals can alleviate negative emotions. *Emotion, 10*, 498–510.

De Houwer, J., & Hermans, D. (Eds.). (2010). *Cognition and emotion: Reviews of current research and theories.* New York: Psychology Press.

Dennis, T. A., & Kelemen, D. A. (2009). Preschool children's views on emotion regulation: Functional associations and implications for social–emotional adjustment. *International Journal of Behavioral Development, 33*, 243–252.

Domitrovich, C. E., Moore, J. E., Thompson, R. A., and the CASEL Preschool to Elementary

School Social and Emotional Learning Assessment Workgroup. (2012). Interventions that promote social–emotional learning in young children. In R. C. Pianta, W. S. Barnett, L. M. Justice, & S. M. Sheridan (Eds.), *Handbook of early childhood education* (pp. 393–415). New York: Guilford Press.

Duncan, G. J., Dowsett, C. J., Claessens, A., Magnuson, K., Huston, A. C., Klebanov, P., et al. (2007). School readiness and later achievement. *Developmental Psychology, 43,* 1428–1446.

Dweck, C. S., Mangels, J. A., & Good, C. (2004). Motivational effects on attention, cognition, and performance. In D. Y. Dai & R. J. Sternberg (Eds.), *Motivation, emotion, and cognition* (pp. 41–55). Mahwah, NJ: Erlbaum.

Dykas, M. J., & Cassidy, J. (2011). Attachment and the processing of social information across the life span: Theory and evidence. *Psychological Bulletin, 137,* 19–46.

Eich, E., Kilhstrom, J. F., Bower, G. H., Forgas, J. P., & Niedenthal, P. M. (Eds.). (2000). *Cognition and emotion.* New York: Oxford University Press.

Feldman Barrett, L., & Bar, M. (2009). See it with feeling: Affective predictions during object perception. *Philosophical Transactions of the Royal Society of London B (Biological Sciences), 364,* 1325–1334.

Fox, N. A., Henderson, H. A., Marshall, P. J., Nichols, K. E., & Ghera, M. M. (2005). Behavioral inhibition: Linking biology and behavior within a developmental framework. *Annual Review of Psychology, 56,* 235–262.

Frijda, N. H. (1987). *The emotions.* New York: Cambridge University Press.

Gallagher, K. C. (2002). Does child temperament moderate the influence of parenting on adjustment? *Developmental Review, 22,* 623–643.

Garner, P. W., & Spears, F. M. (2000). Emotion regulation in low-income preschoolers. *Social Development, 9,* 246–264.

Giles, J. W., & Heyman, G. D. (2005). Preschoolers use trait-relevant information to evaluate the appropriateness of an aggressive response. *Aggressive Behavior, 31,* 498–509.

Goodvin, R., Meyer, S., Thompson, R. A., & Hayes, R. (2008). Self-understanding in early childhood: Associations with attachment security and maternal emotional risk. *Attachment and Human Development, 10*(4), 433–450.

Gunnar, M. R., Fisher, P. A., & the Early Experience, Stress, and Prevention Network. (2006). Bringing basic research on early experience and stress neurobiology to bear on preventive interventions for neglected and maltreated children. *Development and Psychopathology, 18,* 651–677.

Gunnar, M. R., & Vazquez, D. (2006). Stress neurobiology and developmental psychopathology. In D. Cicchetti & D. Cohen (Eds.), *Developmental psychopathology: Vol. III. Risk, disorder, and adaptation* (2nd ed., pp. 533–577). New York: Wiley.

Harris, P. L. (2007). Trust. *Developmental Science, 10,* 135–138.

Harris, P. L. (2008). Children's understanding of emotion. In M. Lewis, J. M. Haviland-Jones, & L. Feldman Barrett (Eds.), *Handbook of emotions* (3rd ed., pp. 320–331). New York: Guilford Press.

Heckman, J. J. (2007). The economics, technology, and neuroscience of human capital formation. *Proceedings of the National Academy of Sciences, 104,* 13250–13255.

Hendrix, R., & Thompson, R. A. (2011). Development of self-produced locomotion in the first year: Changes in parent perceptions and infant behavior. *Infant and Child Development, 20,* 288–300.

Heyman, G. D., & Gelman, S. A. (1999). The use of trait labels in making psychological inferences. *Child Development, 70,* 604–619.

Howe, M. L., & Courage, M. L. (1997). The emergence and early development of autobiographical memory. *Psychological Review, 104*(3), 499–523.

Izard, C. E. (2010). The many meanings/aspects of emotion: Definitions, functions, activation, and regulation. *Emotion Review, 2,* 363–370.

Izard, C. E., Kagan, J., & Zajonc, R. B. (1984). *Emotions, cognition, and behavior.* New York: Cambridge University Press.

Izard, C. E., King, K. A., Trentacosta, C. J., Morgan, J. K., Laurenceau, J., Krauthamer-Ewing, E. S., et al. (2008). Accelerating the development of emotion competence in Head Start children: Effects on adaptive and maladaptive behavior. *Development and Psychopathology, 20,* 369–397.

Kober, H., Feldman Barrett, L., Joseph, J., Bliss-Moreau, E., Lindquist, K., & Wager, T. D. (2008). Functional grouping and cortical–subcortical interactions in emotion: A meta-analysis of neuroimaging studies. *NeuroImage, 42,* 998–1031.

Kochanska, G. (1991). Socialization and temperament in the development of guilt and conscience. *Child Development, 62,* 1379–1392.

Kochanska, G. (1997). Multiple pathways to conscience for children with different temperaments: From toddlerhood to age 5. *Developmental Psychology, 33*, 228–240.

Lagattuta, K. H., & Thompson, R. A. (2007). The development of self-conscious emotions: Cognitive processes and social influences. In L. J. Tracy, R. W. Robins, & J. P. Tangney (Eds.), *The self-conscious emotions: Theory and research* (2nd ed., pp. 91–113). New York: Guilford Press.

Lagattuta, K. H., & Wellman, H. M. (2001). Thinking about the past: Young children's knowledge about links between past events, thinking, and emotion. *Child Development, 72*, 82–102.

Laible, D., & Thompson, R. A. (2007). Early socialization: A relationship perspective. In J. E. Grusec & P. D. Hastings (Eds.), *Handbook of socialization: Theory and research* (pp. 181–207). New York: Guilford Press.

Lemerise, E. A., & Arsenio, W. F. (2000). An integrated model of emotion processes and cognition in social information processing. *Child Development, 71*, 107–118.

Lewis, M. (2008). Self-conscious emotions: Embarrassment, pride, shame, and guilt. In M. Lewis, J. M. Haviland-Jones, & L. Feldman Barrett (Eds.), *Handbook of emotions* (3rd ed., pp. 742–756). New York: Guilford Press.

Lewis, M., & Brooks-Gunn, J. (1979). *Social cognition and the acquisition of self.* New York: Plenum Press.

MacTurk, R. H., & Morgan, G. A. (1995). *Mastery motivation: Origins, conceptualizations, and applications.* Norwood, NJ: Ablex.

Magnuson, K., Duncan, G., Lee, Y.-G., & Metzger, M. (2009, April). *Early school adjustment and high school dropout.* Paper presented at the biennial meetings of the Society for Research in Child Development, Denver, CO.

McClelland, M. M., Morrison, F. J., & Holmes, D. L. (2000). Children at risk for early academic problems: The role of learning-related social skills. *Early Childhood Research Quarterly, 15*, 307–329.

Meltzoff, A. N. (2007). The "like me" framework for recognizing and becoming an intentional agent. *Acta Psychologica, 124*, 26–43.

Mischel, W., Shoda, Y., & Rodriguez, M. L. (1989). Delay of gratification in children. *Science, 244*, 933–938.

Moses, L. J., Baldwin, D. A., Rosicky, J. G., &

Tidball, G. (2001). Evidence for referential understanding in the emotions domain at twelve and eighteen months. *Child Development, 72*, 718–735.

National Scientific Council on the Developing Child. (2005). *Excessive stress disrupts the architecture of the developing brain* (Working Paper #3). Available at *www.developingchild. net.*

Nelson, K., & Fivush, R. (2004). The emergence of autobiographical memory: A social–cultural developmental theory. *Psychological Review, 111*, 486–511.

Ochsner, K. N., Ray, R. R., Hughes, B., McRae, K., Cooper, J. C., Weber, J., et al. (2009). Bottom-up and top-down processes in emotion generation: Common and distinct neural mechanisms. *Psychological Science, 20*, 1322–1331.

Owens, E. B., & Shaw, D. S. (2003). Predicting growth curves of externalizing behavior across the preschool years. *Journal of Abnormal Child Psychology, 31*, 575–590.

Pollak, S. D. (2002). Effects of early experience on children's recognition of facial displays of emotion. *Developmental Psychology, 38*, 784–791.

Pollak, S. D. (2008). Mechanisms linking early experience and the emergence of emotions: Illustrations from the study of maltreated children. *Current Directions in Psychological Science, 17*, 370–375.

Pollak, S. D., & Kistler, D. J. (2002). Early experience is associated with the development of categorical representations for facial expressions of emotion. *Proceedings of the National Academy of Sciences, 99*, 9072–9076.

Pollak, S. D., Klorman, R., Thatcher, J. E., & Cicchetti, D. (2001). P3b reflects maltreated children's reactions to facial displays of emotion. *Psychophysiology, 38*, 267–274.

Pollak, S. D., & Tolley-Schell, S. A. (2003). Selective attention to facial emotion of physically abused children. *Journal of Abnormal Psychology, 113*, 323–338.

Power, M. J., & Dalgleish, T. (2008). *Cognition and emotion: From order to disorder.* New York: Psychology Press.

Raikes, H. A., & Thompson, R. A. (2008). Attachment security and parenting quality predict children's problem-solving, attributions, and loneliness with peers. *Attachment and Human Development, 10*, 1–26.

Raver, C. C., Garner, P. W., & Smith-Donald, R. (2007). The roles of emotion regulation and emotion knowledge for children's academic readiness: Are the links causal? In R. C. Pianta, M. J. Cox, & K. L. Snow (Eds.), *School readiness and the transition to kindergarten in the era of accountability* (pp. 121–147). Baltimore, MD: Brookes.

Raver, C. C., Jones, S. M., Li-Grining, C., Zhai, F., Bub, K., & Pressler, E. (2011). CSRP's impact on low-income preschoolers' preacademic skills: Self-regulation as a mediating mechanism. *Child Development, 82*, 362–378.

Repacholi, B. M., & Gopnik, A. (1997). Early reasoning about desires: Evidence from 14– and 18–month-olds. *Developmental Psychology, 33*, 12–21.

Rothbart, M. K. (2011). *Becoming who we are: Temperament and personality in development.* New York: Guilford Press.

Saarni, C., Campos, J., Camras, L., & Witherington, D. (2006). Emotional development: Action, communication, and understanding. In N. Eisenberg (Vol. Ed.), & W. Damon & R. M. Lerner (Eds.), *Handbook of child psychology: Vol. 3. Social, emotional and personality development* (6th ed., pp. 226–299). New York: Wiley.

Schweinhart, L. J., Montie, J., Xiang, Z., Barnett, W. S., Belfield, C. R., & Nores, M. (2005). Lifetime effects: The HighScore Perry Preschool study through age 40. *Monographs of the HighScore Educational Research Foundation, 14.*

Shackman, J. E., & Pollak, S. D. (2005). Experiential influences on multimodal perception of emotion. *Child Development, 76*, 1116–1126.

Shaw, D. S., Miles, G., Ingoldsby, E. M., & Nagin, D. S. (2003). Trajectories leading to school-age conduct problems. *Developmental Psychology, 39*, 189–200.

Smetana, J. G. (1989). Toddlers' social interactions in the context of moral and conventional transgressions in the home. *Developmental Psychology, 25*, 499–508.

Smiley, P. A., & Dweck, C. S. (1994). Individual differences in achievement goals among young children. *Child Development, 65*, 1723–1743.

Spinrad, T. L., Stifter, C. A., Donelan-McCall, N., & Turner, L. (2004). Mothers' regulation strategies in response to toddlers' affect: Links to later emotion self-regulation. *Social Development, 13*, 40–55.

Stipek, D., Recchia, S., & McClintic, S. (1992).

Self-evaluation in young children. *Monographs of the Society for Research in Child Development, 57* (Serial No. 226).

Surguladze, S. A., Brammer, M. J., Young, A. W., Andrew, C., Travis, M. J., Williams, S. C. R., et al. (2003). A preferential increase in the extrastriate response to signals of danger. *NeuroImage, 19*, 1317–1328.

Thompson, R. A. (1990). Emotion and self-regulation. In R. A. Thompson (Ed.), *Socioemotional development. Nebraska Symposium on Motivation* (Vol. 36, pp. 383–483). Lincoln: University of Nebraska Press.

Thompson, R. A. (2001). Childhood anxiety disorders from the perspective of emotion regulation and attachment. In M. W. Vasey & M. R. Dadds (Eds.), *The developmental psychopathology of anxiety* (pp. 160–182). Oxford, UK: Oxford University Press.

Thompson, R. A. (2006a). Conversation and developing understanding: Introduction to the special issue. *Merrill–Palmer Quarterly, 52*, 1–16.

Thompson, R. A. (2006b). The development of the person: Social understanding, relationships, self, conscience. In N. Eisenberg (Vol. Ed.) & W. Damon & R. M. Lerner (Eds.), *Handbook of child psychology: Vol. 3. Social, emotional, and personality development* (6th ed., pp. 24–98). New York: Wiley.

Thompson, R. A. (2010). Feeling and understanding through the prism of relationships. In S. D. Calkins & M. A. Bell (Eds.), *Child development at the intersection of emotion and cognition* (pp. 79–95). Washington, DC: American Psychological Association.

Thompson, R. A. (2011a). Emotion and emotion regulation: Two sides of the developing coin. *Emotion Review, 3*, 53–61.

Thompson, R. A. (2011b). The emotionate child. In D. Cicchetti & G. I. Roissman (Eds.), *The origins and organization of adaptation and maladaptation: Minnesota Symposium on Child Psychology* (Vol. 36, pp. 13–54). New York: Wiley.

Thompson, R. A., & Goodman, M. (2010). Development of emotion regulation: More than meets the eye. In A. M. Kring & D. M. Sloan (Eds.), *Emotion regulation and psychopathology: A transdiagnostic approach to etiology and treatment* (pp. 38–58). New York: Guilford Press.

Thompson, R. A., & Goodvin, R. (2007). Taming the tempest in a teapot: Emotion regulation in toddlers. In C. A. Brownell & C. B. Kopp

(Eds.), *Transitions in early socioemotional development: The toddler years* (pp. 320–341). New York: Guilford Press.

Thompson, R. A., & Lagatutta, K. (2006). Feeling and understanding: Early emotional development. In K. McCartney & D. Phillips (Ed.), *The Blackwell handbook of early childhood development* (pp. 317–337). Oxford, UK: Blackwell.

Thompson, R. A., & Nelson, C. A. (2001). Developmental science and the media: Early brain development. *American Psychologist, 56,* 5–15.

Thompson, R. A., & Raikes, H. A. (2007). The social and emotional foundations of school readiness. In D. F. Perry, R. F. Kaufmann, & J. Knitzer (Eds.), *Social and emotional health in early childhood* (pp. 13–35). Baltimore, MD: Brookes.

Thompson, R. A., Thompson, J. E., & Winer, A. C. (2012). Establishing the foundations: Prosocial education in early childhood development. In P. M. Brown, M. W. Corrigan, & A. Higgins-D'Alessandro (Eds.), *The handbook of prosocial education* (Vol. 2, pp. 525–544). New York: Roman & Littlefield.

Thompson, R. A., Virmani, E., Waters, S. F., Meyer, S., & Raikes, A. (2013). The development of emotion regulation: The whole and the sum of the parts. In K. Barrett, N. A. Fox, G. A. Morgan, D. J. Fidler, & L. A. Daunhauer (Eds.), *Handbook of self-regulatory processes in development: New directions and inter-* national perspectives (pp. 5–26). New York: Taylor & Francis.

Thompson, R. A., Winer, A. C., & Goodvin, R. (2011). The individual child: Temperament, emotion, self, and personality. In M. H. Bornstein & M. E. Lamb (Eds.), *Developmental psychology: An advanced textbook* (6th ed., pp. 427–468). Hillsdale, NJ: Erlbaum.

Trentacosta, C. J., & Izard, C. E. (2007). Kindergarten children's emotion competence as a predictor of academic competence in first grade. *Emotion, 7*(1), 77–88.

Trentacosta, C. J., Mostow, A. J., & Izard, C. E. (2005, April). *Emotion knowledge and social skills in middle childhood as predictors of academic competence in later childhood.* Poster presented at the meeting of the Society for Research in Child Development, Atlanta, GA.

Wareham, P., & Salmon, K. (2006). Mother–child reminiscing about everyday experiences: Implications for psychological interventions in the preschool years. *Clinical Psychology Review, 26,* 535–554.

Wellman, H. M. (2002). Understanding the psychological world: Developing a theory of mind. In U. Goswami (Ed.), *Blackwell handbook of childhood cognitive development* (pp. 167–187). London: Blackwell.

Wright, J. C., & Bartsch, K. (2008). Portraits of early moral sensibility in two children's everyday conversations. *Merrill–Palmer Quarterly, 54,* 56–85.

CHAPTER 17

Affective Personality Traits and Cognition

Interactions between Extraversion/Neuroticism, Affect, and Cognition

Adam A Augustine, Randy J. Larsen, and Hwaryung Lee

The interplay between affect and cognition has received a massive amount of attention across several distinct literature areas (see Robinson, Watkins, & Harmon-Jones, Chapter 1, this volume). Indeed, mounting evidence suggests that affect (i.e., emotions and moods) and cognition are, in the least, dependent on one another (Storbeck & Clore, 2007), or at most, not treated differently by the brain (Duncan & Feldman Barrett, 2007). As individuals seek to process their surroundings and make decisions, affect serves as a constant source of information, especially when deliberative thinking is either not possible or not appropriate. As Slovic and Peters (2006) stated, "Although analysis is certainly important in some decision-making tasks circumstances, reliance on affect is generally a quicker, easier, and more efficient way to navigate in a complex, uncertain, and sometimes dangerous world" (p. 322).

Just as state affect exerts a momentary influence on cognition and serves as a momentary source of quick and (usually) efficient information, trait affect may exert a stable influence and serve as a constant source of information. In other words, trait affect may influence cognition in a stable and global manner. Given their strong links

to a variety of affective processes, the personality traits of extraversion and neuroticism have received a relatively large amount of attention in regard to links with cognition (but see also Harmon-Jones, Price, Peterson, Gable, & Harmon-Jones, Chapter 18; Graziano & Tobin, Chapter 19; and Brackett et al., Chapter 20, this volume). In this chapter we review the links between extraversion and neuroticism, affect, and cognition. As we discuss in the ensuing sections, these personality traits exert an influence on a variety of cognitive processes and also interact with affective processes to predict cognition. The role of extraversion and neuroticism in affect–cognition interactions is consistent with the strong links between these traits and affective experience.

Extraversion is a personality trait comprised of enthusiasm, assertiveness, friendliness, gregariousness, activity level, excitement seeking, and cheerfulness; this trait is predictive of both unique positive emotion/mood states (e.g., happiness, gratitude, excitement) and amalgamated measures of positive emotion/mood, or positive affect. Neuroticism is a trait characterized by volatility, withdrawal, anxiety, anger, depression, self-consciousness, immoderation, and vulnerability; this trait is predictive of both unique negative emotion/mood states (e.g., sadness, anxiety, annoyance) and amalgamated measures of negative emotion/mood, or negative affect. The personality traits of extraversion and neuroticism have been consistently linked in correlational studies with trait measures of positive and negative affect, respectively (Costa & McCrae, 1980; Eysenck & Eysenck, 1985). Extraversion and neuroticism also predict state, or momentary, measures of affect; those higher in extraversion experience more frequent and intense positive affect, whereas those higher in neuroticism experience more frequent and intense negative affect (Gross, Sutton, & Ketelaar, 1998). These traits also predict a number of the temporal features of affect, such as rate of change, variance, patterns of change over time, etc. (Hemenover, 2003; Kuppens, Oravecz, & Tuerlinckx, 2010; for a review, see Augustine & Larsen, 2012b). In addition, extraversion and neuroticism predict affect reactivity, or the degree to which one reacts to a given stimulus; extraversion predicts the magnitude of affective reactions to positive stimuli, and neuroticism predicts the magnitude of affective reactions to negative stimuli (Rusting & Larsen, 1997, 1999; Zelenski & Larsen, 1999). Finally, these traits predict a number of components of the affect regulation process (see Suri, Sheppes, & Gross, Chapter 11, this volume), including the choice of affect regulation strategies (Larsen & Prizmic, 2004), affect regulation goals (Augustine, Hemenover, Larsen, & Shulman, 2010), affect regulation ability (Augustine & Hemenover, 2008; Hemenover, Augustine, Shulman, Tran, & Barlett, 2008), and the ability to understand affect (Swinkels & Guiliano, 1995). In the following sections, we discuss the role of extraversion and neuroticism in relation to affect and cognition.

Extraversion

Research examining relationships between extraversion and cognition can be largely organized by theoretical models regarding the core of extraversion. In this section, we rely on the two dominant theories of extraversion—Eysenck and Gray's—and examine studies within these two theoretical traditions that focus on cognitive and affective hypotheses derived from these theories. We also cover some of the more recent work on extraversion and affect regulation.

Eysenck's Theory of Extraversion

One of the first scientific approaches to extraversion is found in the biological theory proposed by Hans Eysenck (1967). This theory of extraversion was based on the then-popular notions of inhibition and excitation and held that introverts were higher in cortical arousal than extraverts. Extraverts, Eysenck proposed, were chronically underaroused relative to introverts. Moreover, assuming people seek an optimal level of arousal, extraverts need more objective stimulation to reach that level than introverts (Eysenck, 1967). Extraverts are extraverted precisely because they need the heightened levels of stimulation provided by high levels of socializing, heightened activity levels, and the seeking out of stimulating activities.

This parsimonious theory has generated several testable predictions about cognition and emotion related to the trait of extraversion. Regarding cognitive activity, because extraverts are relatively underaroused, they should perform better on demanding tasks, especially under arousing conditions (e.g., under high cognitive load), compared to introverts. Alternatively, introverts should perform tasks that require sustained attention in low-demand situations better, because extraverts would be bored or distractible in such conditions.

An example of research testing these deductions from Eysenck's arousal theory of extraversion is that of Revelle, Humphreys, Simon, and Gilliland (1980). In this series of experiments, Revelle and colleagues manipulated arousal with caffeine administration and examined performance on a difficult cognitive test (similar to the verbal test of the Graduate Record Examination) as the dependent variable. They found that administration of a moderate dose of caffeine hindered the performance of introverts. In other words introverts are already overaroused relative to extraverts, and further arousal (due to caffeine administration) pushed them beyond the optimal level of arousal for performance on this demanding task (resulting in decreased performance). They also documented time-of-day effects, with extraverts showing highest arousal levels in the evening and introverts in the morning, a finding that is highly replicable (Larsen, 1985).

Caffeine administration was also used to manipulate physiological arousal in an experiment on cognitive performance conducted by Smillie and Gökçen (2010). In a randomized double-blind placebo-controlled design, they examined the effects of caffeine on working memory (N-back task) as a function of extraversion. Participants received 200 mg of caffeine (equivalent to about three cups of strong coffee). Consistent with the notion that extraverts are underaroused relative to introverts, this dose of caffeine (compared to placebo) improved performance on the working memory task, but only for extraverts.

Other researchers have manipulated arousal with demanding tasks. For example, Lieberman (2000) used a memory scanning paradigm, which is a difficult task tapping the central executive component of working memory. He found that extraversion predicted better performance on this task, consistent with the notion that for introverts (who are already higher in arousal compared to extraverts), the task demands pushed them beyond the optimal level of arousal for performing this task. In a later study, Lieberman and Rosenthal (2001) used a multitasking paradigm to increase task demands, and hence the arousal potential, of the experimental situation. In three experiments they found that introverts performed more poorly than extraverts on a nonverbal decoding task, but only when this task was embedded within the multitasking context. They discuss these results as consistent with Eysenck's arousal theory of extraversion, in that the multitasking environment overstimulated introverts, leading to a decrement in performance relative to extraverts.

While Eysenck's original theory of extraversion proposed individual differences in resting or characteristic levels of arousal, a large body of research now shows that the difference is mainly in arousability, or the arousal response to stimulation. For example, Gale (1983, 1986) provides reviews of studies using moderate levels of stimulation, which show that introverts react with stronger or faster arousal responses than extraverts (i.e., response, rather than resting, differences). This is a subtle, though

important, distinction because of its implications for when we would expect individual differences in extraversion to make a difference. Data such as these led Eysenck to revise his theory of extraversion to implicate arousability, not resting arousal level, as the underlying mechanism (Eysenck & Eysenck, 1985). Extraverts and introverts do not differ, for example, in their level of brain activity while sleeping, or while lying quietly in a darkened room with their eyes shut (Stelmack, 1990). When presented with moderate levels of stimulation, however, introverts show an enhanced physiological reactivity, relative to extraverts (Bullock & Gilliland, 1993).

The development of functional magnetic resonance imaging (fMRI) has allowed researchers to directly test Eysenck's cortical arousability model of extraversion by assessing activity in specific brain regions during task performance. For example, Kumari, Ffytche, Williams, and Gray (2004) used fMRI to assess activity in the dorsolateral prefrontal cortex and the anterior cingulate cortex during performance on an N-back task under varying memory loads (0, 1-, 2-, and 3-back conditions). As predicted by Eysenck's theory, they found that the higher the extraversion score, the greater the increase in fMRI signal from rest to the 3-back condition in these brain areas (but not the lowest-challenge task condition). Interestingly, they also found that extraversion was negatively related to resting brain activity (in the thalamus and Broca's area). Extraverts showed larger increases in brain activation as the task became more demanding, mainly because they started at a lower level of activity in these brain areas than the introverts. In other words, extraverts required a greater level of neurological arousal to perform the task.

An interesting motivational and affective corollary of this individual difference in reactivity, or arousal response to stimulation, results when combined with the notion of optimal level of arousal (Hebb, 1955). Here the idea is that, for any task, there exists an optimal level of arousal, a level at which performance is maximal. If a person is underaroused relative to the optimal level (such as an extravert), then an increase in stimulation will be pleasing and will be sought out. On the other hand, if a person is overaroused relative to the optimal level (such as an introvert), then a decrease in stimulation will be pleasing and the person will seek to avoid or withdraw from stimulation. Consequently, when given a choice, extraverts should prefer higher levels of stimulation relative to introverts. A clever study by Russel Geen (1984) examined choice of level of auditory stimulation while performing a difficult paired-associates learning task. Extraverts consistently chose a higher level of noise than introverts. Moreover, when paired with the level of stimulation chosen by the opposite group, both introverts and extraverts performed worse than the level chosen by their own group (presumably because the level was underarousing for extraverts and overarousing for introverts, a conclusion supported by physiological data).

Because of their diminished reactivity to stimulation, extraverts should be more susceptible to boredom and find boring situations more aversive than introverts. Larsen and Zarate (1991) used a boredom induction (having to perform simple addition and subtraction tasks for a long period of time) and a measure of reducing–augmenting (strongly related to extraversion–introversion, with extraverts scoring in the reducing direction, with a reduced responsiveness to sensory stimulation) to test this hypothesis. During the boredom induction, extraverted participants showed diminished productivity relative to the introverts. Afterward the extraverts rated the activity as significantly more aversive than the introverts, were more likely to choose to undergo a negative mood induction rather than engage in a similarly boring task than the introverts, and were less likely to volunteer for similar experiments in the future. Anecdotally, several of the extraverted subjects engaged in spontaneous self-stimulation during this experiment (e.g., singing, pacing, while working on the problems). Also, two subjects fell asleep during the study (both extraverts).

In sum, several reviews of Eysenck's theory of extraversion (e.g., Matthews & Gilliland, 1999; Wilt & Revelle, 2009; Zelenski, 2007) conclude that the arousal theory of extraversion has received a moderate amount of support, with introverts displaying more reactivity to stimulation, and hence more stimulation avoidance, than extraverts. After more than a half century

since it was proposed, this theory is finding some support using modern imaging methods to directly assess brain reactivity under various cognitive conditions. Nevertheless, in the 1970s and 1980s, another prominent researcher proposed an alternative causal theory of extraversion. This theory, which is also parsimonious, has likewise generated much research on the topic.

Gray's Theory of Extraversion

An influential alternative theory of extraversion is that proposed by Jeffrey Gray (1970, 1981, 1982), which is today referred to as *reinforcement sensitivity theory* (Beattie & Corr, 2010; Corr, 2009). Gray based his theory on studies of brain function in animals, and he constructed a model of human personality based on hypothesized biological systems in the brain. He called these systems the *behavioral activation system* (BAS) and the *behavioral inhibition system* (BIS). Measures of these two systems map closely onto measures of extraversion and neuroticism, respectively (e.g., Elliot & Thrash, 2010; Rusting & Larsen, 1997, 1999; Smits & Boeck, 2006). Indeed, several questionnaire measures of BAS (e.g., Carver & White, 1994) are found to load highly on a dimension defined by extraversion measures (Zelenski & Larsen, 1999). Results such as these led Gray to revise his model and acknowledge that BAS and extraversion were very nearly the same psychometric construct (Pickering, Corr, & Gray, 1999), but differ in terms of the proposed causal mechanism. Gray proposed sensitivity to reward cues as the underlying cause of this individual difference, whereas Eysenck proposed arousability.

The BAS is the hypothetical brain circuit that Gray proposed was responsive to incentives and reward, such as cues of positive reinforcement, and is thought to underlie and motivate approach behavior. Moreover, people differ in the sensitivity of their BAS, and hence differ in their sensitivity to reward cues and in their responsiveness to positive reinforcement. Using fMRI methods, Canli and colleagues (2001) showed that the brains of extraverts (compared to introverts) were more reactive to pleasant, rewarding images. Some people are more reactive to reward, and have stronger positive emotional responses to pleasant stimuli, because, Gray would argue, they have a relatively sensitive behavioral activation system.

This theory generates predictions about emotional reactivity and extraversion, suggesting that it should be easier to evoke positive emotions in extraverts compared to introverts. Although numerous studies have shown reliable correlations between extraversion and positive affect (e.g., Costa & McCrae, 1980), Larsen and colleagues (Larsen & Ketelaar, 1989, 1991; Rusting & Larsen, 1998; Zelenski & Larsen, 1999) were the first to demonstrate this relation experimentally. In these studies, positive affect was manipulated in the laboratory and affective response was measured. The studies differ with respect to how affect was manipulated and how positive affect was measured. Nevertheless, they all converge on the finding that extraverts show a significantly larger positive affect response than introverts, a finding that has been replicated in numerous other laboratories (e.g., Canli et al., 2001; McNiel, Lowman, & Fleeson, 2010).

Because positive affect influences several cognitive activities, individual differences in positive affect reactivity (i.e., BAS or extraversion) should be associated with those cognitive activities. This line of research has grown into a very large literature, and we review only a handful of studies here. For example, Robinson, Moeller, and Ode (2010) found, across four experiments, that extraversion correlated with the magnitude of affective priming effects, but only for positive primes, suggesting that the activation of positive associations in people's memories is stronger for extraverts than introverts. Gomez, Gomez, and Cooper (2002) found that extraversion predicted more efficient information processing, but only when the information was positive (compared to negative and neutral information). Stafford, Ng, Moore, and Bard (2010) examined the interaction of extraversion and a positive mood induction and found that performance on a creativity task improved in the positive mood induction (compared to the negative induction), but mainly for extraverted subjects (compared to introverts). A similar finding was obtained by Hirsh, Guindon, Morisano, and Peterson (2010) using delay discounting as the dependent variable; posi-

tive mood was associated with a preference for more immediate rewards, especially if subjects were high on extraversion. A similarly designed study by Rafienia, Azadfallah, Fathi-Ashtiani, and Rasoulzadeh-Tabatabaiei (2008) showed that a positive mood induction influenced subjects to make more positive judgments and interpretations of an ambiguous story, but only more extraverted subjects.

Other studies have demonstrated that, even controlling for current mood, extraverts tend to show positive affect-like effects on cognitive processing. For example, Uziel (2006) showed that extraversion was associated with more positive ratings of a variety of life events, even after controlling for current levels of positive affect. Rusting and Larsen (1998) showed, in Study 1, that extraversion was associated with several positive cognitive effects: for example, faster reaction time to judge positive words, fewer errors in processing positive words, and more accurate memory for positive words. Moreover, in Study 2, Rusting and Larsen showed that such findings remained intact after controlling for current levels of positive affect, suggesting that extraversion is associated with a bias for processing positive material that goes beyond the influence of that expected from their generally heightened levels of positive emotion. Rusting (1999) went on to demonstrate similar effects of extraversion on higher-level cognitive processing using a series of memory and judgment tasks, finding that extraversion (in interaction with positive affect) predicted the retrieval of positive memories and the tendency to make positive judgments.

Researchers using functional brain imaging have also been active in investigating predictions from Gray's theory of extraversion. For example, Amin, Constable, and Canli (2004) used fMRI while participants were engaged in an attentional task to identify brain regions that are involved in attentional bias in processing words that are positive or negative. They found that activation in the fusiform gyrus was significantly correlated with extraversion, especially when participants were searching for positive words in sections of the visual field least likely to be attended to. Canli, Amin, Haas, Omura, and Constable (2004) used fMRI while participants completed an emotional Stroop task and found that activation in the anterior cingulate increased while processing positive words as a function of extraversion. In a review of extraversion and neuroscience, Canli (2004) discusses numerous brain regions (e.g., amygdala, caudate, mediofrontal gyrus, right fusiform gyrus) in which extraversion predicts activation during certain cognitive and positive affective tasks. Based on these results, Canli concludes that extraversion refers to individual differences that are widely distributed across brain areas, and that they are tuned to process stimuli associated with positive incentives.

In summary, a great deal of research supports Gray's reinforcement sensitivity theory of extraversion. Extraverts consistently show more reactivity to positive mood inductions, have chronically higher levels of positive affect, and show a number of cognitive biases in the processing of positive stimuli. While Eysenck and Gray's theories are often viewed as competing theoretical positions, it is actually possible that both may be at least partially correct. That is, extraverts may be both lower in general arousability than introverts *and* more sensitive to positive stimuli and incentives. Major reviews of these two theoretical traditions (e.g., Matthews & Gilliland, 1999; Wilt & Revelle, 2009) conclude that both have received moderate levels of support. A particularly interesting line of research comes from studies that consider the interaction of extraversion and neuroticism in predicting outcomes (e.g., Robinson, Wilkowski, & Meier, 2008), though a review of this area is beyond the scope of this chapter.

Extraversion and Emotion Regulation

Many investigators have shown that extraversion is consistently related to long-term measures of happiness, well-being, and trait pleasant affect (e.g., Costa & McCrae, 1980). Understanding the mechanisms underlying this effect has been the object of recent research on mood or affect regulation. For example, Larsen and Prizmic (2004) discuss a detailed taxonomy, and present a related measure, of a variety of specific affect regulation strategies and behaviors, ranging from helping others and counting one's blessings to the seeking out of pleasure and spending time with others. They speculated that individual differences in either the frequency or effectiveness of specific affect regulation attempts would relate to affectively relevant personality traits, such as extraversion. Other studies have shown direct correlations between extraversion and specific affect regulation strategies. For example, Augustine and Hemenover (2008) showed that extraversion predicted affect repair when alone, and that social interaction—something for which extraverts are known—helped all participants repair their negative moods.

Lischetzke and Eid (2006) present a series of studies that ask the question: Why are extraverts happier than introverts? Their conclusion, based on three studies employing multiple methods, is that, even though extraverts are more reactive to positive events, they also maintain their positive affect longer following those events compared to introverts. That is, extraversion is related to mood maintenance, or the continuation of positive affect after it is evoked. This specific form of affect regulation is distinguished from affect repair, which did not relate strongly to extraversion in the studies reported by Lischetzke and Eid. Instead, extraversion related to longer duration of positive affect, with multimethod evidence that extraverts show a slower decay of positive affect. Such findings are consistent with Larsen and Prizmic's (2007) contention that strategies to repair negative affect are distinct from strategies to promote positive affect, and that neuroticism predicts the former, whereas extraversion predicts the latter. This is also consistent with Eysenck's theory of extraversion; seeking to extend positive affect through mood maintenance may be yet another way that the extraverted individual increases arousal levels.

Other researchers are investigating cognitive mechanisms underlying affect regulation in extraverts. For example, Tamir, Robinson, and Clore (2002) showed that, when in a positive mood, extraverts were faster to link their personal motives to events, suggesting that trait-consistent moods (positive for extraverts) have a pragmatic benefit for processing motivation-relevant stimuli. Other studies, discussed above in the section on Gray's theory, suggest that, for extraverts, positive mood promotes the kind of cognitive activity that can, in turn, further promote positive mood. For example, Tamir and Robinson (2004) showed that positive mood promotes selective attention and preferential processing of rewarding and other positive stimuli. Tamir (2009) has shown that extraversion is related to a motive toward happiness and that preferences for happiness-inducing activities were correlated with extraversion scores. Thus, extraverts, more so than introverts, demonstrate the types of cognitive activities that promote positive feelings, which, in turn, promote the kinds of cognitive activities that maintain those feelings.

Neuroticism

Findings concerning neuroticism and cognition span a number of literatures, but can generally be organized into four different levels of processing. First, neuroticism predicts both the ways in which individuals perceive and react to various types of stimuli. Second, neuroticism predicts broad cognitive patterns; it is indicative of a cognitive style. Third, differences in the ways in which individual encode and recall information is related to neuroticism. Finally, differences in judgments and decision making are related to neuroticism.

Stimulus Reactivity

When presented with a negative stimulus, those higher in neuroticism tend to have a stronger negative affective reaction to that stimulus, or a greater degree of negative affect reactivity. These reactivity effects have been observed with both affective and non-affective stimuli. Indeed, it may be this reactivity that underlies the status of neuroticism as a risk factor for various forms of psychopathology (for a review, see Kotov, Gamez, Schmidt, & Watson, 2010). In regard to affective stimuli, the process of affect reactivity has been widely replicated with a variety of stimulus types. Those higher in neuroticism show greater affect reactivity to a number of negative (but not positive) affect induction procedures, including guided imagery (Larsen & Ketelaar, 1991), false performance feedback (Larsen & Ketelaar, 1989), viewing affective images (Augustine & Larsen, 2011; Zelenski & Larsen, 2000),

and viewing affective films (Hemenover, 2003; Hemenover et al., 2008).

Affect reactivity findings for neuroticism have also been extended into nonlaboratory settings using experience sampling designs. Individuals high in neuroticism experience more negative health symptoms (Larsen & Kasimatis, 1991), undesirable events (David, Green, Martin, & Suls, 1997), and general problems (Suls & Martin, 2005). They also react more strongly when these troubles arise. For instance, neuroticism predicts greater reactivity to interpersonal conflicts (Suls, Martin, & David, 1998) and negative stress appraisals (Cimbolic Gunthert, Cohen, & Armeli, 1999).

Differential reactions to negative affective stimuli can also be observed at a physiological level. Neuroticism predicts the magnitude of facial emotional responses to negative stimuli (Berenbaum & Williams, 1995). In addition, neuroticism predicts greater skin conductance reactivity (as well as a more prolonged response) to negative stimuli (Norris, Larsen, & Cacioppo, 2007). Neuroticism also predicts heightened, nonspecific spontaneous electrodermal activity at rest, suggesting hyperactivity of the sympathetic nervous system on the part of those higher in neuroticism (Larsen & Cruz, 1995). At a neural level, neuroticism predicts neural activation in response to negative stimuli; this effect is observable across a number of different brain regions (Canli et al., 2001). Finally, the frontal brain asymmetries associated with neuroticism are also predictive of differential reactions to negative affect (Wheeler, Davidson, & Tomarken, 1993; but see Schmidtke & Heller, 2004, for a discussion of frontal vs. posterior activation and neuroticism). Thus, neuroticism predicts the degree to which individuals respond to negative affective stimuli, such that those higher in neuroticism display greater negative affect reactivity. Those higher in neuroticism also show differential responses to stimuli that are not purely affective, but merely possess affective connotations (e.g., threatening or punishment-related stimuli).

Although findings concerning neuroticism and the ability to detect threatening stimuli have been mixed, recent research indicates that those higher in neuroticism react more strongly to signals of punishment (Moeller & Robinson, 2010). At a broad level, trait negative affect is related to cognitive control, such that those higher in trait negative affect (e.g., those high in neuroticism) show lessened cognitive control, or a lessened ability to inhibit dominant responses (i.e., attend to negative stimuli; Moriya & Tanno, 2008). The effects of this lack of control on stimulus reactivity can be observed by measuring individuals' reaction to errors. There are two primary ways of encapsulating cognitive error reactivity: posterror adjustment and the tendency to make errors in strings.

In standard cognitive tasks (e.g., the Stroop task), some individuals show greater posterror slowing, or the tendency to slow down on the trial following a trial on which an error was committed. This slowing tendency is thought to represent the ability to detect threats (i.e., negative stimuli) as they occur. Although this slowing tendency or threat detection ability does not relate directly to neuroticism, posterror slowing interacts with neuroticism, such that those high in neuroticism and high in posterror slowing show lower levels of daily distress (Robinson, Ode, Wilkowski, & Amodio, 2007). In other words, those higher in neuroticism who have a greater tendency to down-regulate threats/punishment/errors show better affective outcomes. Consistent with this finding, those who are higher in neuroticism and also better at threat identification show better affective outcomes (Tamir, Robinson, & Solberg, 2006). In addition to posterror slowing, some individuals also display posterror behavioral adjustments. However, those relatively higher in neuroticism are more likely to make these posterror behavioral adjustments when they are told that they have committed an error (Moeller & Robinson, 2010). In other words, those higher in neuroticism are more sensitive to error feedback and more likely to change their behavior when they receive error feedback. Although posterror slowing and behavioral adjustment may not directly relate to neuroticism, the second error reactivity measure—the tendency to make errors in strings—is directly related to neuroticism.

Some individuals show a tendency to make errors in strings in standard cognitive tasks; they are likely to make more than one error in a row (Compton et al., 2008), and this tendency (measured using the AX-CPT and *N*-back) is directly related to neuroti-

cism (Augustine, 2011). The link between neuroticism and the tendency to make errors in strings may be due to the anxiety component of neuroticism; the tendency to make errors in strings shows stronger relationships with the anxiety subfacet of neuroticism (Augustine, 2011) and moderates the relationships between daily stress and anxiety, such that those who are more likely to make errors in strings show a stronger relationship between daily stress and anxiety (Compton et al., 2008). The tendency to make errors in strings also predicts health in a similar manner as does neuroticism; those higher in neuroticism and those who are more likely to make errors in strings report more intense daily health symptoms (Augustine, 2011).

At a neurological level, error regulation and affective functioning are associated with activation in the same brain regions. The anterior cingulate cortex is thought to be involved in emotion regulation (Hajcak & Foti, 2008; Ochsner & Gross, 2005). This region has also been shown to be involved in error avoidance and monitoring (Brown & Braver, 2005). In addition, this brain region shows a response when errors are made, the degree of this response predicts the magnitude of negative reaction to the error, and this response is modulated by affective variables (Hajcak & Foti, 2008). Thus, the individual high in neuroticism shows deficits in both affect regulation (Hemenover et al., 2008) and error regulation (Augustine, 2011), and these two processes are associated with activation in the same neurological structures.

Cognitive Style

Neuroticism predicts a number of broad patterns in cognition, or a cognitive style (e.g., Shapiro, 1965). These neuroticism-based patterns can be detected by examining the ways in which individuals focus their attention on negative stimuli, the degree of variation in response to stimuli, and the manner in which individuals allocate effort in response to varying task demands. In general, these processing patterns paint a picture of the highly neurotic individual as a negatively focused, cognitively erratic, and mentally depleted individual.

Research examining the attentional focus of those higher in neuroticism indicates that neurotics are relatively high in self-focused attention/cognition (Field, Joudy, & Hart, 2010). Given that those higher in neuroticism experience a larger number of negative events (Suls & Martin, 2005), it is not surprising that this increased self-focus results in higher levels of negative affect (Field et al., 2010). Consistent with this increased and relatively negative self-focus, those higher in neuroticism are also more likely to ruminate on negative events and occurrences. Findings have consistently indicated that neurotics are higher in both trait and daily ruminative patterns (Augustine et al., 2010; Hankin, Fraley, & Abela, 2005; Larsen & Prizmic, 2004), whereby these individual spend more time thinking about negative events. This increase in negative self-focused attention and rumination may also explain links between neuroticism and depression. The inability to inhibit negative cognition/attention and ruminate on negative occurrences is a hallmark of the depressed individual (Joormann & Gotlib, 2010) and this cognitive style is also indicative of the highly neurotic individual. Indeed, the tendency to ruminate on negative events has been found to mediate the relationship between neuroticism and both vulnerability to depression (Roberts, Gilboa, & Gotlib, 1998) and current depressive symptoms (Hankin et al., 2005; Muris, Roelofs, Rassin, Franken, & Mayer, 2005; Roelefs, Huibers, Peeters, & Arntz, 2008). Thus, the neurotic individual has a relatively negative and self-focused cognitive style, and this cognitive style explains the links between neuroticism and depression.

In addition to a negative cognitive style, those who are higher in neuroticism also display a more variant pattern of cognition, also known as the *mental noise hypothesis* (Robinson & Tamir, 2005). Across a variety of experimental tasks, Robinson and Tamir (2005) found that neuroticism predicted variance in reaction times, such that those who were higher in neuroticism displayed more variability in the speed of their responses. In other words, effort (speed) should be allocated on a fairly even basis, peaking at the point of decision or reaction in one of these tasks. However, those higher in neuroticism do not show the appropriate allocation of effort. Consistent with this notion, those higher in neuroticism show

more sustained neural activity (in the anterior cingulate cortex) during a speeded reaction tasks (the N-back); this is essentially wasted energy, as activation should peak at the time of decision/reaction, as is the case for those lower in neuroticism (Gray et al., 2005). This increased mental noise and wasted effort also has negative affective consequences, as those higher in neuroticism and higher in mental noise experience more distress and negative affect (Robinson, Wilkowski, & Meier, 2006).

The relatively high mental noise of the neurotic individual can also be seen during periods of changing demands. Negative affect is more highly related to neuroticism when an individual is also higher in response inflexibility/perseveration (Robinson, Wilkowski, Kirkeby, & Meier, 2006). Findings such as these may stem from the general lack of cognitive control expressed by the highly neurotic individual (Moriya & Tanno, 2008) and the tendency for those higher in neuroticism to ruminate (Augustine et al., 2010; Hankin et al., 2005; Larsen & Prizmic, 2004). In line with this possibility, Flehmig, Steinborn, Langner, and Westhoff (2007) found that those higher in neuroticism experienced more cognitive failures. These cognitive failures came in the form of the intrusion of task-irrelevant cognitions, the inability to encode–retrieve task-relevant content, and the inability to detect task-relevant features. However, the variant nature of neurotic cognitions and the inability to vary effort according to task demands can have some benefits for the neurotic individual.

As tasks become more difficult, those higher in neuroticism may actually increase in their performance (Smillie, Yeo, Furnham, & Jackson, 2006). However, this increase in performance as difficulty increases is not necessarily a broad effect for neuroticism; the nature of these benefits depends on certain aspects of neuroticism. When examined at the level of aspects (e.g., DeYoung, Quilty, & Peterson, 2007), the costs and benefits of cognitive inflexibility diverge. Those who are higher in the withdrawal (e.g., depression/worry) aspect of neuroticism do experience an increase in performance as difficulty increases, possibly due to a decrease in intrusive cognitions. On the other hand, those higher in the volatility (i.e., affect reactivity) aspect of neuroticism decrease in performance as difficulty increases, possibly due to frustration with increasing task demands (van Doorn, & Lang, 2010).

Encoding and Recall

Not only does neuroticism predict the ways in which individuals respond to and process stimuli, it also impacts the manner in which experiences are stored in and retrieved from memory. These effects may arise, in part, due to basic differences in working memory. Those with larger working memory capacities are better able to regulate their automatic behavioral and affective responses (Hofmann, Gschwendner, Friese, Wiers, & Schmitt, 2008). In other words, larger working memory capacities may facilitate behavioral self-regulation. In line with this proposal, working memory capacity predicts individuals' ability to engage in affect regulation, and these increased abilities lead to improved regulatory outcomes (i.e., more positive and less negative affect; Schmeichel, Volokhov, & Demaree, 2008). Those higher in neuroticism also show a wide range of regulatory deficits (e.g., Compton et al., 2008; Hemenover et al., 2008) and thus may have some deficit in working memory capacity or flexibility.

Indeed, affective information takes up space in working memory and affect regulation may, in part, function by interrupting the maintenance of this information. With a larger working memory capacity, more space would be available for the deployment of a regulation attempt. In other words, those with smaller working memory capacities could have such a large portion of their cognitive resources engaged by the affective experience itself that no resources are available for regulation. Working memory may also possess a uniquely affective component, and individuals with deficits in the affective components of working memory may show a decreased ability to repair affect (Mikels, Reuter-Lorenz, Beyer, & Fredrickson, 2008). Although research into the relation among neuroticism, self-regulation, and working memory is just beginning, it is possible that there are neuroticism-related differences in working memory. Although this research is at a rather tentative stage, a number of findings suggest that neuroticism is related to differences in long-term storage and retrieval.

In addition to working memory differences, those higher in neuroticism may possess associative networks (e.g., Bower & Forgas, 2001) containing broader and more densely interconnected negative affective information (Robinson, Ode, Moeller, & Goetz, 2007). This is consistent with both the daily experiences of the highly neurotic individual and with the types of information those higher in neuroticism encode and recall. Given their relatively negative experiences (Suls & Martin, 2005), those higher in neuroticism have more negative events/experiences to encode. In line with this, those higher in neuroticism (and other negative affect-laden traits) recall more negative memories under a variety of experimental conditions (e.g., Bradley & Mogg, 1994; Lyubomirsky, Caldwell, & Nolen-Hoeksema, 1998). Not only does the highly neurotic individual recall more negative memories, but focusing on these negative memories can lead to a negativity bias when interpreting a number of neutral events for those higher in negative affect (Lyubomirsky & Nolen-Hoeksema, 1995; see also Watkins, Chapter 21, this volume), and this bias exists at both the encoding level and at the recall level of events (Larsen, 1992). Thus, the highly neurotic individual should possess a broad and densely interconnected associative network for negative information. With more negative experiences and a bias toward interpreting events as negative, those higher in neuroticism possess memory systems that are relatively awash with negative affective information.

Judgments and Decision Making

Given that neuroticism predicts cognitive processes ranging from attention up through memory recall, it would be reasonable to assume that neuroticism would predict higher-level cognitive processes, such as complex judgment and decision making. Indeed, a number of findings indicate that neuroticism is related to higher-level cognitions. For instance, neuroticism predicts broad decision patterns: Those higher in neuroticism are more likely to rely on the recognition heuristic (Hilbig, 2008). Neuroticism also predicts cognitions regarding decisions, with neurotics (vs. emotionally stable individuals) showing lower confidence in their responses to general knowledge questions (Hancock, Moffoot, & O'Carroll, 1996). In addition, neuroticism predicts response speed. When they are experiencing negative affect, those higher in neuroticism are faster to categorize words (Tamir & Robinson, 2004). Finally, neuroticism predicts the types of risks individuals are willing to take: Those higher in neuroticism are apt to make less risky decisions to achieve gains, but more risky decisions to avoid losses (Lauriola & Levin, 2001).

Although not an exhaustive review, these findings are fairly representative of research relating neuroticism to judgments and decision making. In general, these findings are relatively scattered and inconsistent (Oreg & Bayazit, 2009). This is rather surprising given the broad pattern of effects relating neuroticism to lower-level cognitive processes. However, this inconsistency may be due to some basic issues regarding both experimental design and research examining the effect of momentary affect on judgments and decision making.

A massive amount of attention has been paid to the impact of momentary affect on cognition. Indeed, it can be relatively easy to change individuals' decision-making patterns, requiring only minor affective information. As an example, Augustine and Larsen (2012a) inserted a single affect adjective into a lengthy vignette describing a potential outcome and had participants judge the probability that the described event would actually occur. Probability judgments varied based on which affect adjective had been inserted into the vignette, with affects indicative of approach motivations (e.g., *happy, angry*) leading to higher probability estimates than those indicative of avoidance motivations (e.g., *sad, scared*).

Despite the relative ease of obtaining effects for momentary affective information and decision making, affect does not show consistent effects across different tasks and outcomes (Chepenik, Cornew, & Farah, 2007). These inconsistencies could be due to two factors. First, condition (positive or negative affective information) is usually taken as a proxy for actual affective experience. However, and as was previously described, individual differences exist in the degree to

which one responds to affective stimuli (i.e., *affect reactivity*; Larsen & Ketelaar, 1991). Second, these studies often fail to take into account individual difference variables, such as neuroticism. As described in a recent theory regarding personality and decision making (Oreg & Bayazit, 2009), individual difference variables, such as neuroticism, should be related to decision processes in a number of domains.

To gain a more detailed understanding of the influence of personality on decision making, we (Augustine & Larsen, 2011; Augustine, Larsen, & Elliot, in press) conducted a series of studies examining the ways in which affective stimuli, state affect, and trait affect (i.e., neuroticism) jointly influence decision making. If all of these sources of affective information can predict decision making, then it follows that they may do so in a synergistic manner. In other words, if all of these sources of affect are taken into account, then the inconsistencies in research relating affect and personality to higher-level cognition may disappear.

In our first examination of this possibility (Augustine & Larsen, 2011), we evaluated the influence of primed, induced, and experienced affect, as well as neuroticism, on temporal discounting (the tendency to choose a small immediate, rather than a large delayed, reward). Our results indicated that primed affect (positive or negative affect adjective primes), experienced affect, and neuroticism interacted to predict temporal discounting rates (Augustine & Larsen, 2011, Study 1). In addition, induced affect (positive or negative affect induction), experienced affect, and neuroticism interacted to predict temporal discounting rates (Augustine & Larsen, 2011, Study 2). Moreover, the nature of these interactions differed between studies. With less intense negative affective information available in the priming study, those higher in neuroticism were less likely to choose the regulatory option of receiving an immediate reward. With more intense negative affective information in the induction study, those higher in neuroticism were actually more likely to choose the regulatory option.

The influence of affective information on higher-level judgments may also function in an additive manner. In a second examination, we (Augustine et al., in press) found that primed affect (affect adjective and affective picture primes) and experienced affect predicted evaluative judgments of ambiguous stimuli (Arabic characters and Rorschach figures) in an additive manner, while neuroticism interacted with the valence of experimental affective information to predict these judgments (e.g., was only predictive in the negative priming condition). The results indicate that, unlike our findings for temporal discounting, these sources of affective information tend to function in a more additive manner. In other words, evaluative decisions become more negative when an individual has access to more sources (e.g., environmental/experimental, state, trait), or more intense sources of negative affective information, be it in the form of experimental stimuli or experience; neuroticism adds to this predictive power for negative, but not positive, informational loads. Thus, neuroticism can consistently predict higher-level cognitive processes, such as judgments and decision making. However, one must also take into account other sources of affective information that can impact those decisions.

Conclusions

In this chapter we provide a review of research relating the "Big Two" personality variables—extraversion and neuroticism—to cognition and emotion. Of all the individual difference factors, at least outside of the ability domain, these two personality variables have seen the most research related to cognition and emotion. Consequently, our review was meant to be illustrative rather than exhaustive, with our goal to provide a sampling of findings that illustrate how emotion, cognition, and their interaction are related to these two fundamental dispositions.

Allport (1937) taught that personality was a self-maintaining system that functioned to provide consistency over time and situation. Indeed, the cognitive underpinnings of neuroticism and extraversion may partially account for this consistency. Looking over our discussion of neuroticism and extraversion, we can see hints of the homeostatic nature of personality traits. Neuroticism is related to negative affect, which in turn promotes the kinds of cognitive activities that

reinforce or promote further negative affect, hence perpetuating the individual difference over time and situation. Extraversion relates to positive affect in a similar manner, with associated cognitive activities that promote the further experience or maintenance of positive emotion. Understanding the intervening processes—both cognitive and affective, as well as their interactions—has provided an exciting avenue of research on these two basic dimensions of personality.

Acknowledgments

During the preparation of this chapter, Adam A Augustine was supported by a National Research Service Award (No. T32 GM081739) to Randy J. Larsen. Preparation of this work was also supported by Grant No. R01 AG028419 to Randy J. Larsen.

References

Allport, G. W. (1937). *Personality: A psychological interpretation.* New York: Henry Holt.
Amin, Z., Constable, R., & Canli, T. (2004). Attentional bias for valenced stimuli as a function of personality in the dot-probe task. *Journal of Research in Personality, 38,* 15–23.
Augustine, A. A (2011). *Personal cognition and the affect regulation process: Affect reactivity, affect regulation ability, and responses to cognitive errors.* Unpublished doctoral dissertation. Washington University in St. Louis, MO.
Augustine, A. A, & Hemenover, S. H. (2008). Extraversion and the consequences of social interaction on affect repair. *Personality and Individual Differences, 44,* 1151–1161.
Augustine, A. A, Hemenover, S. H., Larsen, R. J., & Shulman, T. E. (2010). Composition and consistency of the desired affective state: The role of personality and motivation. *Motivation and Emotion, 34,* 133–143.
Augustine, A. A, & Larsen, R. J. (2011). Affect regulation and temporal discounting: Interactions between primed, state, and trait affect, *Emotion, 11,* 403–412.
Augustine, A. A, & Larsen, R. J. (2012a). *Affective influences on probability judgments.* Manuscript in preparation.
Augustine, A. A, & Larsen, R. J. (2012b). Emotion research. In M. R. Mehl & T. S. Conner (Eds.), *Handbook of research methods for*

studying daily life (pp. 497–510). New York: Guilford Press.

Augustine, A. A, Larsen, R. J., & Elliot, A. J. (in press). Affect is greater than, not equal to, condition: Condition and person effects in affective priming paradigms. *Journal of Personality.*

Beattie, E. K., & Corr, P. J. (2010). Reinforcement, arousal and temporal factors in procedural learning: A test of Eysenck's and Gray's personality theories. *Journal of Individual Differences, 31,* 167–177.

Berenbaum, H., & Williams, M. (1995). Personality and emotional reactivity. *Journal of Research in Personality, 29,* 24–34.

Bower, G. H., & Forgas, J. P. (2001). Affect, memory, and social cognition. In E. Eich (Ed.), *Cognition and emotion* (pp. 87–168). Oxford, UK: Oxford University Press.

Bradley, B., & Mogg, K. (1994). Mood and personality in recall of positive and negative information. *Behavior Research and Therapy, 32,* 137–141.

Brown, J. W., & Braver, T. S. (2005). Learned predictions of error likelihood in the anterior cingulate cortex. *Science, 307,* 1118–1121.

Bullock, W. A., & Gilliland, K. (1993). Eysenck's arousal theory of introversion–extraversion: A converging measures investigation. *Journal of Personality and Social Psychology, 64,* 113–123.

Canli, T. (2004). Functional brain mapping of extraversion and neuroticism: Learning from individual differences in emotion processing. *Journal of Personality, 72*(6), 1105–1132.

Canli, T., Amin, Z., Haas, B., Omura, K., & Constable, R. (2004). A double dissociation between mood states and personality traits in the anterior cingulate. *Behavioral Neuroscience, 118*(5), 897–904.

Canli, T., Zhao, Z., Desmond, J. E., Kang, E., Gross, J. J., & Gabrieli, J. D. E. (2001). An fMRI study of personality influences on brain reactivity to emotional stimuli. *Behavioral Neuroscience, 115,* 33–42.

Carver, C. S., & White, T. L. (1994). Behavioral inhibition, behavioral activation, and affective responses to impeding reward and punishments: The BIS/BAS scales. *Journal of Personality and Social Psychology, 67,* 319–333.

Chepenik, L. G., Cornew, L. A., & Farah, M. J. (2007). The influence of sad mood on cognition. *Emotion, 7,* 802–811.

Cimbolic Gunthert, K., Cohen, L. H., & Armeli, S. (1999). The role of neuroticism in daily stress and coping. *Journal of Personality and Social Psychology, 77,* 1087–1100.

Compton, R. J., Robinson, M. D., Ode, S., Quandt, L. C., Fineman, S. L., & Carp, J. (2008). Error-monitoring ability predicts daily stress regulation. *Psychological Science, 19,* 702–708.

Corr, P. J. (2009). The reinforcement sensitivity theory of personality. In P. J. Corr & G. Matthews (Eds.), *The Cambridge handbook of personality psychology* (pp. 347–376). New York: Cambridge University Press.

Costa, P. T., & McCrae, R. R. (1980). Influence of extraversion and neuroticism on subjective well-being: Happy and unhappy people. *Journal of Personality and Social Psychology, 36,* 668–678.

David, J. P., Green, P. J., Martin, R., & Suls, J. (1997). Differential roles of neuroticism, extraversion, and event desirability for mood in daily life: An integrative model of top-down and bottom-up influences. *Journal of Personality and Social Psychology, 73,* 149–159.

DeYoung, C. G., Quilty, L. C., & Peterson, J. B. (2007). Between facets and domains: 10 aspects of the Big Five. *Journal of Personality and Social Psychology, 93,* 880–896.

Duncan, S., & Feldman Barrett, L. (2007). Affect is a form of cognition: A neurobiological analysis. *Cognition and Emotion, 21,* 1184–1211.

Elliot, A. J., & Thrash, T. M. (2010). Approach and avoidance temperament as basic dimensions of personality. *Journal of Personality, 78*(3), 865–906.

Eysenck, H. J. (1967). *The biological basis of personality.* Springfield, IL: Charles C Thomas.

Eysenck, H. J., & Eysenck, M. W. (1985). *Personality and individual differences.* New York: Plenum Press.

Field, N. P., Joudy, R., & Hart, D. (2010). The moderating effect of self-concept valence on the relationship between self-focused attention and mood: An experience sampling study. *Journal of Research in Personality, 44,* 70–77.

Flehmig, H. C., Steinborn, M., Langner, R., & Westhoff, K. (2007). Neuroticism and the mental noise hypothesis: Relationships to lapses of attention and slips of action in everyday life. *Psychology Science, 49,* 343–360.

Gale, A. (1983). Electroencephalographic studies of extraversion–introversion: A case study in the psychophysiology of individual differences. *Personality and Individual Differences, 4,* 371–380.

Gale, A. (1986). Extraversion–introversion and

spontaneous rhythms of the brain: Retrospect and prospect. In J. Strelau, F. Farley, & A. Gale (Eds.), *The biological basis of personality and behavior* (Vol. 2). Washington, DC: Hemisphere.

Geen, R. G. (1984). Preferred stimulation levels in introverts and extroverts: Effects of arousal and performance. *Journal of Personality and Social Psychology, 46*(6), 1303–1312.

Gomez, R., Gomez, A., & Cooper, A. (2002). Neuroticism and extraversion as predictors of negative and positive emotional information processing: Comparing Eysenck's, Gray's and Newman's theories. *European Journal of Personality, 16*, 333–350.

Gray, J. A. (1970). The psychophysiological basis of introversion–extraversion. *Behaviour Research and Therapy, 8*, 249–266.

Gray, J. A. (1981). A critique of Eysenck's theory of personality. In H. J. Eysenck (Ed.), *A model for personality* (pp. 246–277). Berlin: Springer-Verlag.

Gray, J. A. (1982). *Neuropsychological theory of anxiety: An investigation of the septal-hippocampal system.* Cambridge, UK: Cambridge University Press.

Gray, J. R., Burgess, G. C., Schaefer, A., Yarkoni, T., Larsen, R. J., & Braver, T. S. (2005). Affective personality differences in neural processing efficiency confirmed using fMRI. *Cognitive, Affective, and Behavioral Neuroscience, 5*, 182–190.

Gross, J. J., Sutton, S. K., & Ketelaar, T. V. (1998). Relations between affect and personality: Support for the affect-level and affective-reactivity views. *Personality and Social Psychology Bulletin, 24*, 279–288.

Hajcak, G., & Foti, D. (2008). Errors are aversive: Defensive motivation and the error-related negativity. *Psychological Science, 19*, 103–108.

Hancock, J., Moffoot, A., & O'Carroll, R. (1996). "Depressive realism" assessed via confidence in decision-making. *Cognitive Neuropsychiatry, 1*, 213–220.

Hankin, B. L., Fraley, R. C., & Abela, J. R. (2005). Daily depression and cognitions about stress: Evidence for a trait-like depressogenic cognitive style and the prediction of depressive symptoms in a prospective daily diary study. *Journal of Personality and Social Psychology, 88*, 673–685.

Hebb, D. O. (1955). Drives and the CNS (conceptual nervous system). *Psychological Review, 62*, 243–259.

Hemenover, S. H. (2003). Individual differences in rate of affect change: Studies in affective chronometry. *Journal of Personality and Social Psychology, 85*, 121–131.

Hemenover, S. H., Augustine, A. A, Shulman, T. E., Tran, T. Q., & Barlett, C. (2008). Individual differences in negative affect repair. *Emotion, 8*, 468–478.

Hilbig, B. E. (2008). Individual differences in fast-and-frugal decision making: Neuroticism and the recognition heuristic. *Journal of Research in Personality, 42*, 1641–1645.

Hirsh, J. B., Guindon, A., Morisano, D., & Peterson, J. B. (2010). Positive mood effects on delay discounting. *Emotion, 10*(5), 717–721.

Hofmann, W., Gschwendner, T., Friese, M., Wiers, R. W., & Schmitt, M. (2008). Working memory capacity and self-regulatory behavior: Toward an individual differences perspective on behavior determination by automatic versus controlled processes. *Journal of Personality and Social Psychology, 95*, 962–977.

Joormann, J., & Gotlib, I. H. (2010). Emotion regulation in depression: Relation to cognitive inhibition. *Cognition and Emotion, 24*, 281–298.

Kotov, R., Gamez, W., Schmidt, F., & Watson, D. (2010). Linking "big" personality traits to anxiety, depressive, and substance use disorder. *Psychological Bulletin, 136*, 768–821.

Kumari, V., Ffytche, D. H., Williams, S. R., & Gray, J. A. (2004). Personality predicts brain responses to cognitive demands. *Journal of Neuroscience, 24*, 10636–10641.

Kuppens, P., Oravecz, Z., & Tuerlinckx, F. (2010). Feelings change: Accounting for individual differences in the temporal dynamics of affect. *Journal of Personality and Social Psychology, 99*, 1024–1060.

Larsen, R. J. (1985). Individual differences in circadian activity rhythm and personality. *Personality and Individual Differences, 6*, 305–311.

Larsen, R. J. (1992). Neuroticism and selective encoding and recall of symptoms: Evidence from a combined concurrent–retrospective study. *Journal of Personality and Social Psychology, 62*, 480–488.

Larsen, R. J., & Cruz, M. H. (1995). Personality correlates of individual differences in electrodermal lability. *Social Behavior and Personality, 23*, 93–104.

Larsen, R. J., & Kasimatis, M. (1991). Day-to-day physical symptoms: Individual differences in the occurrence, duration, and emotional concomitants of minor daily illnesses. *Journal of Personality, 59,* 387–423.

Larsen, R. J., & Ketelaar, T. (1989). Extraversion, neuroticism, and susceptibility to positive and negative mood induction procedures. *Personality and Individual Differences, 10,* 1221–1228.

Larsen, R. J., & Ketelaar, T. (1991). Personality and susceptibility to positive and negative emotional states. *Journal of Personality and Social Psychology, 61,* 132–140.

Larsen, R. J., & Prizmic, Z. (2004). Affect regulation. In K. D. Vohs & R. F. Baumeister (Eds.), *Handbook of self-regulation: Research, theory, and applications* (pp. 40–61). New York: Guilford Press.

Larsen, R. J., & Prizmic, Z. (2007). Regulation of emotional well-being: Overcoming the hedonic treadmill. In M. Eid & R. J. Larsen (Eds.), *The science of subjective well-being* (pp. 258–289). New York: Guilford Press.

Larsen, R. J., & Zarate, M. (1991). Extending reducer/augmenter theory into the emotion domain: The role of emotion in regulating stimulation level. *Personality and Individual Differences, 12,* 713–722.

Lauriola, M., & Levin, I. P. (2001). Personality traits and risky decision making in a controlled experimental task: An exploratory study. *Personality and Individual Differences, 31,* 215–226.

Lieberman, M. D. (2000). Introversion and working memory: Central executive differences. *Personality and Individual Differences, 28(3),* 479–486.

Lieberman, M. D., & Rosenthal, R. (2001). Why introverts can't always tell who likes them: Multitasking and nonverbal decoding. *Journal of Personality and Social Psychology, 80(2),* 294–310.

Lischetzke, T., & Eid, M. (2006). Why extraverts are happier than introverts: The role of mood regulation. *Journal of Personality, 74,* 1127–1161.

Lyubomirsky, S., Caldwell, N., & Nolen-Hoeksema, S. (1998). Effects of ruminative and distracting responses to depressed mood on retrieval of autobiographical memories. *Journal of Personality and Social Psychology, 75,* 166–177.

Lyubomirsky, S., & Nolen-Hoeksema, S. (1995). Effects of self-focused rumination on negative thinking and interpersonal problem solving. *Journal of Personality and Social Psychology, 69,* 176–190.

Matthews, G., & Gilliland, K. (1999). The personality theories of H. J. Eysenck and J. A. Gray: A comparative review. *Personality and Individual Differences, 26,* 583–626.

McNiel, J., Lowman, J. C., & Fleeson, W. (2010). The effect of state extraversion on four types of affect. *European Journal of Personality, 24,* 18–35.

Mikels, J. A., Reuter-Lorenz, P. A., Beyer, J. A., & Fredrickson, B. L. (2008). Emotion and working memory: Evidence for domain-specific processes for affective maintenance. *Emotion, 8,* 256–266.

Moeller, S. K., & Robinson, M. D. (2010). Cognitive sources of evidence for neuroticism's link to punishment-reactivity processes. *Cognition and Emotion, 24,* 741–759.

Moriya, J., & Tanno, Y. (2008). Relationships between negative emotionality and attentional control in effortful control. *Personality and Individual Differences, 44,* 1348–1355.

Muris, P., Roelofs, J., Rassin, E., Franken, I., & Mayer, B. (2005). Mediating effects of rumination and worry on the links between neuroticism, anxiety, and depression. *Personality and Individual Differences, 39,* 1105–1111

Norris, C. J., Larsen, J. T., & Cacioppo, J. T. (2007). Neuroticism is associated with larger and more prolonged electrodermal responses to emotionally evocative pictures. *Psychophysiology, 44,* 823–826.

Ochsner, K. N., & Gross, J. J. (2005). The cognitive control of emotion. *Trends in Cognitive Sciences, 9,* 242–249.

Oreg, S., & Bayazit, M. (2009). Prone to bias: Development of a bias taxonomy from an individual differences perspective. *Review of General Psychology, 13,* 175–193.

Pickering, A. D., Corr, P. J., & Gray, J. A. (1999). Reply to Rusting and Larsen (1999). *Personality and Individual Differences, 26,* 357–365.

Rafienia, P., Azadfallah, P., Fathi-Ashtiani, A., & Rasoulzadeh-Tabatabaiei, K. (2008). The role of extraversion, neuroticism, and positive and negative mood in emotional information processing. *Personality and Individual Differences, 44,* 392–402.

Revelle, W., Humphreys, M. S., Simon, L., & Gilliland, K. (1980). The interactive effect of personality, time of day, and caffeine: A test of the arousal model. *Journal of Experimental Psychology: General, 109,* 1–31.

Roberts, J. E., Gilboa, E., & Gotlib, I. H. (1998). Ruminative response style and vulnerability to episodes of dysphoria: Gender, neuroticism, and episode duration. *Cognitive Therapy and Research, 22*(4), 401–423.

Robinson, M. D., Moeller, S. K., & Ode, S. (2010). Extraversion and reward-related processing: Probing incentive motivation in affective priming tasks. *Emotion, 10*, 615–626.

Robinson, M. D., Ode, S., Moeller, S. K., & Goetz, P. W. (2007). Neuroticism and affective priming: Evidence for a neuroticism-linked negative schema. *Personality and Individual Differences, 42*, 1221–1231.

Robinson, M. D., Ode, S., Wilkowski, B. M., & Amodio, D. M. (2007). Neurotic contentment: A self-regulation view of neuroticism linked distress. *Emotion, 7*, 579–591.

Robinson, M. D., & Tamir, M. (2005). Neuroticism as mental noise: A relation between neuroticism and reaction time standard deviations. *Journal of Personality and Social Psychology, 89*, 107–114.

Robinson, M. D., Wilkowski, B. M., Kirkeby, B. S., & Meier, B. P. (2006). Stuck in a rut: Perseverative response tendencies and the neuroticism–distress relationship. *Journal of Experimental Psychology: General, 135*, 78–91.

Robinson, M. D., Wilkowski, B. M., & Meier, B. P. (2006). Unstable in more ways than one: Reaction time variability and the neuroticism/distress relationship. *Journal of Personality, 74*(2), 311–343.

Robinson, M. D., Wilkowski, B. M., & Meier, B. P. (2008). Approach, avoidance, and self-regulatory conflict: An individual differences perspective. *Journal of Experimental Social Psychology, 44*, 65–79.

Roelofs, J., Huibers, M., Peeters, F., & Arntz, A. (2008). Effects of neuroticism on depression and anxiety: Rumination as a possible mediator. *Personality and Individual Differences, 44*, 576–586.

Rusting, C. L. (1999). Interactive effects of personality and mood on emotion-congruent memory and judgment. *Journal of Personality and Social Psychology, 77*, 1073–1086.

Rusting, C. L., & Larsen, R. J. (1997). Extraversion, neuroticism, and susceptibility to positive and negative affect: A test of two theoretical models. *Personality and Individual Differences, 22*, 607–612.

Rusting, C. L., & Larsen, R. J. (1998). Personality and cognitive processing of affective information. *Personality and Social Psychology Bulletin, 24*, 200–213.

Rusting, C. L., & Larsen, R. J. (1999). Clarifying Gray's theory of personality: A response

to Pickering, Corr, and Gray. *Personality and Individual Differences, 26*, 367–372.

Schmeichel, B. J., Volokhov, R. N., & Demaree, H. A. (2008). Working memory capacity and the self-regulation of emotional expression and experience. *Journal of Personality and Social Psychology, 95*, 1526–1540.

Schmidtke, J. I., & Heller, W. (2004). Personality, affect, and EEG: Predicting patterns of regional brain activity related to extraversion and neuroticism. *Personality and Individual Differences, 36*, 717–732.

Shapiro, D. (1965). *Neurotic styles.* New York: Basic Books.

Slovic, P., & Peters, E. (2006). Risk perception and affect. *Current Directions in Psychological Science, 15*, 322–325.

Smillie, L. D. (2008). What is reinforcement sensitivity?: Neuroscience paradigms for approach–avoidance process theories of personality. *European Journal of Personality, 22*, 359–384.

Smillie, L. D., & Gökçen, E. (2010). Caffeine enhances working memory for extraverts. *Biological Psychology, 85*, 496–498.

Smillie, L. D., Yeo, G. B., Furnham, A. F., & Jackson, C. J. (2006). Benefits of all work and no play: The relationship between neuroticism and performance as a function of resource allocation. *Journal of Applied Psychology, 91*, 139–155.

Smits, D. M., & Boeck, P. D. (2006). From BIS/BAS to the Big Five. *European Journal of Personality, 20*(4), 255–270.

Stafford, L. D., Ng, W., Moore, R. A., & Bard, K. A. (2010). Bolder, happier, smarter: The role of extraversion in positive mood and cognition. *Personality and Individual Differences, 48*, 827–832.

Stelmack, R. M. (1990). Biological basis of extraversion: Psychophysiological evidence. *Journal of Personality, 58*, 293–311.

Storbeck, J., & Clore, G. L. (2007). On the interdependence of cognition and emotion. *Cognition and Emotion, 21*, 1212–1237.

Suls, J., & Martin, R. (2005). The daily life of the garden-variety neurotic: Reactivity, stressor exposure, mood spillover, and maladaptive coping. *Journal of Personality, 73*, 1–25.

Suls, J., Martin, R., & David, J. P. (1998). Person–environment fit and its limits: Agreeableness, neuroticism, and emotional reactivity to interpersonal conflict. *Personality and Social Psychology Bulletin, 24*, 88–98.

Swinkels, A., & Giuliano, T. A. (1995). The

measurement and conceptualization of mood awareness: Monitoring and labeling one's mood states. *Personality and Social Psychology Bulletin, 21,* 934–949.

Tamir, M. (2009). Differential preferences for happiness: Extraversion and trait-consistent emotion regulation. *Journal of Personality, 77*(2), 447–470.

Tamir, M., & Robinson, M. D. (2004). Knowing good from bad: The paradox of neuroticism, negative affect, and evaluative processing. *Journal of Personality and Social Psychology, 87,* 913–925.

Tamir, M., Robinson, M. D., & Clore, G. L. (2002). The epistemic benefits of trait-consistent mood states: An analysis of extraversion and mood. *Journal of Personality and Social Psychology, 83,* 663–677.

Tamir, M., Robinson, M. D., & Solberg, E. C. (2006). You may worry, but can you recognize threats when you see them?: Neuroticism, threat identification, and negative affect. *Journal of Personality, 74,* 1481–1506.

Uziel, L. (2006). The extraverted and the neurotic glasses are of different colors. *Personality and Individual Differences, 41,* 745–754.

van Doorn, R. R. A., & Lang, J. W. B. (2010). Performance differences explained by the neuroticism facets withdrawal and volatility, variations in task demand, and effort allocation. *Journal of Research in Personality, 44,* 446–452.

Wheeler, R. E., Davidson, R. J., & Tomarken, A. J. (1993). Frontal brain asymmetry and emotional reactivity: A biological substrate of affective style. *Psychophysiology, 30,* 82–89.

Wilt, J., & Revelle, W. (2009). Extraversion. In M. R. Leary & R. H. Hoyle (Eds.), *Handbook of individual differences in social behavior* (pp. 27–45). New York: Guilford Press.

Zelenski, J. M. (2007). Experimental approaches to individual differences and change: Exploring the causes and consequences of extraversion. In A. D. Ong & M. van Dulmen (Eds.), *Handbook of methods in positive psychology* (pp. 205–219). New York: Oxford University Press.

Zelenski, J. M., & Larsen, R. J. (1999). Susceptibility to affect: A comparison of three personality taxonomies. *Journal of Personality, 67,* 761–791.

Zelenski, J. M., & Larsen, R. J. (2000). The distribution of emotions in everyday life: A state and trait perspective from experience sampling data. *Journal of Research in Personality, 34,* 178–197.

The Influence of Behavioral Approach and Behavioral Inhibition Sensitivities on Emotive Cognitive Processes

Eddie Harmon-Jones, Tom F. Price, Carly K. Peterson, Philip A. Gable, and Cindy Harmon-Jones

Individual differences in the sensitivity of the behavioral inhibition system (BIS) and the behavioral approach system (BAS) (Gray, 1970) have been found to influence a number of cognitive processes related to emotive responding. In this chapter we review evidence suggesting that BIS–BAS sensitivities influence how individuals attend to, process, remember, learn, and react to emotional events, measured physiologically and behaviorally. Also, we review evidence suggesting that BAS sensitivity is associated with cognitive dissonance reduction and aggressive cognitions following interpersonal insults.

Conceptual Overview of BIS and BAS from Reinforcement Sensitivity Theory

One of the most fundamental motivational properties in living organisms is that of motivational direction—the urge to move toward or approach versus the urge to move away or withdraw from stimuli. Various theories have been advanced to address issues surrounding approach and withdrawal motivation, and one of the most productive theories is the reinforcement sensitivity theory, proposed by Jeffrey Gray (1970), concerning a BAS and BIS. Although this theory emerged

in the animal learning literature, it soon became an important theory concerned with individual differences in humans. Here we review research that has examined the relationship of individual differences in BIS–BAS with psychological and physiological variables that test some of the fundamental predictions of BIS–BAS theorizing.

Originally, Gray's (1970) reinforcement sensitivity theory posited that the BAS was sensitive to signals of conditioned reward (i.e., stimuli associated with learned rewards), nonpunishment, and escape from punishment. The activation of the BAS was proposed to cause movement toward goals. Thus, it is involved in the generation of anticipatory positive affect. BAS sensitivity should be associated with personality characteristics related to optimism, reward responsiveness, and impulsiveness, which relate to clinical problems such as addictive behaviors, high-risk impulsive behaviors, and mania. Low levels of BAS sensitivity were posited to predispose individuals toward unipolar depression.

The BIS, on the other hand, was proposed to be sensitive to signals of conditioned punishment (i.e., stimuli associated with punishment), nonreward, novelty, and innate fear stimuli. Accordingly, the BIS inhibited behavior, increased arousal, prepared the organism for vigorous behavior, and increased attention to aversive stimuli. The BIS was posited to be associated with negative affect, and high levels of BIS sensitivity were posited to predispose individuals toward anxiety disorders. A third system, the fight–flight system (FFS), was also advanced in Gray's original theory as responsive to unconditioned punishment, although it received less research attention than the other two systems.

In 2000, Gray and McNaughton revised the reinforcement sensitivity theory: They retained basic three systems (BIS, BAS, FFS) but revised the functions of the systems and how they interacted. The BAS remained essentially the same as in the earlier conceptions, but the other systems were revised substantially. The fight–flight–freeze system (FFFS) was proposed to mediate reactions to all aversive stimuli. This differs from the original theory that proposed that the BIS mediated reactions to conditioned aversive stimuli, and the FFS mediated reactions to unconditioned aversive stimuli. The revised FFFS is posited to mediate fear but not anxiety, and it is designed to reduce the discrepancy between the immediate threat and the desired state of safety. The FFFS should be associated with personality characteristics related to fear proneness and avoidance, which relate to clinical disorders such as phobia and panic.

The BIS received the most substantial revision. Instead of mediating reactions to conditioned aversive stimuli and innate fear stimuli, it is now posited to be responsible for the resolution of goal conflict in general. Conflicts may be between BAS and FFFS, or BAS and BAS, or FFFS and FFFS reactions to specific but different stimuli that may be mediated by the same system (e.g., "Which car should I purchase?"). That is, the BIS should inhibit conflict behaviors, scan for possible conflicts, and help resolve conflicts. BIS resolves conflict by increasing the negative valence of the stimuli. Ultimately, behavioral conflict resolution is achieved through approach or avoidance. BIS activity is subjectively experienced as worry or rumination. BIS should be associated with personality characteristics involving worry and anxious rumination, which relate to clinical problems such as generalized anxiety disorder and obsessive–compulsive disorder. See Table 18.1.

Although beyond the scope of the current chapter, it is important to note that reinforcement sensitivity theory has been applied to understanding psychological disorders. For instance, BIS has been related to generalized anxiety disorder and obsessive–compulsive disorder (Zinbarg & Yoon, 2008). The FFFS has been related to phobia and panic (McNaughton & Corr, 2008). And BAS has been related to high-risk impulsive behaviors, unipolar depression, and bipolar depression (Alloy et al., Chapter 26, this volume).

TABLE 18.1. Overview and Differences between 1982 and 2000 Versions of Reinforcement Sensitivity Theory

	Version of the theory	
	Gray (1982)	Gray & McNaughton (2000)
BIS		
• Eliciting stimuli	Conditioned punishment, nonreward, novelty, and innate fear stimuli	Conflicts between motivations
• Emotions	Fear, anxiety	Anxiety
BAS		
• Eliciting stimuli	Conditioned reward, nonpunishment, and escape from punishment	Added unconditioned appetitive stimuli
• Emotions	Anticipatory positive affect	Added unconditioned appetitive stimuli
FFFS		
• Eliciting stimuli	Unconditioned punishment	All aversive stimuli
• Emotions	Rage, panic	Fear

Gray's theory has been evaluated using various personality measures, such as measures of extraversion and neuroticism. However, Gray (1970) posited that extraversion and neuroticism should be rotated approximately 30 degrees to form more causally efficient axes of punishment sensitivity (BIS) reflecting anxiety, and reward sensitivity (BAS) reflecting impulsivity. Furthermore, he claimed that extraversion and neuroticism were derivative, secondary factors of the more fundamental BAS and BIS. In Gray's theory, BAS was considered to be a combination of neuroticism and extraversion, whereby individuals high in BAS are neurotic extraverts, and individuals low in BAS are stable/non-neurotic introverts (Gray, 1970). Later, Gray (1987) revised his position on the relationship of BIS–BAS and neuroticism–extraversion because Eysenck's psychoticism scale, assessed with items related to aggressiveness and interpersonal hostility, was found to relate to BAS. It was then posited that neuroticism did not contribute to BAS (Pickering & Gray, 1999). Because extraversion and neuroticism are considered by Augustine, Larsen, and Lee (Chapter 17, this volume), we do not review research on these traits. Also, to make this review more manageable, we focus on the most widely used measure of BIS–BAS: the BIS–BAS questionnaire developed by Carver and White (1994). This questionnaire was based on the original version of the reinforcement sensitivity theory. To date, no questionnaires have been used extensively to test the revised version of the theory.

Carver and White's (1994) BIS–BAS questionnaire is designed to assess individual differences in BIS and BAS sensitivity. It consists of 20 items, and responses to the items are expressed on 4-point scales (1 = strongly disagree, 4 = strongly agree). It is comprised of three BAS subscales and one BIS subscale. The BAS subscales are Reward-Responsiveness, which contains "items that focus on positive responses to the occurrence of anticipation of reward" (Carver & White, 1994, p. 322); Drive, which contains "items pertaining to the persistent pursuit of desired goals" (Carver & White, 1994, p. 322); and Fun-Seeking, which contains "items reflecting both a desire for new rewards and a willingness to approach a potentially rewarding event on the spur of the moment" (Carver & White, 1994, p. 322). BAS-Total, calculated as the sum of all BAS items, is most often used in research, though the subscales are occasionally used as well. The BIS subscale contains "items referencing reactions to the anticipation of punishment" (Carver & White, 1994, p. 322). Thus, the BIS scale was based on the original version of reinforcement sensitivity theory and measures punishment sensitivity.

The Emotive Psychophysiology of BIS–BAS

One of the fundamental predictions of BIS–BAS theorizing concerns the relationship of BIS with punishment sensitivity and anxiety-related responses, and of BAS with reward sensitivity and responses. Research has tested these predictions using a variety of methods, and below we review research that examined relationships between individual differences in BIS–BAS and emotive psychophysiological responses associated with punishment–reward sensitivities. One key advantage of testing such relationships using psychophysiological responses instead of self-report measures of emotions is that any observed relationships will not be due to overlap in semantic meaning or participants' implicit theories between self-reported BIS–BAS individual differences measures and psychophysiological responses, because psychophysiological responses are very unlikely to be influenced by semantic meaning.

Asymmetric Frontal Cortical Activity

One of the first forays into linking individual differences in BIS–BAS with psychophysiological variables involved asymmetric frontal cortical activity. The impetus for attempting to link BIS–BAS with this physiological variable was the fact that activity in the left- and right-frontal cortical regions had been found to be involved in positive affect/approach motivation and negative affect/withdrawal motivation, respectively, for over 70 years with a variety of methods (e.g., Goldstein, 1939; Rossi & Rosadini, 1967). Subsequent studies confirmed these early results and found that persons who had suffered left-hemisphere lesions showed depressive symptoms (Gainotti, 1972; Robinson & Price, 1982), whereas persons who had suffered right-hemisphere lesions showed manic symptoms (Gainotti, 1972; Robinson & Price, 1982). Other research revealed asymmetries underlying appetitive and avoidant behaviors in a number of non-human animal species (for a review, see Vallortigara & Rogers, 2005).

Research with humans suggests these asymmetric activations are specific to the frontal cortex. This research uses asymmetric activity in right- versus left-frontal cortical areas as a variable, usually assessed by electroencephalographic (EEG) recordings, often alpha frequency band activity derived from the EEG. Research has revealed that alpha power is inversely related to regional brain activity using hemodynamic measures (Cook, O'Hara, Uijtdehaage, Mandelkern, & Leuchter, 1998) and behavioral tasks (Davidson, Chapman, Chapman, & Henriques, 1990). Frontal cortical asymmetry is assessed by comparing activity levels between comparable areas in the left and right hemispheres. Difference scores are often used in this research; their use is consistent with the early amytal and lesion research that suggests that asymmetry may be the key variable, with one hemisphere inhibiting the opposite one.

In 1997 two studies observed that individual differences in BAS related to greater left- than right-frontal activity at resting baseline (Harmon-Jones & Allen, 1997; Sutton & Davidson, 1997). One of these studies found that individual differences in BIS related to greater right- than left-frontal activity at baseline (Sutton & Davidson, 1997), whereas the other found no relationship between BIS and asymmetric frontal activity (Harmon-Jones & Allen, 1997). Subsequent studies have found BAS to be associated with greater relative left-frontal activity at baseline and have found no relationship between BIS and asymmetric frontal activity (Amodio, Master, Yee, & Taylor, 2008; Coan & Allen, 2003).

Another study extended this line of research by relating BIS–BAS with neural excitability of the left and right primary motor cortex as assessed by transcranial magnetic stimulation (TMS; Schutter, de Weijer, Meuwese, Morgan, & van Honk, 2008). Moreover, this study provided a better understanding of the physiological meaning of the previous EEG asymmetry findings. Neural excitability of left and right primary motor cortex was measured by applying TMS of increasing intensity over the primary motor cortex and measuring thumb twitches. The lowest TMS pulse intensity that evokes a motor response is thus a measure of cortical excitability; this is called the *motor threshold*. The motor threshold reflects the excitability of axonal fibers of corticospinal neurons and interneurons that act on the output cells in the motor cortex (Moll et al., 1999), and research has revealed a very strong relationship between cortical responses obtained from the motor cortex and the prefrontal cortex (Kähkönen, Komssi, Wilenius, & Ilmoniemi, 2005). As Schutter and colleagues (2008) predicted, greater left over right motor cortical excitability measured using this TMS method was associated with greater BAS relative to BIS.

Affective Modulated Startle Eyeblink Responses

Another measure that has been widely used in emotive psychophysiology is the startle eyeblink reflex. It is typically measured by assessing the electromyography (EMG) to a startling noise from two sensors placed over the orbicularis oculi muscle underneath the eye. This startle eyeblink reflex is modulated by motivationally significant stimuli (i.e., stimuli rated high in arousal and valence). In the standard paradigm, participants view pictures that range from affectively pleasant (e.g., erotica, windsailing) to affectively unpleasant (e.g., severed hand, snakes), while bursts of 100 decibel white noise are presented intermittently during picture presentation (Vrana, Spence, & Lang, 1988). Because the startle eyeblink itself is a defensive response generated by neurons within the amygdala, it is larger when elicited during arousing unpleasant emotional states and inhibited when elicited during arousing pleasant emotional states (Lang, 1995).

Hawk and Kowmas (2003) found that individual differences in BAS sensitivity predicted startle eyeblink responses during affective pictures. Specifically, as compared to low-BAS individuals, high-BAS individuals were more responsive to pleasant stimuli (i.e., they exhibited smaller startle eyeblinks), consistent with Lang's (1995) model of motivational priming as well as other work linking trait approach emotions to an approach motivational startle response pattern (Amodio & Harmon-Jones, 2011).

Unexpectedly, individual differences in BIS sensitivity did not relate to startle eyeblink responses to unpleasant pictures. Hawk and Kowmas (2003) suggested that this result may have been due to the specific unpleasant stimuli used in their study. In particular, most of the unpleasant pictures used in Hawk and Kowmas did not depict human and animal attacks, the categories of unpleasant pictures found to evoke the strongest startle potentiation (Bradley, Codispoti, Cuthbert, & Lang, 2001). Other research using an individual differences questionnaire closely related to BIS (i.e., sensitivity to punishment) found greater startle potentiation in high-BIS individuals, but only during fear and not blood–disgust pictorial stimuli (Caseras et al., 2006). That is, both low- and high-BIS individuals demonstrated greater startle eyeblink responses to blood–disgust than to neutral pictures, but only high-BIS individuals demonstrated greater startle eyeblink responses to fear as compared to neutral pictures (low-BIS individuals showed no differences between fear and neutral pictures). These results suggest that both personality and stimulus type influence the startle reflex (Caseras et al., 2006).

Event-Related Potentials to Startle Probes

In an extension of previous work investigating asymmetric frontal cortical activity and individual differences in BIS–BAS, Peterson, Gable, and Harmon-Jones (2008) related individual differences in BIS–BAS to asymmetric frontal event-related potentials (ERPs) to emotive stimuli. An ERP is an electrical brain response directly related to the onset of a stimulus and is assessed with and extracted from the EEG (see Weinberg, Ferri, & Hajcak, Chapter 3, this volume, for more information on ERPs). Although ERPs are often investigated in relation to cognitive processes such as attention, language, and decision making (Brandeis & Lehmann, 1986), research in the last decade has implicated some ERPs, such as the N1 and P3, in affective processes (Cuthbert, Schupp, Bradley, McManis, & Lang, 1998; Schupp, Cuthbert, Bradley, Birbaumer, & Lang, 1997).

The N1 is a negative-going brain response approximately 100 milliseconds (ms) after event onset and is associated with selective attention (Hillyard, Hink, Schwent, & Picton, 1973), whereas the P3 is a positive-going response about 300 ms after event onset and is related to updating of working memory (Donchin & Coles, 1988). Potentiated N1s, indicative of greater selective attention, occur in response to startle probes presented during negative stimuli, whereas inhibited P3s occur in response to probes during both positive and negative stimuli, reflective of the use of greater working memory processes activated by the motivationally significant stimuli (Cuthbert et al., 1998).

Because several studies had implicated frontal brain asymmetry in emotive processes, Peterson and colleagues (2008) examined asymmetric frontal N1 and P3 amplitudes in relation to BIS–BAS. Using the startle eyeblink picture-viewing paradigm described earlier, greater BIS sensitivity was associated with greater relative right frontal N1 amplitude to startle probes during both negative and positive stimuli; BIS was not associated with P3 amplitude. Such findings suggested that high-BIS individuals are more likely to selectively process emotional stimuli, whether positive or negative, a notion consistent with the idea that anxious individuals respond strongly to both negative and positive stimuli (Martin, Williams, & Clark, 1991). The localization of this effect to the right frontal region is consistent with some research linking BIS to the right prefrontal cortex (Sutton & Davidson, 1997). In contrast, BAS sensitivity was related to reduced left frontal P3 amplitude to startle probes only during positive stimuli, suggesting that these individuals dedicated more working memory processes to appetitive stimuli. That this effect was localized in the left frontal region is consistent with previous research linking the left prefrontal cortex to approach motivation (Harmon-Jones & Allen, 1997; Sutton & Davidson, 1997). BAS sensitivity did not relate to N1 amplitude.

ERPs to Affective Pictures

The study by Peterson and colleagues (2008) examined the N1 ERP response to the startle noise probe during the midst of affective picture viewing. This was done to follow up on previous research by Cuthbert and colleagues (1998). In addition, the number of picture trials used in Peterson and colleagues was not sufficient to examine ERPs to picture onset, as a large number of pictures is needed for signal averaging ERPs to complex stimuli such as affective pictures.

In more recent research using a larger number of affective pictures, ERPs starting at picture onset were examined and related to trait BIS–BAS (Gable & Harmon-Jones, in press). One of the earliest ERPs modulated by the affective or motivational significance of stimuli is the N1 (Keil et al., 2001). The N1 is larger in amplitude to affective than to neutral pictures (Foti, Hajcak, & Dien, 2009). Similarly, individuals show greater N1 activation to food-related words when they are in a food-deprived state, as opposed to a satiated state (Plihal, Haenschel, Hachl, Born, & Pietrowsky, 2001). This early modulation of the N1 by emotional stimuli has been proposed to be associated with the early allocation of attention for emotional stimuli, such that these stimuli are more motivationally relevant and thus capture greater attentional resources (Keil et al., 2001).

In a study designed to test the prediction that individual differences in BAS influence N1 amplitudes to appetitive pictures, participants viewed appetitive (delicious desserts) or neutral (rock) pictures (Gable & Harmon-Jones, in press). Overall, the N1 was larger to appetitive pictures than to neutral pictures. More importantly, individual differences in BAS related to larger N1 amplitudes to appetitive pictures but not larger N1 amplitudes to neutral pictures. BIS was unrelated to N1 amplitude to either picture type. These results indicate that very early neurophysiological processes related to attention toward appetitive stimuli are driven by individual differences in BAS.

ERPs to Errors

The previously reviewed studies examined ERPs during the processing of affective pictures. But emotive responses occur in a variety of situations that can be easily evoked in the lab and examined with ERPs. For instance, after individuals commit an error, a negative deflection in the ERP occurs approximately 50–100 ms later. The tasks used in this type of research are typically speeded reaction time tasks, such as the flankers or Stroop task. In these types of tasks, individuals respond to high- and low-conflict trials. High-conflict trials involve incongruent or competing stimuli; low-conflict trials do not. For example, on a flankers task in which individuals are asked to indicate as quickly and accurately as possible which direction the middle arrow is pointing, a high-conflict trial appears as <<><<, whereas a low-conflict trial appears as <<<<<. In these tasks, a large number of high-conflict trials are included, which, unsurprisingly, causes participants to make a number of errors.

The ERP component associated with these errors, the error-related negativity (ERN), is maximal at frontal-central sites (Fz, FCz, Cz). The main neural generator of the ERN is thought to be the anterior cingulate cortex (ACC; Dehaene, Posner, & Tucker, 1994; Holroyd, Dien, & Coles, 1998; van Veen & Carter, 2002). Larger ERNs have been associated with increased conflict-related ACC activity (Yeung, Botvinick, & Cohen, 2004) and psychiatric internalizing disorders such as obsessive–compulsive disorder and depression (Olvet & Hajcak, 2008). Larger ERNs are associated with larger startle responses, that is, more defensive responses, following the commission of errors (Hajcak & Foti, 2008).

With regard to individual differences, the ERN has been associated with BIS and trait anxiety. For example, Hajcak, McDonald, and Simons (2004) found that individuals with higher trait negative affect have larger ERNs on incorrect trials on a Stroop task. Similarly, individuals who score higher in BIS have larger ERN amplitudes following errors (Amodio et al., 2008; Boksem, Tops, Wester, Meijman, & Lorist, 2006) as well as greater task absorption (Tops & Boksem, 2010). In these studies, BAS did not relate to ERNs.

Hormonal Levels

BIS–BAS have also been associated with hormonal levels (see Wirth & Gaffey, Chapter 5, this volume, for more information on hormones). The association between testosterone, trait BAS, and BAS-related constructs is complex and still not fully understood (Vermeersch, T'Sjoen, Kaufman, & Vincke, 2009). Researchers, however, have noted that administering the hormone cortisol to individuals high (but not low) in trait BIS increases their physiological attention and behavioral avoidance toward threatening stimuli (van Peer et al., 2007). In this experiment, participants were presented with approach-oriented happy, and threat-oriented angry, faces. Participants were asked to indicate, as quickly and accurately as possible, whether a presented face was happy or angry. Participants made these responses by pressing one of three buttons, which were arranged vertically. One button was above (top) and another button was below (bottom) the middle start point. Thus, when pressing the top button, participants made an arm-flexion pose indicative of pulling something toward them (approach). When pressing the bottom button, however, participants made an arm-extension pose indicative of pushing something away (avoidance). In addition, participants were told either congruent ("Press the top button to indicate a happy face and the bottom to indicate an angry face") or incongruent (the reverse) instructions for the task.

Results indicated that participants were faster to respond to happy faces with approach as compared to avoidant arm movements (van Peer et al., 2007). In addition, participants were faster to respond to angry-threat faces with avoidant as compared to approach arm movements. High-trait BIS participants given cortisol versus placebo, additionally, were faster to respond to angry faces with avoidant as compared to approach movements. In addition, these participants had larger P3s to angry threat faces as compared to happy faces when making avoidant arm movements. These results suggest that cortisol might enhance the processing of threat stimuli in high-trait BIS individuals, as well as their avoidance reactions to these stimuli.

Functional Magnetic Resonance Imaging

Other research has examined fMRI responses (which detect changes in blood oxygenation and blood flow responses associated with metabolic activity required by certain populations of neurons) during tasks that should be of relevance to BIS–BAS sensitivities (see Pessoa & Pereira, Chapter 4, this volume, for more information on fMRI). In one study using a monetary incentive delay task (Simon et al., 2010), individuals high in BAS sensitivity showed more activation of the ventral striatum during the receipt of a reward, and more medial orbitofrontal activity during both the receipt and omission of a reward. In contrast, individuals high in BIS sensitivity showed less activation in the ventral striatum during the receipt of a reward. Based on much research linking ventral striatum activation with reward processing (see Nikolova, Bogdan & Hariri, Chapter 2, this volume), these results suggest that individuals high in BAS sensitivity are more responsive to positive outcomes, whereas individuals low in BAS sensitivity and those high in BIS sensitivity show a blunted response to rewards.

Based on research suggesting that individuals high in BAS have more frequent and intense food cravings and are more likely to be overweight or develop eating disorders associated with excessive food intake (Franken & Muris, 2005), a study examined fMRI responses to pictures of appetizing foods (e.g., chocolate cake, pizza; Beaver et al., 2006). Results indicated that individual differences in BAS correlated with greater activation to the pictures of appetizing foods in a frontal–striatal–amygdala–midbrain network, which has been implicated in reward processing. Also, consistent with the previously reviewed research on asymmetric frontal cortical activity and motivation, increased left anterolateral orbitofrontal cortical activation occurred in response to appetizing foods relative to nonfood objects (and increased right orbitofrontal cortical activation occurred in response to disgusting foods relative to nonfood objects). Moreover, BAS correlated with greater left anterolateral orbitofrontal cortical activation in response to appetizing foods.

Consistent with other work linking BAS to anger (see below and Carver & Harmon-Jones, 2009), Beaver, Larwence, Passamonti, and Calder (2008) found that trait BAS predicted activation in neural regions implicated in aggression when individuals viewed facial expressions of anger. That is, greater BAS drive was associated with increased amygdala activation and decreased ventral anterior cingulate and ventral striatal activation to facial expressions of anger, relative to sad and neutral expressions. In contrast, greater BIS was associated with increased activation in the dorsal anterior cingulate, a region involved in the perception of fear and threat. These results suggest that trait BAS constitutes a significant factor governing the function of neural regions implicated in aggression, and is consistent with other research suggesting that BAS is related to angry responses.

The Effects of BIS–BAS on Behavioral Measures

Individual differences in BIS–BAS sensitivities have also been linked with a variety of behavioral measures of emotive cognitive processing. Trait BIS–BAS influences how individuals attend to, process, remember, learn, and react to emotional events. BAS also influences cognitive dissonance reduction and aggressive cognitions following insults. We review this research below.

Selective Attention

A large body of research has suggested that trait anxiety is associated with selective attention or vigilance toward threatening cues (for reviews, see MacLeod & Clarke, Chapter 29, this volume; Morrison, Gordon, & Heimberg, Chapter 23, this volume). Other research has suggested that angry and/or dominant individuals show vigilant responding to angry faces (van Honk et al., 1999; van Honk, Tuiten, de Haan, van den Hout, & Stam, 2001), even when controlling for anxiety. These latter results have been interpreted in line with the social signal function of angry expressions; that is, aggressive or dominant individuals will perceive an angry facial expression as a dominance clash and will be provoked to retaliate rather than avoid this social challenge. Consistent with the idea that anger is related to approach motivation, research has found that trait BAS relates to vigilant attention toward angry faces (Putman, Hermans, & van Honk, 2004). In this study, trait BIS–BAS was measured, and an emotional Stroop task was performed in which neutral, angry, and happy faces were displayed and

colored with transparent red, blue, or yellow. The faces were presented for only 25 ms each, and they were backward-masked with a contrast-rich masking pattern in the same color as the face. Participants were instructed to say the color of the mask as quickly as possible, and reaction times to name the color were measured. Interference scores were calculated by subtracting mean latencies to neutral faces from mean latencies to emotional faces, so that scores greater than 0 represented a slowed response to name the color of the mask of the emotional faces. Results revealed that trait BAS (as well as trait anger) related to more interference to masked angry faces, consistent with the social dominance clash interpretation.

This research was recently extended by showing that trait BAS predicted gaze responses to masked angry faces in a saccade latency paradigm (Terburg, Hooiveld, Aarts, Kenemans, & van Honk, 2011). In this more ecologically valid paradigm, color-masked emotional and neutral faces were presented and then participants had to respond by looking, as quickly as possible, away from the mask to a dot that was the same color as the preceding face. The logic behind the test was this: If participants are attentionally engaged or vigilant toward the masked angry face, they should be slower to look away from it. Thus, the difference between latencies on angry-face trials and other-face trials provides a measure of implicit dominance motivation. The results link BAS with vigilance toward masked angry faces, suggesting that implicit and reflexive mechanisms underlie dominant gaze behavior in face-to-face confrontations.

Attentional Scope

A large body of research suggests that affective states influence the breadth of attention or attentional scope (see reviews by Fredrickson, 2001). In most previous work on the attentional consequences of affect, researchers focused on the valence dimension, that is, whether the affect was positive or negative, and they suggested that positive affect broadened attention, whereas negative affect narrowed attention. An examination of this past work, however, suggested that these differences in attentional scope were likely caused by the motivational intensity of the affective state. That is, this past research primarily tested positive affective states low in approach motivation and negative affective states high in withdrawal motivation (Harmon-Jones & Gable, 2008). For example, positivity was created by giving participants gifts (Isen & Daubman, 1984), having them watch a funny film (Fredrickson & Branigan, 2005), listen to pleasant music (Rowe, Hirsh, & Anderson, 2007), or recall pleasant memories (Gasper & Clore, 2002). These manipulations likely evoked low-approach motivation; the manipulations involved affect that is postgoal or not goal-relevant. On the other hand, in this research, negative affect was created by electric shock (Wachtel, 1968), scary novel situations (Weltman & Egstrom, 1966), faces expressing negative emotion (Fenske & Eastwood, 2003), difficult ego-threatening tasks, and noise stimuli (Chajut & Algom, 2003). These manipulations likely evoked high-withdrawal motivation; the manipulations involved affective states associated with an urge to avoid stimuli.

Affective states vary in motivational intensity. For example, some positive affective states are relatively low in approach motivation (e.g., joy after watching a funny film), whereas others are relatively high in approach motivation (e.g., enthusiasm while approaching a desirable object). Although positive affective states that are low in approach motivation tend to broaden attention, positive affective states high in approach motivational intensity may narrow attention, as organisms shut out irrelevant perceptions and cognitions as they approach and attempt to acquire the desired objects. This cognitive narrowing associated with positive affect high in approach motivation may assist in the tenacious pursuit of desired goals. During goal pursuit, broadening of attention might prove maladaptive as it may lead one away from the current goal pursuit. Easterbrook's (1959) thesis that emotional arousal causes a reduction in the "range of cue utilization" is consistent with these ideas. However, Easterbrook's model referred to drive, "a dimension of emotional arousal or general covert excitement, the innate response to a state of biological deprivation or noxious stimulation. . . . The emotional arousal is greater in neurotic than in normal subjects" (p. 184). Easterbrook

clearly viewed this aroused state as negative. More recent models of emotion assume arousal can be either positive or negative and that arousal reflects motivational activation (Bradley & Lang, 2007).

Based on the preceding ideas, high-approach positive affect should narrow attentional scope (Harmon-Jones & Gable, 2008). To this end, a series of experiments tested this prediction and found that whereas low-approach positive affect broadened attentional scope (Gable & Harmon-Jones, 2008, Study 1; Gable & Harmon-Jones, 2011, Studies 1 and 2), high-approach positive affect narrowed attentional scope (Gable & Harmon-Jones, 2008, Studies 2–4; Gable & Harmon-Jones, 2011, Studies 1 and 2; Harmon-Jones & Gable, 2009).

Individual differences in BAS were found to predict attentional narrowing following the evocation of high-approach positive affect. In this study (Gable & Harmon-Jones, 2008, Study 3), participants viewed either appetitive (dessert or cute baby animals) or neutral (rocks or office supplies) pictures. After each affective or neutral picture, a Navon (1977) letter was presented to assess attentional breadth. In this Navon task, pictures of a large letter composed of smaller letters are presented. The large letters are made up of closely spaced smaller letters (e.g., an *H* made of small *F*'s). Individuals are asked to respond to particular individual letters throughout the task (e.g., *T* or *H*). If the response letters were *T* and *H*, global targets would be those in which a *T* or an *H* is composed of different smaller letters. Local targets would be those where a large letter is composed of smaller *T*'s or *H*'s. Faster responses to the large letters indicate a global (broad) focus, whereas faster responses to the small letters indicate a local (narrow) focus.

As predicted, reaction times to global targets were slower after appetitive pictures than after neutral pictures. In contrast, reaction times to local targets were faster after appetitive pictures than after neutral pictures. In addition, individuals higher in BAS responded with more narrowed attention following approach/motivating stimuli (controlling for responses to neutral pictures). BIS was not related to attentional scope to appetitive pictures (Gable & Harmon-Jones, 2008, Study 3). This study provided convergent evidence supportive of the hypothesis that attentional narrowing caused by appetitive stimuli is due to approach motivation, as individuals high in BAS showed more narrowed attention following appetitive stimuli.

Extending this work with attention, other experiments have found that positive affects differing in motivational intensity influence cognitive categorization (Price & Harmon-Jones, 2010) and memory for verbal information presented in central versus peripheral visual space (Gable & Harmon-Jones, 2010). Research has yet to test whether individual differences in BAS moderate these effects. Based on the results with attentional scope, however, we would predict that high-BAS compared to low-BAS individuals are more prone to narrowly categorize information and have better memory for centrally presented information when in approach-motivated positive affective states.

Memory for Emotional Events

BIS–BAS also influences memories for emotional events (Lench & Levine, 2010). In the first of these studies, participants reported their goals before completing an anagram task that, they were told, measured verbal intelligence. With regard to goals, participants indicated to what extent they wanted to succeed on the anagram task (approach goals) and to what extent they wanted to avoid errors on the task (avoidance goals). Based on these responses, participants were placed into one of four groups for the purpose of analysis: high BIS with avoidance goals, high BIS with approach goals, high BAS with avoidance goals, and high BAS with approach goals. Afterward, participants completed 21 anagrams; the first 7 were insolvable, followed by 14 solvable anagrams. Participants were given 25 minutes to complete these anagrams and, at the end of each one, they rated how happy or anxious they felt. Following the completion of this task, participants completed a distracter task and then they recalled the average intensities of happiness and anxiety they had experienced during the anagram task. Results indicated that trait BIS or BAS as well as personal goals related to memory biases for emotions experienced during the anagram task. More specifically, the rela-

tionship between peak (highest rating during the anagram task) and remembered happiness was strongest for participants with BAS and approach goals. On the other hand, the relationship between peak and remembered anxiety was strongest for participants with BIS and avoidance goals.

A second study replicated these results using a manipulation of approach and avoidance goals (Lench & Levine, 2010). In the approach condition, the anagrams were described as a measure of the strength of verbal intelligence, and participants were told to try and succeed. In the avoidance condition, the anagrams were described as a measure of the weakness of verbal intelligence, and participants were told to try and avoid failure. Results indicated that high-BIS participants with avoidance goals exaggerated their experienced anxiety on the anagram task, whereas high-BAS participants with approach goals exaggerated their experienced happiness on the anagram task. Thus, these findings support the idea that BIS–BAS relate to memory for emotional experiences.

Gomez and Gomez (2002) also found that trait BIS–BAS was associated with memory for emotional events. In this study, participants completed a word fragment task, in which half of a list of incomplete words could be completed to form words with neutral or negative meanings (e.g., *ang_ _*), and half could be completed to form words with neutral or positive meanings (e.g., *e_ a_ed*). Participants also completed a word recognition task wherein they saw 20 positive (e.g., *calm*), 20 negative (e.g., *afraid*), and 20 neutral words (e.g., *circle*). Word order was randomized and each word was presented individually; participants indicated via key press whether they thought the words were positive, negative, or neutral in meaning. Finally, participants completed a free recall task wherein they were given 4 minutes to remember as many words as possible from the previous word recognition test. Results indicated that individual differences in BAS positively correlated with the number of word fragments completed to form positive meanings, the number of positive words correctly identified in the word recognition task, and the number of positive words recalled in the free recall task. On the other hand, individual differences in BIS positively correlated with the number of word fragments completed to form negative meanings, the number of correct identifications of negative words, and the number of negative words recalled in the free recall task.

Affective Learning

Consistent with the idea that BIS relates to anxiety-related responses, individuals high in trait BIS develop aversive learning more quickly than individuals lower in trait BIS. In a study testing this notion, Zinbarg and Mohlman (1998, Study 2) had participants complete a discrimination learning task, in which they learned, across several blocks of trials, whether repeated numeric cues (e.g., 22) were associated with losses or gains. In a monetary incentive condition, participants won 25¢ by pressing a computer key after randomly designated reward cues. They lost 25¢ by pressing the key to designated loss cues. In order to test the idea that individuals with high BIS sensitivity are more responsive to internal threats than to external threats (e.g., electric shock), participants were also randomly assigned to an ego-threat condition. In this condition, participants completed the same task. They were told, however, that it measured their intelligence. Pressing the key to reward cues resulted in the gain of 2 bogus IQ points, whereas pressing it to loss cues resulted in the loss of 2 points. Additionally, participants in this condition completed the discrimination task while a nearby researcher took bogus notes (making the participant feel as if his or her performance were being evaluated). In both conditions, blocks of trials ended with participants seeing the cues again and indicating whether they thought pressing the computer key to that cue would be associated with a loss or gain. In other words, participants provided both reward and punishment expectancies throughout the task. Results indicated that, in the ego-threat condition only, BIS scores were positively correlated with faster acquisition of punishment expectancies. In order words, individuals with higher BIS scores learned more quickly that certain cues were associated with the loss of IQ points and the associated ego threat.

Guilt and Shame Responses

BIS–BAS have been found to relate to whether individuals react to negative events with shame or guilt, which are distinct psychological constructs (Tangney & Dearing, 2002). Whereas guilt may be associated with the need to rectify one's behavior and, consequently, with increased approach motivation (Amodio, Devine, Harmon-Jones, 2007), shame may be associated with the need to hide because this state is more associated with the person's (negative) self-concept. As a consequence, guilt may be linked to BAS, whereas shame may be linked to BIS. For example, Sheikh and Janoff-Bulman (2010, Study 1) had participants fill out BIS and BAS scales before completing a task assessing proneness to shame and guilt. Results indicated that participants with a strong BIS orientation were more likely to report greater levels of shame, whereas participants with a strong BAS orientation were more likely to report greater levels of guilt. Thus, BIS–BAS might also predict how individuals react to negative emotional events.

Aggressive Cognitions

The BAS items all measure responses to rewarding situations, such as, "When I get something I want, I feel excited and energized." There is no semantic overlap between BAS items and items found on anger and aggression measures. Despite the bias against BAS items relating to angry affect, attitudes, or behaviors, several studies have shown that Carver and White's (1994) BAS scale relates positively to self-reported anger and/or aggression (Carver, 2004; Cooper, Gomez, & Buck, 2008; Harmon-Jones, 2003; Smits & Kuppens, 2005). More recently, Harmon-Jones and Peterson (2008) examined the interactional effects of trait and state BAS on aggressive cognitions. In the study, participants listened to an ostensible pilot radio broadcast that was designed to be insulting and has been found to elicit anger in previous studies (Harmon-Jones, Harmon-Jones, Abramson, & Peterson, 2009). Afterward, participants completed one of three questionnaires designed to manipulate their mindset: positive-high-approach (steps to obtain a desired goal), positive-low-approach (a positive event happened without the participant's action), or neutral (an ordinary day). They then indicated how likely it was that they would recommend future radio jobs for the person who spoke in the broadcast, which was considered indicative of aggressive inclinations, given that the participants were told the feedback would be provided to the radio station. As expected, trait BAS sensitivity and approach mindset interacted to predict aggressive thoughts, so that participants in the high-approach mindset who were also high in BAS sensitivity were less likely to like the speaker or recommend the speaker for future jobs. These results show the interactive effects of BAS personality and situationally induced approach motivation on aggressive inclinations.

Cognitive Dissonance Reduction

The influence of BAS on cognitive dissonance processes has recently been examined (Harmon-Jones, Schmeichel, Inzlicht, & Harmon-Jones, 2011). This integration of BAS with cognitive dissonance theory was suggested by the action-based model of dissonance (Harmon-Jones, Amodio, & Harmon-Jones, 2009).

The original theory of cognitive dissonance predicted that when an individual holds two or more elements of knowledge that are relevant to each other but inconsistent with one another, a state of discomfort or dissonance is created (Festinger, 1957). This dissonance was posited to motivate organisms to engage in psychological work to decrease the discrepancy between cognitions. Although research on cognitive dissonance theory has spanned more than five decades, theoretical revisions to dissonance theory had said little about why organisms experience dissonance and are motivated to reduce it.

The action-based model of dissonance was proposed to address these issues. It begins by assuming that many perceptions and cognitions activate action tendencies. Moreover, when cognitions or perceptions with action implications come into conflict, a negative affective state of dissonance is aroused, because conflicting action-based cognitions have the potential to interfere with effective action (Harmon-Jones, Amodio, & Har-

mon-Jones, 2009). This conflict activates the ACC, a region involved in negative affective responses to the detection of basic cognitive conflicts (Hajcak & Foti, 2008) and to the types of conflict aroused by typical dissonance manipulations (van Veen, Krug, Schooler, & Carter, 2009). When conflict is detected or dissonance is aroused, dissonance reduction is likely to occur. According to the action-based model, individuals change their cognitions to reduce dissonance because this assists in behaving effectively. Consequently, dissonance reduction is proposed to be an approach-motivated process aimed at translating a behavioral intention into effective action. Dissonance reduction is posited to be an adaptive, approach-related process (Harmon-Jones, Amodio, et al., 2009) present in a number of species (Egan, Bloom, & Santos, 2010).

According to the action-based model, dissonant cognitions can interfere with effective action particularly when the cognitions have competing action tendencies. Dissonance reduction causes the individual to bring the cognitions in line with behavioral intentions, which assists in furthering goal-directed behavior (Harmon-Jones & Harmon-Jones, 2002).

Dissonance reduction typically occurs following a behavioral commitment (Beauvois & Joule, 1999; Brehm & Cohen, 1962), when the individual is prepared to act (Beckmann & Irle, 1985; Gollwitzer, 1990; Kuhl, 1984). This state has been referred to as an *action-oriented state*, or *implemental mindset*, and it is one in which intentions are formed to execute behaviors associated with a commitment (Gollwitzer & Sheeran, 2006). That is, the individual is approach motivated to behave effectively with regard to the commitment.

To test the prediction that state approach motivation would increase dissonance reduction, Harmon-Jones and Harmon-Jones (2002) manipulated the degree of action-orientation that participants experienced following a decision. In the experiment, participants first made an easy or a difficult decision regarding which of several physical exercises they would perform while at the experiment. Next, participants were randomly assigned one of two conditions. In the action-oriented mindset condition, participants listed seven things they could do to perform well on the exercise they had chosen. In the neutral mindset condition, participants listed seven things they did in a typical day. Participants then reevaluated the exercises. Among participants who made a difficult decision, those in the action-oriented condition demonstrated more spreading of alternatives than those in the neutral mindset condition. In other words, these participants spread their evaluations of the decision alternatives further apart or demonstrated a greater increase in preference for the chosen over the rejected exercise after the decision. No spreading of alternatives occurred in either easy decision condition.

Harmon-Jones, Harmon-Jones, Fearn, Sigelman, and Johnson (2008) conceptually replicated the above experiment, with the addition of a more general action-oriented (implemental) mindset condition (see Gollwitzer & Sheeran, 2006) and a condition intended to evoke low-approach positive affect. In this latter condition, participants wrote about a time when something had happened that made them feel very good, but was not caused by their own actions. EEG activity was measured. As predicted, the action-oriented mindset increased left frontal cortical activity and spreading of alternatives, compared to the low-approach positive affect condition and the neutral condition.

These results are consistent with the action-based model prediction that dissonance reduction is facilitated by state approach motivation. Because they are all based on experiments in which action orientation was manipulated and/or asymmetric frontal cortical activity was assessed, one could question whether approach motivation was the key construct manipulated or measured. The prediction that dissonance reduction is facilitated by approach motivation was tested more directly by examining the relationship between trait BAS and dissonance reduction. Doing so also integrates two major motivational theories that have yet to be integrated: dissonance theory and reinforcement sensitivity theory.

Two studies were designed to test the prediction that individuals who are dispositionally high in BAS should engage in more dissonance reduction (Harmon-Jones et al., 2011). Study 1 found that trait BAS was associated with more spreading of alternatives (more liking for the chosen over the rejected decision alternative) following a difficult decision. Study 2 found that trait BAS was associated with attitudes being more consistent with recent induced compliance behavior. In Study 1 but not Study 2, BIS was related inversely with dissonance reduction (as measured by attitudes). These studies suggest that BAS contributes to dissonance reduction, as predicted by the action-based model. Moreover, they connect two major motivational theories that emerged from very different traditions—reinforcement sensitivity theory and cognitive dissonance theory—showing how basic motivational dimensions influence cognition–emotion interactions.

Summary and Conclusion

Individual differences in the sensitivity of BIS and BAS have been found to influence a number of cognitive processes related to emotive responding. For example, BIS–BAS sensitivities influence how individuals attend to, process, remember, learn, and react to emotional events, measured physiologically and behaviorally. Also, BAS sensitivity is associated with dissonance reduction and aggressive cognitions following interpersonal insults.

One particularly interesting aspect of much of the reviewed research is that it has gone beyond "zero-variable" theorizing (Wicklund, 1990) of assessing behavioral responses obviously associated with trait BIS–BAS. Instead, much of the research has illustrated how individual differences in BIS–BAS sensitivities relate to variables not obviously measured by the BIS–BAS questionnaire, thus digging deeper into the psychology of BIS–BAS. For instance, items assessing BAS sensitivity focus on positive reactions to rewards, but research has demonstrated that BAS sensitivity also relates to attentional engagement with angry faces (Putman et al., 2004) and to more aggressive cognitions following the situational activation of approach motivation (Harmon-Jones & Peterson, 2008). Similarly, BAS sensitivity was found to relate to cognitive dissonance reduction, an emotive cognitive process that is also unrelated to items on the BAS questionnaire. In addition, much of the reviewed research illustrates the consideration of contextual variables in how trait BIS–BAS relates to psychophysiological processes. For instance, trait BAS interacted with situationally aroused approach motivation to influence attentional scope (Gable & Harmon-Jones, 2008), memory (Lench & Levine, 2010), and aggressive cognitions (Harmon-Jones & Peterson, 2008). Finally, the reviewed research demonstrates how reinforcement sensitivity theory has been effectively integrated with cognitive dissonance theory to better understand how individuals respond to dissonance arousing situations. We hope this review assists in advancing theory and research on BIS–BAS.

References

Amodio, D. M., Devine, P. G., & Harmon-Jones, E. (2007). A dynamic model of guilt: Implications for motivation and self-regulation in the context of prejudice. *Psychological Science, 18*, 524–530.

Amodio, D. M., & Harmon-Jones, E. (2011). Trait emotions and affective modulation of the startle eyeblink: On the unique relationship of trait anger. *Emotion, 11*, 47–51.

Amodio, D. M., Master, S. L., Yee, C. M., & Taylor, S. E. (2008). Neurocognitive components of the behavioral inhibition and activation systems: Implications for theories of self-regulation. *Psychophysiology, 45*, 11–19.

Beauvois, J. L., & Joule, R. V. (1999). A radical point of view on dissonance theory. In E. Harmon-Jones & J. Mills (Eds.), *Cognitive dissonance: Progress on a pivotal theory in social psychology* (pp. 43–70). Washington, DC: American Psychological Association.

Beaver, J. D., Lawrence, A. D., Passamonti, L., & Calder, A. J. (2008). Appetitive motivation predicts the neural response to facial signals of aggression. *Journal of Neuroscience, 28*, 2719–2725.

Beaver, J. D., Lawrence, A. D., van Ditzhuijzen, J., Davis, M. H., Woods, A., & Calder, A. J. (2006). Individual differences in reward drive predict neural responses to images of food. *Journal of Neuroscience, 26*, 5160–5166.

Beckmann, J., & Irle, M. (1985). Dissonance and action control. In J. Kuhl & J. Beckmann (Eds.), *Action control: From cognition to behavior* (pp. 129–150). Berlin: Springer-Verlag.

Boksem, M. A., Tops, M., Wester, A. E., Meijman, T. F., & Lorist, M. M. (2006). Error-related ERP components and individual differences in punishment and reward sensitivity. *Brain Research, 1101*, 92–101.

Bradley, M. M., Codispoti, M., Cuthbert, B. N., & Lang, P. J. (2001). Emotion and motivation: I. Defensive and appetitive reactions in picture processing. *Emotion, 1*, 276–298.

Bradley, M. M., & Lang, P. H. (2007). Emotion and motivation. In J. T. Cacioppo, L. G. Tassinary, & G. Berntson (Eds.), *Handbook of psychophysiology* (3rd ed., pp. 581–607). New York: Cambridge University Press.

Brandeis, D., & Lehmann, D. (1986). Event-related potentials of the brain and cognitive processes: Approaches and applications. *Neuropsychologia, 24*, 151–168.

Brehm, J. W., & Cohen, A. R. (1962). *Explorations in cognitive dissonance*. New York: Wiley.

Carver, C. S. (2004). Negative affects deriving from the behavioral approach system. *Emotion, 4*, 3–22.

Carver, C. S., & Harmon-Jones, E. (2009). Anger is an approach-related affect: Evidence and implications. *Psychological Bulletin, 135*, 183–204.

Carver, C. S., & White, T. L. (1994). Behavioral inhibition, behavioral activation, and affective responses to impending reward and punishment: The BIS/BAS scales. *Journal of Personality and Social Psychology, 67*, 319–333.

Caseras, F. X., Fullana, M. A., Riba, J., Barbanoj, M. J., Aluja, A., & Torrubia, R. (2006). Influence of individual differences in the behavioral inhibition system and stimulus content (fear vs. blood–disgust) on affective startle reflex modulation. *Biological Psychology, 72*, 251–256.

Chajut, E., & Algom, D. (2003). Selective attention improves under stress: Implications for theories of social cognition. *Journal of Personality and Social Psychology, 85*, 231–248.

Coan, J. A., & Allen, J. J. B. (2003). Frontal EEG asymmetry and the behavioral activation and inhibition systems. *Psychophysiology, 40*, 106–114.

Cook, I. A., O'Hara, R., Uijtdehaage, S. H. J., Mandelkern, M., & Leuchter, A. F. (1998). Assessing the accuracy of topographic EEG mapping for determining local brain function. *Electroencephalography and Clinical Neurophysiology, 107*, 408–414.

Cooper, A., Gomez, R., & Buck, E. (2008). The relationship between the BIS and BAS, anger, and responses to anger. *Personality and Individual Differences, 44*, 403–413.

Cuthbert, B. N., Schupp, H. T., Bradley, M. M., McManis, M., & Lang, P. J. (1998). Probing affective pictures: Attended startle and tone probes. *Psychophysiology, 35*, 344–347.

Davidson, R. J., Chapman, J. P., Chapman, L. J., & Henriques, J. B. (1990). Asymmetric brain electrical activity discriminates between psychometrically-matched verbal and spatial cognitive tasks. *Psychophysiology, 27*, 528–543.

Dehaene, S., Posner, M. I., & Tucker, D. M. (1994). Localization of a neural system for error detection and compensation. *Psychological Science, 5*, 303–305.

Donchin, E., & Coles, M. G. H. (1988). Is the P300 component a manifestation of context updating? *Behavioral and Brain Sciences, 11*, 355–372.

Easterbrook, J. A. (1959). The effect of emotion on cue utilization and the organization of behavior. *Psychological Review, 66*, 183–201.

Egan, L., Bloom, P., & Santos, L. R. (2010). Choice-induced preferences in the absence of choice: Evidence from a blind two choice paradigm with young children and capuchin monkeys. *Journal of Experimental Social Psychology, 46*, 204–207.

Fenske, M. J., & Eastwood, J. D. (2003). Modulation of focused attention by faces expressing emotion: Evidence from flanker tasks. *Emotion, 3*, 327–343.

Festinger, L. (1957). *A theory of cognitive dissonance*. Evanston, IL: Row, Peterson.

Foti, D., Hajcak, G., & Dien, J. (2009). Differentiating neural responses to emotional pictures: Evidence from temporal–spatial PCA. *Psychophysiology, 46*, 521–530.

Franken, I. H. A., & Muris, P. (2005). Individual differences in reward sensitivity are related to food craving and relative body weight in healthy women. *Appetite, 45*, 198–201.

Fredrickson, B. L. (2001). The role of positive emotions in positive psychology: The broaden-and-build theory of positive emotions. *American Psychologist, 56*, 218–226.

Fredrickson, B. L., & Branigan, C. (2005). Positive emotions broaden the scope of attention and thought–action repertoires. *Cognition and Emotion, 19*, 313–332.

Gable, P. A., & Harmon-Jones, E. (2008). Approach-motivated positive affect reduces breadth of attention. *Psychological Science, 19*, 476–482.

Gable, P. A., & Harmon-Jones, E. (2010). The effect of low vs. high approach-motivated positive affect on memory for peripherally vs. centrally presented information. *Emotion, 10*, 599–603.

Gable, P. A., & Harmon-Jones, E. (2011). Attentional consequences of pre-goal and post-goal positive affects. *Emotion, 11*, 1358–1367.

Gable, P. A., & Harmon-Jones, E. (in press). Trait behavioral approach sensitivity (BAS) relates to early (< 150 ms) electrocortical responses to appetitive stimuli. *Social Cognitive Affective Neuroscience*.

Gainotti, G. (1972). Emotional behavior and hemispheric side of the lesion. *Cortex, 8*, 41–55.

Gasper, K., & Clore, G. L. (2002). Attending to the big picture: Mood and global versus local processing of visual information. *Psychological Science, 13*, 34–40.

Goldstein, K. (1939). *The organism: An holistic approach to biology, derived from pathological data in man*. New York: American Book.

Gollwitzer, P. M. (1990). Action phases and mind-sets. In E. T. Higgins & R. M. Sorrentino (Eds.), *Handbook of motivation and cognition: Vol. 2. Foundations of social behavior* (pp. 53–92). New York: Guilford Press.

Gollwitzer, P. M., & Sheeran, P. (2006). Implementation intentions and goal achievement: A meta-analysis of effects and processes. In M. P. Zanna (Ed.), *Advances in experimental social psychology* (Vol. 38, pp. 69–119). San Diego, CA: Elsevier Academic Press.

Gomez, A., & Gomez, R. (2002). Personality traits of the behavioral approach and inhibition systems: Associations with processing of emotional stimuli. *Personality and Individual Differences, 32*, 1299–1316.

Gray, J. A. (1970). The psychophysiological basis of introversion–extraversion. *Behaviour Research and Therapy, 8*, 249–266.

Gray, J. A. (1982). *The neuropsychology of anxiety: An enquiry into the functions of the septo-hippocampal system*. Oxford, UK: Oxford University Press.

Gray, J. A. (1987). *The psychology of fear and stress* (2nd ed.). Cambridge, UK: Cambridge University Press.

Gray, J. A., & McNaughton, N. (2000). *The neuropsychology of anxiety: An enquiry into the functions of the septo-hippocampal sys-*

tem (2nd ed.). Oxford, UK: Oxford University Press.

Hajcak, G., & Foti, D. (2008). Errors are aversive: Defensive motivation and the error-related negativity. *Psychological Science, 19*, 103–108.

Hajcak, G., McDonald, N., & Simons, R. F. (2004). Error-related psychophysiology and negative affect. *Brain and Cognition, 56*, 189?197.

Harmon-Jones, C., Schmeichel, B. J., Inzlicht, M., & Harmon-Jones, E. (2011). Trait approach motivation relates to dissonance reduction. *Social Psychological and Personality Science, 2*, 21–28.

Harmon-Jones, E. (2003). Anger and the behavioral approach system. *Personality and Individual Differences, 35*, 995–1005.

Harmon-Jones, E., & Allen, J. J. B. (1997). Behavioral activation sensitivity and resting frontal EEG asymmetry: Covariation of putative indicators related to risk for mood disorders. *Journal of Abnormal Psychology, 106*, 159–163.

Harmon-Jones, E., Amodio, D. M., & Harmon-Jones, C. (2009). Action-based model of dissonance: A review, integration, and expansion of conceptions of cognitive conflict. In M. P. Zanna (Ed.), *Advances in experimental social psychology* (Vol. 41, pp. 119–166). San Diego, CA: Academic Press.

Harmon-Jones, E., & Gable, P. A. (2008). Incorporating motivational intensity and direction into the study of emotions: Implications for brain mechanisms of emotion and cognition–emotion interactions. *Netherlands Journal of Psychology, 64*, 132–142.

Harmon-Jones, E., & Gable, P. A. (2009). Neural activity underlying the effect of approach-motivated positive affect on narrowed attention. *Psychological Science, 20*, 406–409.

Harmon-Jones, E., & Harmon-Jones, C. (2002). Testing the action-based model of cognitive dissonance: The effect of action-orientation on post-decisional attitudes. *Personality and Social Psychology Bulletin, 28*, 711–723.

Harmon-Jones, E., Harmon-Jones, C., Abramson, L. Y., & Peterson, C. K. (2009). PANAS positive activation is associated with anger. *Emotion, 9*, 183–196.

Harmon-Jones, E., Harmon-Jones, C., Fearn, M., Sigelman, J. D., & Johnson, P. (2008). Action orientation, relative left frontal cortical activation, and spreading of alternatives: A test of the action-based model of dissonance.

Journal of Personality and Social Psychology, 94, 1–15.

Harmon-Jones, E., & Peterson, C. K. (2008). Effect of trait and state approach motivation on aggressive inclinations. *Journal of Research in Personality, 42*, 1381–1385.

Hawk, L. W., & Kowmas, A. D. (2003). Affective modulation and prepulse inhibition of startle among undergraduates high and low in behavioral inhibition and approach. *Psychophysiology, 40*, 131–138.

Hillyard, S. A., Hink, R. F., Schwent, V. L., & Picton, T. W. (1973). Electrical signs of selective attention in the human brain. *Science, 182*, 177–180.

Holroyd, C. B., Dien, J., & Coles, M. G. (1998). Error-related scalp potentials elicited by hand and foot movements: Evidence for an output-independent error processing system in humans. *Neuroscience Letters, 242*, 65–68.

Isen, A. M., & Daubman, K. A. (1984). The influence of affect on categorization. *Journal of Personality and Social Psychology, 47*, 1206–1217.

Kähkönen, S., Komssi, S., Wilenius, J., & Ilmoniemi, R. J. (2005). Prefrontal TMS produces smaller EEG responses than motor-cortex TMS: Implications for rTMS treatment in depression. *Psychopharmacology, 181*, 16–20.

Keil, A., Muller, M. M., Gruber, T., Wienbruch, C., Stolarova, M., & Elbert, T. (2001). Effects of emotional arousal in the cerebral hemispheres: A study of oscillatory brain activity and event-related potentials. *Clinical Neurophysiology, 112*, 2057–2068.

Kuhl, J. (1984). Volitional aspects of achievement motivation and learned helplessness: Toward a comprehensive theory of action-control. In B. A. Maher (Ed.), *Progress in experimental personality research* (Vol. 13, pp. 99–171). New York: Academic Press.

Lang, P. J. (1995). The emotion probe: Studies of motivation and attention. *American Psychologist, 50*, 372–385.

Lench, H. C., & Levine, L. J. (2010). Motivational biases in memory for emotions. *Cognition and Emotion, 24*, 401–418.

Martin, M., Williams, R. M., & Clark, D. M. (1991). Does anxiety lead to selective processing of threat-related information? *Behaviour Research and Therapy, 29*, 147–160.

McNaughton, N., & Corr, P. J. (2008). The neuropsychology of fear and anxiety: A foundation for reinforcement sensitivity theory. In P. J. Corr (Ed.), *The reinforcement sensitivity theory of personality* (pp. 44–94). Cambridge, UK: Cambridge University Press.

Moll, G. H., Heinrich, H., Wischer, S., Tergau, F., Paulus, W., & Rothenberger, A. (1999). Motor system excitability in healthy children: Developmental aspects from transcranial magnetic stimulation. *Electroencephalography and Clinical Neurophysiology, 51,* 243–249.

Navon, D. (1977). Forest before trees: The precedence of global features in visual perception. *Cognitive Psychology, 9,* 353–383.

Olvet, D. M., & Hajcak, G. (2008). The error-related negativity (ERN) and psychopathology: Toward an endophenotype. *Clinical Psychology Reviews, 28,* 1343–1354.

Peterson, C. K., Gable, P., & Harmon-Jones, E. (2008). Asymmetrical frontal ERPs, emotion, and behavioral approach/inhibition sensitivity. *Social Neuroscience, 3,* 113–124.

Pickering, A. D., & Gray, J. A. (1999). The neuroscience of personality. In L. Pervin & O. P. John (Eds.), *Handbook of personality* (2nd ed., pp. 277–299). New York: Guilford Press.

Plihal, W., Haenschel, C., Hachl, P., Born, J., & Pietrowsky, R. (2001). The effect of food deprivation on ERP during identification of tachistoscopically presented food-related words. *Journal of Psychophysiology, 15,* 163–172.

Price, T. F., & Harmon-Jones, E. (2010). The effect of embodied emotive states on cognitive categorization. *Emotion, 10,* 934–938.

Putman, P., Hermans, E., & van Honk, J. (2004). Emotional Stroop performance for masked angry faces: It's BAS, not BIS. *Emotion, 4,* 305–311.

Robinson, R. G., & Price, T. R. (1982). Poststroke depressive disorders: A follow-up study of 103 patients. *Stroke, 13,* 635–641.

Rossi, G. F., & Rosadini, G. R. (1967). Experimental analyses of cerebral dominance in man. In D. H. Millikan & F. L. Darley (Eds.), *Brain mechanisms underlying speech and langauge* (pp. 167–184). New York: Grune & Stratton.

Rowe, G., Hirsh, J. B., & Anderson, A. K. (2007). Positive affect increases the breadth of attentional selection. *Proceedings of the National Academy of Sciences of the United States of America, 104,* 383–388.

Schupp, H. T., Cuthbert, B. N., Bradley, M. M., Birbaumer, N., & Lang, P. J. (1997). Probe P3 and blinks: Two measures of affective startle modulation. *Psychophysiology, 34,* 1–6.

Schutter, D. J., de Weijer, A. D., Meuwese, J. D., Morgan, B., & van Honk, J. (2008). Interre-

lations between motivational stance, cortical excitability, and the frontal electroencephalogram asymmetry of emotion: A transcranial magnetic stimulation study. *Human Brain Mapping, 29,* 574–580.

Sheikh, S., & Janoff-Bulman, R. (2010). The "should" and "should nots" of moral emotions: A self-regulatory perspective on shame and guilt. *Personality and Social Psychology Bulletin, 36,* 213–224.

Simon, J. J., Walther, S., Fiebach, C. J., Friederich, C. J., Stippich, C., Weisbrod, M., et al. (2010). Neural reward processing is modulated by approach- and avoidance-related personality traits. *NeuroImage, 49,* 1868–1874.

Smits, D. J. M., & Kuppens, P. (2005). The relations between anger, coping with anger, and aggression, and the BIS–BAS system. *Personality and Individual Differences, 39,* 783–793.

Sutton, S. K., & Davidson, R. J. (1997). Prefrontal brain asymmetry: A biological substrate of the behavioral approach and inhibition systems. *Psychological Science, 8,* 204–210.

Tangney, J. P., & Dearing, R. L. (2002). *Shame and guilt.* New York: Guilford Press.

Terburg, D., Hooiveld, N., Aarts, H., Kenemans, J. L., & van Honk, J. (2011). Eye tracking unconscious face-to-face confrontations: Dominance motives prolong gaze to masked angry faces. *Psychological Science, 22,* 314–319.

Tops, M., & Boksem, M. A. (2010). Absorbed in the task: Personality measures predict engagement during task performance as tracked by error negativity and asymmetrical frontal activity. *Cognitive, Affective, and Behavioral Neuroscience, 10,* 441–453.

Vallortigara, G., & Rogers, L. J. (2005). Survival with an asymmetrical brain: Advantages and disadvantages of cerebral lateralization. *Behavioral and Brain Sciences, 28,* 575–633.

van Honk, J., Tuiten, A., de Haan, E., van den Hout, M., & Stam, H. (2001). Attentional biases for angry faces: Relationships to trait anger and anxiety. *Cognition and Emotion, 15,* 279–299.

van Honk, J., Tuiten, A., Verbaten, R., van den Hout, M., Koppeschaar, H., Thijssen, J., et al. (1999). Correlations among salivary testosterone, mood, and selective attention to threat in humans. *Hormones and Behavior, 36,* 17–24.

van Peer, J. M., Roelofs, K., Rotteveel, M., van Dijk, J. G., Spinhoven, P., & Ridderinkhof, K. R. (2007). The effects of cortisol administration on approach–avoidance behavior: An event-related potential study. *Biological Psychology, 76,* 135–146.

van Veen, V., & Carter, C. S. (2002). The timing of action-monitoring processes in the anterior cingulate cortex. *Journal of Cognitive Neuroscience, 14,* 593–602.

van Veen, V., Krug, M. K., Schooler, J. W., & Carter, C. S. (2009). Neural activity predicts attitude change in cognitive dissonance. *Nature Neuroscience, 12,* 1469–1474.

Vermeersch, H., T'Sjoen, G., Kaufman, J.-M., & Vincke, J. (2009). The relationship between sex steroid hormones and behavioural inhibition (BIS) and behavioural activation (BAS) in adolescent boys and girls. *Personality and Individual Differences, 47,* 3–7.

Vrana, S. R., Spence, E. L., & Lang, P. J. (1988). The startle probe response: A new measure of emotion? *Journal of Abnormal Psychology, 97,* 487–491.

Wachtel, P. L. (1968). Anxiety, attention, and coping with threat. *Journal of Abnormal Psychology, 73,* 137–143.

Weltman, G., & Egstrom, G. H. (1966). Perceptual narrowing in novice diver. *Human Factors, 8,* 499–506.

Wicklund, R. A. (1990). *Zero-variable theories and the psychology of the explainer.* New York: Springer-Verlag.

Yeung, N., Botvinick, M. M., & Cohen, J. D. (2004). The neural basis of error detection: Conflict monitoring and the error-related negativity. *Psychological Review, 111,* 931–959.

Zinbarg, R. E., & Mohlman, J. (1998). Individual differences in the acquisition of affectively-valenced associations. *Journal of Personality and Social Psychology, 74,* 1024–1040.

Zinbarg, R. E., & Yoon, K. L. (2008). RST and clinical disorders: Anxiety and depression. In P. J. Corr (Ed.), *The reinforcement sensitivity theory of personality* (pp. 360–397). Cambridge, UK: Cambridge University Press.

CHAPTER 19

The Cognitive and Motivational Foundations Underlying Agreeableness

William G. Graziano and Renée M. Tobin

Interpersonal accommodation is a process central to social psychology. G. W. Allport (1968) defined social psychology in terms of the adjustments in thoughts, feelings, and behavior that individuals make as a result of the actual, imagined, or implied presence of other people. In line with this perspective, *agreeableness* refers to the motivation to accommodate to other people with the goal of maintaining smooth interpersonal relationships (Graziano & Eisenberg, 1997; Graziano & Habashi, 2010). More formally, agreeableness is defined as a superordinate summary term for a set of interrelated dispositions and characteristics, manifested as differences in being likable, pleasant, and harmonious in relations with others. Agreeableness can be indexed through individual differences, but it is a larger construct presumably reflecting underlying psychological processes. Research shows that persons who are described by others as *trusting* are also described as *kind* and *warm*. Taken together, this combination of characteristics points toward a dimension that we now know to be relatively stable over time (Hair & Graziano, 2003; Shiner, Masten, & Roberts, 2003).

Using an astronomical metaphor, agreeableness can be likened to the Jupiter of a Big Five solar system. Because it is seen as distant from the center of the action, researchers find it easier to gaze at it than to explore empirically. It seems different from the other planets, perhaps a giant bag of vapor with no clear hard core. It certainly has sufficient gravity to attract eccentrically orbiting clutter. Getting past its vaporous outer edges, at its core is it hot or cold? Nevertheless, despite these questions, serious observers of the system find it hard to ignore. Leaving this metaphorical flight of fancy, agreeableness is arguably the largest dimension of the five-factor approach to personality (Digman & Takemoto-Chock, 1981). It is concerned with how individuals orient toward interpersonal relationships.

Well before scientific psychology appeared, writers commented on agreeableness in emotional life (e.g., Ricord, 1840). In modern scientific research, agreeableness has an unusual history relative to other recognized dimensions of personality. Unlike the "super traits" of extraversion and neuroticism, agreeableness did not initially receive attention because of deductive top-down theorizing about its link to biology or to especially conspicuous processes such as anxiety. It was not tied to distinctive psychological processes of brain activity in the way that extraversion or neuroticism was. Instead, systematic agreeableness research was stimulated by observable regularities arising in descriptions of others, and later in self-descriptions (Digman & Takemoto-Chock, 1981). A literature search with the keyword *agreeableness* identified a minimum of 2,402 peer-reviewed journal articles written in English through a PsycINFO search from 1965 to June 2011. Notably, more than 99% of these articles were written after 1995.

In modern psychology, agreeableness is usually described in behavioral terms, not in terms of underlying affective or cognitive processes. That is, agreeableness is described as differences in behavior characterizing people who score high versus people who score low on agreeableness measures. From extreme group (high vs. low) behavioral differences, researchers can and do make inferences about underlying processes, but rarely test them directly. For example, agreeableness is presumed to be related to the cognitive and affective processes of prejudice because persons who score high on agreeableness are more positive about most social groups and are less negative about outgroup members and traditional targets of prejudice, than are persons who score low on agreeableness (Graziano, Bruce, Sheese, & Tobin, 2007; Graziano & Habashi, 2010). A similar logic could be used to connect agreeableness to empathy (Graziano, Habashi, Sheese, & Tobin, 2007). Agreeableness has also been linked to other overt behaviors, such as effective conflict resolution (Graziano, Jensen-Campbell, & Hair, 1996; Jensen-Campbell, Gleason, Adams, & Malcolm, 2003; Jensen-Campbell & Graziano, 2001) and cooperation (Graziano, Hair, & Finch, 1997; see Graziano & Tobin, 2009, for a review). Because of its behavioral and empirical origins, controversies appeared about its sources within human psychology, its correlates, and even a suitable label for this hypothetical construct. Alternative labels used to describe the dimension are *friendly compliance versus hostile noncompliance, tender mindedness, likeability, communion,* and even *love versus hate.*

Verbal labels such as *friendly compliance* have led to misunderstandings about agreeableness. For example, the term *compliance* has a process-based meaning in social psychology that often places it on a continuum of social influence with internalization and identification (e.g., Petty & Wegener, 1999). That variety of compliance is considerably

different from the one used more casually in personality to imply tendencies to follow rules and norms. *Friendly compliance* might imply a generally conforming personality, but we know of no experimental or even correlational evidence that persons high in agreeableness are more responsive to persuasive communications or to social influence than individuals low in agreeableness (Kassner, 2011; but see Carlo, Okun, Knight, & de Guzman, 2005, p. 1302; Erdheim, Wang, & Zichar, 2006; Habashi & Wegener, 2008; see Parks, 2011, "Conformity," pp. 530–531).

Measurement methods have also contributed to skepticism about agreeableness. Agreeableness has been measured through observation by knowledgeable informants such as spouses (Costa & McCrae, 1988), employment supervisors (Hogan, Hogan, & Roberts, 1996), and teachers/child care supervisors (e.g., Digman & Takemoto-Chock, 1981; Tobin & Graziano, 2011), but self-report measures continue to be the most commonly used method (Costa & McCrae, 1988; Goldberg, 1992; Goldberg et al., 2006; John & Srivastava, 1999). (See Finch, Panter, & Caskie, 1999; Graziano & Tobin, 2009, for a more thorough discussion of agreeableness assessment.) Because self-report is the most common way of measuring agreeableness, it is reasonable to ask questions about self-favoring biases emerging from self-report.

Examination of the items assessing agreeableness has raised social desirability concerns, given that words and descriptions indicative of high agreeableness (e.g., *friendly, likes to cooperate with others*) are considered more favorable than those indicating low agreeableness (e.g., *cool and aloof, unkind*). Observations of these measures have generated suspicions that agreeableness scores may simply reflect responsiveness to the direction of the prevailing social wind. If this is true, then an individual's standing on agreeableness could be manipulated by telling that individual it was good or bad to be agreeable. Both correlational and experimental data, however, do not support this alternative explanation for agreeableness findings. Finch and colleagues (1999) conducted both joint and interbattery factor analyses of the Big Five, as measured with NEO (Costa & McCrae, 1988) and Murray's needs, as measured with the Personality Research Form (PRF; Jackson, 1984). Both methods produced a large factor for agreeableness (and for each of the other Big Five dimensions), but both analyses failed to find evidence that needs related to social desirability such as Abasement, Defendence, Succorance, or Desirability loaded on the agreeableness factor. Taking a more focused experimental approach, Graziano and Tobin (2002) tested directly the social desirability hypothesis in a three-study set. They found no evidence that agreeableness could be manipulated through random assignment to various kinds of social pressure conditions. Graziano and Tobin found that self-ratings of agreeableness actually increased for participants who were randomly assigned to an experimental condition in which they were told it was bad to be agreeable. Furthermore, they found that other dimensions of the Big Five (i.e., neuroticism and conscientiousness) had stronger correlations with measures of social desirability than did agreeableness. Taken together, these and other findings suggest that agreeableness effects are probably not merely artifacts of social desirability.

Consistent with the material outlined previously, Graziano and Tobin (2009) argued that major instruments for measuring agreeableness assess a genuine, organized aspect of psychological functioning. This happy message requires qualification in light of recent studies using abbreviated instruments. First, perhaps in an effort to reduce measurement load and to be more efficient, some researchers have adopted abbreviated measures of the Big Five in general, and of agreeableness in particular. These short measures may be well suited for certain hypotheses and methodological constraints (e.g., time-limited surveys). Nevertheless, when a study uses an agreeableness instrument consisting of no more than two self-report items, generating low internal consistency reliabilities (e.g., alpha values of < .60), then failures to find effects for agreeableness hardly provide fair tests of hypotheses.

Other measurement issues have implications for agreeableness as a predictor. In analyzing agreeableness, it may be misleading to ignore other aspects of personality, whether or not they are correlated with agreeableness. Research showed that agreeableness was related (inversely) to retaliatory aggression (Gleason, Jensen-Campbell, & Richardson, 2004) and its facets (inversely) to vengefulness (Bellah, Bellah, & Johnson, 2003), but there may be a configural aspect to this story. Using a rationale derived from an interactive theoretical perspective, Ode, Robinson, and Wilkowski (2008) showed that at higher levels of agreeableness, the anger–neuroticism link was considerably reduced. In another set of studies, Ode and Robinson (2008) found a similar moderating effect for agreeableness on the relation between neuroticism and depressive symptoms.

Using a different rationale in a resistance-to-temptation study, Jensen-Campbell and Graziano (2005) showed that higher levels of conscientiousness could partially compensate for lower levels of agreeableness in predicting cheating in adolescents. Interestingly, in each of these cases the substantive concern was affect regulation. The configuration of personality patterns (vs. one personality dimension at a time) is a cutting-edge issue in personality theory and measurement, generally under the rubric of the *abridged Big Five circumplex* (AB5C), but it suggests avenues for refinement of links among personality dimensions and their collective relation with behavior (De Raad, 2000, p. 83; De Raad, Hendriks, & Hofstee, 1994). The configuration issue will become important in the subsequent discussion of our opponent process approach to agreeableness (Graziano & Habashi, 2010; Graziano & Tobin, 2009).

From a validity perspective, the process of searching for measurement artifacts could be endless but for the guideposts provided by relevant theory on social and personality development. Agreeableness may be tied distinctively to systems of self-regulation, especially as they apply to frustration regulation in social relations (Cumberland-Li, Eisenberg, & Reiser, 2004; Jensen-Campbell & Graziano, 2005; Jensen-Campbell & Malcolm, 2007; Laursen, Pulkkinen, & Adams, 2002; Tobin & Graziano, 2011). Consistent with these findings, Smits and Boeck (2006) found that agreeableness had a positive relation with the behavioral inhibition system (BIS) and a negative one with the drive scale of the behavioral approach system (BAS).

Ahadi and Rothbart (1994) theorize that an early appearing temperamental variable, effortful control, lays the developmental foundation for subsequent personality structure in children, adolescents, and adults. They propose that effortful control is part of a common developmental system underlying two of the major dimensions in the Big Five structural model of personality, namely agreeableness and conscientiousness. Specifically, Rothbart and her colleagues (e.g., Rothbart & Bates, 2006; Rothbart & Posner, 1985) propose that effortful control modulates other temperament systems as the frontal cortex matures. Effortful control is related to early-appearing differences in the ability to sustain and shift attention, and the ability to initiate and inhibit action voluntarily (e.g., Kochanska & Knaack, 2003; Kochanska, Murray, & Coy, 1997). Effortful control seems to be related to the ability to suppress a dominant behavior to perform a subdominant response or even an opposing dominant response, as is commonly the case for agreeableness.

Consistent with this theoretical connection, Jensen-Campbell and colleagues (2002) found that both agreeableness and conscientiousness were associated with traditional assessments of self-regulation (e.g., Stroop, Wisconsin Card Sorting Task). Furthermore, Haas, Omura, Constable, and Canli (2007) found that agreeableness is related to activation of the right lateral prefrontal cortex following exposure to negative emotional stimuli. These results suggest that individuals high in agreeableness automatically engage in emotion regulation processes when exposed to negative stimuli. Consistent with these results, Tobin, Graziano, Vanman, and Tassinary (2000) found that individuals high in agreeableness reported experiencing stronger emotional reactions to evocative stimuli and exerted greater efforts to regulate these emotions than their peers. Similarly, Tobin and Graziano (2011) found a significant relation between agreeableness and negative affect regulation in school-age children using the disappointing gift paradigm (Cole, 1986; Saarni, 1984). In this study, each child who helped an experimenter with a task was provided with a gift-wrapped box containing an undesirable toy (in most cases, a broken baby rattle), and the child's reaction to the toy was videotaped for later observational coding. Independent observers rated the negative emotion dis-

plays of children low in agreeableness as significantly greater than the negative displays of children high in agreeableness. Thus, individual differences in agreeableness have been linked to negative affect regulation in school-age children.

Laursen and colleagues (2002) reported a 25-year prospective longitudinal study of regulation-related behaviors. Specifically, they tracked 194 individuals, measuring teacher and peer reports of aggression, compliance, and self-control beginning at age 8. These same variables distinguished high-agreeable from low-agreeable adults at age 33. Profile analyses revealed two behavioral types in childhood and two personality types in adulthood, with considerable continuity in the composition of these high- and low-agreeable types over time. High-agreeable childhood types had fewer disobedience and concentration problems than low-agreeable childhood types, and among boys, high-agreeable childhood types had better school grades and fewer behavior problems than their low-agreeable counterparts. High-agreeable adulthood types reported less alcoholism and depression, fewer arrests, and more career stability than did low-agreeable adulthood types. From these patterns, Laursen and colleagues inferred that agreeableness was related to important regulatory processes that appear in childhood and seem to confer advantages to those children, relative to their peers.

Agreeableness may not be highly related to other major structural dimensions of personality, but it is probably related to other dispositions, perhaps due to overlapping regulatory processes (e.g., Finch et al., 1999). Intuitively, one might expect empathy to be a component of agreeableness. Studies show that agreeableness is related to dispositional empathy. Persons high in agreeableness report greater ease in seeing the world through others' eyes (perspective taking) and feeling the suffering of others (empathic concern), but not necessarily in experiencing self-focused negative emotions (personal distress) when observing victims in sorrow. Past research showed that these cognitive and emotional processes are related to overt helping, so we might expect persons high in agreeableness to offer more help and aid to others, even to strangers, than do their peers. Recent empirical research supports the claim that agreeableness is related to both empathy and helping (e.g., Graziano, Habashi, et al., 2007). We discuss this line of research in more detail subsequently.

Agreeableness as a Complex of Motivational and Cognitive Processes

In the first comprehensive review of agreeableness as a distinct, psychological construct, Graziano and Eisenberg (1997) proposed that agreeableness could be defined in motivational terms. Specifically, they proposed that agreeableness was a summary label for individual differences in the motivation to maintain positive relations with others. Twelve years later, Graziano and Tobin (2009) observed that the agreeableness literature had identified some reliable behavioral differences, that motivational processes could be implicated, but that research is still needed to dig deeper to uncover the psychological processes and mechanisms generating the diverse phenomena. Graziano and Tobin took a step in the direction of identifying psychological processes in noting parallels in the way agreeableness related to the two outwardly opposite social behaviors of prejudice and helping. As philosopher of science Wesley C. Salmon (1984) observed, these parallels are "damn strange coincidences" (see also Meehl, 1997).

Despite behavioral genetic evidence that prosocial and antisocial systems may be different (e.g., Krueger, Hicks, & McGue, 2001), Graziano and Tobin noted that the specific behaviors of prejudice and helping are not merely Salmonian coincidences: Underlying both are accommodative processes with approach and avoidance elements. One implication is that a common motivational regulatory system linking approach, avoidance, and agreeableness may underlie both forms of behavior, and probably others. Agreeableness and social accommodation might be tied closely to self-regulation in general and to balancing approach and avoidance tendencies in particular.

Building on that rationale, Graziano and Habashi (2010) proposed that a *dual-process model* may explain some anomalies and curiosities within the two research literatures of prejudice and helping. One component of their dual-process model was agreeableness. We discuss the dual-process model to explicate further the affective, cognitive, and behavioral components underlying social accommodation. Dual- and multiprocess models are prominent in the literatures on prejudice (Pryor, Reeder, Yeadon, & Hesson-McInnis, 2004) and on helping (Batson, 1991; Dijker & Koomen, 2007). Indeed, these processes may be more general than previously recognized. We believe some clarification of the apparent inconsistencies in the literatures on social accommodation can be obtained using a dual-process, sequential opponent motivational system that incorporates agreeableness. Before we proceed further, we discuss two related issues that bear on this explication of processes underlying agreeableness. These are contextual elicitation and temporal course of processes. (For a related discussion of empathy and antisocial tendencies controlled by two different cognitive–motivational complexes, see Baron-Cohen [2011] and Billington, Baron-Cohen, and Wheelwright [2007]. Baron-Cohen [2011] proposes that "zero empathy" can be related to both negative and positive outcomes. Negative outcomes associated with low empathy are narcissism, antisocial tendencies, and prejudice. Less intuitive are positive outcomes such as skills in removing the self from here-and-now contexts and in detecting patterns of cause and effect.)

Contextual Influences in the Expression of Social Accommodation: The Case of Interpersonal Conflict

If persons differ in their motivation to maintain positive relationships with others, then we can expect agreeableness to covary with their efforts to obtain certain goals and to avoid other goals. Persons high in dispositional agreeableness should approach goals that permit them to promote and retain positive relations with others. They should perform more positive, prosocial, constructive behaviors in various behavioral domains than their peers. We should also expect them to approach prosocial goals with great intensity and to persist in seeking prosocial goals when such goals are not achieved initially. This goal-seeking approach was a reasonable starting place for beginning a program of scientific work, and it helped uncover several important behavioral differences, which in turn implicated emotion, motivation, and cognition.

The approach has some limitations, however, as a means for linking agreeableness to psychological processes in general and to interpersonal behaviors in particular. First, interpersonal behaviors are determined to a large extent by expectations about the likely reactions of interaction partners (Kelley et al., 2003). However highly motivated Person A might be to cooperate, when A develops expectations that cooperative behaviors will be met by exploitation from Person B, expectations can redirect the underlying cooperative motivation (e.g., Graziano et al., 1997; Savani, Morris, Naidu, Kumar, & Berlia, 2011).

Second, personality can operate indirectly through its potent influence on the self-selection of situations. Self-selection processes should be especially striking for interpersonal behaviors, even to the point of masking potential moderation by personality variables. These considerations apply directly to agreeableness. Persons high in agreeableness are well liked and popular with their peers, in part because they project positivity onto others and make excuses for others' shortcomings (Graziano, Bruce, et al., 2007; Graziano & Tobin, 2002; Jensen-Campbell et al., 2002). Persons high in agreeableness enter encounters with the expectation that others will be pleasant and likable, and appear to elicit such behavior from their partners. This pattern is consistent with the reciprocity-of-attraction principle, but it suggests the need to look past a simple personality moderator approach. In particular, it points to the need for attention to social interdependence and to other social-cognitive processes underlying interpersonal interaction. The person × situation approach is a step in that direction (Graziano, Habashi, et al., 2007). That is, rather than treating agreeableness as a variable that merely raises or lowers the level of situational effects, agreeableness enters the stage as part of an ensemble of cognitive, affective, and interpersonal elements. In some cases, the presence of persons at different levels of agreeableness can fundamentally alter the situations themselves (cf. Moskowitz, Ho, & Turcotte-Tremblay, 2007).

Time in the Expression of Social Accommodation: The Case of Interpersonal Conflict

Let us turn now to the general issue of time in the expression of social accommodation. Time is the stage upon which context can exert its influence. Time may be a less critical variable in interpreting lab-based experimental research, but it looms much larger in more naturalistic research. To illustrate, we selected an anomaly from the research on agreeableness and interpersonal conflict. Intuitively, it would seem that agreeableness would be related to affect and cognition surrounding interpersonal conflict. If agreeableness is defined in terms of motivation to maintain positive relations with others, then conflict represents a threat to that goal. Goal blockage should lead to distinctive emotions and thoughts. Precisely what behavioral differences should we expect? On the one hand, persons low in agreeableness should find conflicts less distressing than their peers because they are not particularly motivated to maintain positive relations with others. In terms of social cognition, their expectations about conflict and its disruptive consequences for interpersonal harmony may be lower. In terms of emotions, they may experience less frustration. On the other hand, one could make the case that persons high in agreeableness might find conflicts less distressing because they have acquired skills for handling them, have a more diverse, flexible tool kit for dealing with conflict, have better relationships initially, have peer allies in case conflicts do escalate, etc. Which of these two seemingly opposite options is correct?

Graziano and colleagues (1996) found that when middle school students provided self-reports on their reactions to interpersonal conflict, persons high in agreeableness reported greater distress when they experienced interpersonal conflict. This makes sense, yet when teachers of these same students rated how each of their students reacted to conflict, teachers reported that students high in agreeableness experience *less* emotional distress during conflict. One simplistic interpretation is that self-ratings and ratings by knowledgeable informants do not meet a minimum standard to converge across method, casting doubt on the reliability, much less the validity, of a link between agreeableness and conflict. Another interpretation involves time and regulation: Like many other important social behaviors, conflict is a sequence of interrelated events that unfolds over time. If conflict is defined in terms of initial overt reactions only, we would find one pattern of data. If we focused on events later in the sequence, defining in terms of resolution processes only, we would find an entirely different pattern. The bigger picture lies in the dynamic unfolding of emotion and cognition over time.

To exactly what event should the assessment of emotional distress refer? Because Graziano and colleagues (1996) had conceptualized the question as one single event narrowly circumscribed in time, they did not collect data that might have shown differences over time. In the absence of data, we must speculate on time-related differences. From the students' perspective, the salient aspect of the conflict was probably the events that brought it into being. It is plausible that students' self-ratings were evaluating distress early in the conflict episode, close to the time of detecting the interpersonal conflict. Teacher ratings were probably based on events later in the episode, perhaps the sequelae of conflict, including efforts to restore peace following the conflict. In these circumstances, students high in agreeableness probably showed better emotional control, appeared less distressed, and were engaged in more constructive action.

The timing issues described to this point may have larger implications for understanding not only agreeableness, but also the dynamics of social accommodation. First, complex social behaviors are almost certainly influenced by multiple components and mechanisms. In the case of social accommodation, we have already seen social-cognitive components and emotional components. It is unlikely that these components will be activated by the same cues or at the same time. By overlooking the time dimension, we may be missing opportunities to see how components combine to create behavioral differences. There is more to it, of course, than the quasi-voyeuristic satisfaction from merely observing covariation in components. A more penetrating theoretical analysis becomes possible. Why, for example, do certain components appear together, but not others? Second, the choice of units of time will be determined by the nature of the components under investigation. Units for perceptual aspects of social cognition might be defined in milliseconds, but units for the planning aspects of social cognition will almost certainly be longer. Third, if we have learned anything in the last 60 years of behavioral research, it is that the actual and expected consequences following behavior leave a residue. By including time, we are exposing the components to the risk of consequences. That is, by including time we can observe the impact of consequences on actions, processes, and choices. Anticipated consequences will surely affect social accommodation activities. Fourth, by including time it is easier to see why agreeableness has been harder to study than other major dimensions of personality (e.g., Gosling, 2008, "blob analysis" of agreeableness, p. 186). Studies can generate contradictory outcomes because they may be assessing the operation of potentially conflicting motives of approach and avoidance differentially within the larger framework of interpersonal accommodation.

Time in the Expression of Social Accommodation: Anomalies of Prejudice and Helping

Graziano and Habashi (2010) framed their temporal sequential model with an eye to finding underlying order beneath some apparent anomalies. In particular, they concentrated on anomalies in prejudice and helping, two interpersonal behaviors seemingly at opposite ends of the prosocial continuum. In practical terms, the two literatures live in isolation from each other. This makes sense intuitively. Prejudice is generally seen as a negative, even antisocial behavior, whereas helping is a positive, constructive, prosocial activity. With closer inspection, however, the presumed polarity, much less the separation, is harder to justify. Prejudice and helping are both affective, presumably motivated phenomena with implications for accommodation, usually operating at the initiation phase of interpersonal attraction, at least as investigated by social psychologists (Graziano & Bruce, 2008).

Perhaps such similarities are mere super-ficial coincidences, like a tennis ball and a planet both being spheres. The trick is finding the deeper connection, if any. The deeper connection may lie with elements of both approach and avoidance (e.g., Pur-sell, Laursen, Rubin, Booth-LaForce, & Rose-Krasnor, 2008). Within the helping literature, research indicates that "messy victims" (e.g., bleeding) seem to activate avoidance that interferes with helping (e.g., Piliavin, Callero, & Evanset, 1982). In Bat-son's (1991) empathy–altruism model, self-focused personal distress seems to interfere with helping, especially when escape from the helping situation is relatively easy (Bat-son, Duncan, Ackerman, Buckley, & Birch, 1981). At the other end of the prosocial con-tinuum, Pryor and colleagues (2004) found that people often have an initially negative reflexive reaction to outgroup members, but that corrective reflective processes can come online and suppress the avoidance within 500 milliseconds. The Pryor paradigm makes it clear that both reflexive avoidance and reflective approach are operative.

In Batson's empathy–altruism approach, the self-focused emotion of personal dis-tress undermines helping, whereas the victim-focused emotion of empathic con-cern promotes helping. This relation has been demonstrated in experimental studies that manipulate perspective taking. For-mally, empathy refers to a set of related components that include personal distress, empathic concern, and perspective taking (Davis, 1996). The last of these three pro-vides a distinctively cognitive process that is relatively easy to manipulate experimentally. In experiments using the Batson paradigm, the affective processes of empathic concern are elicited from research participants opera-tionally by manipulating their focus of atten-tion (e.g., Coke, Batson, & McDavis, 1978; Toi & Batson, 1982). More specifically, to manipulate that focus Batson and colleagues randomly assign participants to one of two conditions. In one condition, they are asked to try to imagine how the person telling the story feels, to put themselves in her shoes. In the other condition, participants are asked to attend to the technical details of the broadcast, ignoring its substantive content. Studies containing manipulation checks on this operationalization (e.g., Graziano,

Habashi, et al., 2007) show that it is effec-tive in manipulating perspective taking.

This line of reasoning implies that the emo-tion of personal distress would be correlated negatively with the emotion of empathic concern and the cognitive processes of per-spective taking. Virtually all studies that have measured both personal distress and empathic concern find that they are corre-lated positively, not negatively (e.g., Batson, O'Quin, Fultz, Vanderplas, & Isen, 1983; Graziano, Habashi, et al., 2007). Batson and colleagues (1983) attempted to address this problem by assigning participants to conditions based on their single-most domi-nant motive (see pp. 711–712). Thus, Batson and his colleagues recognize the operation of two potentially opposing motives linked to avoidance and approach.

That there are many individual differences in moderating helping or prejudice is no lon-ger controversial (Dovidio, Piliavin, Schro-eder, & Penner, 2006). What is controversial is the generality of the influence of any given individual difference. Pryor and colleagues (2004) found that prejudice toward an HIV victim was moderated by individual differ-ences on Heterosexual Attitudes Toward Homosexuals (Larson, Reed, & Hoffman, 1980), but there was no evidence that this individual difference moderated prejudice against ex-convicts. Are various prejudices tightly segregated, or do they shake hands with each other? Part of the problem is theo-retical. It is not clear precisely what mecha-nisms are responsible for differences. Gra-ziano and colleagues (Graziano & Habashi, 2010; Graziano & Tobin, 2009) thought that they had found a single set of motives that cut across substantive topic areas and provided a unifying thread, namely agree-ableness.

Toward a Resolution of Anomalies in Social Accommodation

One important step toward organizing these divergent issues comes from Dijker and Koomen (2007), who outlined an inte-grative perspective to stigmatization that includes two evolved, preverbal systems of motivation. Each system reflects a different aspect of human evolutionary history. The first and older component is a fight–flight system that is part of our paleoreptilian heritage. Encounters with what Dijker and Koomen term *deviance* activate this system without conscious deliberation, driving the individual to flee from danger, or to fight, if necessary. The second system, added more recently in our evolutionary history, is connected to the parental care system associated with kin selection (Hamilton, 1964; Trivers, 1972). These two motivational systems can elicit characteristic emotions when exposed to specific environmental cues. Because humans evolved in small groups of genetically related individuals, reproductive advantages accrued to individual genetic lines that inhibited aggressive reactions to unusual cases. Some of the anomalies probably involved kin for whom repair of deviance would be more beneficial than would responses of aggression or exclusion. The care component can suppress the fight–flight system.

The system proposed by Dijker and Koomen (2007) can be expanded conceptually toward social accommodation and agreeableness. Let us assume that agreeableness is one psychological manifestation of the care system. If so, then it may relate not only to sympathetic care given to the weak and disadvantaged. More importantly, it may also operate to inhibit the reactions generated by the more primitive fight–flight system. From this perspective some agreeableness correlates may be fairly direct expressions of care, whereas others may be a combination of care-based inhibition of fight–flight. Turning to specifics, persons high in agreeableness feel empathic concern directly for victims of misfortune (Graziano, Habashi, et al., 2007), but they may also inhibit (with effort?) negative reactions originating in their fight–flight system toward traditional targets of prejudice (Graziano, Bruce, et al., 2007). In line with our earlier discussion of time, initial reactions in conflict episodes may reflect fight–flight, whereas late reactions may include the active, effortful suppression of destructive conflict tactics.

There is biobehavioral support for claims that the two systems operate both separately and also in concert. In their discussion of the evolution of caregiving, Porges and Carter (2012) note that the traditional model of the mammalian nervous system subdivides the arrangement into two systems, namely sympathetic and parasympathetic. The former is related to the activation of behavior for tasks such as fight or flight, whereas the later is related to the restoration of physiological functions such as promoting immune function. In his polyvagal theory, Porges (1995) challenges this view, proposing instead a three component, hierarchical structure. The first component includes the sympathetic circuits for fight–flight responses, but the second and third components involve a functional reassembly of the parasympathetic circuits. The second component includes circuits that coordinate the activities of the face and head, but also the restorative processes above the diaphragm. The third component is ancient in evolutionary terms and contains vagal circuits that control autonomic states below the diaphragm, permitting immobilization when environmental cues signal mortal danger. In this polyvagal model, the hierarchy of adaptive responses activates the newest branch of circuits first, namely those involving the parasympathetic systems controlling the face and head (and social communication). If the newer circuits fail to provide safety, the older systems are recruited sequentially. Porges and Carter argue that social communication and visceral homeostasis controlled by the newer circuits are inherently incompatible with neurophysiological states that support defensive behaviors of fight–flight and immobilization. The circuits are related to the distribution of receptor cites for oxytocin and arginine vasopressin, neuropeptides that are related to the expression and inhibition of fear in mammals (Viviani & Stoop, 2008).

Porges and Carter described these patterns in process terms, but individual variations can be especially informative about those basic processes (e.g., Porges & Carter, "experiments of nature," 2012, p. 55). For example, effects of oxytocin levels appear to be moderated by individual differences. Rockliff and colleagues (2011) manipulated, through nasal spray, levels of oxytocin in 44 human volunteers. Then they measured a form of introspective social cognition: the ease with which volunteers could imagine others being compassionate to them. Relative to placebo controls, oxytocin increased imagined compassion, but participants higher in self-criticism and lower in self-assurance, social safeness, and attachment security had less positive experiences following oxytocin than placebo.

Taken together, several pieces of a complex puzzle seem to come into a pattern. Separate neurophysiological systems regulate fight–flight and restorative functions. These systems seem to produce incompatible behaviors and may operate in sequence. The systems are related to the operation of neuropeptides such as oxytocin, which are related to caregiving behaviors in mammals. Individual differences moderate the way neuropeptides influence caregiving-related social cognition.

Let us readjust the logic outlined previously, assuming further some connections between the fight–flight and care systems of potential relevance to agreeableness. If both fight–flight and care systems are present in virtually all people (but to different degrees) and fight–flight occurs faster than care upon exposure to an environmental oddity, the two may operate as opponents to each other's preponderant responsive activation tendencies. Adding these simple assumptions, we can offer explanations for apparent paradoxes and anomalies. In the helping context, personal distress may inhibit prosocial acts because it is part of fight–flight, not care. Empathic concern promotes helping because it is part of care. They seem to have opposite effects on helping, but both personal distress and empathic concern are present in most people, explaining the positive correlation. If we view the process from a temporal perspective, we can see that personal distress is the first response to a victim because it is connected to the faster fight–flight system. If there is a chance for easy escape from the victim when personal distress is high, then the victim will not receive help. If escape cannot occur quickly, or if the observer must remain in proximity to the victim, then enough time may pass for the slower empathic concern system to come on line. This passing of time is merely the stage through which the two processes unfold. Time allows empathic concern to suppress the fight–flight system and to increase chances the victim would receive help. This approach explains why outcomes of research on ease–difficulty of escape are unstable. In this case, the critical variable—the time

interval between exposure to the victim and opportunity for escape—is unmeasured.

An Opponent-Process Approach to Social Accommodation

Going one step further, the system we describe may be a case of the opponent-process model of motivation presented by Solomon and his colleague (Solomon, 1980; Solomon & Corbit, 1974). In a search of the published literature, Graziano and Habashi (2010) could locate only two applications of the Solomon opponent-process model to interpersonal conflict, helping, or prejudice. Both (Baumeister & Campbell, 1999; Piliavin et al., 1982) focused on Solomon's explanation for addictive cycles of behavior.

Our version of the opponent approach is presented in Figure 19.1. The first process activated is labeled *Process A;* its activation is automatic. In keeping with Solomon's model, it is a kind of unconditioned response to the onset of an environmental stimulus. It remains active while the evocative stimulus is present and ends when the stimulus is removed. The second process activated is an opponent, labeled *Process B*. It is slower to come online, yet persists well after Process A ends. Processes A and B are opponents, but A is activated first and more quickly in response to an environmental event. Initially, for a brief part of the sequence, Process A

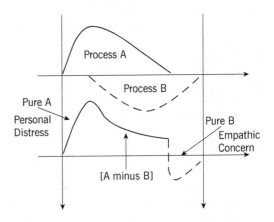

FIGURE 19.1. Opponent-process model of motivation. Adapted from Solomon and Corbit (1974). Copyright 1974 by the American Psychological Association. Adapted by permission.

operates in almost pure form (without an opponent). Applying the model to helping, if Process A is personal distress and Process B is empathic concern, then the initial response to a victim would be unopposed personal distress. If escape is possible in this interval, the victim will not receive help. Using the same logic, first reactions to unusual cases (e.g., victims of misfortune) as well as to members of outgroups would be personal distress and avoidance. As time passes these processes have the opportunity to unfold: Process B can be activated, opposing Process A. These opponent processes may be what Pryor and colleagues (2004) index in their behavior correction research in which initial negative reactions are replaced by more positive ones.

Comparisons with the QUAD Model

Graziano and Habashi (2010) note that the opponent-process model offers a useful approach to examine complex social-psychological phenomenon relative to other process models. In particular, they review adjustment/correction models in social-cognitive psychology (e.g., Martin's [1986] set–reset model), the flexible correction model (FCM; Petty, Brinol, Tormala, & Wegener, 2007; Wegener & Petty, 1997), automatic versus controlled processes (Chaiken & Trope, 1999), and multiprocess models (e.g., the QUAD model; Sherman et al., 2008). Among these models, the QUAD model warrants special attention in the present discussion.

The QUAD model (Sherman et al., 2008) is one of the most comprehensive multiprocess social-cognitive models to date, so direct comparisons between it and the opponent model are instructive. The four processes in the QUAD model are activation, detection, overcoming bias, and guessing. A "shooter bias" example is often used to illustrate the operation of QUAD. That is, the four processes of QUAD are used to predict correct or incorrect responses to situations in which respondents pull the trigger on a gun in response to a black suspect, even when the suspect holds a harmless object. In this situation, there is a correct response—shoot only when the suspect has a gun and is

pointing it at police—and a final structural component is added, namely, guessing. If no response is activated and a correct response cannot be determined, then the perceiver must guess.

The opponent-process model, unlike the QUAD model, does not offer clear correct and incorrect responses in helping that are analogous to the shooter bias. The opponent-process model also proposes a specific temporal sequence, with an explicit pattern to the onset and offset of each of the two processes. The first, Process A, is tied more closely to the onset and offset of an environmental trigger, whereas the second, Process B, is not.

There are, however, several points of congruity between the two models. Neuroimaging data suggest that the activation process described in QUAD is connected to activity in the amygdala and insula, areas of the brain that are involved in emotional processing and arousal (Eisenberger, Lieberman, & Satpute, 2005). Such a pattern of activation is what we would expect from the activation of the fight–flight component described by Dijker and Koomen (2007), and perhaps feelings of personal distress in the opponent process model. Similarly, the detection process described in QUAD is associated with activity in the dorsal anterior cingulate cortex and the dorsolateral prefrontal cortex. These are areas that have been linked to inhibitory control over prepotent responses. We would expect this pattern of activation from the care component in Dijker and Koomen, and perhaps from the feeling of empathic concern in the opponent-process model.

Sherman and colleagues (2008) did not discuss the domains of helping and prosocial behavior; however, they did single out one prosocial domain for special attention: individual differences in motivation to respond without prejudice. As discussed by Graziano and Habashi (2010), this particular domain illustrates the difference in the ways QUAD characterizes the key variables in comparison with the opponent-processes model. Sherman and colleagues applied the QUAD model to data from a weapons identification study by Amodio, Devine, and Harmon-Jones (2008), using a preponderant motive approach in which participants were classified into one of four quadrants in a two (internal vs. external source) by two (low vs. high intensity) design. Participants who were high in internal motivation and also low in external motivation to avoid prejudice showed less implicit bias than did other participants. The QUAD analyses showed that these high internal–low external participants showed less activation of biased association and were better able to detect appropriate and inappropriate responses in overcoming bias.

The opponent-process model offers a different approach. First, individual differences in motivation may be related to prejudice, but those differences would not necessarily require two different dimensions working in configuration or even preponderance. The predictive dimension would be agreeableness and its associated motives for maintaining positive relations with others. In terms of process, prejudice toward outgroup members originates in an initial negative reaction to unusual or unexpected cases, and in fight–flight. This Process A reaction would characterize all participants, not just those who were low in internal motivation to inhibit prejudice. Because the opponent-process model is sequential, Process B is triggered before Process A runs it full course, and the sooner it is activated following the onset of Process A, the less prejudice will be expressed, at least in its pure, unopposed form.

Implications for Social Accommodation

The opponent-process approach raises important questions about the nature of social accommodation. First, how wide is the window for the expression of social accommodation? It seems that if the window is too narrow, we could miss the dynamic processes underlying accommodation, and perhaps the accommodation phenomena we wish to study. The expression of complex social behavior such as helping or prejudice is almost certainly the outcome of several different but related systems. When the systems operate at the same time, one system may reduce the influence of another. In the opponent-process model, the influence of Process A is much reduced once Process B is activated. From observing a single episode

of helping or prejudice, a researcher might conclude that a single process is operative, but it is likely that the process is better studied only by observing the operation of the components over time.

Second, what is the conceptual status of individual differences such as agreeableness, empathic concern, personal distress, and internal–external motivation to control prejudice? One approach to individual differences is to regard them as proxies or markers of differences in cognitive or emotional processes. Then the question becomes one of identifying processes. Temperament researchers (e.g., Rueda, Posner, & Rothbart, 2005) argue that each individual is born with an emotional core and is prepared for a life trajectory by a set of inherited tendencies and motivation systems. The emotional core interacts with the social learning environment, leaving residues such as internal working models, social learning histories, as well as aspects of personality. People learn about others (including outgroup members) as they move through these trajectories, but what exactly are they learning (Biesanz, West, & Millevoi, 2007)? Evidence suggests that most people are selective in their information processing in these situations.

Several theorists (Brown & Brown, 2006; Dijker & Koomen, 2007; Eastwick, 2009; Porges & Carter, 2012) have proposed that evolution left humans with two powerful motive systems in *fight–flight* and *care*, but there are probably individual differences in the relative strength of these motivations. In terms of overt behaviors, observers might notice and label these socially important behavioral differences as neuroticism and agreeableness, respectively (Graziano & Habashi, 2010). We might be satisfied to build structural models or collect data showing intercorrelations among variables such as care, agreeableness, and some other disposition (e.g., empathy or self-esteem). However, this approach would greatly underestimate the dynamic quality of the processes, their major dispositional inputs, and probably the range of influence of the individual difference under consideration. Nevertheless, repeated exposure to certain kinds of environmental events could change the basic parameters of the inherited dispositions and motives. Perhaps this dynamism was the deeper message of Solomon and Corbit.

Linking the affective components of empathy and the personality dimension of agreeableness to interpersonal behaviors and to more general self-regulatory processes (Graziano & Tobin, 2009) is novel. Many questions remain unanswered. Is agreeableness tied to the care system only or to fight–flight as well? Is it tied to both personal distress and empathic concern, to both prejudice and the suppression of prejudice, or to just one of these elements in each pair? We believe that the opponent-process approach to agreeableness allows us to anticipate phenomena that cannot be found elsewhere. Graziano and Habashi (2010) offered a few tentative ideas.

One issue that is worthy of special attention is delayed helping (see Penner, Fritzsche, Craiger, & Freifeld, 1995). In general, a common assumption is that the influence of a manipulation of victim need, mood state, or empathic concern will dissipate for most or all people over time. That is, rates of helping are affected by the time interval between the request for help and the opportunity to provide it. Note the analogue to the correction of prejudice outcomes reported by Pryor and colleagues (2004).

If the opponent-process system operates roughly as described here, then some forms of helping may be greater after a short delay than they are following an immediate request. The initial fight–flight reaction may come under the control of the opponent care system, in effect disinhibiting helping with time. Undoubtedly, we would also see characteristic emotions, such as relief at finally having an opportunity to provide assistance. Based on the previous rationale, we would also expect persons high in agreeableness to offer more help, sooner and with less influence of delay, than persons low in agreeableness. At this point, such conjectures are speculative. Whatever outcomes do appear, it is clear that major motives underlie helping and prejudice, and that they are linked to dispositional variables associated with social accommodation and maintaining positive relationships with others. Understanding the dynamics of these motives will play a role in our deeper understanding of interpersonal processes.

One final point bears comment. It could be argued that it is misleading to describe agreeableness as a one-dimensional individual difference. Inevitably, say critics, persons low in agreeableness are defined by default, as simply lacking qualities that are possessed by persons high in agreeableness. If persons high in agreeableness show empathic concern, willingness to accommodate to the goals of others, and a desire to minimize conflict with others, then do persons low in agreeableness simply lack these qualities? By implication, some of the distinctiveness of persons low in agreeableness might be lost. We offer several responses in rebuttal.

First, available evidence supports the claim that all of the Big Five structural dimensions of personality, including agreeableness, are better represented conceptually as a set of continuous variables than as categories (e.g., Finch et al., 1999). These are major dimensions of personality, whose function is to describe larger patterns and trends in thoughts, feelings, and behaviors. The dimensions may be less well suited to predicting specific unique, one-time behaviors such as preferring spinach over broccoli on Tuesday. It is intriguing, of course, to learn that one study found that children lower in agreeableness like to play chess more than children higher in agreeableness (e.g., Bilalic, McLeod, & Gobet, 2007). If this empirical link is replicated, it gains importance not for its uniqueness but because it implicates a more general process (e.g., most children perceive chess not as a friendly game, but as an exercise in dominance and conflict). That is not to say that a major dimension of personality such as agreeableness is unrelated to daily behaviors such as music preferences (e.g., Gosling, 2008, pp. 51–52; Rentfrow, Goldberg, & Levitin, 2011). Just as group means purchase generality at the price of each individual's unique properties, the assumption of unidimensionality is built on the quest for general patterns and connections, not uniqueness.

Second, the process model outlined here suggests that agreeableness is a proxy for describing a larger underlying process of social accommodation. It is a verbal label for a social construction, not less real than other social constructions, such as extraversion, but still a social construction. That there are noticeable individual differences suggests that the accommodation process itself operates with different settings for different persons (e.g., Pursell et al., 2008). We infer that variability in agreeableness means that both distal evolution processes and more proximal social systems can find uses for persons at most levels along a continuum of social accommodation.

Third, we offer pragmatic reasons for maintaining a single continuum perspective. Much is to be gained by comparing individuals who are located at different places along a single continuum. The comparison can implicate processes underlying the dimension as a whole. Our opponent-process model is a product of these comparisons. Subsequent research may corroborate or refute such inferences, but we are optimistic that further gold remains to be mined.

Acknowledgments

We wish to thank Meara Habashi, Daniel Ozer, Craig Parks, David Tobin, and Laura Vander-Drift for their valuable comments on an earlier version of this chapter.

References

Ahadi, S. A., & Rothbart, M. K. (1994). Temperament, development, and the Big Five. In C. F. Halverson, Jr., G. A. Kohnstamm, & R. P. Martin (Eds.), *The developing structure of temperament and personality from infancy to adulthood* (pp. 189–207). Hillsdale, NJ: Erlbaum.

Allport, G. W. (1968). The historical background of modern social psychology. In G. Lindsey & E. Aronson (Eds.), *The handbook of social psychology* (2nd ed., Vol. 1, pp. 1–80). Reading, MA: Addison-Wesley.

Amodio, D. M., Devine, P. G., & Harmon-Jones, E. (2008). Individual differences in the regulation of intergroup bias: The role of conflict monitoring and neural signals for control. *Journal of Personality and Social Psychology, 94*, 60–74.

Baron-Cohen, S. (2011). *The science of evil: On empathy and the origins of cruelty.* New York: Basic Books.

Batson, C. D. (1991). *The altruism question: Toward a social-psychological answer.* Hillsdale, NJ: Erlbaum.

Batson, C. D., Duncan, B. D., Ackerman, P., Buckley, T., & Birch, K. (1981). Is empathic emotion a source of altruistic motivation?

Journal of Personality and Social Psychology, 40, 290–302.

Batson, C. D., O'Quin, K., Fultz, J., Vanderplas, M., & Isen, A. M. (1983). Influence of self-reported distress and empathy on egoistic versus altruistic motivation to help. *Journal of Personality and Social Psychology, 45*, 706–718.

Baumeister, R. F., & Campbell, W. K. (1999). The intrinsic appeal of evil: Sadism, sensational thrills, and threatened egotism. *Personality and Social Psychology Review, 3*, 210–221.

Bellah, C. G., Bellah, L. D., & Johnson, J. L. (2003). A look at dispositional vengefulness from the three and five-factor models of personality. *Individual Differences Research, 1*, 6–16.

Biesanz, J. C., West, S. G., & Millevoi, A. (2007). What do we learn about someone over time?: The relationship between length of acquaintance, consensus, and self–other agreement in judgments of personality. *Journal of Personality and Social Psychology, 92*, 119–135.

Bilalic, M., McLeod, P., & Gobet, F. (2007). Personality profiles of young chess players. *Personality and Individual Differences, 42*, 901–910.

Billington, J., Baron-Cohen, S., & Wheelwright, S. I. J. (2007). Cognitive style predicts entry into physical sciences and humanities. *Learning and Individual Differences, 17*, 260–268.

Brown, S. L., & Brown, R. M. (2006). Selective investment theory: Recasting the functional significance of close relationships. *Psychological Inquiry, 17*, 1–29.

Carlo, G., Okun, M. A., Knight, G. P., & de Guzman, M. R. T. (2005). The interplay of traits and motives on volunteering: Agreeableness, extraversion, and prosocial value motivation. *Personality and Individual Differences, 38*, 1293–1305.

Chaiken S., & Trope, Y. (Eds.). (1999). *Dual-process theories in social psychology.* New York: Guilford Press.

Coke, J. S., Batson, C. D., & McDavis, K. (1978). Empathic mediation of helping: A two-stage model. *Journal of Personality and Social Psychology, 36*, 752–766.

Cole, P. M. (1986). Children's spontaneous control of facial expression. *Child Development, 57*, 1309–1321.

Costa, P. T., & McCrae, R. R. (1988). Personality in adulthood: A six-year longitudinal study of self-reports and spouse ratings on the NEO Personality Inventory. *Journal of Personality and Social Psychology, 54*, 853–863.

Cumberland-Li, A., Eisenberg, N., & Reiser, M. (2004). Relations of young children's agreeableness and resiliency to effortful control and impulsivity. *Social Development, 13*, 193–212.

Davis, M. H. (1996). *Empathy: A social psychological approach*. Boulder, CO: Westview Press.

De Raad, B. (2000). *The Big Five personality factors: The psycholexical approach to personality*. Seattle, WA: Hogrefe & Huber.

De Raad, B., Hendriks, A. A. J., & Hofstee, W. K. B. (1994). The Big Five: A tip of the iceberg of individual differences. In C. F. Halverson, Jr., G. A. Kohnstamm, & R. P. Martin (Eds), *The developing structure of temperament and personality from infancy to adulthood* (pp. 91–109). Hillsdale, NJ: Erlbaum.

Digman, J. M., & Takemoto-Chock, N. K. (1981). Factors in the natural language of personality: Re-analysis, comparison, and interpretation of six major studies. *Multivariate Behavioral Research, 16*, 149–170.

Dijker, A. J. M., & Koomen, W. (2007). *Stigmatization, tolerance, and repair: An integrative psychological analysis of responses to deviance*. New York: Cambridge University Press.

Dovidio, J., Piliavin, J. A., Schroeder, D. A., & Penner, L. A. (2006). *The social psychology of prosocial behavior*. Mahwah, NJ: Erlbaum.

Eastwick, P. W. (2009). Beyond the Pleistocene: Using phylogeny and constraint to inform the evolutionary psychology of human mating. *Psychological Bulletin, 135*, 794–821.

Eisenberger, N. I., Lieberman, M. D., & Satpute, A. B. (2005). Personality from a controlled processing perspective: An fMRI study of neuroticism, extraversion, and self-consciousness. *Cognitive, Affective, and Behavioral Neuroscience, 5*, 169–181.

Erdheim, J., Wang, M., & Zichar, M. J. (2006). Linking the Big Five personality constructs to organizational commitment. *Personality and Individual Differences, 41*, 959–970.

Finch, J. F., Panter, A. T., & Caskie, G. I. L. (1999). Two approaches to identifying personality dimensions across method. *Journal of Personality, 67*, 407–438.

Gleason, K. A., Jensen-Campbell, L. A., & Richardson, D. S. (2004). Agreeableness as a predictor of aggression in adolescence. *Aggressive Behavior, 30*, 43–61.

Goldberg, L. R. (1992). The development of markers of the Big Five factor structure. *Psychological Assessment, 4*, 26–42.

Goldberg, L. R., Johnson, J. A., Eber, H. W., Hogan, R., Ashton, M. C., Cloninger, C. R., et al. (2006). The International Personality Item Pool and the future of public-domain personality measures. *Journal of Research in Personality, 40*, 84–96.

Gosling, S. (2008). *Snoop: What your stuff says about you*. New York: Basic Books.

Graziano, W. G., & Bruce, J. W. (2008). Attraction and the initiation of relationships: A review of the empirical literature. In S. Sprecher, A. Wenzel, & J. Harvey (Eds.), *Handbook of relationship initiation* (pp. 269–295). New York: Psychology Press.

Graziano, W. G., Bruce, J. W., Sheese, B. E., & Tobin, R. M. (2007). Attraction, personality, and prejudice: Liking none of the people most of the time. *Journal of Personality and Social Psychology, 93*, 565–582.

Graziano, W. G., & Eisenberg, N. (1997). Agreeableness: A dimension of personality. In R. Hogan, J. Johnson, & S. Briggs (Eds.), *Handbook of personality psychology* (pp. 795–824). San Diego, CA: Academic Press.

Graziano, W. G., & Habashi, M. M. (2010). Motivational processes underlying both prejudice and helping. *Personality and Social Psychology Review, 14*, 313–331.

Graziano, W. G., Habashi, M. M., Sheese, B. E., & Tobin, R. M. (2007). Agreeableness, empathy, and helping: A person × situation perspective. *Journal of Personality and Social Psychology, 93*, 583–599.

Graziano, W. G., Hair, E. C., & Finch, J. F. (1997). Competitiveness mediates the link between personality and group performance. *Journal of Personality and Social Psychology, 73*, 1394–1408.

Graziano, W. G., Jensen-Campbell, L. A., & Hair, E. C. (1996). Perceiving interpersonal conflict and reacting to it: The case for agreeableness. *Journal of Personality and Social Psychology, 70*, 820–835.

Graziano, W. G., & Tobin, R. M. (2002). Agreeableness: Dimension of personality or social desirability artifact? *Journal of Personality, 70*, 695–727.

Graziano, W. G., & Tobin, R. M. (2009). Agreeableness. In M. R. Leary & R. H. Hoyle

(Eds.), *Handbook of individual differences in social behavior* (pp. 46–61). New York: Guilford Press.

Haas, B. W., Omura, K., Constable, R. T., & Canli, T. (2007). Is automatic emotion regulation associated with agreeableness?: A perspective using a social neuroscience approach. *Psychological Science, 18*, 130–132.

Habashi, M. M., & Wegener, D. (2008). *Preliminary evidence that agreeableness is more closely related to responsiveness than conformity.* Unpublished manuscript, Purdue University, West Lafayette, IN.

Hair, E. C., & Graziano, W. G. (2003). Self-esteem, personality, and achievement in high school: A prospective longitudinal study in Texas. *Journal of Personality, 71*, 971–994.

Hamilton, W. D. (1964). The genetical evolution of social behaviour: I and II. *Journal of Theoretical Biology, 7*, 1–32.

Hogan, R., Hogan, J., & Roberts, B. W. (1996). Personality measurement and employment decisions: Questions and answers. *American Psychologist, 51*, 469–477.

Jackson, D. F. (1984). *Personality Research Form.* Port Huron, MI: Sigma Assessment Systems.

Jensen-Campbell, L. A., Gleason, K. A., Adams, R., & Malcolm, K. T. (2003). Interpersonal conflict, agreeableness, and personality development. *Journal of Personality, 71*, 1059–1086.

Jensen-Campbell, L. A., & Graziano, W. G. (2001). Agreeableness as a moderator of interpersonal conflict. *Journal of Personality, 69*, 323–361.

Jensen-Campbell, L. A., & Graziano, W. G. (2005). Two faces of temptation: Differing motives for self-control. *Merrill–Palmer Quarterly, 51*, 287–324.

Jensen-Campbell, L. A., & Malcolm, K. T. (2007). The importance of conscientiousness in adolescent interpersonal relationships. *Personality and Social Psychology Bulletin, 33*, 368–383.

Jensen-Campbell, L. A., Rosselli, M., Workman, K. A., Santisi, M., Rios, J. D., & Bojan, D. (2002). Agreeableness, conscientiousness, and effortful control processes. *Journal of Research in Personality, 36*, 476–489.

John, O. P., & Srivastava, S. (1999). The Big Five trait taxonomy: History, measurement, and theoretical perspectives. In L. A. Pervin &

O. P. John (Eds.), *Handbook of personality: Theory and research* (2nd ed., pp. 102–138). New York: Guilford Press.

Kassner, M. (2011). *Personality moderators of the door-in-the-face compliance technique.* Unpublished master's thesis, Purdue University, West Lafayette, IN.

Kelley, H. H., Holmes, J. G., Kerr, N. L., Reis, H. T., Rusbult, C. E., & Van Lange, P. A. M. (2003). *An atlas of interpersonal situations.* New York: Cambridge University Press.

Kochanska, G., & Knaack, A. (2003). Effortful control as a personality characteristic of young children: Antecedents, correlates, and consequences. *Journal of Personality, 71*, 1087–1112.

Kochanska, G., Murray, K., & Coy, K. C. (1997). Inhibitory control as a contributor to conscience in childhood: From toddler to early school age. *Child Development, 68*, 263–277.

Krueger, R. F., Hicks, B. N., & McGue, M. (2001). Altruism and antisocial behavior: Independent tendencies, unique personality correlates, distinct etiologies. *Psychological Science, 12*, 397–402.

Larson, K. S., Reed, M., & Hoffman, S. (1980). Attitudes of heterosexuals toward homosexuals: A Likert-type scale and construct validity. *Journal of Sex Research, 16*, 245–257.

Laursen, B., Pulkkinen, L., & Adams, R. (2002). The antecedents and correlates of agreeableness in adulthood. *Developmental Psychology, 38*, 591–603.

Martin, L. L. (1986). Set/reset: Use and disuse of concepts in impression formation. *Journal of Personality and Social Psychology, 51*, 493–504.

Meehl, P. E. (1997). The problem is epistemology, not statistics: Replace significance tests by confidence intervals and quantify accuracy of risky numerical predictions. In L. L. Harlow, S. A. Muliak, & J. H. Steiger (Eds.), *What if there were no significance tests?* (pp. 393–426). Mahwah, NJ: Erlbaum.

Moskowitz, D. S., Ho, M. R., & Turcotte-Tremblay, A. (2007). Contextual influences on interpersonal complementarity. *Personality and Social Psychology Bulletin, 33*, 1051–1063.

Ode, S., & Robinson, M. D. (2008). Can agreeableness turn gray skies blue?: A role for agreeableness in moderating neuroticism-linked depression. *Journal of Social and Clinical Psychology, 28*, 436–462.

Ode, S., Robinson, M. D., & Wilkowski, B. M. (2008). Can one's temper be cooled?: A role for agreeableness in moderating neuroticism's influence on anger and aggression. *Journal of Research in Personality, 42*, 295–311.

Parks, C. D. (2011). Personality influences on group processes: The past, present, and future. In M. Snyder & K. Deaux (Eds.), *Handbook of social and personality psychology* (pp. 517–544). New York: Oxford University Press.

Penner, L. A., Fritzsche, B. A., Craiger, J. P., & Freifeld, T. S. (1995). Measuring the prosocial personality. In J. N. Butcher & C. D. Spielberger (Eds.), *Advances in personality assessment* (Vol. 10, pp. 147–163). Hillsdale, NJ: Erlbaum.

Petty, R. E., Brinol, P., Tormala, Z. L., & Wegener, D. T. (2007). The role of metacognition in social judgment. In A. W. Kruglanski & E. T. Higgins (Eds.), *Social psychology: Handbook of basic principles* (2nd ed., pp. 254–284). New York: Cambridge University Press.

Petty, R. E., & Wegener, D. T. (1999). The elaboration likelihood model: Current status and controversies. In S. Chaiken & Y. Trope (Eds.), *Dual-process theories in social psychology* (pp. 41–72). New York: Guilford Press.

Piliavin, J. A., Callero, P. L., & Evanset, D. E. (1982). Addiction to altruism?: Opponent-process theory and habitual blood donation. *Journal of Personality and Social Psychology, 43*, 1200–1213.

Porges, S. W. (1995). Orienting in a defensive world: Mammalian modifications of our evolutionary heritage. A polyvagal theory. *Psychophysiology, 49*, 12–21.

Porges, S. W., & Carter, C. S. (2012). Mechanisms, mediators, and adaptive consequences of caregiving. In S. L. Brown, R. M. Brown, & L. A. Penner (Eds.), *Moving beyond self-interest: Perspectives from evolutionary biology, neuroscience, and social science* (pp. 53–74). New York: Oxford University Press.

Pryor, J. B., Reeder, G. D., Yeadon, C., & Hesson-Mclnnis, M. (2004). A dual-process model of reactions to perceived stigma. *Journal of Personality and Social Psychology, 87*, 436–452.

Pursell, G. R., Laursen, B., Rubin, K. H., Booth-LaForce, C., & Rose-Krasnor, L. (2008). Gender differences in patterns of association between prosocial behavior, personality, and externalizing behavior. *Journal of Research in Personality, 42*, 472–481.

Rentfrow, P. J., Goldberg, L. R., & Levitin, D. J. (2011). The structure of musical preferences: A five-factor model. *Journal of Personality and Social Psychology, 100*, 1139–1157.

Ricord, E. (1840). *Elements of the philosophy of mind applied to the development of thoughts and feelings.* New York: John N. Bogert.

Rockliff, H., Karl, A., McEwan, K., Gilbert, J., Matos, M., & Gilbert, P. (2011). Effects of intranasal oxytocin on "compassion-focused imagery." *Emotion, 11*, 1388–1396.

Rothbart, M. K., & Bates, J. E. (2006). Temperament. In N. Eisenberg, W. Damon, & R. M. Lerner (Eds.), *Handbook of child psychology: Vol. 3. Social, emotional, and personality development* (6th ed., pp. 99–166). Hoboken, NJ: Wiley.

Rothbart, M. K., & Posner, M. I. (1985). Temperament and the development of self-regulation. In L. C. Hartlage & C. F. Telzrow (Eds.), *The neuropsychology of individual differences: A developmental perspective* (pp. 93–123). New York: Plenum Press.

Rueda, M. R., Posner, M. I., & Rothbart, M. K. (2005). The development of executive attention: Contributions to the emergence of self-regulation. *Developmental Neuropsychology, 28*, 573–594.

Saarni, C. (1984). An observational study of children's attempts to monitor their expressive behavior. *Child Development, 55*, 1504–1513.

Salmon, W. C. (1984). *Scientific explanation and the causal structure of the world.* Princeton, NJ: Princeton University Press.

Savani, K., Morris, M. W., Naidu, N. V. R., Kumar, S., & Berlia, N. V. (2011). Cultural conditioning: Understanding interpersonal accommodation in India and the United States in terms of modal characteristics of interpersonal influence situations. *Journal of Personality and Social Psychology, 100*, 84–104.

Sherman, J. W., Gawronski, B., Gonsalkorale, K., Hugenberg, K., Allen, T. J., & Groom, C. J. (2008). The self-regulation of automatic associations and behavioral impulses. *Psychological Review, 115*, 314–335.

Shiner, R. L., Masten, A. S., & Roberts, J. M. (2003). Childhood personality foreshadows adult personality and life outcomes two decades later. *Journal of Personality, 71,* 1145–1170.

Smits, D. J. M., & Boeck, P. D. (2006). From BIS/BAS to the Big Five. *European Journal of Personality, 20,* 255–270.

Solomon, R. L. (1980). The opponent-process theory of acquired motivation: The costs of pleasure and the benefits of pain. *American Psychologist, 35,* 691–712.

Solomon, R. L., & Corbit, J. D. (1974). An opponent-process theory of motivation: I. Temporal dynamics of affect. *Psychological Review, 57,* 119–145.

Tobin, R. M., & Graziano, W. G. (2011). The disappointing gift: Dispositional and situational moderators of emotional expressions. *Journal of Experimental Child Psychology, 110,* 227–240.

Tobin, R. M., Graziano, W. G., Vanman, E. J., & Tassinary, L. G. (2000). Personality, emotional experience, and efforts to control emotions. *Journal of Personality and Social Psychology, 79,* 656–669.

Toi, M., & Batson, C. D. (1982). More evidence that empathy is a source of altruistic motivation. *Journal of Personality and Social Psychology, 43,* 281–292.

Trivers, R. (1972). Parental investment and sexual selection. In B. Campbell (Ed.), *Sexual selections and the descent of man: 1871–1971* (pp. 136–179). Chicago: Aldine.

Viviani, D., & Stoop, R. (2008). Opposite effects of oxytocin and vasopressin on the emotional expression of the fear response. *Progress in Brain Research, 170,* 207–218.

Wegener, D. T., & Petty, R. E. (1997). The flexible correction model: The role of naïve theories of bias in bias correction. In M. Zanna (Ed.), *Advances in experimental social psychology* (Vol. 29, pp. 141–208). Mahwah, NJ: Erlbaum.

CHAPTER 20

Emotional Intelligence

Reconceptualizing the Cognition–Emotion Link

*Marc A. Brackett, Michelle Bertoli, Nicole Elbertson, Elise Bausseron,
Ruth Castillo, and Peter Salovey*

Historically, cognition and emotion were viewed as oppositional processes (Lloyd, 1979), an idea infused into the Western worldview by the stoics of Ancient Greece (Lyons, 1999). As recently as the middle of the 20th century, scholars warned that emotions were mentally destabilizing forces (Young, 1943) that prevented logical reasoning (Lefford, 1946). Formalizing the ways in which emotion and thought could work in concert was no small feat—it required overcoming centuries of collective wariness toward "the passions."

Beginning in the late 1970s, a conceptualization of emotion and cognition as interactive forces began to take shape. Increasing frustration with the inability of IQ to explain differences among individuals led to the development of "elasticized" theories of intelligence, including Gardner's multiple intelligence theory (1983/1993) and Sternberg's triarchic theory of intelligence (1985). At the same time, investigators began to examine the impact of moods and emotions on thought processes. Isen, Shalker, Clark, and Karp (1978), for instance, proposed the existence of a "cognitive loop" between mood and judgment. Bower (1981) demonstrated that positive and negative feelings could activate positive and negative memories. It was in this context that the concept of emotional intelligence (EI) emerged.

EI was first introduced to the scientific literature in 1990 by psychologists Salovey and Mayer. They defined EI as "the ability to monitor one's own and others' feelings and emotions, to discriminate among them and to use this information to guide one's thinking and actions" (p. 189). They proposed that emotions facilitate cognitive processes and demonstrated empirically how aspects of EI might be measured as a mental ability.

In the wake of Salovey and Mayer's initial conceptualization of EI, myriad interpretations of the construct were proposed in both academic and popular literatures. The year 1995 saw the popularization of EI with the international success of Goleman's book, *Emotional Intelligence: Why It Can Matter More Than IQ*. His book quickly captured the interest of the media and the general public and resonated powerfully in education and management circles (Mayer, Salovey, & Caruso, 2000). Goleman's (1995, 1998) discourse, often criticized for embracing claims not rooted in research (e.g., Lindebaum, 2009), extended EI well beyond its initial definition. Goleman described EI as an array of traits and dispositions such as self-confidence, optimism, adaptability, and achievement motivation that could account for significant aspects of work performance and success in life.

Today the field of EI is replete with varying definitions, claims, and measurement tools. Many scholars lament that conflicting interpretations have engendered confusion and controversy with regard to what exactly EI is and is not, and what it can and cannot predict (e.g., Daus & Ashkanasy, 2003; Mayer, Salovey, & Caruso, 2008; Zeidner, Roberts, & Matthews, 2004). In this chapter we briefly outline the definitional and measurement issues that have arisen around different conceptions of EI, and then explore the applications of EI, in theory and in practice, in workplace and educational settings.

Models and Measurement of EI

Four primary models of EI exist today (Cherniss, 2010): the Mayer–Salovey ability or four-branch model (Mayer & Salovey, 1997; Salovey & Mayer, 1990), the Bar-On model of emotional–social intelligence (Bar-On, 2006), the Boyatzis–Goleman model (Boyatzis & Sala, 2004), and the trait EI model (Petrides & Furnham, 2003). These models are categorized into two scientific approaches: ability models and mixed models (Mayer, Caruso, & Salovey, 2000). Proponents of ability models have traditionally supported the use of performance measures to assess EI, whereas advocates of mixed models have preferred self-report or multirater assessment methods. The models and their associated approaches to measurement are described briefly below. (For a more thorough discussion of EI models and measures, including psychometrics, please see Mayer, Roberts, & Barsade, 2008.)

The Four-Branch Ability Model and Performance Assessments

Mayer and Salovey's model of EI conceives of the construct as a set of four mental abilities, also referred to as branches: (1) perception of emotion, (2) use of emotion to facilitate thought, (3) understanding of emotion, and (4) management of emotion. These four abilities are arranged hierarchically, with perception of emotion at the base of the model and management of emotion at the top. Here, we give an overview of the four abilities.

Perception of Emotion

This branch of EI refers to the accuracy with which individuals can identify emotions in themselves and others through facial expressions, tone of voice, and body language, as well as in abstract objects, such as works of art. Those skilled in the perception of emotion are able to express emotion appropriately and to articulate emotional needs adaptively. They also are able to determine the authenticity of the emotions expressed by others. Perception of emotion is the foundational skill of the four-branch model of EI.

Use of Emotion to Facilitate Thinking

The ability to use emotion to enhance cognitive activities and to guide attention to salient environmental cues falls under the second branch. People who are skilled in using emotions to facilitate thought understand that certain emotions are relevant to specific tasks or goals. Thus, they may generate moods to support certain types of thinking or to communicate more effectively with others.

Understanding of Emotion

The third branch of EI involves correctly labeling emotions experienced by oneself and others, and understanding how emotions differ from one another. Understanding emotion also involves an awareness of the causes and trajectories of different emotions (e.g., sadness results from a loss; unattended irritation may escalate into anger and then fury). People who are skilled in understanding emotion also are aware of how multiple emotions can "blend" to produce another; for instance, anger and disgust combine to form contempt. Research has shown that being able to label discrete negative emotions correctly can lead to the selection of effective emotion management strategies (Feldman Barrett, Gross, Christensen, & Benvenuto, 2001).

Management of Emotion

The fourth branch of EI describes more complex emotional processes. Individuals skilled in emotion management are able to remain open to both pleasant and unpleasant emotions. They also are able to recognize the value of feeling certain emotions in specific situations, and to understand which short- and long-term strategies work best for enhancing or reducing particular emotions (see Gross, 1998). Emotion regulation efforts benefit from developed skills on the other three branches of EI.

The authors of the ability model have illustrated that EI meets the criteria for a standard intelligence in that it can be operationalized as a set of abilities that (1) are intercorrelated, (2) relate to other extant intelligences, and (3) develop with age and experience (Mayer, Caruso, & Salovey, 1999; Mayer, Salovey, Caruso, & Sitarenios, 2003). As such, the authors assert that EI is a construct best measured by performance assessments requiring respondents to solve emotion-related problems that have correct answers, such as the Mayer–Salovey–Caruso Emotional Intelligence Test (MSCEIT; Mayer, Salovey, & Caruso, 2002). The MSCEIT is a 141-item test comprised of a total of eight tasks. Each of the four emotion abilities is measured with two tasks. Unlike self-report measures of EI, the MSCEIT does not ask respondents to rate their emotion skills; rather, the test asks them to *demonstrate* these skills. For example, emotion management is assessed by the test taker's ability to identify the effectiveness of various emotion management strategies to achieve a specified intrapersonal goal in a given situation (e.g., reducing an unpleasant emotion). Respondents read a short, emotionally charged vignette and then evaluate the effectiveness of four different courses of action to cope with emotions in the story. A comprehensive review of the MSCEIT and other performance assessment tools is available elsewhere (see Rivers, Brackett, Salovey, & Mayer, 2007).

Mixed and Trait Models and Self-Report Assessments

Mixed models of EI are so called because they define EI broadly as a combination of mental abilities and traditional personality traits and dispositions such as optimism, motivation, and stress tolerance (see Cherniss, 2010, for a review). The two

mixed models that have garnered the most attention are the Boyatzis–Goleman model (Boyatzis & Sala, 2004) and the Bar-On model of emotional–social intelligence (Bar-On, 2006). The Boyatzis–Goleman model divides EI competencies into four groups that the authors assert are particularly important for success in the workplace: self-awareness, self-management, social awareness, and relationship management. The Bar-On model proposes five main components of EI: intrapersonal skills, interpersonal skills, adaptability, stress management, and mood.

The trait EI model (Petrides & Furnham, 2003) is another proposed alternative to the Mayer–Salovey ability model. This model offers a framework that encompasses all of the personality traits that share intimate connections with affect (Mikolajczak, Luminet, Leroy, & Roy, 2007). For instance, individuals who are considered to be cheerful, confident, reflective, and driven, among other things, would ostensibly score highly on trait EI. The developers of this model argue that emotions are subjective, and so models of EI should be broad enough to capture accurately the essence of this subjectivity. Not surprisingly, highly significant correlations have been reported between trait EI and other personality traits, but only modest ones, often nonsignificant, between trait EI and ability measures of EI (Petrides, Furnham, & Mavroveli, 2007).

The measurement methods associated with mixed and trait models are mainly self-report assessments. Others are multi-rater scales (e.g., the Emotional Competence Inventory [ECI]; Sala, 2002) that combine various external observers' (e.g., work associates, family members) assessments of an individual's EI into one overall score. Self-report measures have some advantages. For instance, they are relatively quick, easy, and inexpensive to administer. However, they are problematic in that they are vulnerable to social desirability biases and faking (Day & Carroll, 2008) as well as to respondents' inaccurate judgments of their own abilities (e.g., Paulhus, Lysy, & Yik, 1998). Self-report measures of EI also have been found to lack discriminant validity from existing personality measures (Brackett & Mayer, 2003; Brackett, Rivers, Shiffman, Lerner, & Salovey, 2006). Mayer and colleagues (2008) note that some of the scales associated with mixed models do have good reliability, standardization, and factorial validity, but only as measures of *other* constructs, not as measures of EI as a mental ability.

Which Model?

The authors of the Mayer–Salovey model have noted that the EI construct is threatened less by its critics than by those who apply the term haphazardly to a variety of other variables (Mayer, Salovey, & Caruso, 2008). Although the personality and dispositional attributes targeted by the mixed and trait models certainly are important, they should not be confused with EI, a discrete and measurable mental ability. EI, when conceptualized as an ability, elucidates the relationship between cognition and emotion in a meaningful way—one that accounts for variance in individual outcomes beyond what can be explained by cognitive intelligence or personality traits alone (e.g., O'Boyle, Humphrey, Pollack, Hawver, & Story, 2010).

By assessing EI as a construct distinct from personality traits, as the ability model does, we can better understand its unique impact on important outcomes and more easily target the skills that improve these outcomes. Because the ability model, with its associated performance measures, assesses an information-processing capacity that is distinct from other measures of personality, we assert that it is preferable to the mixed and trait models of EI. Furthermore, self-estimates of performance measures are found to correlate only weakly ($r = .19$) with actual performance (Brackett et al., 2006). For these reasons, the rest of this chapter focuses on ability EI and the ways in which it applies in professional and academic settings.

EI in Applied Settings

Since the popularization of EI in the mid-1990s, interest in the real-world applications and implications of the construct has flourished. Researchers have examined—and found positive links between—EI and a number of important outcomes for individuals across the lifespan, including work performance, mental and physical health, social relationships, and academic achievement.

The next sections of the chapter describe in greater detail how ability EI functions in both organizational and educational settings to improve adjustment, performance, and well-being.

EI in the Workplace: An Affective Revolution

Until recently, the organizational behavior literature has neglected to consider seriously the role of emotion in the workplace (e.g., Ashforth & Humphrey, 1995; George, 2000). Emotions traditionally have been perceived as too unpredictable and interfering to warrant reflection outside the personal sphere. It has been asserted, however, that an "affective revolution" is underway in organizational behavior research (Barsade, Brief, & Spataro, 2003). As such, it is proposed that emotions permeate all levels of an organization and critically influence strategic decision making, creativity, prosocial behavior, successful negotiation, productivity, efficiency, and task quality and performance (e.g., Ashton-James & Ashkanasy, 2008; Mayer, Roberts, & Barsade, 2008).

This shift in understanding about the influence of emotions in the workplace arose from findings highlighting the role affect plays in cognitive functioning, and the effect that this connection may have on many work-related outcomes (Forgas & George, 2001). Affective events theory (Weiss & Cropanzano, 1996) and the affect infusion model (Forgas, 1995; also see Forgas & Koch, Chapter 13, this volume) both shed light on the mechanisms by which affect influences cognition and performance in organizations. The affective events theory posits that events that occur at work trigger emotional responses in employees, which, in turn, impact employees' performance, job satisfaction, and attitudes (Weiss & Cropanzano, 1996). An empathic boss, for instance, may recognize accomplishments and facilitate access to resources, leading to feelings of empowerment and competence among employees and, in turn, increased performance and satisfaction. This event–response relationship is hypothesized to be moderated by individual employees' overall affective tendencies and personality traits.

Based on empirical evidence (e.g., Forgas & Moylan, 1991), the affect infusion model asserts that the influence of affect on information processing becomes increasingly determinative as tasks or decisions grow in complexity. According to this theory, managers who engage in strategy development that is risky, highly complex, and that demands an advanced level of information analysis (Ashton-James & Ashkanasy, 2008) will harness affective experiences to make decisions that require heuristic or substantive reasoning (Forgas, 1995). This model suggests that the ability to recognize and regulate affective experiences has a direct impact on tough decisions made at work. Taken together, these theories and their associated research emphasize that emotional experiences at work cannot be ignored; in fact, they can be leveraged to produce better results within the organization as a whole.

Numerous studies have been conducted on the relationship between EI and various workplace outcomes. Evidence related to three of these outcomes—job performance, occupational well-being, and leadership effectiveness—is presented here.

EI and Job Performance

A number of laboratory and field-based studies have examined the link between EI and job performance. In one study, EI was associated with important indicators of job performance, including company rank, percent merit increase, ratings of interpersonal facilitation, and affect and attitudes at work (Lopes, Grewal, Kadis, Gall, & Salovey, 2006). EI also has been found to correlate positively with performance in a variety of managerial simulations involving problem solving, determining employee layoffs, adjusting claims, and negotiating successfully (Day & Carroll, 2004; Feyerherm & Rice, 2002; Mueller & Curhan, 2006). Côté and Miners (2006) proposed and tested a "compensatory model" of ability EI, cognitive intelligence, and performance at work, wherein they hypothesized that, as cognitive intelligence decreased, the association between EI and job performance would become more positive. Their results supported this hypothesis: Employees with lower cognitive intelligence performed tasks correctly (as assessed by managers) when they had higher EI. Most of these studies controlled for personality and general intelligence.

Emotion regulation ability appears to be another key to understanding how EI impacts job performance (O'Boyle et al., 2010). Of course, successfully regulating emotion depends, in great measure, on one's ability to accurately perceive and understand emotions in the self and others (see Joseph & Newman, 2010, for an explanation of "the cascading model of EI," which aligns with the conceptualization of EI skills as hierarchical). Although we cannot consider emotion regulation ability completely apart from other EI skills, it is arguably the skill that we most easily see affecting job performance.

Service-oriented jobs provide a particularly good illustration of the impact of emotion regulation ability on job performance. We tend to expect a specific emotional timbre from individuals in service positions, and the expected tone can vary depending on the service or good that is sought. For example, we generally would not be pleased with a funeral director who was too animated and enthusiastic, but would appreciate one who was sympathetic and reserved. Expressing the emotion deemed necessary for a successful service interaction is called *emotional labor* (Hochschild, 1979). It is not difficult to imagine that someone higher in EI would likely be better able both to understand the need for the particular affective display and to regulate the other, potentially conflicting, emotions felt in order to evoke—or at least produce the facial and bodily indications of—the target emotion. Indeed, recent meta-analyses (Joseph & Newman, 2010; O'Boyle et al., 2010) have found that ability EI has incremental validity over personality and cognitive ability for predicting success in jobs with high emotional labor demands.

Another potential explanation for EI's link to job performance has to do with the allocation of cognitive resources. According to neurological measures, individuals higher in EI exert less effort when solving emotional problems (Jausovec & Jausovec, 2005). Specifically, brain scans of individuals high in EI showed more synchronization and less desynchronization while identifying emotions in pictures than did individuals with average EI. According to the authors, this finding indicates that individuals higher in EI use superior emotion problem-solving strategies that require less cognitive energy. If less energy is expended solving problems related to emotion, more cognitive resources should be available to devote to the completion of tasks. However, this relationship is not simple. It has been argued that, in itself, the process of regulating emotions drains cognitive resources, making task performance more difficult (Joseph & Newman, 2010). For instance, suppression and rumination draw largely upon cognitive resources and impede the processing of incoming information. On the contrary, reappraisal and acceptance are helpful strategies that allow an individual to return attention more quickly to the task at hand (Gross, 1998; see Suri, Sheppes, & Gross, Chapter 11, and Watkins, Chapter 21, this volume, for further discussion of emotion regulation and repetitive thought). More emotionally intelligent individuals actually choose more effective emotion regulation strategies (Ciarrochi, Chan, & Caputi, 2000). Thus, it is reasonable to imagine that EI skills can improve job performance by contributing to the more strategic allocation of cognitive resources.

EI and Occupational Well-Being

Evidence indicates that EI impacts how individuals perform at work, but does it influence how they *feel* at work? Interest in occupational well-being has increased as the impacts of job-related stress have become better understood. Stress at work has been found to trigger many negative outcomes, including aggressive behaviors (Miguel-Tobal & Gonzales Ordi, 2005). This is true especially for emotionally vulnerable individuals who experience long-term, repeated exposure to workplace stressors (Fisher, 2000). EI, and particularly emotion regulation ability, have been argued to bolster resilience and to protect individuals against engaging in risky behaviors (Ciarrochi, Chan, & Bajgar, 2001; Rivers et al., in press) when pressures, work-related or otherwise, build. EI may not only mitigate the harmful effects of work-related stress, it also may facilitate the achievement of emotional well-being (Schutte, Malouff, Simunek, McKenley, & Hollander, 2002). According to EI theory, people with higher EI have a larger "inventory" of strategies for main-

taining desirable emotions and preventing or changing unwanted emotions in themselves and others (Gross & John, 2002; Mayer & Salovey, 1997). Indeed, MSCEIT scores correlate negatively with depression, anxiety, burnout, and stress, and positively with self-esteem and job and life satisfaction (Brackett et al., 2006; Ciarrochi et al., 2000).

EI and Leadership Effectiveness

Employees can benefit not only from their own exercise of emotion regulation strategies, but also from the practices of leaders with high EI who nurture emotional well-being in the workplace (Humphrey, 2002). Many experts in the field of organizational behavior are gravitating toward a conception of leadership as a process of social interactions whereby leaders motivate, influence, guide, and empower followers to achieve organizational goals (e.g., Bass & Riggio, 2006). Transformational leadership (Bass, 1985), a leading articulation of this management style, is characterized by creating a vision and then inspiring others to work toward it. This leadership style is understood in some measure of contrast to transactional leadership, in which leaders offer something followers want in exchange for the successful completion of tasks (Kuhnert & Lewis, 1987).

The use of transformational methods has been shown to predict business-unit performance positively and significantly (Howell & Avolio, 1993). What is more, EI appears to facilitate transformational leadership. In a sample of 24 managers, EI (as measured by the MSCEIT) correlated positively with the *idealized influence* and *individual consideration* dimensions of transformational leadership (Leban & Zulauf, 2004). A study of 177 managers from a U.S.-based global corporation found that the facial recognition scores in the Diagnostic Analysis of Nonverbal Accuracy Scale (Nowicki & Duke, 1994), which are similar to the *perception of emotion* branch of the MSCEIT, correlated with transformational leadership as rated by 480 subordinates (Rubin, Munz, & Bommer, 2005).

Additional research—including a meta-analysis of 48 studies (Mills, 2009)—has supported a positive link between EI and effective leadership. Managers' EI scores have been found to correlate positively with supervisees' ratings of overall managerial performance (Kerr, Garvin, Heaton, & Boyle, 2006) and with subordinates', peers', and direct supervisors' assessments of managers' successful achievement of business goals and effective interpersonal behaviors (Rosete, 2007). Among 41 Australian executives, scores on the *perception of emotion* and *use of emotion* branches of the MSCEIT correlated with their ability to cultivate productive relationships with others and to display greater personal drive and integrity (Rosete & Ciarrochi, 2005). The associations in the above three studies range from *r* = .26 to .52. With the exception of the study by Kerr and colleagues (2006), the correlations reported remained statistically significant after controlling for cognitive ability and personality. Additional research found that EI predicted leadership emergence in groups after controlling for cognitive ability, personality, and gender (Côté, Lopes, Salovey, & Miners, 2010).

Enhancing EI in the Workplace

It is clear that EI has utility for effecting positive outcomes at work, but how can organizations enhance the EI of their members? Like "traditional" intelligence, EI is not necessarily malleable enough that reading one or two books or attending a workshop on the topic can promise to change an individual's competencies dramatically. However, in that EI is a set of four abilities that include targetable skills (e.g., the ability to perceive emotion can be enhanced by building an emotions vocabulary to increase expressive capacities), it is probable that an individual's emotion knowledge base can be expanded and that useful approaches to dealing with emotions at work can be taught and successfully learned.

The EI Skills Group—headed by one of the three authors of the MSCEIT (Caruso)—has led efforts to bring training on the ability model of EI to organizations across the globe. These trainings target everyone from entry-level employees to top decision makers and consist of assessing EI with the MSCEIT, illustrating how EI skills function in the workplace, and teaching specific methods for developing and then applying EI skills. At this time, there is little empirical evidence

of the effectiveness of workplace EI interventions based on the ability model. As such, this is an area that would benefit greatly from future research. In the meantime, evidence that emotional skills can be learned has been accumulating in educational settings (Durlak, Weissberg, Dymnicki, Taylor, & Schellinger, 2011), to which we now turn our attention.

Emotions and EI in Educational Settings

Similar to traditional views of emotions in the workplace, historically, emotions were thought to have no place in the classroom (Sutton & Wheatley, 2003). Still today, many educators see the expression of emotion as juvenile, unprofessional, or uncivilized, and the suppression of emotion as mature, professional, and sophisticated (Ashforth & Humphrey, 1995). Yet, neuroscientific evidence demonstrates that affective and cognitive processes are integrated (Dolan, 2002). Emotions focus attention (Compton, 2003); drive decision making (Damasio, 1994); and impact perception, motivation, critical thinking, and behavior (Lazarus, 1991; Mayer & Salovey, 1997). These relationships between affect and cognition have important implications for the significance of EI in the classroom.

Teaching is considered one of the most emotionally demanding professions (Hargreaves, 2000). Throughout the day, as they plan lessons, instruct, grade student work, and attend meetings with parents and staff, teachers experience a range of pleasant and unpleasant emotions (Sutton & Wheatley, 2003). Teachers report feeling enthusiasm, pride, and satisfaction when witnessing student success or receiving support from parents, administrators, and other teachers (Emmer, 1994). They report feeling angry or frustrated with misbehaving or failing students (Reyna & Weiner, 2001), uncooperative colleagues and administrators (Bullough, Knowles, & Crow, 1991), irresponsible or uncaring parents (Lasky, 2000), and themselves when they feel unable to achieve their goals (Liljestrom, Roulston, & deMarrais, 2007). They experience guilt when feeling ineffective in their teaching roles (Hargreaves & Tucker, 1991), anxiety from the uncertainties and complexities of teaching (Sutton & Wheatley, 2003), and disillusionment with the teaching field (Huberman, 1993).

If not managed well, the negative emotions teachers experience can contaminate the classroom dynamic and hinder student learning (Travers, 2001). The abilities to perceive, use, understand, and regulate emotions are integral to effective teaching (Hargreaves, 2001). In fact, emotion regulation ability among teachers has been associated with positive affect, principal support, job satisfaction, and feelings of personal accomplishment (Brackett, Palomera, Mojsa-Kaja, Reyes, & Salovey, 2010). Teachers with higher EI can create a more supportive, stable, and productive classroom environment—one that encourages learning and achievement among students.

In addition to teacher EI, student EI can impact the learning environment in various ways. Children with higher EI skills tend to experience higher academic achievement than children with lower EI skills (Eisenberg, Fabes, Guthrie, & Reiser, 2000; Gil-Olarte Marquez, Palomera Martin, & Brackett, 2006). The ability to regulate emotions can help students focus in class, adapt to the school environment, and deal with academic anxiety (Lopes & Salovey, 2004; Mestre, Guil, Lopes, Salovey, & Gil-Olarte, 2006). Students with higher EI also tend to behave less aggressively and more prosocially at school, and they tend to be more secure and popular (Denham et al., 2003; Nellum-Williams, 1997; Rubin, 1999). Lower EI has been linked to poor physical and psychological health (Southam-Gerow & Kendall, 2000), alcohol and tobacco use (Trinidad & Johnson, 2002), anxiety and depression (e.g., Rottenberg, Kasch, Gross, & Gotlib, 2002), impulsive and aggressive behavior (Brackett, Mayer, & Warner, 2004; Winters, Clift, & Dutton, 2004), and suicidal ideation and attempts (Cha & Nock, 2009). In contrast, students who can recognize emotions accurately interact more positively with others (Izard et al., 2001). Additionally, children skilled in communicating their emotions tend to adhere well to societal rules and cultural norms for expressing how they feel (Saarni, 1999). When students have the ability to develop quality relationships with their teachers and peers, they feel more comfortable at school, receive more support, and form healthier attachments to school (Agos-

tin & Bain, 1997; O'Neil, Welsh, Parke, Wang, & Strand, 1997).

Though copious research lends support for the role of EI in educational settings, until recently, there has been no systematic approach to developing these crucial life skills in teachers or students. Providing training in EI to both educators and students is one way to assure that student learning and achievement are optimized (Salovey & Sluyter, 1997; Zins, Weissberg, Wang, & Walberg, 2004).

The RULER Approach: A School-Based Intervention for Enhancing EI

Although the traditional emphasis in schools has been on academic instruction, the last few decades have seen growing efforts toward a more holistic approach that incorporates the social and emotional aspects of learning. In the early 1990s, the field of social and emotional learning was introduced as a framework for providing opportunities for young people to acquire the skills necessary for attaining and maintaining personal well-being and positive relationships across the lifespan (see Elbertson, Brackett, & Weissberg, 2010). Working within this framework, a school-based program grounded in the ability model of EI was developed. This program, The RULER Approach ("RULER"), is based on decades of research evidencing that the knowledge and skills associated with recognizing, understanding, labeling, expressing, and regulating emotion (i.e., the RULER skills) are essential to teaching, learning, and positive development in both students and adults (Brackett et al., 2009; Rivers & Brackett, 2011).

RULER focuses on the development of these EI skills in both the adult stakeholders in students' education (i.e., teachers, parents, administrators, and other school staff) as well as the students themselves. First, adults are educated on the role of emotion skills in enhancing their relationships at school and the educational, social, and personal lives of their students. Adults develop their own EI and learn how to foster an emotionally supportive learning environment though the use of program tools, including collaborative mission statements for learning environments and visual aids such as the "Mood

Meter" for enhancing self-awareness and emotion regulation (Brackett, Elbertson, Alster, Kremenitzer, & Caruso, 2011). Then, classroom teachers are trained on the Feeling Words Curriculum for students, a vocabulary-based program aimed at helping children from kindergarten through eighth grade acquire EI. This curriculum helps children develop a sophisticated understanding of terms such as *alienation, commitment, elation*, and *empathy* (see Brackett et al., 2011, for a review of the lesson plans). These feeling words are the vehicle by which children learn to identify, evaluate, and understand their own and others' feelings and behavior, and to develop strategies for managing the emotions they experience in their daily lives.

RULER improves both academic outcomes and the social and emotional climate of classrooms. In a recent clustered, randomized control trial in 62 schools, classrooms that implemented RULER, as compared to standard-of-care classrooms, were rated as more emotionally supportive using an objective measurement tool, the Classroom Assessment Scoring System (CLASS; Pianta, La Paro, & Hamre, 2008). Specifically, RULER classrooms were rated by trained, naïve coders as having (1) higher degrees of warmth and connectedness between teachers and students, (2) teachers who focused more on students' interests, and (3) more autonomy and leadership among students. Classrooms using RULER also had more positive learning climates, including more respectful interactions, more prosocial behavior, greater enthusiasm about learning, and fewer occurrences of bullying. Teachers in classrooms using RULER, as compared to control classrooms, also expressed anger and frustration less frequently and were more supportive of students (Reyes, Brackett, Rivers, White, & Salovey, 2012). In a separate study, students in classrooms integrating RULER had higher year-end grades and higher teacher ratings of social and emotional competence (e.g., leadership, social skills, and study skills) compared to students in the comparison classrooms (Brackett, Rivers, Reyes, & Salovey, 2012). Moreover, teachers who implemented RULER with greater quality had students with higher scores on indices of social competencies and EI, as measured by the MSCEIT (Reyes, Brackett, Rivers, Elb-

ertson, & Salovey, 2012). Finally, a recent study showed that after just 1 year, students in RULER classrooms showed greater growth in MSCEIT scores than students in comparison classrooms (Reyes, Brackett, & Rivers, 2011). Together, these findings suggest that RULER enhances students' social and emotional skills as well as classrooms in ways that can promote positive student and teacher development.

Limitations and Future Directions in EI Research

Much remains to be investigated about EI. Most important are necessary developments in the measurement of EI, high-quality theorizing on its development, and further research on the outcomes associated with the construct (Mayer, Salovey, & Caruso, 2008). In regard to measurement, the MSCEIT, which was the first omnibus, performance test of EI, has a number of limitations (see Rivers, Brackett, & Salovey, 2008). For example, the factor structure of the test has not been replicated across studies (Palmer, Gignac, Manocha, & Stough, 2005). The MSCEIT also does not allow for the assessment of several abilities, especially the higher-order skills specified in the Mayer and Salovey (1997) model, including the expression of emotion in the voice and body (e.g., posture) and the ability to monitor and reflect on one's own emotions. Designing measures of these and other, more fluid abilities will require innovative methods. Possibilities include lab-based experiments examining people's real-time behavior after various mood inductions and interactions that mimic real-life encounters in virtual environments, among many others.

On the topic of enhancing EI theory and studies on its outcomes, greater attention should be paid to developmental trajectories, gender and cultural differences, and how EI operates and can be nurtured in workplace and educational settings. Some specific, unanswered research questions include: Do certain EI abilities, such as the language of emotion, influence the development of other EI abilities, such as the perception and management of emotion? Are growth trajectories in EI, across each branch, the same for both males and females? Are interventions universally applicable to both genders? These and many other important questions present exciting opportunities to expand EI research.

Conclusion

The recent decades have unearthed the dynamic and complex relationship between emotion and cognition, bringing to light the importance of EI in harnessing the power of emotion to optimize cognition. Although much about EI is yet to unfold, the research conducted thus far supports a model of EI that defines the construct as a mental ability that is separable from both personality and general intelligence and that is assessed best by performance measures that predict well-being and other significant outcomes in both workplace and educational settings. Findings so far indicate that attention to emotion-related aspects of working and learning environments, and a focus on bolstering the EI skills of individuals within these contexts, can contribute to more productive, supportive, and healthy professional and academic experiences.

References

Agostin, R. M., & Bain, S. K. (1997). Predicting early school success with development and social skills screeners. *Psychology in the Schools, 34,* 219–228.

Ashforth, B. E., & Humphrey, R. H. (1995). Emotion in the workplace: A reappraisal. *Human Relations, 48,* 97–125.

Ashton-James, C. E., & Ashkanasy, N. M. (2008). Affective events theory: A strategic perspective. In W. J. Zerbe, C. E. J. Hartel, & N. M. Ashkanasy (Eds.), *Research on emotion in organizations: Vol. 4. Emotion, ethics, and decision-making* (pp. 1–34). Bingley, UK: Emerald Group/JAI Press.

Bar-On, R. (2006). The Bar-On model of emotional–social intelligence (ESI). *Psicothema, 18*(Suppl.), 13–25.

Barsade, S. G., Brief, A. P., & Spataro, S. E. (2003). The affective revolution in organizational behavior: The emergence of a paradigm. In J. Greenberg (Ed.), *Organizational behavior: The state of the science* (2nd ed., pp. 3–51). Mahwah, NJ: Erlbaum.

Bass, B. M. (1985). *Leadership and performance beyond expectations.* New York: Free Press.

Bass, B. M., & Riggio, R. E. (2006). *Transformational leadership* (2nd ed.). Mahwah, NJ: Erlbaum.

Bower, G. H. (1981). Mood and memory. *American Psychologist, 36,* 129–148.

Boyatzis, R., & Sala, F. (2004). The Emotional Competency Inventory (ECI). In G. Geher (Ed.), *Measuring emotional intelligence: Common ground and controversy* (pp. 143–178). Hauppauge, NY: Nova Science.

Brackett, M. A., Elbertson, N., Alster, B., Kremenitzer, J. P., & Caruso, D. (2011). Emotionally literate teaching. In M. A. Brackett & J. P. Kremenitzer, with M. Maurer, M. Carpenter, S. E. Rivers, & N. Elbertson (Eds.), *Creating emotionally literate classrooms: An introduction to The RULER Approach to social and emotional learning* (pp. 49–68). Port Chester, NY: National Professional Resources.

Brackett, M. A., & Mayer, J. D. (2003). Convergent, discriminant, and incremental validity of competing measures of emotional intelligence. *Personality and Social Psychology Bulletin, 29,* 1147–1158.

Brackett, M. A., Mayer, J. D., & Warner, R. M. (2004). Emotional intelligence and its relation to everyday behaviour. *Personality and Individual Differences, 36,* 1387–1402.

Brackett, M. A., Palomera, R., Mojsa-Kaja, J., Reyes, M. R., & Salovey, P. (2010). Emotion-regulation ability, burnout, and job satisfaction among British secondary-school teachers. *Psychology in the Schools, 47,* 406–417.

Brackett, M. A., Patti, J., Stern, R., Rivers, S. E., Elbertson, N., Chisholm, C., et al. (2009). A sustainable, skill-based model to building emotionally literate schools. In R. Thompson, M. Hughes, & J. B. Terrell (Eds.), *Handbook of developing emotional and social intelligence: Best practices, case studies, and tools* (pp. 329–358). New York: Wiley.

Brackett, M. A., Rivers, S. E., Reyes, M. R., & Salovey, P. (2012). Enhancing academic performance and social and emotional competence with the RULER Feeling Words Curriculum. *Learning and Individual Differences, 22,* 218–224.

Brackett, M. A., Rivers, S. E., Shiffman, S., Lerner, N., & Salovey, P. (2006). Relating emotional abilities to social functioning: A comparison of self-report and performance measures of emotional intelligence. *Journal of Personality and Social Psychology, 91,* 780–795.

Bullough, R. V., Jr., Knowles, J. G., & Crow, N. A. (1991). *Emerging as a teacher*. London: Routledge.

Cha, C., & Nock, M. (2009). Emotional intelligence is a protective factor for suicidal behavior. *Journal of the American Academy of Child and Adolescent Psychiatry, 48*, 422–430.

Cherniss, C. (2010). Emotional intelligence: Toward clarification of a concept. *Industrial and Organizational Psychology, 3*, 110–126.

Ciarrochi, J., Chan, A. Y. C., & Bajgar, J. (2001). Measuring emotional intelligence in adolescents. *Personality and Individual Differences, 31*, 1105–1119.

Ciarrochi, J. V., Chan, A. Y. C., & Caputi, P. (2000). A critical evaluation of the emotional intelligence construct. *Personality and Individual Differences, 28*, 539–561.

Compton, R. (2003). The interface between emotion and attention: A review of evidence from psychology and neuroscience. *Behavioral and Cognitive Neuroscience Reviews, 2*, 115–129.

Côté, S., Lopes, P. N., Salovey, P., & Miners, C. T. H. (2010). Emotional intelligence and leadership emergence in small groups. *Leadership Quarterly, 21*, 496–508.

Côté, S., & Miners, C. T. H. (2006). Emotional intelligence, cognitive intelligence, and job performance. *Administrative Science Quarterly, 51*, 1–28.

Damasio, A. R. (1994). *Descartes' error: Emotion, reason, and the human brain*. New York: Grosset/Putnam.

Daus, C. S., & Ashkanasy, N. M. (2003). Will the real emotional intelligence please stand up?: On deconstructing the emotional intelligence "debate." *Industrial-Organizational Psychologist, 41*, 69–72.

Day, A. L., & Carroll, S. A. (2004). Using an ability-based measure of emotional intelligence to predict individual performance, group performance, and group citizenship behaviours. *Personality and Individual Differences, 36*, 1443–1458.

Day, A. L., & Carroll, S. A. (2008). Faking emotional intelligence (EI): Comparing response distortion on ability and trait-based EI measures. *Journal of Organizational Behavior, 29*, 761–784.

Denham, S. A., Blair, K. A., DeMulder, E., Levitas, J., Sawyer, K., Auerbach-Major, S., et al. (2003). Preschool emotional competence: Pathway to social competence. *Child Development, 74*, 238–256.

Dolan, R. J. (2002). Emotion, cognition, and behavior. *Science, 298*, 1191–1194.

Durlak, J. A., Weissberg, R. P., Dymnicki, A. B., Taylor, R. D., & Schellinger, K. B. (2011). The impact of enhancing students' social and emotional learning: A meta-analysis of school-based universal interventions. *Child Development, 82*, 405–432.

Eisenberg, N., Fabes, R. A., Guthrie, I. K., & Reiser, M. (2000). Dispositional emotionality and regulation: Their role in predicting quality of social functioning. *Journal of Personality and Social Psychology, 78*, 136–157.

Elbertson, N. A., Brackett, M. A., & Weissberg, R. P. (2010). School-based social and emotional learning (SEL) programming: Current perspectives. In A. Hargreaves, M. Fullan, D. Hopkins, & A. Lieberman (Eds.), *The second international handbook of educational change* (pp. 1017–1032). New York: Springer.

Emmer, E. T. (1994). Toward an understanding of the primary of classroom management and discipline. *Teaching Education, 6*, 65–69.

Feldman Barrett, L., Gross, J., Christensen, T. C., & Benvenuto, M. (2001). Knowing what you're feeling and knowing what to do about it: Mapping the relation between emotion differentiation and emotion regulation. *Cognition and Emotion, 15*, 713–724.

Feyerherm, A. E., & Rice, C. L. (2002). Emotional intelligence and team performance: The good, the bad and the ugly. *International Journal of Organizational Analysis, 10*, 343–362.

Fisher, C. D. (2000). Mood and emotions while working: Missing pieces of job satisfaction? *Journal of Organizational Behavior, 21*, 185–202.

Forgas, J. P. (1995). Mood and judgment: The affect infusion model (AIM). *Psychological Bulletin, 117*, 39–66.

Forgas, J. P., & George, J. M. (2001). Affective influences on judgments and behavior in organizations: An information processing perspective. *Organizational Behavior and Human Decision Processes, 86*, 3–34.

Forgas, J. P., & Moylan, S. J. (1991). Affective influences on stereotype judgements. *Cognition and Emotion, 5*, 379–395.

Gardner, H. (1993). *Frames of mind: The theory of multiple intelligences (10th Anniversary Edition)*. New York: Basic Books. (Original work published 1983)

George, J. M. (2000). Emotions and leadership: The role of emotional intelligence. *Human Relations, 53*, 1027–1055.

Gil-Olarte Marquez, P., Palomera Martin, R., & Brackett, M. A. (2006). Relating emotional intelligence to social competence and academic achievement in high school students. *Psicothema, 18,* 118–123.

Goleman, D. (1995). *Emotional intelligence.* New York: Bantam Books.

Goleman, D. (1998). *Working with emotional intelligence.* New York: Bantam Books.

Gross, J. J. (1998). The emerging field of emotion regulation: An integrative review. *Review of General Psychology, 2,* 271–299.

Gross, J. J., & John, O. P. (2002). Wise emotion regulation. In L. Feldman Barrett & P. Salovey (Eds.), *The wisdom in feeling: Psychological processes in emotional intelligence* (pp. 297–319). New York: Guilford Press.

Hargreaves, A. (2000). Mixed emotions: Teachers' perceptions of their interactions with students. *Teaching and Teacher Education, 16,* 811–826.

Hargreaves, A. (2001). The emotional geographies of teachers' relations with colleagues. *International Journal of Educational Research, 35,* 503–527.

Hargreaves, A., & Tucker, E. (1991). Teaching and guilt: Exploring the feelings of teaching. *Teaching and Teacher Education, 7,* 491–505.

Hochschild, A. R. (1979). Emotion work, feeling rules, and social structure. *American Journal of Sociology, 85,* 551–575.

Howell, J. M., & Avolio, B. J. (1993). Transformational leadership, transactional leadership, locus of control, and support for innovation: Key predictors of consolidated-business-unit performance. *Journal of Applied Psychology, 78,* 891–902.

Huberman, M. (1993). Steps toward a developmental model of the teaching career. In L. Kremer-Hayon, H. C. Vonk, & R. Fessler (Eds.), *Teacher professional development: A multiple perspective approach* (pp. 93–118). Amsterdam: Swets & Zeitlinger.

Humphrey, R. H. (2002). The many faces of emotional leadership. *Leadership Quarterly, 13,* 493–504.

Isen, A. M., Shalker, T. E., Clark, M., & Karp, L. (1978). Affect, accessibility of material in memory, and behavior: A cognitive loop? *Journal of Personality and Social Psychology, 36,* 1–12.

Izard, C. E., Fine, S., Schultz, D., Mostow, A., Ackerman, B., & Youngstrom, E. (2001). Emotion knowledge as a predictor of social behavior and academic competence in children at risk. *Psychological Science, 12,* 18–23.

Jausovec, N., & Jausovec, K. (2005). Differences in induced gamma and upper alpha oscillations in the human brain related to verbal/performance and emotional intelligence. *International Journal of Psychophysiology, 56,* 223–235.

Joseph, D. L., & Newman, D. A. (2010). Emotional intelligence: An integrative meta-analysis and cascading model. *Journal of Applied Psychology, 95,* 54–78.

Kerr, R., Garvin, J., Heaton, N., & Boyle, E. (2006). Emotional intelligence and leadership effectiveness. *Leadership Organization Development Journal, 27,* 265–279.

Kuhnert, K. W., & Lewis, P. (1987). Transactional and transformational leadership: A constructive developmental analysis. *Academy of Management Review, 12,* 648–657.

Lasky, S. (2000). The cultural and emotional politics of teacher–parent interactions. *Teaching and Teacher Education, 16,* 843–860.

Lazarus, R. S. (1991). *Emotion and adaptation.* New York: Oxford University Press.

Leban, W., & Zulauf, C. (2004). Linking emotional intelligence abilities and transformational leadership styles. *Leadership Organization Development Journal, 25,* 554–564.

Lefford, A. (1946). The influence of emotional subject matter on logical reasoning. *Journal of General Psychology, 34,* 127–151.

Liljestrom, A., Roulston, K., & deMarrais, K. (2007). "There is no place for feeling like this in the workplace": Women teachers' anger in school settings. In P. A. Schutz & R. Pekrun (Eds.), *Emotion in education* (pp. 275–292). San Diego, CA: Elsevier.

Lindebaum, D. (2009). Rhetoric or remedy?: A critique on developing emotional intelligence. *Academy of Management Learning Education, 8,* 225–237.

Lloyd, A. C. (1979). Emotion and decision in stoic psychology. In J. M. Rist (Ed.), *The stoics* (pp. 233–246). Los Angeles: University of California Press.

Lopes, P. N., Grewal, D., Kadis, J., Gall, M., & Salovey, P. (2006). Evidence that emotional intelligence is related to job performance and affect and attitudes at work. *Psicothema, 18*(Suppl.), 132–138.

Lopes, P. N., & Salovey, P. (2004). Toward a broader education: Social, emotional, and practical skills. In J. E. Zins, R. P. Weissberg,

M. C. Wang, & H. J. Walberg (Eds.), *Building academic success on social and emotional learning: What does the research say?* (pp. 76–93). New York: Teachers College Press.

Lyons, W. (1999). The philosophy of emotion and cognition. In T. Dalgleish & M. J. Power (Eds.), *Handbook of cognition and emotion* (pp. 21–44). Chichester, UK: Wiley.

Mayer, J. D., Caruso, D. R., & Salovey, P. (1999). Emotional intelligence meets traditional standards for an intelligence. *Intelligence, 27,* 267–298.

Mayer, J. D., Caruso, D. R., & Salovey, P. (2000). Selecting a measure of emotional intelligence: The case for ability scales. In R. Bar-On & J. D. A. Parker (Eds.), *The handbook of emotional intelligence: Theory, development, assessment, and application at home, school, and in the workplace* (pp. 320–342). San Francisco: Jossey-Bass.

Mayer, J. D., Roberts, R. D., & Barsade, S. G. (2008). Human abilities: Emotional intelligence. *Annual Review of Psychology, 59,* 507–536.

Mayer, J. D., & Salovey, P. (1997). What is emotional intelligence? In P. Salovey & D. J. Sluyter (Eds.), *Emotional development and emotional intelligence: Educational implications* (pp. 3–34). New York: Basic Books.

Mayer, J. D., Salovey, P., & Caruso, D. R. (2000). Emotional intelligence as zeitgeist, as personality, and as a mental ability. In R. Bar-On & J. D. A. Parker (Eds.), *The handbook of emotional intelligence: Theory, development, assessment, and application at home, school, and in the workplace* (pp. 92–117). San Francisco: Jossey-Bass.

Mayer, J. D., Salovey, P., & Caruso, D. R. (2002). *The Mayer–Salovey–Caruso Emotional Intelligence Test (MSCEIT), Version 2.0.* Toronto: Multi-Health Systems.

Mayer, J. D., Salovey, P., & Caruso, D. R. (2008). Emotional intelligence: New ability or eclectic traits? *American Psychologist, 63,* 503–517.

Mayer, J. D., Salovey, P., Caruso, D. R., & Sitarenios, G. (2003). Measuring emotional intelligence with the MSCEIT V2.0. *Emotion, 3,* 97–105.

Mestre, J. M., Guil, R., Lopes, P. N., Salovey, P., & Gil-Olarte, P. (2006). Emotional intelligence and social and academic adaptation to school. *Psicothema, 18*(Suppl.), 112–117.

Miguel-Tobal, J. J., & Gonzales Ordi, H. (2005).

The role of emotions in cardiovascular disorders. In A. S. G. Antoniou & C. L. Cooper (Eds.), *Research companion to organizational health psychology* (pp. 455–477). Cheltenham, UK: Edward Elgar.

Mikolajczak, M., Luminet, O., Leroy, C., & Roy, E. (2007). Psychometric properties of the Trait Emotional Intelligence Questionnaire: Factor structure, reliability, construct, and incremental validity in a French-speaking population. *Journal of Personality Assessment, 88,* 338–353.

Mills, L. B. (2009). A meta-analysis of the relationship between emotional intelligence and effective leadership. *Journal of Curriculum and Instruction, 3,* 22–38.

Mueller, J. S., & Curhan, J. R. (2006). Emotional intelligence and counterpart mood induction in a negotiation. *International Journal of Conflict Management, 17,* 110–128.

Nellum-Williams, R. (1997). Educator's commentary. In P. Salovey & D. J. Sluyter (Eds.), *Emotional development and emotional intelligence* (pp. 164–167). New York: Basic Books.

Nowicki, S., & Duke, M. P. (1994). Individual differences in the nonverbal communication of affect: The Diagnostic Analysis of Nonverbal Accuracy Scale. *Journal of Nonverbal Behavior, 18*(1), 9–35.

O'Boyle, E. H., Humphrey, R. H., Pollack, J. M., Hawver, T. H., & Story, P. A. (2010). The relation between emotional intelligence and job performance: A meta-analysis. *Journal of Organizational Behavior, 32,* 788–818.

O'Neil, R., Welsh, M., Parke, R. D., Wang, S., & Strand, C. (1997). A longitudinal assessment of the academic correlates of early peer acceptance and rejection. *Journal of Clinical Child Psychology, 26,* 290–303.

Palmer, B. R., Gignac, G., Manocha, R., & Stough, C. (2005). A psychometric evaluation of the Mayer–Salovey–Caruso Emotional Intelligence Test Version 2.0. *Intelligence, 33,* 285–305.

Paulhus, D. L., Lysy, D. C., & Yik, M. S. M. (1998). Self-report measures of intelligence: Are they useful as proxy IQ tests? *Journal of Personality, 66,* 525–554.

Petrides, K. V., & Furnham, A. (2003). Trait emotional intelligence: Behavioural validation in two studies of emotion recognition and reactivity to mood induction. *European Journal of Personality, 17,* 39–57.

Petrides, K. V., Furnham, A., & Mavroveli, S.

(2007). Trait emotional intelligence: Moving forward in the field of EI. In G. Matthews, M. Zeidner, & R. Roberts (Eds.), *Emotional intelligence: Knowns and unknowns* (pp. 151–166). Oxford, UK: Oxford University Press.

Pianta, R. C., La Paro, K., & Hamre, B. (2008). *Classroom assessment scoring system: K–3.* Baltimore, MD: Brookes.

Reyes, M. R., Brackett, M. A., & Rivers, S. E. (2011, April). *Longitudinal impact of the RULER approach on students' emotional literacy skills, social competence, and academic performance.* Paper presented at the annual meeting of the Society for Research in Child Development, Montreal, Canada.

Reyes, M. R., Brackett, M. A., Rivers, S. E., Elbertson, N., & Salovey, P. (2012). The interaction effects of program training, dosage, and implementation quality on targeted student outcomes for The RULER Approach to social and emotional learning. *School Psychology Review, 41,* 82–99.

Reyes, M. R., Brackett, M. A., Rivers, S. E., White, M., & Salovey, P. (2012). Classroom emotional climate, student engagement, and academic achievement. *Journal of Educational Psychology, 104,* 700–712.

Reyna, C., & Weiner, B. (2001). Justice and utility in the classroom: An attributional analysis of the goals of teachers' punishment and intervention strategies. *Journal of Educational Psychology, 93,* 309–319.

Rivers, S. E., & Brackett, M. A. (2011). Achieving standards in the English language arts (and more) using the RULER Approach to social and emotional learning. *Reading and Writing Quarterly, 27,* 75–100.

Rivers, S. E., Brackett, M. A., Omori, M., Sickler, C., Bertoli, M., & Salovey, P. (in press). Emotion skills as a protective factor for risky behaviors among college students. *Journal of College Student Development.*

Rivers, S. E., Brackett, M. A., & Salovey, P. (2008). Measuring emotional intelligence as a mental ability in adults and children. In G. Boyle, G. Matthews, & D. Saklofske (Eds.), *The Sage handbook of personality theory and assessment* (Vol. 2, pp. 440–460). Thousand Oaks, CA: Sage.

Rivers, S. E., Brackett, M. A., Salovey, P., & Mayer, J. D. (2007). Measuring emotional intelligence as a set of mental abilities. In G. Matthews, M. Zeidner, & R. D. Roberts (Eds.), *The science of emotional intelligence* (pp. 230–257). New York: Oxford University Press.

Rosete, D. (2007). *Does emotional intelligence play an important role in leadership effectiveness?* Unpublished doctoral dissertation, University of Wollongong, Wollongong, New South Wales, Australia.

Rosete, D., & Ciarrochi, J. (2005). Emotional intelligence and its relationship to workplace performance outcomes of leadership effectiveness. *Leadership and Organization Development Journal, 26,* 388–399.

Rottenberg, J., Kasch, K. L., Gross, J. J., & Gotlib, I. H. (2002). Sadness and amusement reactivity differentially predict concurrent and prospective functioning in major depressive disorder. *Emotion, 2,* 135–146.

Rubin, M. M. (1999). *Emotional intelligence and its role in mitigating aggression: A correlational study of the relationship between emotional intelligence and aggression in urban adolescents.* Unpublished dissertation, Immaculata College, Immaculata, PA.

Rubin, R. S., Munz, D. C., & Bommer, W. H. (2005). Leading from within: The effects of emotion recognition and personality on transformational leadership behavior. *Academy of Management Journal, 48,* 845–858.

Saarni, C. (1999). *The development of emotional competence.* New York: Guilford Press.

Sala, F. (2002). *Emotional Competence Inventory: Technical manual.* Philadelphia: McClelland Center for Research and Innovation, Hay Group.

Salovey, P., & Mayer, J. D. (1990). Emotional intelligence. *Imagination, Cognition, and Personality, 9,* 185–211.

Salovey, P., & Sluyter, D. J. (Eds.). (1997). *Emotional development and emotional intelligence: Educational implications.* New York: Basic Books.

Schutte, N. S., Malouff, J. M., Simunek, M., McKenley, J., & Hollander, S. (2002). Characteristic emotional intelligence and emotional well-being. *Cognition and Emotion, 16,* 769–785.

Southam-Gerow, M. A., & Kendall, P. C. (2000). Cognitive-behaviour therapy with youth: Advances, challenges, and future directions. *Clinical Psychology and Psychotherapy, 7,* 343–366.

Sternberg, R. J. (1985). *The triarchic mind: A new theory of human intelligence.* New York: Penguin.

Sutton, R. E., & Wheatley, K. F. (2003). Teachers' emotions and teaching: A review of the literature and directions for future research. *Educational Psychology Review, 15,* 327–358.

Travers, C. J. (2001). Stress in teaching: Past, present, and future. In J. Dunham (Ed.), *Stress in the workplace: Past, present, and future* (pp. 130–163). Philadelphia: Whurr.

Trinidad, D. R., & Johnson, C. A. (2002). The association between emotional intelligence and early adolescent tobacco and alcohol use. *Personality and Individual Differences, 32,* 95–105.

Weiss, H. M., & Cropanzano, R. (1996). Affective events theory: A theoretical discussion of the structure, causes and consequences of affective experiences at work. *Research in Organizational Behavior, 18*(Suppl. 1), 1–74.

Winters, J., Clift, R. J. W., & Dutton, D. G. (2004). An exploratory study of emotional intelligence and domestic abuse. *Journal of Family Violence, 19,* 255–267.

Young, P. T. (1943). *Emotion in man and in animal: Its nature and relation to attitude and motive.* New York: Wiley.

Zeidner, M., Roberts, R. D., & Matthews, G. (2004). The emotional intelligence bandwagon: Too fast to live, too young to die? *Psychological Inquiry, 15,* 239–248.

Zins, J. E., Weissberg, R. P., Wang, M. C., & Walberg, H. J. (Eds.). (2004). *Building academic success on social and emotional learning: What does the research say?* New York: Teachers College Press.

PART VI

PROBLEMS, DISORDERS, AND TREATMENT

CHAPTER 21

Repetitive Thought

Edward R. Watkins

What Is Repetitive Thought?

Segerstrom, Stanton, Alden, and Shortridge (2003, p. 3) defined *repetitive thought* (RT) as the "process of thinking attentively, repetitively or frequently about one's self and one's world," and they proposed that it formed "the core of a number of different models of adjustment and maladjustment." RT is a process common to a number of important constructs in the realms of psychopathology and self-regulation, including worry, rumination, emotional processing, and cognitive processing. RT has both constructive and unconstructive consequences for cognition and emotion, with rumination and worry implicated in exacerbating negative affect and the maintenance of psychiatric disorders, but with RT also implicated in problem solving and recovery from upsetting events (Watkins, 2008). This chapter reviews the evidence concerning the relationship of RT with emotion and associated cognition, considers its role in psychopathology, examines the processes that may underpin the development and maintenance of RT, and finishes with recent treatment developments.

The most studied forms of RT within the clinical field are *rumination* and *worry*. *Depressive rumination* is defined as "passively and repetitively focusing on one's symptoms of distress and the circumstances surrounding these symptoms" (Nolen-Hoeksema, McBride, & Larson, 1997, p. 855). The response styles theory (RST; Nolen-Hoeksema, 1991; Nolen-Hoeksema, Wisco, & Lyubomirsky, 2008) hypothesized, and found supportive empirical evidence that, depressive rumination is a particular response style to depressed mood, which is causally implicated in the onset and maintenance of depression. Within the study of social anxiety, postevent rumination ("postevent processing," "postmortem thinking") has been defined as "repetitive thoughts about subjective experiences during a recent social interaction, including self-appraisals and external evaluations of partners and other details involving the event" (Kashdan & Roberts, 2007, p. 286). Postevent rumination is hypothesized to contribute to the development and maintenance of social anxiety (Clark & Wells, 1995; Rapee & Heimberg, 1997).

However, rumination has been conceptualized more broadly and not necessarily as only a pathological process: Martin and Tesser (1996, p. 7) defined *rumination* as "a class of conscious thoughts that revolve around a common instrumental theme and that recur in the absence of immediate environmental demands requiring the thoughts." Within this conceptualization, rumination is RT on a theme related to unresolved personal goals and concerns, which can have either constructive or unconstructive consequences, depending on whether the RT helps or hinders the progress toward the unattained goal that triggered the rumination. Consistent with the potential adaptive effects of RT, cognitive processing accounts propose that RT about an upsetting event is part of the process of resolving the discrepancy between the stressful event and core beliefs in order to work through, make sense of, and integrate the upsetting experience into one's beliefs and assumptions about the world (Greenberg, 1995; Watkins, 2008).

Worry is defined as "a chain of thoughts and images, negatively affect-laden and relatively uncontrollable," and as "an attempt to engage in mental problem-solving on an issue whose outcome is uncertain but contains the possibility of one or more negative outcomes" (Borkovec, Robinson, Pruzinsky, & Depree, 1983, p. 9). Worry typically involves RT about potential future threat, imagined catastrophes, uncertainties, and risks (e.g., "What if they have an accident?"). It is conceptualized as an attempt to avoid negative events, prepare for the worst, and to problem-solve and is linked to unconstructive outcomes that include increased negative affect (anxiety, depression), interference with cognitive function, and disruptions to physiological processes (Borkovec, Ray, & Stöber, 1998). Chronic worry about a range of problems is a defining component of generalized anxiety disorder (GAD; American Psychiatric Association, 2000). However, worry can also serve constructive functions when it is objective, controllable, and brief (Tallis & Eysenck, 1994), including directing attention to an issue that requires immediate priority, prompting awareness of potential unresolved threats, and preparing an individual for difficulties through adopting adaptive behavior (e.g., studying for an exam).

Thus, RT is hypothesized to be involved in the maintenance of emotional disorders (e.g., major depression, GAD, social anxiety), but it is also hypothesized to have potentially constructive consequences with respect to recovery from upsetting emotional events, planning, and problem solving. Understanding the differential emotional consequences of RT is a key issue addressed later in this chapter.

There is a debate as to whether different conceptualizations of RT reflect distinct but related processes (e.g., Papageorgiou & Wells, 1999) or whether they reflect the same underlying process applied to different disorder-specific contents (Segerstrom, Tsao, Alden, & Craske, 2000; Watkins, 2008), especially for worry and rumination. These constructs are highly related: There is typically a high correlation (.6–.7) between the standardized questionnaire measures of worry and rumination (Penn State Worry Questionnaire [PSWQ] vs. Response Styles Questionnaire [RSQ], respectively). Moreover, structural equation modeling finds that these measures load on a common factor, and that both forms of RT are similarly related to symptoms of anxiety and depression (Fresco, Frankel, Mennin, Turk, & Heimberg, 2002; Segerstrom et al., 2000). Moreover, when individuals rated personal examples of worry and rumination on multiple cognitive dimensions, few differences were found (Papageorgiou & Wells, 1999; Watkins, 2004b; Watkins, Moulds, & Mackintosh, 2005), other than that worry and rumination predominantly focused on the future and past, respectively. There are similar effects of experimentally manipulating worry versus rumination, with both increasing ratings of anxiety and depression, relative to control conditions (e.g., Blagden & Craske, 1996; McLaughlin, Borkovec, & Sibrava, 2007). Thus, the convergent evidence indicates considerable similarities between the processes and consequences of worry and rumination. Although we need to be cautious about reaching a definitive conclusion, the most parsimonious account consistent with the evidence is that worry and rumination share a common underlying RT process that differs in specific content. This account is consistent with goal-based models of RT (e.g., Martin & Tesser, 1989, 1996), which propose that RT occurs in response to an unattained or unresolved goal and persists until the goal is attained or abandoned, with the thought content depending on the unresolved goal. Thus, worry may be triggered by unresolved goals related to threat and focused on the future, whereas depressive rumination may be triggered by unresolved goals related to self-identity and focused on the past.

RT and Emotion: Affective and Cognitive Consequences of RT

RT has significant direct consequences on mood and emotion, as well as on patterns of cognition associated with the onset, maintenance of, or recovery from emotional responses such as attribution, appraisal, memory recall, and problem solving (for detailed reviews, see Nolen-Hoeksema et al., 2008; Watkins, 2008). The main consequences of RT are (1) exacerbation of emotional states such as anxiety and depression; (2) elaborating and polarizing the thought content that is the focus of the RT; (3) influencing problem solving, planning, and associated instrumental action. These effects of RT can result in either constructive or unconstructive consequences, depending on the valence of the thought content within the RT, the intrapersonal and situational context in which the RT occurs, and the mode of processing adopted during RT (Watkins, 2008; also see Table 21.1). RT can enhance/ intensify a negative mood or exacerbate a positive mood, depending on the focus of the RT (Lyubomirsky & Nolen-Hoeksema,

1995). RT can both improve and impair effective social problem solving (Watkins & Baracaia, 2002; Watkins & Moulds, 2005a). This section examines each of these key consequences of RT and reviews those factors that moderate outcome, with reference to experimental studies.

RT as Magnifier: Amplification of Mood and Elaboration of Cognition

The principal action of RT with respect to affect is to magnify, amplify, prolong, and exacerbate existing mood states, as well as to elaborate associated mood-congruent cognition. RT is hypothesized to amplify the reciprocal relationship between cognition and mood state, for example, wherein negative mood increases the accessibility of negative cognition, which in turn, fuels the negative mood (Ciesla & Roberts, 2008; Nolen-Hoeksema, 1991; Teasdale, 1983, 1988). RT amplifies this reciprocal relationship between cognition and mood by increasing self-focus, which makes both mood and cognition more salient, and is demonstrated to amplify the effect of negative mood on

TABLE 21.1. Major Classes of RT Classified by Valence, Context, and Level of Construal

Class of RT	Valence	Context	Construal	Consequence
Depressive rumination	–	–	A	–
Rumination (control theory)	±	±	A/C	±
Worry	–	–	A	–
	–	±	C	+
Perseverative cognition	–	–	A	–
Cognitive–emotional processing	+	–	A	+
	–	–	C	+
Planning/problem solving	–	+	C	+
Counterfactuals	±	±	A/C	±
Defensive pessimism	–	+	C	+
Reflection	+	+	A	+?
Mind wandering	±	±	A/C	±
Postevent rumination	–	–	A	–
Positive rumination	+	+ BD	A?	–
	+	+	A	+
Habitual negative self-thinking	–	–	A	–

Note. Valence, valence of thought content; Context, situational and/or intrapersonal context; Construal, level of construal; Consequence, consequence of RT; – refers to negative valence/context or unconstructive consequence; – refers to negative valence/context or constructive consequence; ± means that valence, context, or consequence is mixed or underspecified (e.g., class of RT can have both constructive and unconstructive consequences); A, abstract level of construal; C, concrete level of construal; ?, unclear/unknown; BD, vulnerability to bipolar disorder.

thinking (Ingram, 1990; Pyszczynski & Greenberg, 1987) and of negative thoughts on mood (Mor & Winquist, 2002). Furthermore, RT serves to focus attention on the discrepancy between the desired goal and the actual situation, making the unresolved discrepancy more salient, perpetuating the unresolved issue, and exacerbating negative affect. RT further elaborates, polarizes, and consolidates the cognitions on which it is focused, with such extensive processing leading to greater mood congruence in cognition (see Forgas & Koch, Chapter 13, this volume). This process of RT amplification thereby exacerbates and prolongs existing mood states and enhances mood-congruent cognition.

Consistent with this magnifying effect of RT, there is extensive experimental evidence that manipulating RT causally exacerbates existing negative affect and increases existing negative cognition. Studies have used a standardized rumination induction, in which participants are instructed to spend 8 minutes concentrating on a series of sentences that involve rumination about themselves, their current feelings and physical state, and the causes and consequences of their feelings (e.g., "Think about the way you feel inside"; Lyubomirsky & Nolen-Hoeksema, 1995). As a control condition, a distraction induction is typically used, in which participants are instructed to spend 8 minutes concentrating on a series of sentences that involve imagining visual scenes that are unrelated to the self or to current feelings (e.g., "Think about a fire darting round a log in a fire place").

Compared to the distraction induction, the rumination induction is reliably found to have negative consequences on mood and cognition. Critically, the differential effects of these manipulations are found only when participants are already in a negative rather than a euthymic mood (e.g., selected dysphoric participants, depressed patients, or following a sad mood induction) before the manipulations, indicating a moderating role for existing mood state. Thus, for participants in a sad mood (but not a happy or neutral mood), compared to distraction, rumination exacerbates negative mood, increases negative thinking about the self, increases negative autobiographical memory recall, reduces the specificity of autobiographical

memory retrieval (see Murray, Holland, & Kensinger, Chapter 9, this volume), increases negative thinking about the future, impairs concentration and central executive functioning, and impairs social problem solving (e.g., Lyubomirsky & Nolen-Hoeksema, 1995; Watkins & Brown, 2002; Watkins & Teasdale, 2001).

These effects of RT on exacerbating affect are also found for emotional states other than sadness. Compared to distraction, rumination exacerbates preexisting anxious mood (Blagden & Craske, 1996), preexisting anger (Rusting & Nolen-Hoeksema, 1998), anger in response to a provocation (Bushman, 2002; Bushman, Bonacci, Pedersen, Vasquez, & Miller, 2005), and negative affect and intrusive memories in response to describing a personally distressing event (Ehring, Fuchs, & Klaesener, 2009). Likewise, studies that experimentally manipulated RT by asking participants to briefly worry about a self-chosen concern, found that worry increases anxiety and depressed mood in normal participants (Borkovec et al., 1998; McLaughlin et al., 2007) and produces a short-term increase in intrusive negative thoughts, relative to relaxation or visual imagery or no instruction conditions (Borkovec et al., 1998).

The aforementioned effects of RT on increasing mood-congruent cognition (negative memories/attributions/predictions) lead to further exacerbation of affect, since these cognitions influence mood state (Teasdale, 1983, 1988). For example, training individuals to adopt thinking patterns characteristic of rumination (e.g., asking "Why?" and focusing on meanings and implications) increases affective reactivity to a subsequent stressor relative to inducing a thinking style inconsistent with rumination (Moberly & Watkins, 2008; Watkins, Moberly, & Moulds, 2008).

However, most experimental studies investigating the consequences of RT are limited because their induction of RT involves asking participants to voluntarily and deliberately ruminate or worry. This approach introduces potential demand effects into the subsequent consequences of RT. Moreover, it may not be ecologically valid, given that much pathological RT is described as passive, involuntary, and uncontrollable. Studies that induce involuntary RT covertly, for example, by priming elements of a ruminative thinking style (see paragraph above and Watkins et al., 2008, for further details) followed by a failure induction that affords an opportunity for self-focused rumination, are necessary to reduce these limitations.

Moderators of the Affective Consequences of RT: Valence of Content and Context

The findings above suggest that *the content of RT* and *the context in which RT occurs* are potential moderators of the consequences of RT: That is, RT can be adaptive or maladaptive depending on the valence of the initial mood state and thought content. Since the thought content during RT is the material that is elaborated and polarized, it will influence the consequence of RT. Thus, for negatively valenced cognitions, RT would amplify the negative consequences of these negative cognitions and exacerbate existing negative mood, potentially resulting in more unconstructive outcomes. Although exacerbating negative mood is not necessarily maladaptive because negative mood can engender constructive consequences (e.g., Forgas & Koch, Chapter 13, this volume), prolonging and exacerbating negative cognition/mood increases the likelihood of clinical levels of distress, anxiety, depression, and dysfunctional cognitive–affective responses. Consistent with this hypothesis, there is evidence that the valence of thought content is a major factor in determining whether RT is helpful or unhelpful. For example, Segerstrom and colleagues (2003) examined the nature of RT and its role in adjustment in women who were exposed to a stressful situation through being identified as being at high risk for breast cancer. The valence of thought content during RT predicted concurrent affect and well-being: Less negative content during RT was associated with less negative affect, more positive affect, better overall mental health, less anxiety, and fewer physical symptoms. In a large meta-analysis of the self-focus literature, attention to negative aspects of the self was strongly related to increased levels of negative affect, whereas attention to positive aspects of the self was related to lower levels of negative affect (Mor & Winquist, 2002).

Likewise, the context in which RT occurs is also an important moderator of its consequences (Watkins, 2008). As reviewed earlier, the presence of a negative affective state (sadness, anger, anxiety) or a focus on negative concerns is a setting condition for RT to produce unconstructive consequences. Likewise, the consequences of worry are moderated by levels of trait anxiety: Worry is associated with more active coping and greater information seeking (Davey, Hampton, Farrell, & Davidson, 1992) and predicts better prospective performance (Siddique, LaSalle-Ricci, Glass, Arnkoff, & Diaz, 2006) when associated trait anxiety is held constant.

Key elements of context are (1) the prevailing valence of the cognitive–affective system of the individual engaged in RT in terms of mood state, self-beliefs, and dispositional traits; and (2) the situation and environment in which RT occurs. Both contexts can range from negatively valenced (e.g., intrapersonal: dysphoric mood, low self-esteem; situational: stressful events) to positively valenced (intrapersonal: positive mood, positive expectations; situational: success events). Both will often determine the valence of thought content during RT. When an individual has low self-esteem or is in a dysphoric mood, negative thoughts, memories, and expectations become more easily accessible and available, as illustrated by the phenomenon of mood-congruent memory (Bower, 1981; see also Murray, Holland, & Kensinger, Chapter 9, this volume). Similarly, a negative, stressful environment will activate negative thoughts and increase the likelihood of negative mood. Thus, by extension, in a negatively valenced intrapersonal or situational context, RT is likely to involve negative content and to further amplify the effect of that context on mood and cognition.

Consistent with this hypothesis, both intrapersonal context such as mood state and beliefs and external context such as the environment influence the consequences of RT. For example, the ability of RT to predict depression is moderated by the degree of negative self-related beliefs, with dysfunctional attitudes and self-esteem moderating the extent to which rumination prospectively predicts (1) the onset of depressive episodes (Robinson & Alloy, 2003) and (2) worse treatment outcome (Ciesla & Roberts,

2002). Likewise, the effects of experimentally manipulating rumination are moderated by the negative self-related beliefs held by individuals (Ciesla & Roberts, 2008).

Moderators of the Consequences of RT: Processing Mode

A further variable influencing the affective and cognitive consequences of RT is the processing mode adopted during RT (Borkovec et al., 1998; Watkins, 2008). There is evidence that RT characterized by an abstract processing mode has more unconstructive consequences than RT characterized by a concrete processing mode, at least when RT is focused on negatively valenced content (see Table 21.1). An abstract processing mode is conceptualized as focusing on general, superordinate, and decontextualized mental representations that convey the essential meaning, causes, and implications of goals and events, including the "why" aspects of an action and the ends consequential to it. In contrast, a concrete processing mode involves a focus on the direct, specific, and contextualized experience of an event, and on the details of goals, events, and actions that denote the feasibility, mechanics, and means of "how" to do the action.

The processing mode account (Watkins, 2008) proposes that the consequences of abstract versus concrete processing are determined by their relative sensitivity to contextual and situational detail. Relative to a concrete mode, an abstract mode (1) insulates an individual from the specific context, making the individual less distractible, less impulsive, and enabling more consistency and stability of goal pursuit across time; (2) allows both gainful and unhelpful generalizations and inferences across different situations; (3) but also makes the individual less responsive to the environment and to any situational change; and (4) provides fewer specific guides to action and problem solving because of its distance from the mechanics of action (Watkins, 2011). Thus, with respect to difficulties and negative events, a concrete processing mode will be adaptive relative to an abstract processing mode because it will result in (1) improved self-regulation focused on the immediate demands of the situation rather than its evaluative implications (Leary, Adams, & Tate, 2006); (2) reduced

negative overgeneralizations to emotional events, wherein a single failure is explained in terms of a global personal inadequacy, which is implicated in increased emotional reactivity (Carver & Scheier, 1982, 1990) and vulnerability to depression (Carver, 1998); and (3) more effective problem solving by providing more elaborated and contextual detail about the specific means and actions by which to best proceed when faced with difficult, novel, or complex situations. Similarly, the reduced concreteness theory of worry proposes that worry is predominantly experienced in a more abstract verbal form than in a more concrete visual imagery form and that this reduced concreteness leads to negative consequences for problem solving and affect regulation (Borkovec et al., 1998; Stöber, 1998; Stöber & Borkovec, 2002; Stöber, Tepperwien, & Staak, 2000).

Consistent with these theories, both worry and rumination are predominantly experienced in a verbal form rather than in images (Borkovec et al., 1998; McLaughlin et al., 2007). Moreover, elaborations of problems about which participants worry or ruminate are independently and blindly rated as more abstract and less concrete than problems about which participants do not worry or ruminate (Stöber, 1998; Stöber & Borkovec, 2002; Watkins & Moulds, 2007).

Using an experience sampling method in 31 undergraduates sampled eight times a day for 1 week, Takano and Tanno (2010) found that individuals with increasing levels of depressive symptoms engaged in more abstract thinking in daily life. Moreover, consistent with the hypothesis that processing mode influences the consequences of RT, self-focused RT was only significantly positively associated with negative affect in the context of elevated abstract thinking.

Experimental studies have further demonstrated that manipulating processing mode influences the consequences of RT, consistent with the processing mode and reduced concreteness theories. Studies adapted the standardized rumination induction to retain the key original element of repetitive focus on self, symptoms, and mood, but with instructions to adopt different processing modes. In depressed patients, a rumination induction encouraging more concrete processing, in which participants were instructed to "focus attention on the experience of" feelings, mood, and symptoms, was compared to a rumination induction encouraging more abstract processing, in which participants were instructed to "think about the causes, meanings, and consequences" of feelings, mood, and symptoms. Compared to abstract rumination, concrete rumination reduced negative global self-judgments such as "I am worthless" (Rimes & Watkins, 2005), improved social problem solving (Watkins & Moulds, 2005a), and increased specificity of autobiographical memory recall (Watkins & Teasdale, 2001). Thus RT focused on the direct concrete experience of moods and feelings reduces patterns of cognitive processing implicated in increased vulnerability for depression, relative to RT focused on the causes, meanings, and consequences of moods and feelings.

Experimental studies have also investigated whether manipulating participants to think repetitively in either an abstract or concrete mode influences the emotional response to analogue loss and trauma events. Relative to manipulations to engage in abstract RT, manipulations that instructed participants to engage in concrete RT produced faster recovery from negative affect and reduced intrusions after a previous negative induction (failure on IQ test, Watkins, 2004a; watching a distressing film, Ehring, Szeimies, & Schaffrick, 2009). Further studies trained participants to think in an abstract or a concrete way, through repeated practice at either abstractly evaluating the causes, meanings, and implications of emotional scenarios, or imagining the concrete details of what is happening in each scenario, prior to an unanticipated failure. Individuals trained to think about emotional events in a concrete way had reduced emotional reactivity to a subsequent experimental stressor relative to those trained to be abstract (Watkins et al., 2008). Thus, processing mode may play a causal role in the outcomes of RT in response to an upsetting or distressing event.

RT, Problem Solving, Planning, and Instrumental Action

RT has been implicated in both effective and ineffective problem solving, reflecting the moderating effects of thought valence and processing mode outlined earlier. On

the one hand, there is evidence that RT (e.g., rumination) can interfere with effective problem solving and instrumental behavior by making individuals more pessimistic and fatalistic, and engendering thinking that is more abstract and distanced from the specific details of how to solve a difficulty (e.g., Lyubomirsky & Nolen-Hoeksema, 1993, 1995; Watkins & Moulds, 2005a). Such RT prevents the resolution of the problems that may have led to anxious and depressed mood, and may potentially produce further increases in stressful circumstances. On the other hand, RT has been found to positively influence social problem solving. Diary measures indicate that a large proportion of worry reflects problem-solving attempts, which are often successful (Szabo & Lovibond, 2006). RT that involves concrete processing tends to produce improved problem solving: Prompting RT focused on causal attributions and abstract evaluations (using questions such as "Why did this problem happen?") impaired social problem solving in a recovered depressed group, who performed as well as never-depressed participants in a no-prompt control condition, whereas prompting RT focused on the concrete process of how to proceed (questions such as "How are you deciding what to do next?") ameliorated the problem-solving deficit normally found in a group of currently depressed patients (Watkins & Baracaia, 2002).

RT, Contextual Insensitivity, and Anhedonia

RT has recently been hypothesized to reduce responsiveness to information that is unrelated to the focus of the RT (Stein, Lehtonen, Harvey, Nicol-Harper, & Craske, 2009; Watkins, 2008, 2011). Preoccupation with the foci of the RT is hypothesized to reduce engagement with the external environment, unless the environment is directly related to the central concerns of the RT, as a function of (1) increased focus and preoccupation on the RT concern at the expense of other information (a focus "in the head" rather than "in the world"), and (2) increased abstract processing focused on evaluating the general implications of events, which is less sensitive to contextual and situational detail. Thus, inducing preoccupation about everyday concerns reduced the processing of interpersonal information in individuals prone to preoccupation (Lehtonen et al., 2009). Similarly, Rottenberg, Gross, and Gotlib (2005) speculated that rumination may partially account for the phenomenon of *emotional context insensitivity*, in which individuals with major depression are characterized by reduced emotional reactivity to both positively and negatively valenced stimuli (Bylsma, Morris, & Rottenberg, 2008).

This reduced responsiveness to the environment could lead to less contact with positive reinforcers and less awareness of positive contingency, contributing to anhedonia. Consistent with this hypothesis, rumination is associated with melancholia, which is characterized by less responsiveness to the environment and increased anhedonia (Nelson & Mazure, 1985). Moreover, RT during a large-scale experience sampling study concurrently and prospectively predicted reduced happiness during activities (Killingsworth & Gilbert, 2010), suggesting that off-task RT interferes with the impact of activities on positive affect.

Effects of Emotion on RT

As well as amplifying existing mood state, RT is itself influenced by mood. The control theory account (Martin & Tesser, 1989, 1996) predicts that RT is triggered by unresolved goals and focuses attention on goal discrepancies as a means to potentially reduce the discrepancy. Because unresolved goals are also implicated in the activation of emotions (Oatley & Johnson-Laird, 1987, e.g., loss of a goal leads to sadness; frustration of a goal leads to anger), RT will often co-occur with negative affect. Moreover, negative affect can act as a signal of an unresolved goal and thereby trigger further RT. Similarly, RST proposes that rumination is a response that is automatically triggered by the context of negative affect (Nolen-Hoeksema, 1991). The RST account therefore predicts that RT will increase when negative affect increases.

Consistent with these accounts, self-reported rumination has both trait-like and state-like components, with endorsement of rumination greater in currently depressed than formerly depressed participants (Rob-

erts, Gilboa, & Gotlib, 1998), and with increasing symptoms prospectively predicting increased rumination (Nolen-Hoeksema, Stice, Wade, & Bohon, 2007). In an experience sampling methodology study, Moberly and Watkins (2008) found that momentary RT prospectively predicted momentary negative affect but that momentary negative affect also prospectively predicted increases in momentary RT at the next sampling point, after controlling for initial RT.

Repetitive Negative Thought as a Transdiagnostic Process

There is emergent evidence that RT focused on negative content (henceforward *repetitive negative thought* [RNT], e.g., worry, depressive rumination) may be a transdiagnostic process—that is, a process present across multiple psychiatric diagnoses that causally contributes to those disorders (Harvey, Watkins, Mansell, & Shafran, 2004). Recent reviews (Ehring & Watkins, 2008; Harvey et al., 2004; Nolen-Hoeksema & Watkins, 2011) have proposed that RNT is a transdiagnostic process based on elevated RNT being found across a range of disorders and predicting symptoms in prospective longitudinal studies.

RNT is involved in the onset and maintenance of depression, with both depressive rumination and other types of RNT (1) predicting future depression in longitudinal prospective studies and (2) increasing negative affect when experimentally induced (see reviews by Nolen-Hoeksema et al., 2008; Watkins, 2008). RNT is a diagnostic component of GAD and a key element within theoretical models of social anxiety and posttraumatic stress disorder (PTSD), which is elevated relative to nonpsychiatric controls in GAD, social anxiety, and PTSD (e.g., Abbott & Rapee, 2004; Borkovec et al., 1998; Clohessy & Ehlers, 1999). RNT is associated with symptoms in eating disorders (e.g., Nolen-Hoeksema et al., 2007), alcohol abuse and dependency (Caselli, Bortolai, Leoni, Rovetto, & Spada, 2008), and psychosis (e.g., Morrison & Wells, 2007). Thus, there is evidence of the presence of RNT for nearly all Axis I disorders compared to nondisordered controls. A recent meta-analysis showed that rumination was significantly related to four distinct symptom types (depression, anxiety, eating disorder, alcohol abuse; Aldao, Nolen-Hoeksema, & Schweizer, 2010).

Longitudinal studies find that RNT prospectively predicts a range of symptoms, indicating that RNT is a vulnerability factor for emotional disorder, rather than only a consequence or associate of psychopathology (Ehring & Watkins, 2008; Nolen-Hoeksema & Watkins, 2011; Watkins, 2008). RNT prospectively predicts the onset of major depressive episodes, the severity of depressive symptoms in nondepressed and currently depressed individuals, and mediates the effects of other risk factors on depression (e.g., Nolen-Hoeksema, 2000; Spasojevic & Alloy, 2001; see meta-analysis by Mor & Winquist, 2002; Watkins, 2008). RNT prospectively predicts symptoms of anxiety after controlling for baseline anxiety in numerous longitudinal studies (Watkins, 2008). For example, RNT predicts the onset and severity of posttraumatic stress symptoms and diagnosis of PTSD up to 3 years after traumatic events (e.g., Ehlers, Mayou, & Bryant, 1998). Moreover, two large-scale longitudinal studies found that RNT explained the concurrent and prospective associations between symptoms of anxiety and depression (McLaughlin & Nolen-Hoeksema, 2011). RNT prospectively predicts substance abuse (Nolen-Hoeksema et al., 2007; Skitch & Abela, 2008), alcohol abuse (Caselli et al., 2010), and eating disorders (Holm-Denoma & Hankin, 2010; Nolen-Hoeksema et al., 2007), after controlling for initial symptoms. In a prospective longitudinal sample of 496 female adolescents over 4 years, rumination predicted future increases in bulimic and substance abuse symptoms, as well as onset of major depression, binge eating, and substance abuse (Nolen-Hoeksema et al., 2007). The experimental studies reviewed earlier further support the hypothesis that RNT may play a causal role in the onset or maintenance of psychopathology.

Why Do People Engage in RT?

Given these well-documented negative consequences, key questions are why individuals engage in RT, why some individuals engage in RT more frequently, and why some individuals get stuck in pathological RNT. It is important to discriminate between a single bout of RT, which is not necessarily pathological and may indeed be adaptive, versus the tendency to repeatedly engage in persistent and chronic RT, which tends to be associated with psychopathology. Nearly everyone will engage in bouts of RT in response to personal difficulties and unexpected setbacks, such as the failure of a romantic relationship or bereavement, but only a subset of individuals consistently and frequently engages in severe RT (worriers, ruminators).

Control Theory Account

The control theory account (Martin & Tesser, 1989, 1996) provides a coherent account for distinct bouts of RT consistent with the extant evidence (Watkins, 2008): RT is hypothesized to be activated by a perceived goal discrepancy and is maintained until the unresolved goal is either achieved or abandoned (see Carver & Scheier, Chapter 10, this volume). Consistent with this account, there is an extensive literature confirming that unresolved and blocked goals increase the priming and accessibility of goal-relevant information, with thoughts relating to unresolved goals persisting longer than those associated with resolved goals (e.g., Zeigarnik, 1938). Moreover, in naturalistic diary and experience sampling studies, unresolved personally important goals are associated with increased RT (Moberly & Watkins, 2010; Gebhardt, Van der Doef, Massey, Verhoeven, & Verkuil, 2010). However, this theory does not provide a full account of individual differences in the tendency toward RT, other than the proposal that individuals prone to more abstract processing will engage in less constructive and more persistent RT (Watkins, 2008).

With respect to explaining individual differences in RT, there are three broad classes of accounts: a learned response account, a functional account, and an information-processing account. These accounts are neither mutually exclusive nor independent, and it is likely that the fullest account of RT will require some integration across them: The learned response and functional accounts overlap in the role of learning and conditioning in the development of RNT.

RNT as Learned Response

The learned response account is exemplified by the RST (Nolen-Hoeksema 1991), which hypothesizes that depressive rumination is a stable trait-like cognitive style of responding to depressed mood. Consistent with this hypothesis, individual differences in rumination are found to be stable across situations and repeated testing (Nolen-Hoeksema, Morrow & Fredrickson, 1993; Nolen-Hoeksema et al., 2008), even when there are changes in the levels of depression. Similar stability is found for worry (Borkovec et al., 1998).

RST and developmental models of worry propose that learning, conditioning, and socialization processes during childhood and adolescence contribute to the development of RNT and implicate the role of parenting behaviors (see reviews by Kertz & Woodruff-Boden, 2011; Nolen-Hoeksema et al., 2008). Depressive rumination is hypothesized to be learned in childhood, because it was modeled by parents who themselves had a passive coping style (Nolen-Hoeksema, 1991); or because the child failed to learn more active coping strategies as a consequence of overcritical, intrusive, and over-controlling parents (Nolen-Hoeksema, Mumme, Wolfson, & Guskin, 1995); or because of early physical/sexual abuse. Similarly, worry is hypothesized to be learned in childhood because it was modeled by anxious parents or it was a response to parental overprotection and overcontrol (Kertz & Woodruff-Boden, 2011). Consistent with this hypothesis, elevated rumination and worry are associated with retrospective self-report of overcontrolling parents (Spasojevic & Alloy, 2002) and of parents with anxious rearing and rejecting styles (Muris, Meesters, Merckelbach, & Hulsenbeck, 2000), respectively. In addition, rumination is associated with reported physical, emotional, and sexual abuse (Conway, Mendelson, Giannopoulos, Csank, & Holm, 2004).

An integration of the RST and control theories can be hypothesized. Individual bouts of rumination are initially triggered by goal discrepancies. However, with repetition in the same context, the ruminative response can become a habit (Wood & Neal, 2007) through a process of automatic association between the RT and the context that occurs repeatedly with performance of the behavior—in this case, the negative affect generated by the goal discrepancy. This account makes explicit that pathological RT can be learned as a habitual response to a mood cue. Consistent with this conceptualization, high ruminators report that they are unable to control rumination, which is compulsive and habitual (Watkins & Baracaia, 2001). Verplanken, Friborg, Wang, Trafimow, and Woolf (2007) found that a self-reported index of the habitual nature of negative thinking—assessing frequency, lack of awareness of initiating negative self-thinking, lack of conscious intent, mental efficiency, and difficulty to control negative thinking—was correlated significantly and positively with behavioral and self-report measures of RNT.

Functional Accounts of RNT

Functional accounts propose that individuals may develop a tendency toward more frequent and extensive RNT because RNT has an instrumental benefit via instrumental learning and the effects of positive and negative reinforcement (e.g., Martell, Addis, & Jacobson, 2001) and/or through explicit metacognitive beliefs about the perceived pros and cons of RNT (e.g., Wells, 1995). Both accounts hypothesize that similar reinforcing functions maintain and exacarbate elevated RNT, but differ in the degree to which individuals are hypothesized to be consciously aware of these functions.

RNT has been conceptualized as an avoidance behavior that is negatively reinforced by the removal of aversive experience (Borkovec & Roemer, 1995; Martell et al., 2001; Watkins et al., 2007). Hypothesized functions include (1) avoiding the risk of failure/humiliation by thinking about rather than implementing behavior; (2) attempting to problem-solve but without a concrete plan of action; (3) avoiding and minimizing criticism by anticipating potential negative responses from others; (4) controlling unwanted feelings; (5) avoiding unwanted attributes by motivating oneself (e.g., "keeping me on my toes"); and (6) trying to understand the reasons why something happened so as to better know what to do and to prevent future problems. There is evidence that worry may avoid intense affect and/

or reduce physiological arousal by distancing an individual from specific details and increasing verbal/conceptual thinking at the expense of emotionally vivid imagery (Borkovec et al., 1998; Stöber & Borkovec, 2002).

Importantly, although RNT may be experienced as aversive to the individual and have demonstrable negative consequences, it could still be reinforced if it avoids an even more aversive condition. For example, if RNT exacerbates sadness but reduces anger in an individual who finds anger more aversive, then it will be reinforced. Moreover, since RNT is often initiated as an attempt at problem solving, the ability to discriminate between helpful versus unhelpful thinking during RNT (e.g., concrete vs. abstract modes) and between soluble problems versus unanswerable questions is critical. Poor discrimination would result in bouts of RT with positive outcomes reinforcing less adaptive RT. In addition, this reinforcement can occur superstitiously if RT does not influence an outcome but is perceived to do so because it is consistently paired with a reinforcing outcome: If worry about a problem was regularly followed by the coincidental removal of the problem, the worry could become reinforced. Finally, the reinforcement of RT probably occurs intermittently, resulting in a pattern of partial reinforcement, which is more resistant to extinction than continuous reinforcement (Jenkins & Stanley, 1950), making it harder to abandon.

Consistent with RNT having an avoidant function, rumination is positively correlated with self-reported avoidance (Cribb, Moulds, & Carter, 2006; Giorgio et al., 2010; Moulds, Kandris, Starr, & Wong, 2007), as well as with greater frequency of escape and avoidance behavior such as cutting, bingeing, and drug and alcohol abuse (Nolen-Hoeksema et al., 2007). Borkevec and Roemer (1995) found that worriers reported that worry distracted them from more bothersome concerns.

Consistent with the functional account, Lyubomirsky and Nolen-Hoeksema (1993) found that after experimentally inducing rumination, dysphoric individuals reported gaining insight into their problems relative to distraction, even though rumination in depressed individuals is associated with poorer problem solving. Watkins and Bara-caia (2001) and Freeston, Rheaume, Letarte, and Dugas (1994) found that high ruminators and high worriers reported perceived advantages of RNT that included increasing understanding and insight of self and depression, solving problems, learning from past mistakes, preventing future mistakes, increasing empathy, and not losing control. Individual differences in worry and rumination are positively associated with beliefs about the importance of understanding and making sense of difficulties and with beliefs that RNT is helpful in understanding problems (e.g., Papageorgiou & Wells, 2003; Watkins & Moulds, 2005b). Positive metacognitive beliefs prospectively predict increased RNT following a laboratory-based stressor (Moulds, Yap, Kerr, Williams, & Kandris, 2010), and perceived instrumental functions for RNT prospectively predict increases in RNT 6–8 weeks later (Kingston, Watkins, & O'Mahen, 2012).

However, a key hypothesis within the functional account—namely, that RNT has reinforcing qualities that causally lead to its further consolidation—has not been directly tested. Experimental studies are required that (1) manipulate RNT and demonstrate that it has an impact on the identified functions (e.g., increases sense of understanding), and then (2) demonstrate that manipulating such functions and perceptions influences the frequency and duration of RNT.

Information-Processing Accounts of RNT

A number of accounts propose that individual differences in RNT arise as a consequence of individual differences in information processing, whether these be deficits such as reduced executive control, impaired inhibitory control, and reduced working memory (Joormann, 2010), or biases in information processing such as an impairment in disengaging attention from negative self-referent information (Koster, De Lissnyder, Derakshan, & De Raedt, 2011). Joormann (2010) proposed that RNT increases in those individuals who are unable to inhibit now irrelevant but previously relevant information in working memory. Consistent with this account, poor inhibitory control, as indexed on a range of experimental tasks, is correlated with RNT (e.g., Gotlib & Joormann,

2010; Joormann, Yoon, & Zetsche, 2007). Zetsche and Joormann (2011) found that impaired interference control for word and face stimuli, assessed on a negative priming task, prospectively predicted rumination 6 months later.

There is emerging evidence consistent with the hypothesis that biases in attention to negative information are involved in RNT. Self-reported rumination is correlated with selective attentional bias toward sad faces (Joormann, Dkane, & Gotlib, 2006) and toward negative words on the dot probe task (Donaldson, Lam, & Mathews, 2007), whereas worry and GAD are associated with an attentional bias toward threat words (MacLeod, Mathews, & Tata, 1986).

A key next step is to look at the causal direction of the relationship between these deficits and the tendency toward RNT: If these biases and deficits cause RNT, then manipulations of these biases via prolonged cognitive bias modification training (see MacLeod & Clarke, Chapter 29, this volume) should reduce RNT. There is recent evidence for such a causal role of attention in maintaining RNT: Training attention to neutral words on a dot probe paradigm (see chapters on attention and CBM for further details) led to fewer negative thought intrusions following instructed worry than a mixed attention control condition in high worriers (Hayes, Hirsch, & Mathews, 2010). However, as noted earlier, these studies only assess voluntary RNT rather than involuntary RNT.

Interventions for RNT

Given that RNT appears to be an important contributor to psychopathology, what treatment approaches are effective in reducing it? Randomized controlled trials demonstrate that cognitive-behavioral therapy (CBT) is an empirically supported treatment for GAD (Newman & Borkovec, 2002) and indicate that CBT can specifically reduce worry (Covin, Ouimet, Seeds, & Dozois, 2008). CBT treatment approaches for GAD include self-monitoring of anxiety cues, applied relaxation, self-controlled desensitization, and cognitive restructuring (Newman & Borkovec, 2002). CBT treatments have also targeted metacognitive beliefs about worry

and cognitive avoidance, with some success (Ladouceur et al., 2000).

Although trials have demonstrated the efficacy of CBT for depression, the majority have not assessed whether CBT reduces depressive rumination, leaving unresolved whether standard CBT for depression is effective at reducing RNT (see Schmaling, Dimidjian, Katon, & Sullivan, 2006, for negative evidence). One treatment designed to explicitly and exclusively target RNT in depression is rumination-focused CBT (RFCBT; Watkins et al., 2007, 2009, 2011). RFCBT is a manualized treatment, theoretically informed by processing mode and functional approaches to RNT, in which patients are coached to shift from unconstructive RT to constructive RT and to reduce avoidant behavior through the use of functional analysis, experiential/imagery exercises, and behavioral experiments, incorporating the functional–analytic and contextual principles and techniques of behavioral activation (BA; Martell et al., 2001). In addition, patients use directed imagery to recreate previous mental states when a more helpful thinking style was active, such as memories of being completely absorbed in an activity (e.g., "flow" or "peak" experiences) and experiences of increased compassion, which act directly counter to RNT. RFCBT significantly reduced rumination and depression in a multiple baseline case series of patients with residual depression (Watkins et al., 2007) and significantly outperformed treatment as usual (continuation antidepressants) in reducing rumination and depression in a Phase II randomized controlled trial (Watkins et al., 2011).

Another treatment hypothesized to reduce RNT is mindfulness-based CBT. Mindfulness-based CBT is a psychosocial group-based relapse prevention program that incorporates meditational practice within the framework of CBT principles as a means to increase resilience against depression (Segal, Williams, & Teasdale, 2012). A key element is mindfulness practice in which participants learn experientially to maintain their attention to their breath, thoughts, and feelings, and to hold such experiences in awareness, in a nonjudgmental and accepting way. These mindfulness skills are proposed to enable individuals to develop alternative responses to negative thoughts and feelings and thereby to step out of habitual patterns of RNT. Mindfulness approaches reduce RNT in experimental analogue studies (e.g., Feldman, Greeson, & Senville, 2010) and in randomized controlled trials (Jain et al., 2007; Ramel, Goldin, Carmona, & McQuaid, 2004). Moreover, mindfulness-based CBT has been demonstrated to be an effective relapse prevention treatment for individuals with three or more episodes of depression (Kuyken et al., 2008; Teasdale et al., 2000).

Consistent with a causal relationship between processing mode and individual differences in RT, a proof-of-principle randomized controlled treatment intervention trial found that training depressed individuals to be more concrete when faced with difficulties reduced depression, anxiety, and rumination relative to a no-treatment control (Watkins, Baeyens, & Read, 2009). The concreteness training involved repeated practice at asking *how* questions and focusing on specific details when thinking about recent difficulties. In a Phase II randomized controlled trial, guided self-help concreteness training was found to be superior to treatment as usual in reducing rumination, worry, and depression in patients with major depression recruited in primary care (Watkins et al., 2012). Thus, shifting depressed patients into a more concrete processing mode reduced RT and associated symptoms.

Conclusion

RT is a universal and common cognitive process that is closely aligned with emotional experience: It tends to be triggered in response to emotionally eliciting events and difficulties in making progress on personally relevant goals, and it can act to either exacerbate the existing emotional state and goal discrepancy or to address the underlying difficulty, leading to improvements in affect. RT focused on negative content, such as past losses, current symptoms, or future threat, tends to amplify the associated negative affect and to elaborate mood-congruent cognitions. As such, it is unsurprising that such RNT is implicated as a transdiagnostic process that causally contributes to depression, anxiety, and other psychiatric disorders. Nonetheless, RT can be adap-

tive, particularly when it is focused on positive content and on the concrete contextual details of situations and on how to move forward. There is evidence indicating that individual differences in RNT are influenced by negative reinforcement, parenting style, early experiences, metacognitive beliefs, and deficits and biases in attentional and inhibitory control, although an integrated model of these variables remains to be developed.

References

Abbott, M. J., & Rapee, R. M. (2004). Post-event rumination and negative self-appraisal in social phobia before and after treatment. *Journal of Abnormal Psychology, 113*, 136–144.

Aldao, A., Nolen-Hoeksema, S., & Schweizer, S. (2010). Emotion regulation strategies across psychopathology: A meta-analytic review. *Clinical Psychology Review, 30*, 217–237.

American Psychiatric Association. (2000). *Diagnostic and statistical manual of mental disorders* (4th ed., text rev.). Washington, DC: Author.

Blagden, J. C., & Craske, M. G. (1996). Effects of active and passive rumination and distraction: A pilot replication with anxious mood. *Journal of Anxiety Disorders, 10*, 243–252.

Borkovec, T. D., Ray, W. J., & Stöber, J. (1998). Worry: A cognitive phenomenon intimately linked to affective, physiological, and interpersonal behavioral processes. *Cognitive Therapy and Research, 22*, 561–576.

Borkovec, T. D., Robinson, E., Pruzinsky, T., & Depree, J. A. (1983). Preliminary exploration of worry: Some characteristics and processes. *Behaviour Research and Therapy, 21*, 9–16.

Borkovec, T. D., & Roemer L. (1995). Perceived functions of worry among generalized anxiety disorder subjects: Distraction from more emotionally distressing topics? *Journal of Behaviour Therapy and Experimental Psychiatry, 26*, 25–30.

Bower, G. H. (1981). Mood and memory. *American Psychologist, 36*, 129–148.

Bushman, B. J. (2002). Does venting anger feed or extinguish the flame?: Catharsis, rumination, distraction, anger, and aggressive responding. *Personality and Social Psychology Bulletin, 28*, 724–731.

Bushman, B. J., Bonacci, A. M., Pedersen, W. C., Vasquez, E. A., & Miller, N. (2005). Chewing on it can chew you up: Effects of rumination on triggered displaced aggression. *Journal of Personality and Social Psychology, 88,* 969–983.

Bylsma, L. M., Morris, B. H., & Rottenberg, J. (2008). A meta-analysis of emotional reactivity in major depressive disorder. *Clinical Psychology Review, 28,* 676–691.

Carver, C. S. (1998). Generalization, adverse events, and development of depressive symptoms. *Journal of Personality, 66,* 607–619.

Carver, C. S., & Scheier, M. F. (1982). Control-theory: A useful conceptual-framework for personality—social, clinical, and health psychology. *Psychological Bulletin, 92,* 111–135.

Carver, C. S., & Scheier, M. F. (1990). Origins and functions of positive and negative affect: A control-process view. *Psychological Review, 97,* 19–35.

Caselli, G., Bortolai, C., Leoni, M., Rovetto, F., & Spada, M. M. (2008). Rumination in problem drinkers. *Addiction Research and Theory, 16,* 564–571.

Caselli, G., Ferretti, C., Leoni, M., Rebecchi, D., Rovetto, F., & Spada, M. M. (2010). Rumination as a predictor of drinking behaviour in alcohol abusers: A prospective study. *Addiction, 105,* 1041–1048.

Ciesla, J. A., & Roberts, J. E. (2002). Self-directed thought and response to treatment for depression: A preliminary investigation. *Journal of Cognitive Psychotherapy: An International Quarterly, 16,* 435–453.

Ciesla, J. A., & Roberts, J. E. (2008). Rumination, negative cognition, and their interactive effects on depressed mood. *Emotion, 7,* 555–565.

Clark, D. M., & Wells, A. (1995). The cognitive model of social phobia. In R. G. Heimberg, M. R. Liebowitz, D. A. Hope, & F. R. Schneier (Eds.), *Social phobia: Diagnosis, assessment, and treatment* (pp. 69–93). New York: Guilford Press.

Clohessy, S., & Ehlers, A. (1999). PTSD symptoms, response to intrusive memories and coping in ambulance service workers. *British Journal of Clinical Psychology, 38,* 251–265.

Conway, M., Mendelson, M., Giannopoulos, C., Csank, P. A. R., & Holm, S. L. (2004). Childhood and adult sexual abuse, rumination on sadness, and dysphoria. *Child Abuse and Neglect, 28,* 393–410.

Covin, R., Ouimet, A. J., Seeds, P. M., & Dozois, D. J. A. (2008). A meta-analysis of CBT for pathological worry among clients with GAD. *Journal of Anxiety Disorders, 22,* 108–116.

Cribb, G., Moulds, M. L., & Carter, S. (2006). Rumination and experiential avoidance in depression. *Behaviour Change, 23,* 165–176.

Davey, G. C. L., Hampton, J., Farrell, J., & Davidson, S. (1992). Some characteristics of worrying: Evidence for worrying and anxiety as separate constructs. *Personality and Individual Differences, 13,* 133–147.

Donaldson, C., Lam, D., & Mathews, A. (2007). Rumination and attention in major depression. *Behaviour Research and Therapy, 45,* 2664–2678.

Ehlers, A., Mayou, R. A., & Bryant, B. (1998). Psychological predictors of chronic posttraumatic stress disorder after motor vehicle accidents. *Journal of Abnormal Psychology, 107,* 508–519.

Ehring, T. A., Fuchs, N., & Klaesener, I. (2009). The effects of experimentally induced rumination versus distraction on analogue posttraumatic stress symptoms. *Behavior Therapy, 40,* 403–413.

Ehring, T. A., Szeimies, A. K., & Schaffrick, C. (2009). An experimental analogue study into the role of abstract thinking in trauma-related rumination. *Behaviour Research and Therapy, 47,* 285–293.

Ehring, T. A., & Watkins, E. R. (2008). Repetitive negative thinking as a transdiagnostic process. *International Journal of Cognitive Therapy, 1,* 192–205.

Feldman, G., Greeson, J., & Senville, J. (2010). Differential effects of mindful breathing, progressive muscle relaxation, and loving-kindness meditation on decentering and negative reactions to repetitive thoughts. *Behaviour Research and Therapy, 48,* 1002–1011.

Freeston, M. H., Rheaume, J., Letarte, H., & Dugas, M. J. (1994). Why do people worry? *Personality and Individual Differences, 17,* 791–802.

Fresco, D. M., Frankel, A. N., Mennin, D. S., Turk, C. L., & Heimberg, R. G. (2002). Distinct and overlapping features of rumination and worry: The relationship of cognitive production to negative affective states. *Cognitive Therapy and Research, 26,* 179–188.

Gebhardt, W. A., Van der Doef, M. P., Massey, E. K., Verhoeven, C. J. M., & Verkuil, B. (2010). Goal commitment to finding a partner and satisfaction with life among female singles: The mediating role of rumination. *Journal of Health Psychology, 15,* 122–130.

Giorgio J. M., Sanflippo, J., Kleiman, E., Reilly, D., Bender, R. E., Wagner, C. A., et al. (2010).

An experiential avoidance conceptualization of depressive rumination: Three tests of the model. *Behaviour Research and Therapy, 48,* 1021–1031.

Gotlib, I. H., & Joormann, J. (2010). Cognition and depression: Current status and future directions. *Annual Review of Clinical Psychology, 6,* 285–312.

Greenberg, M. A. (1995). Cognitive processing of traumas: The role of intrusive thoughts and reappraisals. *Journal of Applied Social Psychology, 25,* 1262–1296.

Harvey, A. G., Watkins, E., Mansell, W., & Shafran, R. (2004). *Cognitive behavioural processes across psychological disorders.* Oxford, UK: Oxford University Press.

Hayes, S., Hirsch, C. R., & Mathews, A. (2010). Facilitating a benign attentional bias reduced negative thought intrusions. *Journal of Abnormal Psychology, 119,* 235–240.

Holm-Denoma, J. M., & Hankin, B. L. (2010). Perceived physical appearance mediates the rumination and bulimic symptom link in adolescent girls. *Journal of Clinical Child and Adolescent Psychology, 39,* 537–544.

Ingram, R. E. (1990). Self-focused attention in clinical disorders: Review and a conceptual model. *Psychological Bulletin, 107,* 156–176.

Jain, S., Shapiro, S. L., Swanick, S., Roesch, S. C., Mills, P. J., Bell, I., et al. (2007). A randomized controlled trial of mindfulness meditation versus relaxation training: Effects on distress, positive states of mind, rumination, and distraction. *Annals of Behavioral Medicine, 33,* 11–21.

Jenkins, W. O., & Stanley, J. C. (1950). Partial reinforcement: A review and critique. *Psychological Bulletin, 47,* 193–234.

Joormann, J. (2010). Cognitive inhibition and emotion regulation in depression. *Current Directions in Psychological Science, 19,* 161–166.

Joormann, J., Dkane, M., & Gotlib, I. H. (2006). Adaptive and maladaptive components of rumination?: Diagnostic specificity and relation to depressive biases. *Behavior Therapy, 37,* 269–281.

Joormann, J., Yoon, K. L., & Zetsche, U. (2007). Cognitive inhibition in depression. *Applied and Preventive Psychology, 12,* 128–139.

Kashdan, T. B., & Roberts, J. E. (2007). Social anxiety, depressive symptoms, and post-event rumination: Affective consequences and social contextual influences. *Journal of Anxiety Disorders, 21,* 284–301.

Kertz, S. J., & Woodruff-Boden, J. (2011). The developmental psychopathology of worry. *Clinical Child Family Psychology Review, 14,* 174–197.

Killingsworth, M. A., & Gilbert, D. T. (2010). A wandering mind is an unhappy mind. *Science, 330,* 932.

Kingston, R., Watkins, E. R., & O'Mahen, H. (2012). *A prospective examination of risk factors for repetitive negative thought.* Manuscript in preparation.

Koster, E. H. W., De Lissnyder, E., Derakshan, N., & De Raedt, R. (2011). Understanding depressive rumination from a cognitive science perspective: The impaired disengagement hypothesis. *Clinical Psychology Review, 31,* 138–145.

Kuyken, W., Byford, S., Taylor, R. S., Watkins, E. R., Holden, E., White, K., et al. (2008). Mindfulness-based cognitive therapy to prevent relapse in recurrent depression. *Journal of Consulting and Clinical Psychology, 76,* 966–978.

Ladouceur, R., Dugas, M. J., Freeston, M. H., Leger, E., Gagnon, F., & Thibodeau, N. (2000). Efficacy of a cognitive-behavioral treatment for generalized anxiety disorder: Evaluation in a controlled clinical trial. *Journal of Consulting and Clinical Psychology, 68,* 957–964.

Leary, M. R., Adams, C. E., & Tate, E. B. (2006). Hypo-egoic self-regulation: Exercising self-control by diminishing the influence of the self. *Journal of Personality, 74,* 1803–1831.

Lehtonen, A., Jakub, N., Craske, M., Doll, H., Harvey, A., & Stein, A. (2009). Effects of preoccupation on interpersonal recall: A pilot study. *Depression and Anxiety, 26,* 1–6.

Lyubomirsky, S., & Nolen-Hoeksema, S. (1993). Self-perpetuating properties of dysphoric rumination. *Journal of Personality and Social Psychology, 65,* 339–349.

Lyubomirsky, S., & Nolen-Hoeksema, S. (1995). Effects of self-focused rumination on negative thinking and interpersonal problem-solving. *Journal of Personality and Social Psychology, 69,* 176–190.

MacLeod, C., Mathews, A., & Tata, P. (1986). Attentional bias in emotional disorders. *Journal of Abnormal Psychology, 95,* 15–20.

Martell, C. R., Addis, M. E., & Jacobson, N. S. (2001). *Depression in context: Strategies for guided action.* New York: Norton.

Martin, L. L., & Tesser, A. (1989). Toward a motivational and structural theory of ruminative thought. In J. S. Uleman & J. A. Bargh (Eds.), *Unintended thought* (pp. 306–326). New York: Guilford Press.

Martin, L. L., & Tesser, A. (1996). Some ruminative thoughts. In R. S. Wyer (Ed.), *Ruminative thoughts. Advances in social cognition* (Vol. 9, pp. 1–47). Hillsdale, NJ: Erlbaum.

McLaughlin, K. A., Borkovec, T. D., & Sibrava, N. J. (2007). The effects of worry and rumination on affect states and cognitive activity. *Behavior Therapy, 38,* 23–38.

McLaughlin, K. A., & Nolen-Hoeksema, S. (2011). Rumination as a transdiagnostic factor in depression and anxiety. *Behaviour Research and Therapy, 49,* 186–193.

Moberly, N. J., & Watkins, E. R. (2008). Ruminative thinking and negative affect: An experience sampling study. *Journal of Abnormal Psychology, 117,* 314–323.

Moberly, N. J., & Watkins, E. R. (2010). Negative affect and ruminative self-focus during everyday goal pursuit. *Cognition and Emotion, 24,* 729–739.

Mor, N., & Winquist, J. (2002). Self-focused attention and negative affect: A meta-analysis. *Psychological Bulletin, 128,* 638–662.

Morrison, A. P., & Wells, A. (2007). Relationships between worry, psychotic experiences and emotional distress in patients with schizophrenia spectrum diagnoses and comparisons with anxious and non-patient groups. *Behaviour Research and Therapy, 45,* 1593–1600.

Moulds, M. L., Kandris, E., Starr, S., & Wong, A. C. M. (2007). The relationship between rumination, avoidance and depression in a non-clinical sample. *Behaviour Research and Therapy, 45,* 251–261.

Moulds, M. L., Yap, C. S. L., Kerr, E., Williams, A. D., & Kandris, E. (2010). Metacognitive beliefs increase vulnerability to rumination. *Applied Cognitive Psychology, 24,* 351–364.

Muris, P., Meesters, C., Merckelbach, H., & Hulsenbeck, P. (2000). Worry in children is related to perceived parental rearing and attachment. *Behaviour Research and Therapy, 38,* 487–497.

Nelson, J. C., & Mazure, C. (1985). Ruminative thinking: A distinctive sign of melancholia. *Journal of Affective Disorders, 9,* 41–46.

Newman, M. G., & Borkovec, T. D. (2002). Cognitive behavioral therapy for worry and generalized anxiety disorder. In G. Simos (Ed.), *Cognitive behaviour therapy: A guide for the practicing clinician* (pp. 150–172). New York: Taylor & Francis.

Nolen-Hoeksema, S. (1991). Responses to depression and their effects on the duration of depressive episodes. *Journal of Abnormal Psychology, 100,* 569–582.

Nolen-Hoeksema, S. (2000). The role of rumination in depressive disorders and mixed anxiety/depressive symptoms. *Journal of Abnormal Psychology, 109,* 504–511.

Nolen-Hoeksema, S., McBride, A., & Larson, J. (1997). Rumination and psychological distress among bereaved partners. *Journal of Personality and Social Psychology, 72,* 855–862.

Nolen-Hoeksema, S., Morrow, J., & Fredrickson, B. L. (1993). Response styles and the duration of episodes of depressed mood. *Journal of Abnormal Psychology, 102,* 20–28.

Nolen-Hoeksema, S., Mumme, D., Wolfson, A., & Guskin, K. (1995). Helplessness in children of depressed and nondepressed mothers. *Developmental Psychology, 31,* 377–387.

Nolen-Hoeksema, S., Stice, E., Wade, E., & Bohon, C. (2007). Reciprocal relations between rumination and bulimic, substance abuse, and depressive symptoms in female adolescents. *Journal of Abnormal Psychology, 116,* 198–207.

Nolen-Hoeksema, S., & Watkins, E. R. (2011). A heuristic for developing transdiagnostic models of psychopathology: Explaining multifinality and divergent trajectories. *Perspectives in Psychological Science, 6,* 589–609.

Nolen-Hoeksema, S., Wisco, B. E., & Lyubomirsky, S. (2008). Rethinking rumination. *Perspectives in Psychological Science, 3,* 400–424.

Oatley, K., & Johnson-Laird, P. N. (1987). Towards a cognitive theory of emotions. *Cognition and Emotion, 1,* 29–50.

Papageorgiou, C., & Wells, A. (1999). Process and meta-cognitive dimensions of depressive and anxious thoughts and relationships with emotional intensity. *Clinical Psychology and Psychotherapy, 6,* 156–162.

Papageorgiou, C., & Wells, A. (2003). An empirical test of a clinical metacognitive model of rumination and depression. *Cognitive Therapy and Research, 27,* 261–273.

Pyszczynski, T., & Greenberg, J. (1987). Self-regulatory perseveration and the depressive self-focusing style: A self-awareness theory of reactive depression. *Psychological Bulletin, 102,* 122–138.

Ramel, W., Goldin, P. R., Carmona, P. E., & McQuaid, J. R. (2004). The effects of mindfulness meditation on cognitive processes and affect in patients with past depression. *Cognitive Therapy and Research, 28*, 433–455.

Rapee, R. M., & Heimberg, R. G. (1997). A cognitive-behavioral model of anxiety in social phobia. *Behaviour Research and Therapy, 35*, 741–756.

Rimes, K. A., & Watkins, E. (2005). The effects of self-focused rumination on global negative self-judgements in depression. *Behaviour Research and Therapy, 43*, 1673–1681.

Roberts, J. E., Gilboa, E., & Gotlib, I. H. (1998). Ruminative response style and vulnerability to episodes of dysphoria: Gender, neuroticism, and episode duration. *Cognitive Therapy and Research, 22*, 401–423.

Robinson, M. S., & Alloy, L. B. (2003). Negative cognitive styles and stress-reactive rumination interact to predict depression: A prospective study. *Cognitive Therapy and Research, 27*, 275–291.

Rottenberg, J., Gross, J. J., & Gotlib, I. H. (2005). Emotion context insensitivity in major depressive disorder. *Journal of Abnormal Psychology, 114*, 627–639.

Rusting, C. L., & Nolen-Hoeksema, S. (1998). Regulating responses to anger: Effects of rumination and distraction on angry mood. *Journal of Personality and Social Psychology, 74*, 790–803.

Schmaling, K. B., Dimidjian, S., Katon, W., & Sullivan, M. (2006). Response styles among patients with minor depression and dysthymia in primary care. *Journal of Abnormal Psychology, 111*, 350–356.

Segal, Z. V., Williams, J. M. G., & Teasdale, J. D. (2012). *Mindfulness-based cognitive therapy for depression* (2nd ed.). New York: Guilford Press.

Segerstrom, S. C., Stanton, A. L., Alden, L. E., & Shortridge, B. E. (2003). A multidimensional structure for repetitive thought: What's on your mind, and how, and how much? *Journal of Personality and Social Psychology, 85*, 909–921.

Segerstrom, S. C., Tsao, J. C. I., Alden, L. E., & Craske, M. G. (2000). Worry and rumination: Repetitive thought as a concomitant and predictor of negative mood. *Cognitive Therapy and Research, 24*, 671–688.

Siddique, H. I., LaSalle-Ricci, V. H., Glass, C. R., Arnkoff, D. B., & Diaz, R. J. (2006). Worry, optimism, and expectations as predictors of anxiety and performance in the first year of law school. *Cognitive Therapy and Research, 30*, 667–676.

Skitch, S. A., & Abela, J. R. Z. (2008). Rumination in response to stress as a common vulnerability factor to depression and substance abuse in adolescence. *Journal of Abnormal Child Psychology, 36*, 1029–1045.

Spasojevic, J., & Alloy, L. B. (2001). Rumination as a common mechanism relating depressive risk factors to depression. *Emotion, 1*, 25–37.

Spasojevic, J., & Alloy, L. B. (2002). Who becomes a depressive ruminator?: Developmental antecedents of ruminative response style. *Journal of Cognitive Psychotherapy: An International Quarterly, 16*, 405–419.

Stein, A., Lehtonen, A., Harvey, A. G., Nicol-Harper, R., & Craske, M. (2009). The influence of postnatal psychiatric disorder on child development: Is maternal preoccupation one of the key underlying processes? *Psychopathology, 42*, 11–21.

Stöber, J. (1998). Worry, problem elaboration and suppression of imagery: The role of concreteness. *Behaviour Research and Therapy, 36*, 751–756.

Stöber, J., & Borkovec, T. D. (2002). Reduced concreteness of worry in generalized anxiety disorder: Findings from a therapy study. *Cognitive Therapy and Research, 26*, 89–96.

Stöber, J., Tepperwien, S., & Staak, M. (2000). Worrying leads to reduced concreteness of problem elaborations: Evidence for the avoidance theory of worry. *Anxiety Stress and Coping, 13*, 217–227.

Szabo, M., & Lovibond, P. F. (2006). Worry episodes and perceived problem solving: A diary-based approach. *Anxiety Stress and Coping, 19*, 175–187.

Takano, K., & Tanno, Y. (2010). Concreteness of thinking and self-focus. *Consciousness and Cognition, 19*, 419–425.

Tallis, F., & Eysenck, M. W. (1994). Worry: Mechanisms and modulating influences. *Behavioural and Cognitive Psychotherapy, 22*, 37–56.

Teasdale, J. D. (1983). Negative thinking in depression: Cause, effect, or reciprocal relationship. *Advances in Behaviour Research and Therapy, 5*, 3–25.

Teasdale, J. D. (1988). Cognitive vulnerability to persistent depression. *Cognition and Emotion, 2*, 247–274.

Teasdale, J. D., Segal, Z. V., Williams, J. M. G., Ridgeway, V. A., Soulsby, J. M., & Lau, M. A. (2000). Prevention of relapse/recurrence in major depression by mindfulness-based cognitive therapy. *Journal of Consulting and Clinical Psychology, 68,* 615–623.

Verplanken, B., Friborg, O., Wang, C. E., Trafimow, D., & Woolf, K. (2007). Mental habits: Metacognitive reflection on negative self-thinking. *Journal of Personality and Social Psychology, 92,* 526–541.

Watkins, E. R. (2004a). Adaptive and maladaptive ruminative self-focus during emotional processing. *Behaviour Research and Therapy, 42,* 1037–1052.

Watkins, E. R. (2004b). Appraisals and strategies associated with rumination and worry. *Personality and Individual Differences, 37,* 679–694.

Watkins, E. R. (2008). Constructive and unconstructive repetitive thought. *Psychological Bulletin, 134,* 163–206.

Watkins, E. R. (2009). Depressive rumination: Investigating mechanisms to improve cognitive-behavioral treatments. *Cognitive Behaviour Therapy, 38,* 8–14.

Watkins, E. R. (2011). Dysregulation in level of goal and action identification across psychological disorders. *Clinical Psychology Review, 31,* 260–278.

Watkins, E. R., Baeyens, C. B., & Read, R. (2009). Concreteness training reduces dysphoria: Proof-of-principle for repeated cognitive bias modification in depression. *Journal of Abnormal Psychology, 118,* 55–64.

Watkins, E. R., & Baracaia, S. (2001). Why do people ruminate in dysphoric moods? *Personality and Individual Differences, 30,* 723–734.

Watkins, E. R., & Baracaia, S. (2002). Rumination and social problem-solving in depression. *Behaviour Research and Therapy, 40,* 1179–1189.

Watkins, E. R., & Brown, R. G. (2002). Rumination and executive function in depression: An experimental study. *Journal of Neurology, Neurosurgery, and Psychiatry, 72,* 400–402.

Watkins, E. R., Moberly, N. J., & Moulds, M. (2008). Processing mode causally influences emotional reactivity: Distinct effects of abstract versus concrete construal on emotional response. *Emotion, 8,* 364–378.

Watkins, E. R., & Moulds, M. (2005a). Distinct modes of ruminative self-focus: Impact of abstract versus concrete rumination on problem solving in depression. *Emotion, 5,* 319–328.

Watkins, E. R., & Moulds, M. (2005b). Positive beliefs about rumination in depression: A replication and extension. *Personality and Individual Differences, 39,* 73–82.

Watkins, E. R., & Moulds, M. (2007). Reduced concreteness in depression. *Personality and Individual Differences, 43,* 1386–1395.

Watkins, E. R., Moulds, M., & Mackintosh, B. (2005). Comparisons between rumination and worry in a non-clinical population. *Behaviour Research and Therapy, 43,* 1577–1585.

Watkins, E. R., Mullan, E. G., Wingrove, J., Rimes, K., Steiner, H., Bathurst, N., et al. (2011). Rumination-focused cognitive behaviour therapy for residual depression: Phase II randomized controlled trial. *British Journal of Psychiatry, 199,* 317–322.

Watkins, E. R., Scott, J., Wingrove, J., Rimes, K., Bathurst, N., Steiner, H., et al. (2007). Rumination-focused cognitive-behaviour therapy for residual depression: A case series. *Behaviour Research and Therapy, 45,* 2144–2154.

Watkins, E. R., Taylor, R. S., Byng, R., Baeyens, C. B., Read, R., Pearson, K., et al. (2012). Guided self-help concreteness training as an intervention for major depression in primary care: A Phase II randomized controlled trial. *Psychological Medicine, 42,* 1359–1373.

Watkins, E., & Teasdale, J. D. (2001). Rumination and overgeneral memory in depression: Effects of self-focus and analytic thinking. *Journal of Abnormal Psychology, 110,* 353–357.

Wells, A. (1995). Meta-cognition and worry: A cognitive model of generalized anxiety disorder. *Behavioural and Cognitive Psychotherapy, 23,* 301–320.

Wood, W., & Neal, D. T. (2007). A new look at habits and the habit–goal interface. *Psychological Review, 114,* 843–863.

Zeigarnik, B. (1938). On finished and unfinished tasks. In W. D. Ellis (Ed.), *A source book of gestalt psychology* (pp. 300–314). New York: Harcourt, Brace & World.

Zetsche, U., & Joormann, J. (2011). Components of interference control predict depressive symptoms and rumination cross-sectionally and at six months follow-up. *Journal of Behavior Therapy and Experimental Psychiatry, 42,* 65–73.

CHAPTER 22

Cognition and Emotion in Posttraumatic Stress Disorder

Thomas Ehring, Birgit Kleim, and Anke Ehlers

Posttraumatic stress disorder (PTSD) is a highly prevalent and disabling disorder with onset after traumatic experiences— for example, disasters, accidents, assaults, war experiences, or child sexual or physical abuse—with an estimated lifetime prevalence of 6–8% in the general population (Keane, Marshall, & Taft, 2006). According to the current classification systems, the disorder is characterized by symptoms of reexperiencing, avoidance, numbness, and hyperarousal (American Psychiatric Association, 2000).

The current volume focuses on the interaction between cognition and emotion. PTSD is an interesting disorder to study in this context as it comprises symptoms indicative of cognitive disturbances (e.g., intrusive memories, concentration problems, problems in recalling aspects of the trauma) as well as symptoms that point toward emotional dysregulation (e.g., emotional numbing, anger/irritability, increased startle responses). A number of cognitive and emotional processes have been suggested to underlie these symptoms. In the first part of this chapter we give an overview of research into PTSD from a cognitive perspective. In the second part results from research investigating emotion functioning and emotion regulation in trauma survivors are summarized. The chapter concludes with suggestions for

future research into cognition and emotion in PTSD. Table 22.1 gives an overview of the cognitive and emotional processes covered in our chapter.

PTSD from a Cognitive Perspective

Characteristics of Trauma Memories

Distressing intrusive memories of parts of the trauma are the most common form of reexperiencing in PTSD. These intrusive memories show a number of interesting characteristics (see Ehlers, Hackmann, & Michael, 2004). They mainly consist of brief sensory fragments of the trauma that pop into trauma survivors' mind unwantedly and often appear to come "out of the blue." Interviews with trauma survivors suggest that the intrusive memories are triggered by a particularly wide range of triggers. Although many characteristics of the intrusive memories do not distinguish between trauma survivors with and without PTSD, some features are associated with greater risk for PTSD (Michael, Ehlers, Halligan, & Clark, 2005). First, the degree to which the content of intrusive memories is experienced as if it were happening in the "here and now" (including the original emotions) predicts PTSD. In the most extreme form of reexperiencing, the dissociative flashback,

TABLE 22.1. Overview of PTSD-Related Cognitive and Emotional Processes

Cognitive processes	Emotional processes

Peritraumatic cognitive processing
  Dissocation
  Data-driven processing
  Lack of self-referential processing
	Peritraumatic emotions
	  Fear, helplessness, and horror
	  Other peritraumatic emotions
	  Arousal and panic symptoms

Trauma memory
  Disorganization and decontextualization
  Priming
	Reaction to emotions
	  Interpretation of symptoms
	  Emotion-based reasoning

Negative appraisals	Emotion regulation Awareness and understanding

Dysfunctional cognitive strategies
  Selective attention to threat
  Thought suppression
  Trauma-related rumination
	Acceptance
	  Impulse control
	  Use of emotion regulation strategies

trauma survivors with PTSD can even lose all contact with current reality and feel and behave as if the trauma were happening at that moment. Second, PTSD is predicted by the extent to which the content of the intrusive memory is experienced as disconnected from its context (Michael, Ehlers, Halligan, & Clark, 2005).

Frequent involuntary reexperiencing is not the only memory-related phenomenon in PTSD. Most trauma survivors with PTSD report some difficulties in remembering details of the event, such as its temporal order (e.g., Zoellner & Bittinger, 2004). Given the prominence of memory-related symptoms, different theorists have characterized PTSD as a "disorder of memory" (Brewin, 2011). It is thus not surprising that characteristics of the trauma memory are a central part of current theoretical models of PTSD (see Ehlers, Ehring, & Kleim, 2012). In the following sections, evidence regarding the role of memory in PTSD is summarized.

Peritraumatic Processing

Cognitive models of PTSD suggest that posttraumatic reexperiencing is due to the way in which the trauma is encoded while the event unfolds. Specifically, a number of theories converge in proposing that strong encoding of perceptual information in combination with relatively weak encoding of contextual information should lead to the development of intrusive memories (e.g., Brewin, Gregory, Lipton, & Burgess, 2010;

Ehlers & Clark, 2000). For example, Brewin and colleagues (2010) suggest that traumatic experiences are laid down in memory in two ways. On the one hand, these are sensation-based representations (termed *situationally accessible memories* in earlier versions of the theory) that are thought to be supported by early sensory cortical and subcortical areas and the insula. On the other hand, the trauma is stored in more abstract, conceptual, and contextually bound memories (formerly termed *verbally accessible memories*), supported by the medial temporal lobe system that stores declarative memory. According to this model, trauma-related flashbacks are due to a strong sensation-based memory representation, a weak contextually bound representation, and an impaired association between the two representations. As a consequence, these sensation-based representations can easily be activated, bottom-up, by situational cues without being inhibited by contextual representations of the trauma.

In a cognitive model Ehlers and Clark (2000) describe peritraumatic cognitive processes that are thought to put trauma survivors at risk for subsequent intrusive memories. These include data-driven processing (i.e., primarily processing sensory impressions) and lack of self-referential processing (i.e., the inability to link the traumatic experience to oneself and other self-referent autobiographical information). Other authors have suggested that peritraumatic dissociation contributes to the development of intrusive memories (e.g., van der Kolk &

Fisler, 1995). The concept of dissociation comprises a range of phenomena, including depersonalization, derealization, altered time perception, and emotional numbing, and it is often defined as a disturbance of the integrated organization of identity, memory, perception, and consciousness (Spiegel, 1997). Although the concept of dissociation has frequently been criticized on conceptual and empirical grounds (e.g., Candel & Merckelbach, 2004), there is extensive research investigating its role in the development of PTSD. Ehlers and Clark suggested that it may overlap at least partly with data-driven processing. From a cognitive perspective, data-driven processing, dissociation, and lack of self-referential processing are due to limited cognitive resources being available at the time of the trauma (Brewin et al., 2010; Ehlers & Clark, 2000).

In line with the theoretical ideas presented above, self-reported peritraumatic dissociation assessed shortly after the trauma has been found to be predict PTSD (for a meta-analysis see Ozer, Best, Lipsey, & Weiss, 2003). Similarly, self-reported levels of peritraumatic data-driven processing and lack of self-referential processing predicted future levels of PTSD in a series of prospective longitudinal studies (e.g., Ehring, Ehlers, Cleare, & Glucksman, 2008; Halligan, Michael, Clark, & Ehlers, 2003). Although these findings support cognitive models of PTSD, a problem with questionnaire measures is that it is unclear to what extent the peritraumatic processes of interest are open to introspection. In addition, as they are taken retrospectively, they may be biased, for example, by current levels of PTSD. Parallel results from analogue studies that induced intrusive memories experimentally are therefore informative. A series of studies using the trauma film paradigm showed that high levels of dissociation or data-driven processing assessed as a trait or state variable predicted more frequent intrusive memories in response to a distressing film (e.g., Halligan, Clark, & Ehlers, 2002; Kindt & van den Hout, 2003).

Holmes and colleagues had participants perform parallel tasks while watching a distressing film (e.g., Holmes, Brewin, & Hennessy, 2004). In line with the hypothesis that high levels of perceptual encoding and low levels of conceptual/contextual encoding lead to intrusive reexperiencing, these studies found that the performance of a concurrent visuospatial task reduced the frequency of subsequent intrusive memories, whereas a concurrent verbal task increased the frequency of intrusions. In subsequent studies, Holmes, James, Coode-Bate, and Deeprose (2009) extended these results by showing that the frequency of intrusive memories about a trauma film could even be modulated by secondary tasks conducted up to 4 hours after the film. A likely explanation for these findings is that the tasks interfered with memory consolidation processes.

Disorganization and Decontextualization of Trauma Memories

Several theorists of PTSD suggest that the peritraumatic cognitive processes described above lead to disturbances in the memory of the trauma, which in turn contribute to the development and maintenance of PTSD (see Brewin, 2011, for a general discussion on the effect of emotion on memory; see also Murray, Holland, & Kensinger, Chapter 9, this volume). The nature of this memory disturbance has been one of the most highly debated topics in the PTSD literature. A large part of this debate has centered around the question whether traumatic events can be completely forgotten (*traumatic amnesia*) but remembered again later on (*recovered memory*) as well as the role that *false memories* may play in this context. These issues are beyond the scope of this chapter (for recent reviews, see Brewin, 2007; Ehlers et al., 2012). Instead, we focus on the role of disturbances in the trauma memory in the development and maintenance of PTSD.

Although the general idea of trauma memory disturbance is part of many information-processing theories of PTSD, theories differ considerably regarding the exact nature and degree of disturbance proposed. In one of the strongest formulations, van der Kolk and Fisler (1995) postulated that trauma memories are fragmented and initially recollected in a sensory form "without any semantic representation" and "experienced primarily as fragments of the sensory components of the event" (p. 513). Other authors refer to milder forms of memory disturbances (often termed *memory disorganization*) that show as gaps in memory, lack of coherence, and/or problems remembering the temporal order of events (e.g., Foa & Riggs, 1993; Halligan et al., 2003). Some authors have questioned the fragmentation and memory disorganization concepts altogether (e.g., Rubin, Berntsen, & Bohni, 2008). They suggest that fragmentation might simply be an artifact of the method used, as every autobiographical memory encoding is incomplete and the recalled memory therefore fragmented in some way. Furthermore, these authors argue that memory characteristics observed in PTSD could instead be accounted for by well-known processes identified in cognitive psychology, such as attentional narrowing as a consequence of stress.

According to Ehlers and Clark (2000) and Brewin and colleagues (2010), both perspectives can be reconciled. Trauma memories in PTSD can indeed be understood by general memory processes identified in cognitive psychology and neuroscience; however, reexperiencing is explained by systematic differences in how the trauma is represented in memory in individuals with versus without PTSD. For example, Ehlers and Clark suggest that a lack of conceptual and self-referent processing during trauma should lead to relatively poor links between the worst moments of the trauma and other relevant information in autobiographical memory. Poor elaboration is thought to contribute to PTSD in three ways. First, it leads to a relative disorganization and confusion in recalling the trauma in some individuals with the disorder. Second, poor elaboration makes reexperiencing more likely as it leads to poor inhibition of cue-driven retrieval. Finally, poor elaboration contributes to problematic appraisals such as "I'm to blame for the event." Importantly, Ehlers and colleagues (2004) emphasized that poor elaboration would not be expected for the whole trauma memory, but mainly for the (subjectively) worst moments of the trauma that are later reexperienced. These moments are thought to include impressions and predictions that were present at the time of the trauma (e.g., "I'm going to die") that are disjointed in memory from other information that could otherwise be used to update or disconfirm these prediction (e.g., "I didn't die"). According to Ehlers and colleagues, the overall disorganization of the trauma memory may influence appraisals about

responsibility for the event, but is thought to be less relevant in predicting reexperiencing symptoms than the disorganization of the worst moments.

The hypothesis that trauma memories in PTSD are fragmented or disorganized has been investigated with a range of methods. A first group of studies used self-report questionnaires and interviews to assess memory fragmentation or disorganization. Most of these studies found associations between the self-reported degree of trauma memory disorganization and a diagnosis of PTSD and/or PTSD symptom severity (e.g., Engelhard, van den Hout, Kindt, Arntz, & Schouten, 2003; Halligan et al., 2003; but see also Berntsen, Willert, & Rubin, 2003, for discrepant results). However, it is unclear whether this higher level of memory disorganization in PTSD is *specific* for the memory of the trauma when compared to nontraumatic memories. Of the three studies that have used a two (trauma memory vs. nontraumatic memory) by two (diagnostic group) design to directly test this issue, none showed a significant interaction that would be expected if memory disorganization were indeed specific to remembering traumatic events (Jelinek, Randjbar, Seifert, Kellner, & Moritz, 2009; Megías, Ryan, Vaquero, & Frese, 2007; Rubin, Boals, & Berntsen, 2008). Studies comparing traumatic versus nontraumatic memories, regardless of participants' PTSD status, have produced inconclusive results (see Ehlers et al., 2012). In sum, the evidence from studies using self-report measures of memory disorganization is mixed. In addition, one may question whether trauma memory disorganization can reliably be assessed via self-report.

A second group of studies has therefore used objective measures to assess memory disorganization. Most studies have used a narrative coding method originally developed by Foa, Molnar, and Cashman (1995) to analyze transcripts of trauma narratives. Narratives are first divided into segments defined as one thought, action, or speech utterance. In a second step, each segment is coded by blind raters for indicators of (dis-)organization. Results from this line of research show that high levels of disorganization coded from the trauma narratives are related to a diagnosis of acute stress disorder (ASD) or PTSD and predict the severity of PTSD symptoms at follow-up (e.g., Halligan et al., 2003; Jones, Harvey, & Brewin, 2007). Similar results emerged in studies using a global observer rating of narrative disorganization (e.g., Buck, Kindt, van den Hout, Steens, & Linders, 2007) or a measure of reading level (Amir, Stafford, Freshman, & Foa, 1998; Gray & Lombardo, 2001), although the latter result may be due to differences in verbal intelligence (see Gray & Lombardo, 2001; for a review of evidence regarding low intelligence as a general risk factor for PTSD, see Buckley, Blanchard, & Neill, 2000). Jelinek and colleagues (2009) tested whether disorganization is specific to trauma memories in PTSD and analyzed narratives of the trauma and other events. In line with the disorganization hypothesis, participants with PTSD in this study showed significantly greater trauma memory disorganization than those without PTSD, whereas no group difference emerged for a nontrauma control narrative. These findings could not be replicated by Rubin (2011). However, it should be noted that the sample size was rather small in this study ($n = 15$ per cell) and comprised undergraduate students, both of which may have led to reduced power.

In sum, there is converging evidence from studies using different types of methodology that PTSD is related to higher levels of trauma memory disorganization. However, it remains unclear whether this is specific for the recollection of the trauma or may be due to third variables, such as general cognitive abilities. Unfortunately, methodological problems inherent in this line of research currently preclude strong conclusions, and different authors have recently made suggestions as to how these could be overcome in future research (see Brewin, 2007; Ehlers et al., 2012). In addition, it may also be necessary to refine the theoretical ideas regarding the nature of trauma recall. As described earlier, Ehlers and colleagues (2004) suggested that trauma memory disorganization and disjointedness of trauma memory from other autobiographical information may not be characteristic for the whole trauma memory, but specifically for the worst moments of the trauma that are later reexperienced in the form of intrusive memories. In line with this hypothesis, Evans, Ehlers, Mezey, and Clark (2007a) found that narratives of the

moments that were reexperienced were more disorganized than other segments of the trauma narrative that were not part of intrusive memories. Even stronger, in 23% of the cases these moments were not included in the narrative at all. This finding was partly replicated by Jelinek and colleagues (2010). Converging evidence comes from a study in which assault survivors with and without PTSD completed an autobiographical memory retrieval task during script-driven imagery of (1) the assault and (2) an unrelated negative event (Kleim, Wallott, & Ehlers, 2008). When listening to a taped imagery script of the worst moment of their assault, survivors with PTSD took longer to retrieve unrelated nontraumatic autobiographical information than those without PTSD, but not when listening to a taped script of the worst moment of another negative life event.

Priming

Intrusive memories of the trauma can be triggered by a wide range of stimuli that often show *perceptual* similarities with the intrusive content or stimuli that signaled the onset of the trauma/its worst moments (Michael, Ehlers, Halligan, & Clark, 2005). According to Ehlers and Clark (2000), implicit memory processes play an important role in this phenomenon. Specifically, the authors suggest that trauma survivors with PTSD show heightened perceptual priming for trauma-related stimuli. Priming is a form of implicit memory that comprises facilitated processing of a stimulus because the same stimulus, or a related one, has been processed before (Schacter, Dobbins, & Schnyder, 2004). High perceptual priming for stimuli that are present during the trauma can be expected to contribute to easy triggering of intrusive memories later on, as priming lowers the perceptual threshold and leads to a processing advantage for similar stimuli. Hence, such stimuli are more likely to be noticed than other stimuli in the environment and can trigger trauma memories through unintentional, cue-driven memory retrieval (Ehlers & Clark, 2000). The hypothesis has been supported by results from a series of experimental analogue studies, in which participants watched trauma and neutral picture stories. Subsequently, a picture identification task was used to assess perceptual priming for visual stimuli that had appeared in these stories. Stimuli that had been embedded in the traumatic picture stories were more strongly primed than those that had been part of the neutral stories (e.g., Ehlers, Michael, Chen, Payne, & Shan, 2006; Michael & Ehlers, 2007). In line with Ehlers and Clark's (2000) hypothesis, the degree of priming for objects from the trauma stories predicted the number of intrusive memories about the pictures stories that were experienced in the weeks following the session (Ehlers et al., 2006; Michael & Ehlers, 2007). Further support for the perceptual priming hypothesis comes from two recent studies with trauma survivors (Kleim, Ehring, & Ehlers, 2012). Accident survivors with PTSD identified trauma-related pictures, but not general threat pictures, with greater likelihood than neutral pictures. These results were replicated in a second study with assault survivors, and the relative processing advantage for trauma-related pictures additionally predicted PTSD 6 months later.

The studies described so far have focused on the role of heightened priming *during* the traumatic event. However, *posttrauma* priming has also been suggested to be relevant, as some trauma survivors may show greater priming for trauma-related cues they encounter in the aftermath of traumas than other survivors (see Ehlers et al., 2012). The enhanced priming would lead to processing advantages for these stimuli and thus extend the range of trauma-related cues that are preferentially processed and may serve as generalized potential triggers for PTSD-related symptoms such as intrusive memories, negative affect, or rumination about the trauma. This hypothesis has been tested in several cross-sectional studies using a range of different paradigms (e.g., word-stem completion test, perceptual word identification paradigm, white noise paradigm, visual clarity rating task). In most of these studies, trauma survivors with PTSD showed greater posttrauma priming for trauma-related stimuli than for neutral stimuli, whereas trauma survivors without PTSD did not show differential priming (e.g., Amir, Leiner, & Bomyea, 2010; Michael, Ehlers, & Halligan, 2005). However, other studies did not find such enhanced priming effects in PTSD (Golier, Yehuda, Lupien, & Harvey, 2003; McNally & Amir, 1996). The inconsistent results may be due in part to differences in the sensitivity of the paradigms used to assess priming. In the two studies with negative findings, standard priming tasks using verbal stimuli were used (e.g., a classic word stem completion task). The studies supporting the perceptual priming hypothesis, on the other hand, have either developed adapted versions of these tasks that can be expected to be more sensitive or used tasks with visual or acoustic instead of verbal stimuli.

Summary and Conclusions

A number of cognitive processes have been suggested to explain intrusive memories in trauma survivors with PTSD. There is converging evidence for the hypothesis that intrusive memories are due to the way in which the trauma is processed while it is unfolding; namely, strong encoding of perceptual information in combination with relatively weak encoding of contextual information. In addition, there is some support for the role of implicit memory processes, especially peritraumatic and posttraumatic perceptual priming, which may contribute to intrusive memories being easily triggered by a wide range of stimuli. The question whether explicit trauma recall is disorganized remains controversial, and more rigorous research on this issue is needed before any firm conclusions can be drawn.

It should be noted that researchers have identified additional memory alterations in PTSD that are not covered in this chapter (e.g., overgeneral autobiographical memory, impaired memory for neutral information; for reviews, see Brewin, 2011; Ehlers et al., 2012). In addition, there is extensive research investigating neural correlates of trauma memory characteristics in PTSD (see Rauch, Shin, & Phelps, 2006). However, these lines of research are beyond the scope of the current chapter.

Negative Appraisal and PTSD

Cognitive theories of PTSD emphasize the role of individual differences in the meanings people ascribe to the trauma as contributing to the development and maintenance of PTSD. Early theories suggested that pre-existing schemas of the world and the self are often shattered in the wake of a trauma, as the traumatic experience is incompatible with the assumptions individuals had before the trauma (e.g., Janoff-Bulman, 1992). Accordingly, posttraumatic stress symptoms are thought to reflect the struggle to reconcile these preexisting models with contradicting information of the traumatic experience. This hypothesis has been challenged by evidence showing that the experience of earlier trauma and prior PTSD are risk factors for the development of the disorder following a new trauma (Ozer et al., 2003). It therefore appears that negative trauma-related cognitions in PTSD may reflect either a confirmation or a shattering of previously held beliefs (see Foa & Riggs, 1993). Foa and colleagues stress two central beliefs shared by PTSD sufferers: namely, the view of the self as entirely incompetent and the world as entirely dangerous (Foa & Riggs, 1993). Ehlers and Clark (2000) suggested that persistent PTSD occurs if individuals process the traumatic experience and/or its consequences in a way that produces a sense of a serious current threat. The threat can be either internal (e.g., "The trauma shows that I'm a bad person"; "My reactions show that I'm going crazy") or external (e.g., "I'm going to be assaulted again"; "I can't trust other people").

The role of problematic appraisals about the meaning of the traumatic event and its aftermath has been tested in three types of studies. In the first and largest group of studies, self-report questionnaires, such as the Posttraumatic Cognitions Inventory (PTCI; Foa, Ehlers, Clark, Tolin, & Orsillo, 1999), were used to assess the individual's view of the self and the world. Results from a series of cross-sectional studies show that excessively negative appraisals of the trauma and/or its sequelae are indeed related to symptom levels and/or to a diagnosis of PTSD (e.g., Dunmore, Clark, & Ehlers, 1999; Foa et al., 1999; Steil & Ehlers, 2000). In addition, prospective longitudinal studies found that dysfunctional trauma-related appraisals measured shortly after the event predicted chronic PTSD (e.g., Ehlers, Mayou, & Bryant, 1998; Kleim, Ehlers, & Glucksman, 2007). Importantly, problematic appraisals were found to predict PTSD over and above initial symptom severity (Dunmore, Clark, & Ehlers, 2001; Ehlers et al., 1998)

and over and above what can be predicted from trauma severity and other known risk factors (e.g., Ehring, Ehlers, & Glucksman, 2008; Halligan et al., 2003).

In recent years, implicit measures have increasingly been used to assess functional appraisals in individuals with emotional disorders (see Wiers, Teachman, & De Houwer, 2007). Although PTSD theorists have emphasized the role of implicit trauma-related appraisals in the maintenance of PTSD, only a few studies have tested this idea. Engelhard, Huijding, van den Hout, and de Jong (2007) used an implicit association test (IAT) to assess implicit assumptions about self as vulnerable in soldiers before and after their deployment to Iraq. In line with cognitive appraisal models, a cross-sectional association between implicit representations of the self as vulnerable and PTSD was found postdeployment. However, IAT scores assessed pretrauma did not predict posttrauma psychopathology. The finding that individuals with PTSD show lower implicit self-evaluations than controls was replicated in a recent study with civilian trauma survivors (Roth, Steffens, Morina, & Stangier, 2012).

A final group of studies in this area investigated interpretation biases in PTSD. Studies asking participants to perform probability estimates found that individuals with PTSD or ASD overestimated the probability and cost of future negative events (e.g., Warda & Bryant, 1998; White, McManus, & Ehlers, 2008). Interestingly, this judgment bias was reduced after successful therapy, and ratings were similar to those of controls (White et al., 2008). A small number of additional studies used objective tasks to assess interpretation bias. Using a sentence completion task, Kimble and colleagues (2002) found that veterans with PTSD produced more trauma-related sentence endings than those without the disorder. In a different study using a homograph task, trauma survivors were found to show less inhibition of threatening meanings of homographs than traumatized participants without PTSD (Amir, Coles, & Foa, 2002).

In sum, there is strong evidence for the hypothesis that threatening appraisals of the trauma and its consequences maintain PTSD. Whereas most studies to date have focused on self-report questionnaires, recent research has additionally included objective or implicit measures of interpretations biases and trauma-related appraisals.

Dysfunctional Cognitive Strategies That Maintain PTSD

Although many trauma survivors experience some posttraumatic stress symptoms shortly after the trauma, most recover within the first weeks or months and only a minority continues to develop chronic PTSD (McFarlane, 2000). How can the maintenance of PTSD symptoms in the latter group be explained? As in other anxiety disorders, selective attention to threat and avoidance of trauma reminders are considered important mechanisms that maintain PTSD. Furthermore, trauma survivors with PTSD also frequently engage in cognitive avoidance strategies such as thought suppression and rumination. From a cognitive perspective, these strategies contribute to the maintenance of PTSD by preventing a modification of the trauma memory as well as a disconfirmation of excessively negative appraisals, which inhibits natural recovery and maintains the sense of current threat (Ehlers & Clark, 2000; Wells & Sembi, 2004).

Selective Attention to Threat in PTSD

Several information-processing theories of PTSD suggest that trauma survivors with PTSD show a selective attentional bias that automatically favors trauma-relevant information. This bias is thought to contribute to the generalized fear responses that people with PTSD show in a wide range of situations (e.g., Chemtob, Roitblat, Hamada, & Carlson, 1988), to make it more likely for the individual to detect potential triggers of intrusive memories (Ehlers & Steil, 1995), and to provide evidence for the individual's appraisal that the world is unsafe (Ehlers & Clark, 2000).

Most studies testing the hypothesis of a PTSD-specific attentional bias have used the emotional Stroop task, in which participants are asked to name the colors of trauma-related and control words. Delayed responses to trauma words are interpreted as an attentional bias to trauma-related material, as such a bias can be expected to interfere with color naming. Most reviews conclude that results from studies using the Stroop task support the presence of an attentional bias; trauma survivors with PTSD show greater interference when color-naming trauma-related words than those without PTSD, but not for other words (see Buckley et al., 2000; Constans, 2005). In addition, there is some evidence for the specificity of the Stroop effect, as only PTSD is related to this type of interference, whereas other disorders are not (e.g., Beck, Freeman, Shipherd, Hamblen, & Lackner, 2001; Sveen, Dyster-Aas, & Willebrand, 2009). A recent review, however, has called for caution regarding the emotional Stroop effect in PTSD (Kimble, Frueh, & Marks, 2009) and concluded that only 44% of the peer-reviewed literature actually find the emotional Stroop effect in PTSD. In addition, the Stroop task has been criticized because color-naming latencies in this task appear to be influenced by multiple processes; the task should therefore not be regarded as a pure measure of attentional processes (see Yiend, Barnicot, & Koster, Chapter 6, this volume).

Another group of studies has used the dot probe task, in which participants are required to respond to probes that occur in the same or a different spatial location as the experimental cues of interest. Attentional bias to threat shows via a faster response to probes that occur in the same spatial location as trauma-related cues. Studies using the dot probe task with trauma survivors have shown mixed results (e.g., Bryant & Harvey, 1997; Elsesser, Sartory, & Tackenberg, 2004). One possible explanation for the inconclusive pattern of results may be that attentional bias appears to be moderated by contextual factors, such as real-life threat (e.g., Constans, Vasterling, McCloskey, Brailey, & Mathews, 2004). In line with this hypothesis, Bar-Haim and colleagues (2010) found that imminence of war-related threat in Israeli participants moderated the results in a dot probe task. Participants who lived in a zone bordering the Gaza Strip, where limited time was available for seeking shelter from rocket attacks, showed an attentional bias away from threat in the dot probe task. Participants living outside this zone, on the other hand, displayed a bias toward threat. Results from a recent follow-up study by the same research group showed that an attentional bias away from threat in participants living in the imminent danger zone was related to PTSD symptom severity 1 year later (Wald et al., 2011).

Only a few studies to date have used eye tracking to assess attentional processes in PTSD. However, in a recent study with Iraq veterans high PTSD symptom severity was found to be associated with a trend for preferential attention to Iraq images compared to negative and neutral pictures (Kimble, Fleming, Bandy, Kim, & Zambetti, 2010).

Attentional biases identified in anxiety disorder include not only enhanced detection of threatening stimuli, but also difficulty disengaging from these stimuli and attentional avoidance (see Cisler & Koster, 2010). In line with these general findings, recent studies using visual search tasks for verbal cues suggest that trauma survivors with PTSD also show difficulty disengaging from trauma-related cues when compared to those without the disorder (e.g., Pineles, Shipherd, Mostoufi, Abramovitz, & Yovel, 2009; Pineles, Shipherd, Welch, & Yovel, 2007).

In sum, the relatively large literature on attentional bias to threat in PTSD has produced somewhat inconsistent findings. Whereas the majority of studies provides evidence for an attentional bias toward threat cues in PTSD, other studies point to avoidance. Recent neuroscience findings appear to suggest a biphasic response with initial attention to threat cues, followed by avoidance (e.g., Adenauer et al., 2010). However, more research is needed to test this idea and disentangle the processes of enhanced detection of, versus difficulty disengaging from, threat cues (for a more detailed discussion of this issue, see Ehlers et al., 2012).

Thought Suppression

Evidence for the hypothesis that the suppression of thoughts and memories related to the trauma is involved in the maintenance of PTSD comes from three lines of research. First, research using self-report measures of thought suppression has shown that PTSD is correlated with self-reported levels of suppressing trauma-related thoughts and memories (e.g., Bennett, Beck, & Clapp, 2009; Vázquez, Hervás, & Pérez-Sales, 2008) as well as a trait tendency to suppress unwanted thoughts in general (e.g., Amstadter & Vernon, 2008; Tull, Gratz, Salters, & Roemer, 2004). In addition, levels of thought suppression predicted PTSD in prospective longitudinal studies (Ehlers et al., 1998; Ehring et al., 2008b).

Second, experimental studies investigating the effects of thought suppression in trauma survivors with ASD or PTSD showed that experimentally induced suppression of trauma-related thoughts and/or memories leads to a rebound in intrusions (e.g., Amstadter & Vernon, 2006; Shipherd & Beck, 2005). There is initial evidence that suppressing neutral thoughts may also lead to an enhancement of trauma-related intrusions (Aikins et al., 2009).

A final group of studies used the trauma film paradigm, exposing healthy nontraumatized individuals to a film depicting traumatic experiences (e.g., accidents, rape). In line with the hypothesis that thought suppression maintains PTSD symptoms, it was found that the self-reported degree of suppressing film-related thoughts and memories was positively correlated with the number of film-related intrusions experienced in the days after the session (Nixon, Nehmy, & Seymour, 2007; Regambal & Alden, 2009). Results from analogue studies experimentally inducing thought suppression related to the film are more mixed. Whereas Davies and Clark (1998) found that participants who were instructed to suppress film-related thoughts subsequently reported significantly more intrusive memories regarding the film than those not suppressing the memories, this was not replicated by Buck, Kindt, and van den Hout (2009). A number of different explanations for these inconsistent findings are conceivable. First, they may be due to different control conditions used in these two studies (recording thoughts vs. conceptual processing). Alternatively, they may suggest that thought suppression is not always equally dysfunctional. Results from a series of studies suggest the presence of a stable individual difference factor regarding an individual's ability to successfully suppress negative thoughts (Nixon, Flood, & Jackson, 2007), which may be related to weak inhibitory control (Wessel, Overwijk, Verwoerd, & de Vrieze, 2008). Converging evidence comes from studies with survivors of real-life traumas, in which PTSD has been found to be related to impaired executive functioning, especially when trauma-related material is used (Polak, Witteveen, Reitsma, & Olff, 2012). Low thought suppression ability and/or weak cognitive control may therefore be a risk factor for the development of PTSD, especially when individuals frequently use this strategy for coping with trauma-related memories.

Trauma-Related Rumination

Trauma survivors with PTSD report frequent ruminative thoughts about the event, such as "Why did it happen to me" or "If only I'd . . ." (see also, Watkins, Chapter 21, this volume, for a general discussion on rumination). There is accumulating evidence that trauma-related rumination is phenomenologically and functionally different from intrusive memories. Intrusive memories are predominantly sensory experiences of short duration that represent the experience of the trauma itself, whereas rumination is predominantly described as a train of thoughts of longer duration that elaborate on the experience (e.g., Evans, Ehlers, Mezey, & Clark, 2007b; Speckens, Ehlers, Hackmann, Ruths, & Clark, 2007). According to cognitive theorists, rumination is seen as a form of cognitive avoidance because it focuses on *why* and *what if* types of questions instead of processing the memory of the trauma itself, and is therefore suggested to lead to the maintenance of PTSD symptoms (Ehlers & Clark, 2000; Wells & Sembi, 2004). This hypothesis is supported by results from cross-sectional studies showing that self-reported levels of trauma-related rumination are associated with PTSD (e.g., Michael, Halligan, Clark, & Ehlers, 2007; Moore, Zoellner, & Mollenholt, 2008). Importantly, results from prospective longitudinal studies show that rumination also predicts future PTSD, even when initial symptom levels are statistically controlled (e.g., Ehring, Frank, & Ehlers, 2008; Michael et al., 2007). This finding is in line with the idea that rumination maintains PTSD. The cross-sectional and prospective association between rumination and PTSD was also replicated when using an objective measure of trauma-related repetitive thinking; namely, the number of steps in an adapted version of the Catastrophizing Interview (CI; Ehring, Frank, & Ehlers, 2008). The CI asks participants to elaborate on a worrisome topic in an iterative procedure, and the degree of repetitive thinking is operationalized as the number of steps completed in the interview.

Results from a series of experimental studies shows that rumination is not just an epiphenomenon of PTSD, but appears to be causally involved in the maintenance of PTSD-like symptoms. The induction of rumination about a traumatically themed film led to significantly more analogue PTSD symptoms and/or a significantly slower recovery from the film than different control conditions (e.g., Wells & Papageorgiou, 1995; Zetsche, Ehring, & Ehlers, 2009). The same results were found when inducing rumination about a real-life distressing event (Ehring, Fuchs, & Kläsener, 2009).

Summary and Conclusions

Intrusive reexperiencing is often regarded as the core symptom cluster of PTSD. Several memory processes appear to be responsible for the easy triggering of intrusive memories in PTSD, especially a strong representation of perceptual information in combination with relatively weak elaboration and contextualization of the trauma memory and high perceptual priming for trauma-related stimuli during and after the trauma.

However, the cognitive processes described above do not account only for the "cognitive symptoms" of PTSD, such as intrusive memories or difficulties remembering parts of the trauma, but they are also thought to be involved in the maintenance of some of the "emotional symptoms" that are part of the PTSD diagnosis. First, many negative emotions experienced by trauma survivor can be expected to be the direct consequence of emotionally laden intrusive memories. Second, there is evidence that excessively negative appraisals of the trauma and/or its sequelae contribute to a sense of current threat and can trigger a range of negative emotions such as anxiety, anger, sadness, shame, or guilt. Finally, converging evidence from correlational and experimental studies suggests that trauma survivors with PTSD engage in dysfunctional cognitive coping strategies, such as thought suppression and rumination, which maintains negative trauma-related emotions. A further factor maintaining excessive levels of fear as well as hyperarousal symptoms in PTSD may be an attentional bias toward trauma-related information, although results on this factor are less clear.

Based on the evidence that cognitive processes play an important role in the maintenance of PTSD, psychological treatment approaches for the disorder focus on modifying these cognitive factors. First, effective treatments for PTSD include interventions aimed at the modification or elaboration of the trauma memory (e.g., via imaginal exposure; see Foa, Keane, & Friedman, 2000) or incorporating information that updates the meanings of the worst moments (Ehlers, Clark, Hackmann, McManus, & Fennell, 2005). In line with the view that a modification of the trauma memory is crucial for recovery from PTSD, trauma-focused treatments have been found to be more effective than non-trauma-focused treatments (Bisson et al., 2007). Second, many evidence-based treatments use cognitive strategies to modify negative trauma-related appraisals (e.g., Ehlers et al., 2005; Resick & Schnicke, 1993). Finally, techniques that directly target dysfunctional cognitive strategies, such as thought suppression or rumination, are part of cognitive therapy (Ehlers et al., 2005) as well as part of metacognitive therapy (Wells & Sembi, 2004) for PTSD.

PTSD from an Emotional Perspective

Overview

Whereas extensive research has examined the role of cognitive factors in PTSD, much less attention has been paid to emotional processes that may contribute to the disorder. One of the reasons may be that most research has focused on explaining reexperiencing symptoms as the core of the disorder. However, there is emerging research into the role of emotional processes in PTSD, to which we now turn.

Peritraumatic Emotions and the Development of PTSD

The DSM-IV definition of PTSD emphasizes the role of emotional responding during the trauma in the development of the disorder, in that PTSD can only be diagnosed if the individual has responded to the event with fear, helplessness, or horror (American Psychiatric Association, 2000). Although this criterion has been criticized on theoretical grounds (e.g., Brewin, Lanius, Novac, Schnyder, & Galea, 2009), results from extensive research show that high levels of negative emotions experienced during the trauma predict future PTSD (e.g., Hathaway, Boals, & Banks, 2011; Olde et al., 2005). In a meta-analysis of risk factors for PTSD, peritraumatic negative emotions showed the second highest effect size of all predictor variables under consideration (Ozer et al., 2003). However, in contrast to the DSM-IV definition, there is no empirical support for a special role of the three emotions (fear, helplessness, and horror) exclusively mentioned in the DSM; instead, other negative emotions, such as anger, shame, or guilt, appear to be equally predictive (see Resick & Miller, 2009).

Different pathways by which peritraumatic emotions may contribute to PTSD have been suggested. First, high levels of anxiety during the trauma are thought to lead to strong conditioned fear responses, which can then trigger anxiety and increased startle responses to trauma reminders (e.g., Keane, Zimering, & Caddell, 1985; Lanius, Frewen, Vermetten, & Yehuda, 2010). Second, trauma survivors often interpret their emotional response during the trauma in a negative way (e.g., feeling shame about not keeping calm but showing strong fear during the event), which in turn may increase the sense of current threat (e.g., "If it happens to me again, I may not be able to cope") (see Ehlers & Clark, 2000). Third, excessive levels of negative emotions and/or arousal during the trauma are thought to impair cognitive processing during the event and increase peritraumatic dissociation, which in turn puts individuals at risk for developing intrusive memories and PTSD (see our description of these processes earlier in this chapter). Whereas some authors suggest peritraumatic dissociation to be a defensive mechanism used by trauma survivors to protect themselves from the experience of negative emotions during trauma (e.g., van der Kolk & van der Hart, 1989), others have put forward more benign interpretations of this process—for example, as a physiological compensatory mechanism for high arousal (e.g., Sterlini & Bryant, 2002). In line with both views, peritraumatic emotions and peritraumatic arousal have been shown to be strongly correlated with levels of peritraumatic dissociation, and there is some evidence that dissociation may mediate the relationship between peritraumatic emotions and PTSD (e.g., Bryant et al., 2011; Olde et al., 2005).

Another line of research has specifically investigated the role of panic symptoms during the traumatic event. Results show that the experience of peritraumatic panic attacks not only increases the risk of developing subsequent panic disorder, but also the risk of developing ASD and/or PTSD (e.g., Bryant & Panasetis, 2001; Nixon, Resick, & Griffin, 2004). In addition, there is evidence that peritraumatic dissociation may be due at least partly to the experience of panic attacks during the trauma (e.g., Bryant & Panasetis, 2005).

Reactions to Emotions and Emotion-Based Reasoning in PTSD

Interview studies and clinical observations suggest that emotional states may be important triggers of intrusive memories (Ehlers et al., 2004). Furthermore, as Ehlers and Clark (2000) suggested, people with PTSD show negative interpretations of their emotional responses in the aftermath of a trauma (e.g., "My reactions since the event mean that I have permanently changed for the worse"; "Anger will make me go off the rails"). Results from a series of studies supported this hypothesis by showing that negative interpretations of symptoms and emotions, assessed via self-report questionnaires, are associated with PTSD cross-sectionally and predict chronic levels of PTSD prospectively (e.g., Ehring, Ehlers, & Glucksman, 2008; Halligan et al., 2003; Steil & Ehlers, 2000).

In two studies, Engelhard and colleagues further showed that trauma survivors with PTSD also make inferences about external threat on the basis of their symptoms (Engelhard, Macklin, McNally, van den Hout, & Arntz, 2001; Engelhard, van den Hout, Arntz, & McNally, 2002). They asked participants to rate the dangerousness of different scenarios, wherein objective danger (danger vs. safety) and individuals' subjective response (anxiety/intrusions present vs.

absent) were varied. Results showed that trauma survivors with PTSD rated scenarios as more dangerous if they were coupled with an anxiety response or intrusions, whereas those without PTSD based their ratings on objective danger only.

Emotion Functioning and Emotion Regulation in Trauma Survivors

In recent years, researchers have increasingly become interested in broader aspects of emotion functioning and emotion regulation in PTSD. One reason for this interest is the fact that a number of PTSD symptoms can be interpreted as consequences of either emotional underregulation (e.g., emotional reactivity to trauma reminders, increased irritability/anger, increased startle response) or emotional overregulation (e.g., emotional numbness). Frewen and Lanius (2006) even suggested that PTSD "is most appropriately conceptualized as a psychobiological disorder involving affect arousal dysregulation" (p. 206). Gratz and Roemer (2004) propose that emotion regulation, as relevant to emotional disorders, comprises four key areas: (1) awareness and understanding of one's emotions, (2) acceptance of negative emotions, (3) the ability to successfully engage in goal-directed behavior and control impulsive behavior when experiencing negative emotions, and (4) the ability to use situationally appropriate emotion regulation strategies. There is increasing evidence that PTSD is related to difficulties in all four areas. First, PTSD has been shown to be related to high levels of alexithymia (i.e., an inability to experience, identify, and express negative emotions; see Frewen, Dozois, Neufeld, & Lanius, 2008). Second, the disorder has been found to be correlated with heightened levels of experiential avoidance, fear of emotions, and lack of emotional acceptance (e.g., Kashdan, Morina, & Priebe, 2009; Tull, Jakupcak, McFadden, & Roemer, 2007). Third, trauma survivors with PTSD consistently report difficulties regulating their emotions and controlling impulsive behavior (e.g., Tull, Barrett, McMillan, & Roemer, 2007; van der Kolk, Roth, Pelcovitz, Sunday, & Spinazzola, 2005). Finally, PTSD is related to a frequent use of emotion regulation strategies that have been found to be dysfunctional (e.g., emotion suppression) and an infrequent use of functional strategies (e.g., cognitive reappraisal) (see Ehring & Quack, 2010; Moore et al., 2008). Deficits in emotion regulation in PTSD on a self-report and/or behavioral level are mirrored by neuroscience findings showing that trauma survivors with PTSD often show increased amygdala activation and decreased activation of areas involved in emotion regulation (see Frewen & Lanius, 2006; Rauch et al., 2006).

Most research into emotion regulation in PTSD points toward an *under*regulation of emotions, resulting in high levels of anxiety, anger, sadness, or shame. However, some PTSD symptoms, especially emotional numbing, are more indicative of an *over*regulation of emotions. Different accounts for processes that may underlie emotional numbing have been put forward. For example, it has been argued that emotional numbing is due to emotional depletion caused by hyperarousal; this view is supported by correlational and experimental evidence supporting a close link between hyperarousal and emotional numbing (see Litz & Gray, 2002). Alternatively, emotional numbing may be due to dissociative strategies individuals actively engage in to regulate their negative emotions (see Lanius, Frewen, et al., 2010; Lanius, Vermetter, et al., 2010). More research is needed to determine which of these alternative explanations is correct.

A number of theorists and clinicians have suggested that clinically relevant levels of emotion regulation difficulties are a specific feature of trauma-related disorders following early interpersonal trauma, which should require an adapted treatment approach for this group of survivors (e.g., van der Kolk et al., 2005). However, the empirical evidence for this hypothesis is mixed (see Ehring & Quack, 2010).

Summary and Conclusions

Research into the effects of emotional processes in trauma survivors is still sparse. However, studies have consistently found that peritraumatic negative emotions predict PTSD and may negatively impact on cognitive processing of the trauma. In addition, there is emerging evidence that negative emotions experienced in the aftermath of traumatic events influence cognitive processes (e.g., negative appraisals) via an emotion-based reasoning bias. Finally, PTSD has been shown to be associated with broad emotion regulation deficits. However, it is important to note that research in this area has mainly been cross-sectional and has almost exclusively used self-report questionnaires to assess characteristics of emotion functioning and emotion regulation. Prospective studies are needed to test whether emotion regulation actually predicts the onset and/or maintenance of PTSD. In addition, emerging lines of research testing trauma survivors' emotion regulation capacities and the effect of different emotion regulation strategies in the laboratory (e.g., Dalgleish, Yiend, Schweizer, & Dunn, 2009) and/or the investigation of emotion regulation in PTSD from a neuroscience perspective (e.g., Frewen, Lanius, et al., 2008) appear especially promising.

Conclusions and Future Directions

As detailed in this chapter, past research has identified a number of cognitive and emotional processes that appear to be involved in the development and maintenance of PTSD. Most of this research has thereby focused on processes that can account for cognitive symptoms in PTSD, especially intrusive reexperiencing. Much less in known about symptoms indicative of emotional dysregulation, such as emotional numbing, increased startle, or heightened irritability. In addition, very few studies have investigated the interaction between cognitive and emotional processes in PTSD. For example, it appears likely that heightened irritability in PTSD is due to a number of interacting processes; First, this may include characteristics of the trauma memory leading to frequent intrusive memories that can, in turn, trigger feelings of irritability and anger. Second, negative appraisals of the trauma and/or its consequences can be expected to contribute to feelings of irritability. Finally, lack of emotional acceptance and engagement in dysfunctional emotion regulation strategies can be expected to maintain symptoms of irritability and anger.

A number of avenues appear promising for future research into the roles of cognition and emotion in PTSD. First, PTSD has originally been conceptualized as an anxiety disorder, which is also reflected by its classification in the DSM-IV. However, there is increasing evidence that emotions other than anxiety play a key role within the disorder (see Resick & Miller, 2009). Future research is needed to identify cognitive processes linked to anxiety versus other emotions in PTSD. Second, there is extensive evidence showing that the individual's peritraumatic response is a strong predictor of future PTSD (Ozer et al., 2003). To date, there is hardly any evidence on how emotional, psychobiological, and cognitive processes interact during the traumatic event (see Ehring, Ehlers, Cleare, & Glucksman, 2008). Research explicitly combining these different areas of research can be expected to further improve our understanding on peritraumatic processes and may even lead to the development of innovative preventive interventions. Third, chronic PTSD has been shown to be related to heightened use of cognitive strategies that maintain the disorder, such as thought suppression and rumination. However, it is still unclear why trauma survivors engage in these strategies despite their clearly negative consequences. One intriguing hypothesis is that thought suppression and rumination may be due to a generalized lack of acceptance of negative emotions or high levels of experiential avoidance. Future research directly testing the interaction between emotional dysregulation and cognitive coping strategies in the maintenance of PTSD therefore appears promising.

Finally, research focusing on the interaction between cognitive and emotional factors in PTSD may also have important clinical implications. For example, it has been argued that anger should be targeted directly in the treatment of combat-related PTSD (e.g., Novaco & Chemtob, 2002). In addition, based on the observation that survivors of chronic interpersonal trauma experienced early in childhood (e.g., sexual or physical abuse) often report difficulties with emotion regulation and impulse control, some researchers and clinicians have suggested that evidence-based treatments for PTSD need to be adapted for this group (e.g., Ford, Courtois, Steele, van der Hart, & Nijenhuis, 2005). Specifically, these authors propose that a phase-based treatment is needed, whereby interventions in the first phase are aimed at improving the individual's emotion regulation capacity before trauma-focused treatment takes place in the second phase. The evidence base for this suggestion is still unsatisfactory (although see Cloitre et al., 2010). More research is needed to investigate the exact nature and extent of emotion regulation difficulties in PTSD as well as their relationship with cognitive processes. This may include an investigation as to whether emotion regulation difficulties reported by trauma survivors should best be conceptualized as broad deficits in regulating negative emotional states in general or as specific deficits in regulating negative emotions triggered by trauma reminders as reflected in the PTSD diagnostic criteria. In addition, research testing the effects of skills training, emotion-focused techniques, imaginal exposure *in vivo* or virtual reality exposure, and cognitive therapy on emotion dysregulation in PTSD is needed.

References

Adenauer, H., Pinösch, S., Catani, C., Gola, H., Keil, J., Kißler, J., et al. (2010). Early processing of threat cues in posttraumatic stress disorder: Evidence for a cortical vigilance–avoidance reaction. *Biological Psychiatry, 68,* 451–458.

Aikins, D. E., Johnson, D. C., Borelli, J. L., Klemanski, D. H., Morrissey, P. M., Benham, T. L., et al. (2009). Thought suppression failures in combat PTSD: A cognitive load hypothesis. *Behaviour Research and Therapy, 47,* 744–751.

American Psychiatric Association. (2000). *Diagnostic and statistical manual of mental disorders* (4th ed., text rev.). Washington, DC: Author.

Amir, N., Coles, M. E., & Foa, E. B. (2002). Automatic and strategic activation and inhibition of threat-relevant information in posttraumatic stress disorder. *Cognitive Therapy and Research, 26,* 645–655.

Amir, N., Leiner, A. S., & Bomyea, J. (2010). Implicit memory and posttraumatic stress symptoms. *Cognitive Therapy and Research, 34,* 49–58.

Amir, N., Stafford, J., Freshman, M. S., & Foa, E. B. (1998). Relationship between trauma narratives and trauma pathology. *Journal of Traumatic Stress, 11,* 385–392.

Amstadter, A. B., & Vernon, L. L. (2006). Suppression of neutral and trauma targets: Implications for posttraumatic stress disorder. *Journal of Traumatic Stress, 19*, 517–526.

Amstadter, A. B., & Vernon, L. L. (2008). A preliminary examination of thought suppression, emotion regulation, and coping in a trauma-exposed sample. *Journal of Aggression, Maltreatment and Trauma, 17*, 279–295.

Bar-Haim, Y., Holoshitz, Y., Eldar, S., Frenkel, T. I., Muller, D., Charney, D. S., et al. (2010). Life-threatening danger and suppression of attention bias to threat. *American Journal of Psychiatry, 167*, 694–698.

Beck, J. G., Freeman, J. B., Shipherd, J. C., Hamblen, J. L., & Lackner, J. M. (2001). Specificity of stroop interference in patients with pain and PTSD. *Journal of Abnormal Psychology, 110*, 536–543.

Bennett, S. A., Beck, J. G., & Clapp, J. D. (2009). Understanding the relationship between posttraumatic stress disorder and trauma cognitions: The impact of thought control strategies. *Behaviour Research and Therapy, 47*, 1018–1023.

Berntsen, D., Willert, M., & Rubin, D. C. (2003). Splintered memories or vivid landmarks?: Qualities and organization of traumatic memories with and without PTSD. *Applied Cognitive Psychology, 17*, 675–693.

Bisson, J. I., Ehlers, A., Matthews, R., Pilling, S., Richards, D., & Turner, S. (2007). Psychological treatments for chronic post-traumatic stress disorder: Systematic review and meta-analysis. *British Journal of Psychiatry, 190*, 97–104.

Brewin, C. R. (2007). Autobiographical memory for trauma: Update on four controversies. *Memory, 15*, 227–248.

Brewin, C. R. (2011). The nature and significance of memory disturbance in posttraumatic stress disorder. *Annual Review of Clinical Psychology, 7*, 203–227.

Brewin, C. R., Gregory, J. D., Lipton, M., & Burgess, N. (2010). Intrusive images in psychological disorders: Characteristics, neural mechanisms, and treatment implications. *Psychological Review, 117*, 210–232.

Brewin, C. R., Lanius, R. A., Novac, A., Schnyder, U., & Galea, S. (2009). Reformulating PTSD for DSM-V: Life after Criterion A. *Journal of Traumatic Stress, 22*, 366–373.

Bryant, R. A., Brooks, R., Silove, D., Creamer, M., O'Donnell, M., & McFarlane, A. C. (2011). Peritraumatic dissociation mediates the relationship between acute panic and chronic posttraumatic stress disorder. *Behaviour Research and Therapy, 49*, 346–351.

Bryant, R. A., & Harvey, A. G. (1997). Attentional bias in posttraumatic stress disorder. *Journal of Traumatic Stress, 10*, 635–644.

Bryant, R. A., & Panasetis, P. (2001). Panic symptoms during trauma and acute stress disorder. *Behaviour Research and Therapy, 39*, 961–966.

Bryant, R. A., & Panasetis, P. (2005). The role of panic in acute dissociative reactions following trauma. *British Journal of Clinical Psychology, 44*, 489–494.

Buck, N., Kindt, M., & van den Hout, M. (2009). The effects of conceptual processing versus suppression on analogue PTSD symptoms after a distressing film. *Behavioural and Cognitive Psychotherapy, 37*, 195–206.

Buck, N., Kindt, M., van den Hout, M., Steens, L., & Linders, C. (2007). Perceptual memory representations and memory fragmentation as predictors of post-trauma symptoms. *Behavioural and Cognitive Psychotherapy, 35*, 259–272.

Buckley, T. C., Blanchard, E. B., & Neill, W. T. (2000). Information processing and PTSD: A review of the empirical literature. *Clinical Psychology Review, 28*, 1041–1065.

Candel, I., & Merckelbach, H. (2004). Peritraumatic dissociation as a predictor of posttraumatic stress disorder: A critical review. *Comprehensive Psychiatry, 45*, 44–50.

Chemtob, C. M., Roitblat, H. L., Hamada, R. S., & Carlson, J. G. (1988). A cognitive action theory of post-traumatic stress disorder. *Journal of Anxiety Disorders, 2*, 253–275.

Cisler, J. M., & Koster, E. H. W. (2010). Mechanisms of attentional biases towards threat in anxiety disorders: An integrative review. *Clinical Psychology Review, 30*, 203–216.

Cloitre, M., Stovall-McClough, K. C., Nooner, K., Zorbas, P., Cherry, S., Jackson, C. L., et al. (2010). Treatment for PTSD related to childhood abuse: A randomized controlled trial. *American Journal of Psychiatry, 167*, 915–924.

Constans, J. I. (2005). Information-processing biases in PTSD. In J. J. Vasterling & C. R. Brewin (Eds.), *Neuropsychology of PTSD: Biological, cognitive, and clinical perspectives* (pp. 105–130). New York: Guilford Press.

Constans, J. I., Vasterling, J. J., McCloskey, M. S., Brailey, K., & Mathews, A. (2004). Suppression of attentional bias in PTSD. *Journal of Abnormal Psychology, 113*, 315–323.

Dalgleish, T., Yiend, J., Schweizer, S., & Dunn, B. D. (2009). Ironic effects of emotion suppression when recounting distressing memories. *Emotion, 9,* 744–749.

Davies, M. I., & Clark, D. M. (1998). Thought suppression produces a rebound effect with analogue post-traumatic intrusions. *Behaviour Research and Therapy, 36,* 571–582.

Dunmore, E., Clark, D. M., & Ehlers, A. (1999). Cognitive factors involved in the onset and maintenance of posttraumatic stress disorder (PTSD) after physical or sexual assault. *Behaviour Research and Therapy, 37,* 809–829.

Dunmore, E., Clark, D. M., & Ehlers, A. (2001). A prospective investigation of the role of cognitive factors in persistent posttraumatic stress disorder (PTSD) after physical or sexual assault. *Behaviour Research and Therapy, 39,* 1063–1084.

Ehlers, A., & Clark, D. M. (2000). A cognitive model of posttraumatic stress disorder. *Behaviour Research and Therapy, 38,* 319–345.

Ehlers, A., Clark, D. M., Hackmann, A., McManus, F., & Fennell, M. (2005). Cognitive therapy for post-traumatic stress disorder: Development and evaluation. *Behaviour Research and Therapy, 43,* 413–431.

Ehlers, A., Ehring, T., & Kleim, B. (2012). Information processing in posttraumatic stress disorder. In J. G. Beck & D. Sloane (Eds.), *The Oxford handbook of traumatic stress disorders* (pp. 119–218). New York: Oxford University Press.

Ehlers, A., Hackmann, A., & Michael, T. (2004). Intrusive re-experiencing in post-traumatic stress disorder: Phenomenology, theory, and therapy. *Memory, 12,* 403–415.

Ehlers, A., Mayou, R. A., & Bryant, B. (1998). Psychological predictors of chronic posttraumatic stress disorder after motor vehicle accidents. *Journal of Abnormal Psychology, 107,* 508–519.

Ehlers, A., Michael, T., Chen, Y. P., Payne, E., & Shan, S. (2006). Enhanced perceptual priming for neutral stimuli in a traumatic context: A pathway to intrusive memories? *Memory, 14,* 316–328.

Ehlers, A., & Steil, R. (1995). Maintenance of intrusive memories in posttraumatic stress disorder: A cognitive approach. *Behavioural and Cognitive Psychotherapy, 23,* 217–249.

Ehring, T., Ehlers, A., Cleare, A. J., & Glucksman, E. (2008). Do acute psychological and psychobiological responses to trauma predict subsequent symptom severities of PTSD and depression? *Psychiatry Research, 161,* 67–75.

Ehring, T., Ehlers, A., & Glucksman, E. (2008). Do cognitive models help in predicting the severity of posttraumatic stress disorder, phobia, and depression after motor vehicle accidents?: A prospective longitudinal study. *Journal of Consulting and Clinical Psychology, 76,* 219–230.

Ehring, T., Frank, S., & Ehlers, A. (2008). The role of rumination and reduced concreteness in the maintenance of posttraumatic stress disorder and depression following trauma. *Cognitive Therapy and Research, 32,* 488–506.

Ehring, T., Fuchs, N., & Kläsener, I. (2009). The effects of experimentally induced rumination versus distraction on analogue posttraumatic stress symptoms. *Behavior Therapy, 40,* 403–413.

Ehring, T., & Quack, D. (2010). Emotion regulation difficulties in trauma survivors: The role of trauma type and PTSD symptom severity. *Behavior Therapy, 41,* 587–598.

Elsesser, K., Sartory, G., & Tackenberg, A. (2004). Attention, heart rate, and startle response during exposure to trauma-relevant pictures: A comparison of recent trauma victims and patients with posttraumatic stress disorder. *Journal of Abnormal Psychology, 113,* 289–301.

Engelhard, I. M., Huijding, J., van den Hout, M. A., & de Jong, P. J. (2007). Vulnerability associations and symptoms of post-traumatic stress disorder in soldiers deployed to Iraq. *Behaviour Research and Therapy, 45,* 2317–2325.

Engelhard, I. M., Macklin, M. L., McNally, R. J., van den Hout, M. A., & Arntz, A. (2001). Emotion- and intrusion-based reasoning in Vietnam veterans with and without chronic posttraumatic stress disorder. *Behaviour Research and Therapy, 39,* 1339–1348.

Engelhard, I. M., van den Hout, M. A., Arntz, A., & McNally, R. J. (2002). A longitudinal study of "intrusion-based reasoning" and posttraumatic stress disorder after exposure to a train disaster. *Behaviour Research and Therapy, 40,* 1415–1424.

Engelhard, I. M., van den Hout, M. A., Kindt, M., Arntz, A., & Schouten, E. (2003). Peritraumatic dissociation and posttraumatic stress after pregnancy loss: A prospective study. *Behaviour Research and Therapy, 41,* 67–78.

Evans, C., Ehlers, A., Mezey, G., & Clark, D. M.

(2007a). Intrusive memories in perpetrators of violent crime: Emotions and cognitions. *Journal of Consulting and Clinical Psychology, 75*, 134–144.

Evans, C., Ehlers, A., Mezey, G., & Clark, D. M. (2007b). Intrusive memories and ruminations related to violent crime among young offenders: Phenomenological characteristics. *Journal of Traumatic Stress, 20*, 183–196.

Foa, E. B., Ehlers, A., Clark, D. M., Tolin, D. F., & Orsillo, S. M. (1999). The Posttraumatic Cognitions Inventory (PTCI): Development and validation. *Psychological Assessment, 11*, 303–314.

Foa, E. B., Keane, T. M., & Friedman, M. J. (Eds.). (2000). *Effective treatments for PTSD: Practice guidelines from the International Society of Traumatic Stress Studies.* New York: Guilford Press.

Foa, E. B., Molnar, C., & Cashman, L. (1995). Change in rape narratives during exposure therapy for posttraumatic stress disorder. *Journal of Traumatic Stress, 8*, 675–690.

Foa, E. B., & Riggs, D. S. (1993). Posttraumatic stress disorder and rape. In J. M. Oldham, M. B. Riba, & A. Tasman (Eds.), *American Psychiatric Press review of psychiatry* (pp. 273–303). Washington, DC: American Psychiatric Association.

Ford, J. D., Courtois, C. A., Steele, K., van der Hart, O., & Nijenhuis, E. R. S. (2005). Treatment of complex posttraumatic self-dysregulation. *Journal of Traumatic Stress, 18*, 437–447.

Frewen, P. A., Dozois, D. J. A., Neufeld, R. W. J., & Lanius, R. A. (2008). Meta-analysis of alexithymia in posttraumatic stress disorder. *Journal of Traumatic Stress, 21*, 243–246.

Frewen, P. A., & Lanius, R. A. (2006). Toward a psychobiology of posttraumatic self-dysregulation: Reexperiencing, hyperarousal, dissociation, and emotional numbing. *Annals of the New York Academy of Sciences, 1071*, 110–124.

Frewen, P. A., Lanius, R. A., Dozois, D. J. A., Neufeld, R. W. J., Pain, C., Hopper, J. W., et al. (2008). Clinical and neural correlates of alexithymia in posttraumatic stress disorder. *Journal of Abnormal Psychology, 117*, 171–181.

Golier, J. A., Yehuda, R., Lupien, S. J., & Harvey, P. D. (2003). Memory for trauma-related information in Holocaust survivors with PTSD. *Psychiatry Research, 121*, 133–143.

Gratz, K. L., & Roemer, L. (2004). Multidimensional assessment of emotion regulation and dysregulation: Development, factor structure, and initial validation of the Difficulties in Emotion Regulation Scale. *Journal of Psychopathology and Behavioral Assessment, 26*, 41–54.

Gray, M. J., & Lombardo, T. W. (2001). Complexity of trauma narratives as an index of fragmented memory in PTSD: A critical analysis. *Applied Cognitive Psychology, 15*, S171–S186.

Halligan, S. L., Clark, D. M., & Ehlers, A. (2002). Cognitive processing, memory, and the development of PTSD symptoms: Two experimental analogue studies. *Journal of Behavior Therapy and Experimental Psychiatry, 33*, 73–89.

Halligan, S. L., Michael, T., Clark, D. M., & Ehlers, A. (2003). Posttraumatic stress disorder following assault: The role of cognitive processing, trauma memory, and appraisals. *Journal of Consulting and Clinical Psychology, 71*, 419–431.

Hathaway, L. M., Boals, A., & Banks, J. B. (2011). PTSD symptoms and dominant emotional response to a traumatic event: An examination of DSM-IV Criterion A2. *Anxiety, Stress, and Coping, 23*, 119–126.

Holmes, E. A., Brewin, C. R., & Hennessy, R. G. (2004). Trauma films, information processing, and intrusive memory development. *Journal of Experimental Psychology: General, 133*, 3–22.

Holmes, E. A., James, E. L., Coode-Bate, T., & Deeprose, C. (2009). Can playing the computer game "Tetris" reduce the build-up of flashbacks for trauma?: A proposal from cognitive science. *PLoS ONE, 4*, e4153.

Janoff-Bulman, R. (1992). *Shattered assumptions: Towards a new psychology of trauma.* New York: Free Press.

Jelinek, L., Randjbar, S., Seifert, D., Kellner, M., & Moritz, S. (2009). The organization of autobiographical and nonautobiographical memory in posttraumatic stress disorder (PTSD). *Journal of Abnormal Psychology, 118*, 288–298.

Jelinek, L., Stockbauer, C., Randjbar, S., Kellner, M., Ehring, T., & Moritz, S. (2010). Characteristics and organization of the worst moment of trauma memories in posttraumatic stress disorder. *Behaviour Research and Therapy, 48*, 680–685.

Jones, C., Harvey, A. G., & Brewin, C. R. (2007). The organisation and content of trauma memories in survivors of road traffic accidents. *Behaviour Research and Therapy, 45*, 151–162.

Kashdan, T. B., Morina, N., & Priebe, S. (2009). Post-traumatic stress disorder, social anxiety disorder, and depression in survivors of the Kosovo War: Experiential avoidance as a contributor to distress and quality of life. *Journal of Anxiety Disorders, 23*, 185–196.

Keane, T. M., Marshall, A. D., & Taft, C. T. (2006). Posttraumatic stress disorder: Etiology, epidemiology, and treatment outcome. *Annual Review of Clinical Psychology, 2*, 161–197.

Keane, T. M., Zimering, R. T., & Caddell, J. M. (1985). A behavioral formulation of posttraumatic stress disorder in Vietnam veterans. *Behavior Therapist, 8*, 9–12.

Kimble, M. O., Fleming, K., Bandy, C., Kim, J., & Zambetti, A. (2010). Eye tracking and visual attention to threating stimuli in veterans of the Iraq war. *Journal of Anxiety Disorders, 24*, 293–299.

Kimble, M. O., Frueh, B. C., & Marks, L. (2009). Does the modified Stroop effect exist in PTSD?: Evidence from dissertation abstracts and the peer-reviewed literature. *Journal of Anxiety Disorders, 23*, 650–655.

Kimble, M. O., Kaufman, M. L., Leonard, L. L., Nestor, P. G., Riggs, D. S., Kaloupek, D. G., et al. (2002). Sentence completion test in combat veterans with and without PTSD: Preliminary findings. *Psychiatry Research, 113*, 303–307.

Kindt, M., & van den Hout, M. (2003). Dissociation and memory fragmentation: Experimental effects on meta-memory but not on actual memory performance. *Behaviour Research and Therapy, 41*, 167–178.

Kleim, B., Ehlers, A., & Glucksman, E. (2007). Early predictors of chronic post-traumatic stress disorder in assault survivors. *Psychological Medicine, 37*, 1457–1468.

Kleim, B., Ehring, T., & Ehlers, A. (2012). Perceptual processing advantages for trauma-related visual cues in post-traumatic stress disorder. *Psychological Medicine, 42*, 173–181.

Kleim, B., Wallott, F., & Ehlers, A. (2008). Are trauma memories disjointed from other autobiographical memories in posttraumatic stress disorder?: An experimental investigation. *Behavioural and Cognitive Psychotherapy, 36*, 221–234.

Lanius, R. A., Frewen, P. A., Vermetten, E., & Yehuda, R. (2010). Fear conditioning and early life vulnerabilities: Two distinct pathways of emotional dysregulation and brain dysfunction in PTSD. *European Journal of Psychotraumatology, 1*, 5467.

Lanius, R. A., Vermetten, E., Loewenstein, R. J., Brand, B., Schmahl, C., Bremner, J. D., et al. (2010). Emotion modulation in PTSD: Clinical and neurobiological evidence for a dissociative subtype. *American Journal of Psychiatry, 167*, 640–647.

Litz, B. T., & Gray, M. J. (2002). Emotional numbing in posttraumatic stress disorder: Current and future research directions. *Australian and New Zealand Journal of Psychiatry, 36*, 198–204.

McFarlane, A. C. (2000). Posttraumatic stress disorder: A model of the longitudinal course and the role of risk factors. *Journal of Clinical Psychiatry, 61*(Suppl. 5), 15–21.

McNally, R. J., & Amir, N. (1996). Perceptual implicit memory for trauma-related information in post-traumatic stress disorder. *Cognition and Emotion, 10*, 551–556.

Megías, J. L., Ryan, E., Vaquero, J. M. M., & Frese, B. (2007). Comparisons of traumatic and positive memories in people with and without PTSD profile. *Applied Cognitive Psychology, 21*, 117–130.

Michael, T., & Ehlers, A. (2007). Enhanced perceptual priming for neutral stimuli occurring in a traumatic context: Two experimental investigations. *Behaviour Research and Therapy, 45*, 341–358.

Michael, T., Ehlers, A., & Halligan, S. L. (2005). Enhanced priming for trauma-related material in posttraumatic stress disorder. *Emotion, 5*, 103–112.

Michael, T., Ehlers, A., Halligan, S. L., & Clark, D. M. (2005). Unwanted memories of assault: What intrusion characteristics are associated with PTSD? *Behaviour Research and Therapy, 43*, 613–628.

Michael, T., Halligan, S. L., Clark, D. M., & Ehlers, A. (2007). Rumination in posttraumatic stress disorder. *Depression and Anxiety, 24*, 307–317.

Moore, S. A., Zoellner, L. A., & Mollenholt, N. (2008). Are expressive suppression and cognitive reappraisal associated with stress-related symptoms? *Behaviour Research and Therapy, 46*, 993–1000.

Nixon, R. D. V., Flood, J., & Jackson, K. (2007). The generalizability of thought suppression ability to novel stimuli. *Personality and Individual Differences, 42*, 677–687.

Nixon, R. D. V., Nehmy, T., & Seymour, M.

(2007). The effect of cognitive load and hyperarousal on negative intrusive memories. *Behaviour Research and Therapy, 45*, 2652–2663.

Nixon, R. D. V., Resick, P. A., & Griffin, M. G. (2004). Panic following trauma: The etiology of acute posttraumatic arousal. *Journal of Anxiety Disorders, 18*, 193–210.

Novaco, R. W., & Chemtob, C. M. (2002). Anger and combat-related posttraumatic stress disorder. *Journal of Traumatic Stress, 15*, 123–132.

Olde, E., van der Hart, O., Kieber, R. J., van Son, M. J. M., Wijnen, H. A. A., & Pop, V. J. M. (2005). Peritraumatic dissociation and emotions as predictors of PTSD symptoms following childbirth. *Journal of Trauma and Dissociation, 6*, 125–142.

Ozer, E. J., Best, S. R., Lipsey, T. L., & Weiss, D. S. (2003). Predictors of posttraumatic stress disorder and symptoms in adults: A meta-analysis. *Psychological Bulletin, 129*, 52–73.

Pineles, S. L., Shipherd, J. C., Mostoufi, S. M., Abramovitz, S. M., & Yovel, I. (2009). Attentional biases in PTSD: More evidence for interference. *Behaviour Research and Therapy, 47*, 1050–1057.

Pineles, S. L., Shipherd, J. C., Welch, L. P., & Yovel, I. (2007). The role of attentional biases in PTSD: Is it interference or facilitation? *Behaviour Research and Therapy, 45*, 1903–1913.

Polak, A. R., Witteveen, A. B., Reitsma, J. B., & Olff, M. (2012). The role of executive function in posttraumatic stress disorder: A systematic review. *Journal of Affective Disorders, 141*, 11–21.

Rauch, S. L., Shin, L. M., & Phelps, E. A. (2006). Neurocircuitry models of posttraumatic stress disorder and extinction: Human neuroimaging research—past, present, and future. *Biological Psychiatry, 60*, 376–382.

Regambal, M. J., & Alden, L. E. (2009). Pathways to intrusive memories in a trauma analogue paradigm: A structural equation model. *Depression and Anxiety, 26*, 155–166.

Resick, P. A., & Miller, M. W. (2009). Posttraumatic stress disorder: Anxiety or traumatic stress disorder? *Journal of Traumatic Stress, 22*, 384–390.

Resick, P. A., & Schnicke, M. K. (1993). *Cognitive processing therapy for rape victims: A treatment manual.* Newbury Park, CA: Sage.

Roth, J., Steffens, M. C., Morina, N., & Stangier, U. (2012). Changed for the worse: Subjective change in implicit and explicit self-esteem in individuals with current, past, and no posttraumatic stress disorder. *Psychotherapy and Psychosomatics, 81*, 64–66.

Rubin, D. C. (2011). The coherence of memories for trauma: Evidence from posttraumatic stress disorder. *Consciousness and Cognition, 20*, 857–865.

Rubin, D. C., Berntsen, D., & Bohni, M. K. (2008). A memory-based model of posttraumatic stress disorder: Evaluating basic assumptions underlying the PTSD diagnosis. *Psychological Review, 115*, 985–1011.

Rubin, D. C., Boals, A., & Berntsen, D. (2008). Memory in posttraumatic stress disorder: Properties of voluntary and involuntary, traumatic and nontraumatic autobiographical memories in people with and without posttraumatic stress disorder symptoms. *Journal of Experimental Psychology: General, 137*, 591–614.

Schacter, D. L., Dobbins, I. G., & Schnyder, D. M. (2004). Specificity of priming: A cognitive neuroscience perspective. *Nature Neuroscience, 5*, 853–862.

Shipherd, J. C., & Beck, J. G. (2005). The role of thought suppression in posttraumatic stress disorder. *Behavior Therapy, 36*, 277–287.

Speckens, A. E. M., Ehlers, A., Hackmann, A., Ruths, F. A., & Clark, D. M. (2007). Intrusive memories and rumination in patients with post-traumatic stress disorder: A phenomenological comparison. *Memory, 15*, 249–257.

Spiegel, D. (1997). Trauma, dissociation, and memory. *Annals of the New York Academy of Sciences, 821*, 225–237.

Steil, R., & Ehlers, A. (2000). Dysfunctional meaning of posttraumatic intrusions in chronic PTSD. *Behaviour Research and Therapy, 38*, 537–558.

Sterlini, G. L., & Bryant, R. A. (2002). Hyperarousal and dissociation: A study of novice skydivers. *Behaviour Research and Therapy, 40*, 431–437.

Sveen, J., Dyster-Aas, J., & Willebrand, M. (2009). Attentional bias and symptoms of posttraumatic stress disorder one year after burn injury. *Journal of Nervous and Mental Disease, 11*, 850–855.

Tull, M. T., Barrett, H. M., McMillan, E. S., & Roemer, L. (2007). A preliminary investigation of the relationship between emotion regulation difficulties and posttraumatic stress symptoms. *Behavior Therapy, 38*, 303–313.

Tull, M. T., Gratz, K. L., Salters, K., & Roemer, L. (2004). The role of experiential avoidance in posttraumatic stress symptoms of depression, anxiety, and somatization. *Journal of Nervous and Mental Disease, 192*, 754–761.

Tull, M. T., Jakupcak, M., McFadden, M. E., & Roemer, L. (2007). The role of negative affect intensity and the fear of emotions in posttraumatic stress symptom severity among victims of childhood interpersonal violence. *Journal of Nervous and Mental Disease, 195*, 580–587.

van der Kolk, B. A., & Fisler, R. (1995). Dissociation and the fragmentary nature of traumatic memories: Overview and exploratory study. *Journal of Traumatic Stress, 8*, 505–525.

van der Kolk, B. A., Roth, S., Pelcovitz, D., Sunday, S., & Spinazzola, J. (2005). Disorders of extreme stress: The empirical foundation of a complex adaptation to trauma. *Journal of Traumatic Stress, 18*, 389–399.

van der Kolk, B. A., & van der Hart, O. (1989). Pierre Janet and the breakdown of adaptation in psychological trauma. *American Journal of Psychiatry, 146*, 1530–1540.

Vázquez, C., Hervás, G., & Pérez-Sales, P. (2008). Chronic thought suppression and posttraumatic symptoms: Data from the Madrid March 11, 2004 terrorist attack. *Journal of Anxiety Disorders, 22*, 1326–1336.

Wald, I., Shechner, T., Bitton, S., Holoshitz, Y., Charney, D. S., Muller, D., et al. (2011). Attention bias away from threat during life threatening danger predicts PTSD symptoms at one-year follow-up. *Depression and Anxiety, 28*, 406–411.

Warda, G., & Bryant, R. A. (1998). Cogni-

tive bias in acute stress disorder. *Behaviour Research and Therapy, 36*, 1177–1183.

Wells, A., & Papageorgiou, C. (1995). Worry and the incubation of intrusive images following stress. *Behaviour Research and Therapy, 33*, 579–583.

Wells, A., & Sembi, S. (2004). Metacognitive therapy for PTSD: A core treatment manual. *Cognitive and Behavioral Practice, 11*, 365–377.

Wessel, I., Overwijk, S., Verwoerd, J., & de Vrieze, N. (2008). Pre-stressor cognitive control is related to intrusive cognition of a stressful film. *Behaviour Research and Therapy, 46*, 496–513.

White, M., McManus, F., & Ehlers, A. (2008). An investigation of whether patients with post-traumatic stress disorder overestimate the probability and cost of future negative events. *Journal of Anxiety Disorders, 22*, 1244–1254.

Wiers, R. W., Teachman, B. A., & De Houwer, J. (2007). Implicit cognitive processes in psychopathology: An introduction. *Journal of Behavior Therapy and Experimental Psychiatry, 38*, 95–104.

Zetsche, U., Ehring, T., & Ehlers, A. (2009). The effects of rumination on mood and intrusive memories after exposure to traumatic material: An experimental study. *Journal of Behavior Therapy and Experimental Psychiatry, 40*, 499–514.

Zoellner, L. A., & Bittinger, J. N. (2004). On the uniqueness of trauma memories in PTSD. In G. M. Rosen (Ed.), *Posttraumatic stress disorder: Issues and controversies* (pp. 147–162). Chichester, UK: Wiley.

CHAPTER 23

Anxiety Disorders

Amanda S. Morrison, Dina Gordon, and Richard G. Heimberg

Two primary perspectives have guided our understanding of cognition–emotion interactions in anxiety: the information-processing perspective and the emotion regulation perspective. We first review the abundant literature on information-processing biases in the anxiety disorders, concluding with a brief review of research on the interrelations among these biases. We then review research on the anxiety disorders emerging from the emotion regulation perspective. Finally, we briefly discuss whether cognitive biases and dysregulated emotions can be effectively mitigated by psychotherapy and whether research on cognition–emotion interactions has translational relevance to clinical practice.

Information-Processing Biases in the Anxiety Disorders

Attention Bias to Threat

A wealth of research has investigated whether anxious individuals exhibit preferential attention toward threat information. Meta-analytic findings clearly support biased attention for threat material in anxiety (Bar-Haim, Lamy, Pergamin, Bakermans-Kranenburg, & van IJzendoorn, 2007). Moreover, the effect sizes of threat-related attention bias do not differ across the anxiety disorders. Therefore, we organize the following section of our review by types of attention bias tasks and methodological issues, rather than by specific disorder.

Attentional Probe Task

Much of the research on attention bias to threat in anxiety has utilized variations on the attentional probe, or dot probe, task (MacLeod, Mathews, & Tata, 1986; see Yiend, Barnicot, & Koster, Chapter 6, this volume). Using this task, attention biases toward threat have been demonstrated in generalized anxiety disorder (GAD; e.g., Bradley, Mogg, White, Groom, & De Bono, 1999), social anxiety disorder (SAD; e.g., Asmundson & Stein, 1994), panic disorder (PD; e.g., Asmundson, Sandler, Wilson, & Walker, 1992), and obsessive–compulsive disorder (OCD; e.g., Tata, Liebowitz, Prunty, Cameron, & Pickering, 1996).

Time Course of Attention Bias to Threat. Despite the relatively robust finding of attention bias to threat using the attentional probe task, there have been discrepant findings. Some studies have found no evidence of bias, and others have demonstrated attentional avoidance of threat (i.e., faster response latencies to probes following *neutral* stimuli than following threat stimuli). These seeming discrepancies led to methodical investigations and, ultimately, richer theoretical explanations. One area of investigation has focused on variation in the duration of threatening stimuli presentation, referred to as *stimulus onset asynchrony* (SOA). When SOA is brief (500 milliseconds [ms] or less), studies typically show attentional vigilance for threat (i.e., initial orientation to threat). In contrast, when stimuli are presented for longer durations, leaving sufficient time for conscious processing, attentional avoidance should be displayed. This vigilance–avoidance hypothesis was first voiced by Mathews and MacLeod (1994) to account for findings that anxious individuals typically exhibit attentional vigilance for threat but often do not exhibit anxiety-related biases for more strategic cognitive processes such as explicit memory. Indeed, the results of several studies using the attentional probe task (e.g., Mogg, Bradley, Miles, & Dixon, 2004) or eye-tracking procedures (e.g., Rohner, 2004) support initial vigilance followed by avoidance of threat-related stimuli. However, other studies showed vigilance for threat at SOAs as long as 1500 ms (e.g., Mogg, Bradley, De Bono, & Painter, 1997). Future research is needed to elucidate the complexities in the temporal sequence of automatic and strategic functions in the processing of threat.

Threat Intensity. Another variable of importance is stimulus threat intensity. Nonanxious individuals exhibit vigilance for highly threatening, but not mildly threatening, material. In contrast, anxious individuals exhibit an attention bias for mildly threatening stimuli. Mogg and Bradley's (1998) cognitive–motivational theory suggests that anxious individuals have a lower threshold for appraising threat. Objectively mild threat is appraised by anxious individuals as having higher subjective threat value, thereby leading to attention bias. Differential exhibition of attention bias across low- and high-trait anxious individuals is posited to be due to threat *evaluation*, rather than to how the attentional system responds to threat. To date, tests of this theory have been few but supportive (e.g., Koster, Crombez, Verschuere, & De Houwer, 2006).

Spatial Cueing Task and Disengagement from Threat

Another interpretive issue in the attentional probe task literature is whether findings of biased attention reflect hypervigilance for threat or difficulty disengaging attention from threat. Several researchers have employed the Posner (1980) spatial cueing task, a single-cue task, to examine this issue, though there is debate over whether this task successfully provides a pure measure of the disengagement component of attention (e.g., Mogg, Holmes, Garner, & Bradley, 2008).

Results to date from the spatial cueing task suggest that SOAs of at least 250 ms result in difficulty disengaging attention from threat but not an initial orienting bias in high state anxiety (Fox, Russo, Bowles, & Dutton, 2001), high trait anxiety (e.g., Fox, Russo, & Dutton, 2002, experiment 1), or SAD (Amir, Elias, Klumpp, & Przeworski, 2003). However, other studies have manipulated SOA and the threat value of stimuli, resulting in findings of both facilitated attention toward threat and difficulty disengaging attention from threat at 100 ms durations, as well as avoidance of threat at longer durations (for a review, see Cisler, Bacon, & Williams, 2009). Given that consensus has not been reached as to whether this task successfully discriminates engagement versus disengagement of attention, results should be considered with caution.

Visual Search Tasks

Visual search tasks have also been used to clarify the aforementioned issues, with the majority of research supporting the existence of both facilitated attention toward threat and difficulty disengaging attention from threat in anxious individuals (Cisler et al., 2009). For example, individuals with SAD show both facilitated attention toward, and difficulty disengaging attention from, threat (Gilboa-Schechtman, Foa, & Amir, 1999). Likewise, in GAD, studies have demonstrated difficulties disengaging attention from threatening lexical stimuli and some support for facilitated attention (e.g., Rinck, Becker, Kellerman, & Roth, 2003; Experiment 2).

Potential Causal Role of Attention Bias to Threat

Although cognitive models assert that attention bias to threat plays a causal role in the maintenance of anxiety, most research has been correlational. In the last few years, researchers have manipulated attention bias using a variation of the attentional probe task to train attention either toward or away from threat stimuli (MacLeod, Rutherford, Campbell, Ebsworthy, & Holker, 2002). After training, participants exhibited attention biases corresponding to their training condition. Moreover, participants trained to attend to threat information reported higher anxiety in response to a subsequent stressor. Researchers have also begun to translate similar procedures into interventions for SAD (Amir, Beard, Taylor, et al., 2009; Schmidt, Richey, Buckner, & Timpano, 2009) and GAD (Amir, Beard, Burns, & Bomyea, 2009; see MacLeod & Clarke, Chapter 29, this volume). Because these studies manipulated attention and anxiety decreased thereafter, there is evidence that attention bias to threat has a causal role in the maintenance of anxiety. However, the magnitude of this effect may be smaller than originally proposed (Hallion & Ruscio, 2011).

Interpretation Bias

Interpretation Bias in GAD

Several studies support a tendency to interpret ambiguous stimuli in a threatening manner in GAD. Eysenck, MacLeod, and Mathews (1987) asked participants to write down auditorially presented homophones that had both neutral and threat meanings (e.g., *die* or *dye*). Trait anxiety correlated with the selection of more threatening interpretations. Similarly, Eysenck, Mogg, May, Richards, and Mathews (1991) asked participants to decide whether threatening or neutral sentences were similar in meaning to previously presented ambiguous sentences. Participants with GAD selected the threatening interpretation more often than nonanxious or recovered anxious participants. Hazlett-Stevens and Borkovec (2004) presented evidence suggesting that GAD may be characterized by increased use of con-textual interpretive cues when facing potentially threatening ambiguous situations but deficient use of such cues in nonthreatening situations.

Interpretation Bias in PD

Cognitive-behavioral models emphasize the role of catastrophic misinterpretation of benign bodily symptoms in the development and maintenance of PD (e.g., Clark, 1986), and research has been consistent with this view. For example, patients with PD were more likely than controls to interpret both internal and external ambiguous stimuli in a negative fashion (McNally & Foa, 1987). Patients with PD were also more likely to interpret ambiguous bodily sensations as signs of impending physical or mental catastrophe (Clark et al., 1997). Self-reported misinterpretations of bodily sensations predict various affective, cognitive, and behavioral components of panic (e.g., Teachman, Smith-Janik, & Saporito, 2007).

Interpretation Bias in SAD

To study interpretation biases in SAD, researchers have often asked participants to rate the likelihood and valence of several possible interpretations of ambiguous scenarios (e.g., Amir, Foa, & Coles, 1998). Despite methodological differences, the overwhelming evidence suggests that socially anxious individuals make less positive and/or more negative interpretations of ambiguous or mildly negative social events than nonsocially anxious individuals. Studies using different methodologies and stimuli, such as videos (Amir, Beard, & Bower, 2005), facial expressions (Heuer, Lange, Isaac, Rinck, & Becker, 2010), electroencephalogram recordings (Moser, Hajcak, Huppert, Foa, & Simons, 2008), and reaction time indices (Hirsch & Mathews, 2000) have also revealed the presence of a negative bias and/or lack of a positive bias for ambiguous material.

Interpretation Bias in OCD

Cognitive models assert that it is the interpretation of intrusive thoughts, rather than the content of intrusions, that leads to the maintenance of OCD (Rachman, 1997). Individuals with OCD scored higher than controls on self-report of Control of Thoughts (i.e., the belief that thoughts must be actively controlled), Importance of Thoughts (i.e., the belief that intrusive thoughts are meaningful and indicative of one's character), and Responsibility (i.e., the idea that one must be vigilant about preventing harm at all times) (Obsessive Compulsive Cognitions Working Group, 2003). Individuals with OCD also scored higher than anxious controls on Control of Thoughts and Responsibility, supporting specificity of these appraisals to OCD. Experimentally induced inflated responsibility has also been shown to increase OCD symptoms such as checking behaviors (Arntz, Voncken, & Goosen, 2007).

Potential Causal Role of Interpretation Biases

Like attention biases, recent research on interpretation biases has provided evidence for their causal role in the maintenance of anxiety. For example, interpretation of ambiguous social situations as negative mediated the effect of social anxiety on state anxiety during a speech (Beard & Amir, 2010). Findings of the efficacy of cognitive bias modification procedures (see MacLeod & Clarke, Chapter 29, this volume) also support the causal role of interpretation biases. For example, an interpretation modification program modified interpretations in GAD and resulted in fewer negative thought intrusions during a breathing focus task (Hayes, Hirsch, Krebs, & Mathews, 2010). The effect size for interpretive bias modification procedures may be larger than the effect size for attention bias modification procedures (Hallion & Ruscio, 2011).

Memory and Imagery Biases

Information-processing models of emotional disorders suggest that anxious individuals may be characterized by a memory bias for threat-relevant information. Both encoding and recall of mood-congruent information should be facilitated when the relevant schema is activated (Beck, Emery, & Greenberg, 1985). Bower's (1981) theory of associative networks similarly proposes

that if mood at recall is the same as it was at encoding, recall of mood-congruent information should be enhanced. Williams, Watts, MacLeod, and Mathews (1988) further propose a distinction between explicit and implicit memory in research on anxiety disorders. Explicit memory represents conscious, effortful retrieval of previously learned information and is typically examined through tests of free recall or recognition. In contrast, implicit memory represents retrieval of information that is learned as an unintended effect of experience and is tested indirectly.

An additional topic that has recently begun to receive empirical attention in anxiety is that of memories of personal events that come to mind with no preceding attempt at retrieval (Berntsen, 1996). Related to this line of research is the study of imagery and visual memories, given that involuntary images figure prominently in the clinical phenomenology of several anxiety disorders. Therefore, the remainder of this section is divided into reviews of research on (1) explicit and implicit memory biases and (2) intrusive imagery and visual memories.

Explicit and Implicit Memory Biases

A recent meta-analysis suggested that high-anxious individuals exhibit better recall for threatening material and poorer recall for positive material than low-anxious individuals (Mitte, 2008). In contrast, there was no difference in the selective recognition of threatening information between high- and low-anxious individuals and no overall relationship between anxiety and implicit memory for threat-related information (Mitte, 2008). However, methodological variability within studies suggests that there are important moderators of each of these results.

Memory Biases in PD

Explicit Memory. Support for an explicit memory bias in PD has been relatively strong, though not unequivocal, and it stands in contrast to the vigilance–avoidance hypothesis introduced above. In an early study, individuals with PD recalled relatively more propositions from passages containing threatening versus neutral information than nonanxious individuals (Nunn, Stevenson, & Whalan, 1984). In a second experiment, individuals with PD recalled more threatening than neutral words, whereas the reverse was true of controls. Several later studies were also supportive. For example, individuals with PD recalled and recognized more panic-relevant than neutral or positive words in a lexical decision task (Cloitre & Liebowitz, 1991). Compared to controls, individuals with PD also exhibited greater recall for threat-relevant than neutral words following a self-referential encoding task (Becker, Roth, Andrich, & Margraf, 1999; Lundh, Czyzykow, & Öst, 1997). Lundh, Thulin, Czyzykow, and Öst (1998) showed that patients with PD who rated faces on whether or not the person could be relied on if help were needed later showed better recognition of safe than unsafe faces. In contrast, several studies have found no evidence of an explicit memory bias for threat in PD (e.g., Beck, Stanley, Averill, Baldwin, & Deagle, 1992). Coles and Heimberg (2002) suggest that null findings may be attributable to insufficient depth of processing during encoding tasks.

Implicit Memory. Fewer studies have examined implicit memory biases in PD, with inconsistent results. Using an implicit word stem completion task, Cloitre, Shear, Cancienne, and Zeitlin (1994) found that patients with PD completed more stems with studied threat words than did clinicians or nonanxious controls. In a white noise judgment paradigm, patients with PD rated the noise accompanying old panic-relevant sentences in the low-noise condition as quieter than the noise accompanying neutral sentences, whereas controls did not (Amir, McNally, Riemann, & Clements, 1996). In contrast, no evidence of an implicit memory bias was found in a word stem completion task (Rapee, 1994) or a self-referent encoding task and word completion test (Lundh et al., 1997). However, patients with PD in the latter study did identify more panic-related words than controls on a tachistoscopic identification task.

In sum, the extant literature generally supports the phenomenon of an explicit memory bias for threat in PD. However, the limited research on implicit memory biases is mixed at best.

Memory Biases in SAD

Explicit Memory. The majority of studies on explicit memory in SAD finds no evidence of bias. For example, Rapee, McCallum, Melville, Ravenscroft, and Rodney (1994) found no evidence of an explicit memory bias for threat in SAD across a wide variety of measures. Similarly, individuals with SAD showed no evidence of a recall or recognition bias for social threat words (Cloitre, Cancienne, Heimberg, Holt, & Liebowitz, 1995), a recall bias for threat words following self-referential encoding (Becker et al., 1999; Lundh & Öst, 1997), or recognition bias of previously heard social threat sentences (Amir, Foa, & Coles, 2000). Several studies using facial rather than linguistic stimuli also found no evidence of explicit memory bias for threat in individuals with SAD (e.g., Coles & Heimberg, 2005).

Two studies have reported an explicit memory bias in SAD, and several others have done so in samples of individuals high in social anxiety. Common to these studies are personally relevant encoding tasks. For example, Lundh and Öst (1996) asked participants to rate faces as critical or accepting; individuals with SAD subsequently recognized more critical than accepting faces, whereas the opposite was true for controls. Likewise, recall was superior in high socially anxious individuals for public self-referent information (O'Banion & Arkowitz, 1977), particularly under threat of social evaluation (Smith, Ingram, & Brehm, 1983). However, Coles and Heimberg (2005) note that such findings may be due to a response bias, and future research should employ signal detection analyses to disentangle these effects.

The most recent studies on explicit memory biases in SAD have examined memory for performance feedback and memory of internal sensations. Socially anxious participants showed more positively biased recognition of feedback provided to a confederate than to their own feedback. Compared to low-anxious participants, they also remembered their own negative feedback as worse and showed diminished recognition of positive feedback 2 days later (Cody & Teachman, 2010). Ashbaugh and Radomsky (2011) used a false physiological feedback paradigm in which participants believed various physiological responses, including heart rate fluctuations, sweating, jerky awkward movements, fluctuations in voice quality, and blushing were being measured. No group differences in free recall or recognition of feedback emerged; however, among participants with SAD only, fear of bodily sensations was associated with enhanced memory for stimuli associated with physiological responses.

Implicit Memory. Fewer studies have examined implicit memory in SAD. No evidence of a threat bias was found on an implicit word completion task (Rapee et al., 1994) or anagram task (Rinck & Becker, 2005). Lundh and Öst (1997) also failed to find evidence for an implicit bias in their entire sample of individuals with SAD, but participants with nongeneralized SAD showed stronger implicit memory for social threat words than controls. Because these results were found with a small sample (n = 11) and in post hoc analyses, they should be interpreted with caution. The two studies that have produced evidence of an implicit memory bias in social anxiety have employed versions of the white noise paradigm (Amir et al., 2000; Amir, Bower, Briks, & Freshman, 2003). Given the paucity of research in this area, it is difficult to make strong conclusions regarding an implicit memory bias in SAD.

Autobiographical Memory. It has also been suggested that social anxiety is associated with biased recall of autobiographical social events. Studies using memory cueing procedures have not produced strong evidence of a memory bias in social anxiety. For example, Rapee and colleagues (1994, Study 4) reported that memories recalled from social word cues were associated with more anxiety but that individuals with SAD did not differ from controls in retrieval. Similarly, individuals with SAD did not differ from controls in the percentage of specific personal memories recalled in response to social threat and neutral cue words (Wenzel, Jackson, & Holt, 2002), the time it took to recall threat-related memories, or the affective content of these memories when accounting for levels of depression (Wenzel, Werner, Cochran, & Holt, 2004).

One exception to these null or weak findings is a study by Wenzel and Cochran

(2006) in which single-word stimuli were replaced with automatic thoughts (i.e., negative cognitions) related to SAD, PD, or normative responses to stressful situations. Participants retrieved the first specific memory that came to mind following presentation of an automatic thought cue. Compared to nonanxious participants, individuals with SAD retrieved more anxious/worried memories and retrieved them more quickly when cued with SAD-related automatic thoughts. Cue relevance may be an important moderator of autobiographical memory biases in SAD.

Research on the properties of anxiety-related versus neutral memories in social anxiety more strongly supports a bias. Erwin, Heimberg, Marx, and Franklin (2006) found that individuals with SAD, but not controls, responded to memories of stressful social events with symptoms of hyperarousal and avoidance typical of posttraumatic stress disorder (PTSD). Individuals with SAD also tended to recall social events with greater self-referential information but less sensory information than controls, whereas no differences were noted for memories of nonsocial events (D'Argembeau, Van der Linden, d'Acremont, & Mayers, 2006). In another study, participants with SAD wrote autobiographical narratives of social memories containing greater self-referential information and greater use of words reflecting anxiety symptoms compared to narratives written by controls (Anderson, Goldin, Kurita, & Gross, 2008). In contrast, McNally, Otto, and Hornig (2001) found that spoken fear memories recalled by individuals with SAD could not be distinguished from those recalled by controls when rated by independent coders on various paralinguistic features.

Research on memory bias in SAD is largely inconsistent. Many studies failed to support an explicit memory bias for threat; however, tasks that used ecologically valid stimuli or fear-relevant encoding tasks did find such evidence. Likewise, implicit memory tasks with more ecologically valid stimuli were more likely to result in positive findings. Finally, studies of autobiographical memory biases largely support a memory bias in the subjective content of the memory (e.g., associated emotions, degree of self-referential information). In contrast, studies of more objective measures (e.g., number of memories recalled, speed of recall) tend to produce null results, though one study that used richer cueing stimuli did find such evidence.

Memory Biases in GAD

The excessive and uncontrollable worry of GAD could result in preferential memory for threat-related material, given the many "rehearsals" of threat-related concerns (Coles & Heimberg, 2002). Most studies of explicit memory and several studies of implicit memory suggest that this may not be the case, but the few that have found evidence of such biases provide information regarding potentially important moderators of memory biases in GAD.

Explicit Memory. In their review, Coles and Heimberg (2002) note that only one of nine studies produced modest support for an explicit memory bias in GAD. Only three studies have since examined explicit memory biases in GAD, but all report supportive findings. In two studies, Friedman, Thayer, and Borkovec (2000) found that individuals with GAD recalled significantly more threat than nonthreat words and more threat words than did controls. Coles, Turk, and Heimberg (2007) used idiographic words and found potential evidence of an explicit memory bias in GAD, as evidenced by an effect size of similar magnitude to previous studies documenting explicit memory biases in PD (e.g., Becker et al., 1999); however, the study was limited by low power. Although replication is necessary, this study suggests that stimulus relevance may be an important moderator of explicit memory biases in GAD.

Implicit Memory. Evidence for an implicit memory bias in GAD has been somewhat stronger, with three of five studies producing support. This pattern is consistent with Mathews, Mogg, May, and Eysenck's (1989) assertion that individuals with GAD would show a bias on implicit but not explicit memory tasks for threat-relevant material. Indeed, individuals with GAD generated more threat completions than controls on a primed word stem completion task following self-referential encoding (Mathews

et al., 1989). In a tachistoscopic identification task, individuals with GAD also identified more old threat words than new threat words compared to controls (MacLeod & McLaughlin, 1995). Individuals with GAD also demonstrated an implicit memory bias for idiographic threat words (Coles et al., 2007). However, patients with GAD did not show biased priming in a lexical decision task (Bradley, Mogg, & Williams, 1995) or in an implicit word stem completion task (Mathews, Mogg, Kentish, & Eysenck, 1995).

Taken together, studies on memory biases for threat in GAD are equivocal, with somewhat greater support for an implicit memory bias. These results should be considered somewhat tenuous, however, given that only one study (Coles et al., 2007) was conducted with individuals meeting DSM-IV diagnostic criteria. Furthermore, only Coles and colleagues (2007) used idiographic stimuli, and this study was one of the few to show support for memory biases. Future research should continue to study the effect of personal threat relevance of stimuli.

Memory Biases in OCD

Many OCD researchers believe that compulsions, and particularly checking, result from memory impairments or deficits. A complete review of this literature is beyond the scope of this chapter. Here we review studies examining whether individuals with OCD are characterized by preferential memory for threat-relevant information compared to neutral information. Research on memory biases in OCD has lagged behind that for other anxiety disorders.

Explicit Memory. Several studies have found support for an explicit memory bias for threat in OCD. In an early study, compulsive checkers showed better recall of their last completed action than controls, but only when that action was anxiety-provoking (Constans, Foa, Franklin, & Mathews, 1995). In a directed forgetting task, patients with OCD showed a deficit in forgetting negative but not positive or neutral words, whereas control participants did not (Wilhelm, McNally, Baer, & Florin, 1996).

Radomsky and Rachman (1999) studied recall and recognition memory for ecologically valid stimuli in contamination-fearful patients with OCD. Participants watched an experimenter touch everyday objects, half with a "clean" tissue and half with a "contaminated" tissue. Individuals with OCD recalled significantly more "contaminated" objects than "clean" objects, whereas controls did not. However, participants were not instructed to recall "contaminated" objects; therefore, results may be indicative of both explicit and implicit memory processes. In contrast, groups did not differ in recognition source memory (i.e., which tissue had been used to touch objects), though there was a trend for threat bias in the OCD group. Ceschi, Van der Linden, Dunker, Perroud, and Brédart (2003) replicated this study but failed to find the recall bias; they did find a recognition bias, in that OCD washers attributed the contamination *origin* more accurately to "contaminated" than to "clean" objects, whereas this was not the case for nonanxious participants or for OCD checkers. However, participants in Ceschi and colleagues' study were receiving treatment at the time of the study, and different objects were used in the two studies.

Radomsky, Rachman, and Hammond (2001) visited the homes of patients with OCD with primarily checking compulsions. Participants completed an initial check and then additional checks of something that would have caused anxiety if left unchecked. They remembered significantly more threat-relevant than threat-irrelevant information, and this difference was greater for a high versus low perceived responsibility check, suggesting that greater personal threat relevance increased the likelihood of memory bias.

Other studies found no evidence of an explicit memory bias. Foa, Amir, Gershuny, Molnar, and Kozak (1997) found no such evidence in individuals with OCD with contamination fears using a white noise paradigm. OCD checkers also showed no evidence of cued recall or recognition bias for threat words (Tuna, Tekcan, & Topçuoğlu, 2005), nor did individuals with OCD show biased recall for idiographically selected "safe," "unsafe," and "neutral" objects (Tolin et al., 2001). Radomsky and Rachman (2004) also failed to find evidence of biased recall of disorderly objects in compulsive orderers and arrangers.

Implicit Memory. Few studies have specifically investigated implicit memory biases in OCD. Individuals with elevated contamination fears did not show an implicit memory bias for disgust words compared to high trait-anxious or nonanxious controls (Charash & McKay, 2009). Similarly, individuals with OCD with contamination concerns did not show a threat bias in a white noise paradigm (Foa et al., 1997). However, modest support for an implicit memory bias for threat was found in the study described above by Radomsky and Rachman (1999).

In summary, the few studies that have examined preferential memory for threat-relevant information in OCD generally support an explicit memory bias, whereas there is only very modest support for an implicit memory bias. Research in OCD is complicated by the heterogeneity of patients' concerns. Therefore, future research should continue to focus on subsamples of individuals with OCD with homogeneous concerns.

Intrusive Imagery and Visual Memories

Much of the research on cognitive processes in the anxiety disorders has focused on negative verbal thoughts rather than visual memories and intrusions. However, negative visual imagery has been documented in several anxiety disorders. In contrast, GAD is characterized by a preponderance of verbal thought, which is posited to circumvent the emotion-inducing qualities of imagery (Borkovec, Alcaine, & Behar, 2004).

Imagery in SAD. Cognitive models of SAD posit that negative self-images play a role in the maintenance of the individual's exaggerated perception of the likelihood of negative evaluation (Heimberg, Brozovich, & Rapee, 2010). The image activated in social situations may be derived from long-term memory of previous interactions and notions of the self. Once activated, this image is continuously updated according to external and internal indicators of threat. Indeed, research to date largely supports these theoretical perspectives.

Individuals with SAD are more likely than nonanxious individuals to imagine recent social interactions from an observer perspective (i.e., as if looking at the self from an observer's point of view) than a field perspective (i.e., seeing the situation as if looking through their own eyes; Wells, Clark, & Ahmad, 1998). In contrast, both socially anxious and nonanxious individuals recall images of past nonsocial, anxiety-provoking situations from a field rather than observer perspective. Individuals with SAD are more likely than nonanxious individuals to report spontaneously occurring images during anxiety-provoking situations; the content of these images is significantly more negative (Hackmann, Surawy, & Clark, 1998), appears to remain relatively stable over time and across situations, and dates to the onset of social anxiety symptoms (Hackmann, Clark, & McManus, 2000).

These studies document a link between the imagery activated during social situations and autobiographical memories and are consistent with research by Coles and colleagues on perspective taking in the cued recall of social interactions. For individuals with SAD, memories of highly anxiety-evoking social situations were recalled from an observer perspective, whereas situations associated with medium or low levels of anxiety were recalled from a field perspective (Coles, Turk, Heimberg, & Fresco, 2001). Individuals with SAD were also more likely than controls to recall a role-played social interaction from an observer perspective, and this difference increased over the following 3-week interval (Coles, Turk, & Heimberg, 2002).

More recent studies have largely corroborated early findings, though rates of imagery reported by socially anxious individuals were lower than in previous studies (Moscovitch, Gavric, Merrifield, Bielak, & Moscovitch, 2011). Despite the lower incidence of intrusive imagery, Moscovitch and colleagues (2011) reported that negative images elicited more negative emotional and cognitive consequences in the high compared to low social anxiety group. Similarly, individuals with SAD exceeded control participants in startle reflex and autonomic responding during imagery of social but not survival threat (McTeague et al., 2009).

There is also empirical support for negative self-imagery as a causal factor in SAD. In a series of studies, Hirsch and colleagues trained participants to hold either a negative or benign self-image in mind while engaging in a social interaction with a confeder-

ate or while giving a speech. In contrast to neutral self-imagery, negative self-imagery elicited higher self-reported anxiety, more observable anxious behaviors, and exaggerated negative self-appraisal of performance in individuals with SAD (Hirsch, Clark, Mathews, & Williams, 2003), individuals high in social anxiety (Hirsch, Meynan, & Clark, 2004), and nonanxious individuals (Hirsch, Mathews, Clark, Williams, & Morrison, 2006).

Imagery in OCD. Only recently has research been conducted on the nature of imagery in OCD. Speckens, Hackmann, Ehlers, and Cuthbert (2007) interviewed patients with OCD, revealing that 81% reported mental images, most of which were associated with earlier adverse events and taken from a field perspective. In addition, patients who reported experiencing images endorsed more OCD symptoms, anxiety, and responsibility beliefs. More recently, Lipton, Brewin, Linke, and Halperin (2010) found that imagery in OCD did not differ in prevalence, number, sensory modality, vividness, associated distress, or interpretation from imagery in the other anxiety disorders. However, imagery was found to occur more frequently, to be more likely from a field than observer perspective, and to have a weaker perceived link with past memories in OCD than other anxiety disorders. Imagery in OCD was also predominantly characterized by "unacceptable ideas of harm." Although future research is needed to investigate the function that images play in OCD, preliminary evidence supports the existence of intrusive imagery as a feature in OCD.

Imagery in GAD. In contrast to the other anxiety disorders, research on imagery in GAD suggests that imaginal processing is specifically avoided. Borkovec and Inz (1990) used a mentation sampling method in individuals with GAD and nonanxious controls. During worry, both groups reported similarly high levels of verbal thought as compared to imagery. During relaxation, the nonanxious group reported higher levels of imagery than verbal thought, whereas the GAD group reported equal levels of imagery and verbal thought. A predominance of verbal over imaginal thought during worry was also reported by Freeston,

Dugas, and Ladouceur (1996) using a questionnaire, as well as by Behar, Zuellig, and Borkovec (2005) using a worry task.

The avoidance theory of worry accounts for this predominance of verbal thought over imagery in its assertion that worry functions as motivated avoidance of emotional imagery and its associated somatic sensations (Borkovec et al., 2004). Because images are avoided and emotional processing is precluded, worry-related thoughts are likely to intrude again later, thus perpetuating the worry cycle and associated tension. Preliminary evidence supports this theory. For example, Freeston and colleagues (1996) found that the number of reported somatic symptoms was positively associated with the percentage of images. Another recent study sought to elucidate whether imagery avoidance might occur during worry by examining the occurrence and duration of imagery during worry and positive thinking (Hirsch, Hayes, Mathews, Perman, & Borkovec, 2012). Imagery occurred less often and for briefer durations during worry than while thinking about a future positive event. Furthermore, the deficit in imagery during worry was more pronounced in individuals with GAD. In addition, the duration of imagery during worry and positive thinking was briefer in the GAD group than the control group. In sum, preliminary evidence suggests that avoidance of negative imagery might circumvent somatic symptoms and that GAD may be characterized by a mentation style that favors verbal over imaginal thought.

Relations among the Cognitive Biases

Cognitive behavioral models of anxiety posit a system of interacting cognitive biases. For example, Heimberg and colleagues (2010) postulate an interaction of biased attention toward threat, negative interpretations of physiological symptoms and ambiguous reactions by others, enhanced memory for anxiety-provoking situations, and observer perspective imagery in SAD. More explicitly, Hirsch, Clark, and Mathews (2006) assert that biases in information processing do not operate in isolation and so should be examined in conjunction with one another.

Although few studies have explicitly sought to test the assumption that cogni-

tive biases interact, research to date has been largely supportive. Several studies have examined interactions of self-imagery with other cognitive biases. In one study, nonanxious individuals in a control task exhibited a typical nonthreat interpretation bias, whereas nonanxious individuals trained to hold a negative self-image in mind lacked this nonthreat interpretation bias (Hirsch, Mathews, Clark, Williams, & Morrison, 2003). Those in the experimental group also reported higher levels of state anxiety, supporting the notion that these cognitive biases may interact to maintain anxiety. Interpretation bias has also been shown to affect imagery. Self-images were more negative and elicited more anxiety following a negative interpretation bias induction than a positive interpretation bias induction (Hirsch, Mathews, & Clark, 2007). Imagery has also been shown to affect memory. Participants were faster to retrieve negative autobiographical memories when they held a negative image in mind and faster to retrieve positive autobiographical memories when they held a positive image in mind (Stopa & Jenkins, 2007). Retrieval of positive memories while holding a negative image in mind was slower than retrieval of both negative and neutral images, suggesting an inhibitory effect of negative self-imagery on positive autobiographical memories.

At least two studies have provided support for a relationship between attention and interpretation biases. White, Suway, Pine, Bar-Haim, and Fox (2011) found that participants trained to attend to threat stimuli were more likely than participants in a control condition to interpret the first of several ambiguous scenarios in a threatening manner. In testing the reverse effect, Amir, Bomyea, and Beard (2010) showed that an interpretation modification program, designed to facilitate more benign interpretations of ambiguous social scenarios, facilitated attention disengagement from social threat cues.

Finally, three studies support a link between interpretation and memory biases. Hertel, Brozovich, Joormann, and Gotlib (2008) found that socially anxious participants were more likely than controls to show memory intrusions consistent with biased interpretations made earlier in the study. Salemink, Hertel, and Mackintosh (2010) found that positive compared to negative interpretation training resulted in remembering earlier scenario outcomes as having been more positive. Tran, Hertel, and Joormann (2011) reported similar findings.

Although the literature on the interrelationships among information-processing biases is in its infancy, there is already consistent support. Future research should extend these findings to clinical samples and expand to include topics beyond those most closely related to SAD. Given that information-processing biases differ somewhat across the anxiety disorders, especially in relation to imagery and memory, future research should examine each of the anxiety disorders before firm conclusions are drawn. Finally, research on the interactions between the information-processing biases may have implications for treatment programs, such as cognitive bias modification procedures (see MacLeod & Clarke, Chapter 29, this volume).

Emotion Regulation in the Anxiety Disorders

Our understanding of cognition–emotion interactions in anxiety has also been driven by the examination of difficulties with emotion regulation, the processes by which an individual influences which emotions he or she experiences, when the emotions are experienced, and how the emotions are experienced and expressed (Gross, 1998). Difficulties with emotion regulation have been found in the majority of anxiety disorders (Cisler, Olatunji, Feldner, & Forsyth, 2010); the current review is limited to studies of GAD and SAD. See Suri, Sheppes, and Gross (Chapter 11, this volume) for a more general review of emotion regulation research.

Emotion Regulation in GAD

Mennin, Heimberg, Turk, and Fresco (2005) present an emotion dysregulation model of GAD, which expands upon the avoidance theory of worry and GAD (Borkovec et al., 2004) by specifying four aspects of the relationship of individuals with GAD to their emotional experience: (1) heightened emotional intensity, (2) poor emotional under-

standing, (3) negative reactivity to emotions, and (4) maladaptive management of emotions. *Heightened intensity of emotions* refers to the proneness of individuals with GAD to experience emotions more readily and intensely than others and to have difficulty suppressing the expression of negative affect. *Poor understanding of emotions* entails difficulties describing and identifying emotions, making it difficult for individuals with GAD to identify and glean important information from their emotional experience. *Negative reactivity to emotions* is characterized by anxiety and discomfort in the face of strong emotions, a consequence of their being intense and poorly understood. Finally, individuals with GAD utilize *poor coping skills*, such as controlling, avoiding, or suppressing their emotional experiences. In this context, worry functions as a maladaptive emotional avoidance strategy. Mennin and colleagues (2005) assert that worry interrupts emotional processing and amplifies emotion dysregulation, creating a pathological feedback loop.

The emotion dysregulation model has been consistently supported (Mennin et al., 2005). Both undergraduates with GAD symptoms and patients with GAD reported experiencing the four components of emotion dysregulation to a greater degree than controls, and a composite score based on these components predicted GAD beyond the variance contributed by trait anxiety, worry, and depressive symptoms. In another study, participants with analogue GAD had more difficulty managing emotional reactions and experienced greater increases in self-reported somatic distress than a control group after a negative mood induction (Mennin et al., 2005). Further evidence linked deficits in emotion regulation with chronic worry and GAD in a nonclinical sample (Salters-Pedneault, Roemer, Tull, Rucker, & Mennin, 2006). In contrast to control participants, individuals with analogue GAD endorsed deficits in emotional clarity, difficulty engaging in goal-directed behaviors when distressed, trouble accepting emotions, impulse control deficits, and limited access to effective regulation strategies, controlling for general affective distress.

In a recent paper, Newman and Llera (2011) introduced the contrast avoidance model of worry, theorizing that worry serves to preserve a chronic state of negative emotionality so as to avoid an unexpected emotional shift from a positive or euthymic state to a negative one. This perspective is consistent with the notion that individuals with GAD are overly sensitive to emotional vulnerability and unexpected negative events. Newman and Llera suggest that experiential avoidance in GAD is founded in the belief that chronic distress allows an individual to brace for the worst-case scenario (i.e., the primary focus of threat). Llera and Newman (2010a) exposed students with and without analogue GAD to emotion-inducing film clips following worry, relaxation, and neutral inductions. Worry led to reduced vagal tone for the GAD group, as well as higher negative affect levels for both groups. Additionally, prior worry resulted in less physiological and subjective responding to the fearful film clip, suggesting that worry may have served to prevent a negative emotional contrast. Furthermore, when rating the extent to which the various inductions helped them cope with their emotions during the film clips, participants with analogue GAD were more likely than controls to rate prior worry helpful and the relaxation and neutral inductions as unhelpful, whereas the opposite pattern was observed among the controls (Llera & Newman, 2010b, as cited in Newman & Llera, 2011).

Emotion Regulation in SAD

SAD has also been characterized by emotional hyperreactivity and emotion regulation deficits. Spokas, Luterek, and Heimberg (2009) examined the self-reported suppression of emotional expression and beliefs about emotional suppression in a socially anxious sample. Compared to controls, the socially anxious group reported greater use of emotional suppression and greater ambivalence about expressing emotions. Additionally, they endorsed the beliefs that it is important to have control of emotional expressions, that emotional expression may lead to social rejection, and that expressing one's emotions communicates weakness. These beliefs mediated the association between social anxiety and expressive suppression (Spokas et al., 2009).

Werner, Goldin, Ball, Heimberg, and Gross (2011) developed an interview to measure emotion regulation deficits according to Gross's (1998) process model of emotion regulation. Patients with SAD were interviewed about their use of emotion regulation skills during a speech task and two recent social situations. Compared with controls, patients reported the more frequent use of situation selection (i.e., avoidance) and suppression of emotional expression as well as less self-efficacy in engaging in cognitive reappraisal and expressive suppression. The findings regarding expressive suppression support those of Spokas and colleagues (2009).

In an investigation of the neural mechanisms of emotion regulation in SAD, Goldin, Manber, Hakimi, Canli, and Gross (2009) used functional magnetic resonance imaging (fMRI) to examine emotional reactivity and cognitive regulation (i.e., strategy selection, implementation, monitoring) in patients with SAD and controls. Patients were less likely than controls to recruit cognitive and attention regulation brain networks in response to social threat stimuli, but not physical threat images, suggesting that emotion regulation deficits are specific to social stimuli.

Specificity of Emotion Regulation Deficits across SAD and GAD

Emotion regulation deficits have also been examined across commonly comorbid anxiety disorders, particularly SAD and GAD, to elucidate the degree of overlap and uniqueness of these dimensions across disorders. Using an undergraduate sample, Turk, Heimberg, Luterek, Mennin, and Fresco (2005) compared individuals with analogue GAD, SAD, and controls on self-reported emotion regulations deficits. Individuals in the GAD group reported greater emotion intensity and negative reactivity to sadness than socially anxious individuals or controls. Socially anxious participants indicated being less attentive to their emotions, having more trouble describing emotions (i.e., poor understanding of emotions), and engaging in more expressive suppression of positive emotions than the other two groups. The emotion measures were able to accurately discriminate among the three groups, suggesting specificity of facets of emotion dysregulation to different anxiety disorders. Mennin, McLaughlin, and Flanagan (2009) extended these findings in a clinical sample of individuals with GAD, SAD, or both disorders. Emotional intensity and impaired regulation strategies best discriminated among groups and predicted a GAD diagnosis, regardless of SAD comorbidity. Poor emotional understanding best predicted a SAD diagnosis, regardless of GAD comorbidity.

Mennin, Holaway, Fresco, Moore, and Heimberg (2007) examined the four emotion regulation factors across analogue SAD, GAD, and major depressive disorder (MDD) in an undergraduate sample. All factors displayed specific and common relationships with self-reported symptoms of the three disorders. Specifically, emotional intensity and maladaptive management of emotions uniquely predicted symptoms of GAD, beyond variance shared with symptoms of SAD and MDD. Furthermore, heightened intensity of emotions negatively predicted SAD symptoms, suggesting that "pure" SAD is associated with reduced emotionality. SAD symptoms did, however, remain significantly related to poor understanding of emotions after overlap with symptoms of the other two disorders was considered. Negative reactivity to emotions was associated with SAD, but not GAD. It may be that this factor is better accounted for in GAD by the overlapping of symptoms with other disorders (Mennin et al., 2007).

Psychotherapy, Cognitive Biases, and Emotion Dysregulation in the Anxiety Disorders

An important question is whether cognitive biases can be mitigated by effective psychotherapy. Several early studies suggested that this might be so for attentional biases toward threat. Foa and McNally (1986) examined change in response to a dichotic listening task before and after exposure and response prevention for patients with OCD. After treatment, no differences were found between responses to fear-relevant and neutral targets in unattended passages. Mattia, Heimberg, and Hope (1993) demonstrated increased speed of color-naming social threat words among patients with SAD who responded to cognitive-behavioral treatment

(CBT), but not among nonresponders. Most recently, Tobon, Ouimet, and Dozois (2011) reviewed the literature on the effects of CBT on attentional bias toward threat and found that 10 of 13 studies demonstrated a reduction in bias as a result of treatment.

CBT also appears to be associated with reductions in interpretive biases. In studies of patients with SAD by both Foa, Franklin, Perry, and Herbert (1996) and McManus, Clark, and Hackmann (2000), overestimates of both the probability and cost of negative social events were reduced with CBT. Furthermore, Clark and colleagues (1994) demonstrated that reductions in catastrophic interpretations of bodily sensations at posttreatment predicted positive follow-up outcomes in patients with PD. In a more recent study of patients with PD (Teachman, Marker, & Clerkin, 2010), change in catastrophic misinterpretations predicted subsequent reductions in overall symptom severity, panic attack frequency, distress/apprehension, and avoidance behavior. Future research should examine the effects of CBT on other biases and the potential mediational role of changes in these biases on treatment outcomes.

Recent research (e.g., Roemer & Orsillo, 2008) suggests the efficacy of an acceptance-based intervention for GAD. Treanor, Erisman, Salters-Pedneault, Roemer, and Orsillo (2011) demonstrated that this intervention was associated with significant reductions in difficulties with emotion regulation.

Translational Relevance of Cognition–Emotion Research to Clinical Practice

Translational relevance has been well demonstrated in the early returns on cognitive bias modification procedures (see MacLeod & Clarke, Chapter 29, this volume). However, there are other important areas to examine. These include the utility of mindfulness-based interventions in the treatment of anxiety disorders and the role of imagery-related interventions in clinical practice.

Mindfulness-Based Interventions

Mindfulness interventions, which target the focus of attention, have recently been applied to the treatment of anxiety. Kabat-

Zinn (2003, p. 145) defines mindfulness as "the awareness that emerges through paying attention on purpose, in the present moment, and nonjudgmentally to the unfolding of experience moment by moment." Several open trials have suggested the efficacy of mindfulness-based interventions for SAD, mostly mindfulness-based stress reduction (MBSR; Goldin & Gross, 2010; Goldin, Ramel, & Gross, 2009). Following MBSR, patients demonstrated increased endorsement of positive traits and decreased endorsement of negative traits (Goldin et al., 2009). These changes were associated with increased activity in brain areas indicative of attention to a stimulus and decreased activity in brain areas associated with self-referential processing and language. Goldin and Gross (2010) also demonstrated increased brain activation in areas related to attention as well as decreased activation in the amygdala. One additional study compared MBSR to CBT for SAD (Koszycki, Benger, Shlik, & Bradwejn, 2007). Patients who received CBT showed greater reductions in fear of negative evaluation and behavioral avoidance and were more likely to be classified as responders at posttreatment compared to those who received MBSR. However, both groups demonstrated improvements in mood, well-being, and quality of life. Although it was somewhat less efficacious than CBT, MBSR appeared to produce meaningful improvements for socially anxious patients and therefore appears worthy of further investigation.

Imagery-Related Interventions in CBT

We have reviewed the important role that spontaneously occurring negative self-imagery or holding a negative self-image in mind may have in the anxiety disorders, most notably, in SAD. It is also well documented (see Rapee & Lim, 1992) that persons with SAD view their performance in social situations vastly more poorly than do objective raters. These laboratory observations have given rise to two therapeutic techniques that are often used as part of larger CBT packages: imagery rescripting and video feedback.

Imagery rescripting procedures are well delineated in a recent paper by Wild and Clark (2011). An imagery rescripting session begins with a period of cognitive restructuring focusing on the negative belief reflected in the spontaneous and recurring image reported by the patient. Rescripting itself involves repeated evocation of the socially traumatic memory, insertion of corrective information into the image, and a compassionate stance toward the self in imagery. Patients first imagine that they are the age at which the event occurred and relive it as if it were happening again. They then relive the memory at their current age, watching what happened to their younger self and intervening, if they wish, often conveying to the younger self the alternative perspective derived during cognitive restructuring. Finally, they relive it from the perspective of their younger self with their adult self in the room with them, intervening as before. This time the younger self is also asked what else would need to happen for him or her to feel better, and this material is incorporated into the image as well. Wild, Hackmann, and Clark (2007, 2008) examined imagery rescripting in the treatment of SAD. In an open trial, imagery rescripting was associated with improvements in patients' negative beliefs, the vividness and distress of their image and early memory, and self-reported anxiety (Wild et al., 2007). A session of imagery rescripting was compared with a control session (Wild et al., 2008). The rescripting session was associated with greater improvement in negative beliefs, image and memory distress and vividness, fear of negative evaluation, and anxiety in feared social situations.

Video feedback was initially intended to correct faulty self-perception by providing contrasting evidence of the adequacy of one's performance. However, several experiments with socially anxious undergraduates in public speaking situations demonstrated that the addition of a period of cognitive preparation was necessary (Harvey, Clark, Ehlers, & Rapee, 2000). During cognitive preparation, participants who had just given a videotaped speech were asked to (1) rate from memory several specific behaviors they displayed during their speech, define what the rating meant to them, and specify what they expected to see on the videotape in reference to each behavior; (2) imagine their performance from beginning to end as best they could; and (3) then view the videotape of their speech as if watching the video of a stranger. These studies demonstrated rather robust effects on self-perceptions of performance, and the magnitude of the discrepancy between self-ratings and observer ratings predicted responses to video feedback (e.g., Rodebaugh & Rapee, 2005). However, there was little impact on social anxiety, confidence, or willingness to approach a subsequent public speaking task.

Rodebaugh, Heimberg, Schultz, and Blackmore (2010) tested video feedback with cognitive preparation among treatment-seeking participants with SAD. In Session 1, participants gave an extemporaneous speech and either received the intervention or not. In Session 2, 6–14 days later, participants gave a second extemporaneous speech. The intervention improved self-perceptions of performance. In addition, the intervention reduced anticipatory anxiety for the second speech for participants with high self-observer discrepancy. These findings extend previous results regarding video feedback and suggest that the intervention may be useful for people with SAD and higher self-observer discrepancies for a specific task.

Concluding Comments

A variety of deficits in information processing and emotion regulation underpin the distress and impairment associated with the anxiety disorders. The overall conclusion is that these processes represent a common core of the anxiety disorders. Not surprisingly, many similarities exist among cognitive-behavioral therapies for the various anxiety disorders, with most current treatments focusing on exposure to feared situations often in conjunction with restructuring of maladaptive cognitions that arise within, in anticipation of, or in response to confrontation with these situations. Consistent with this premise is the development and evaluation of "transdiagnostic" (Harvey, Watkins, Mansell, & Shafran, 2004) or "unified" (Barlow, Allen, & Choate, 2004) protocols for the emotional disorders (i.e., anxiety and depressive disorders). These protocols converge on the notion that patients with different disorders may be treated with the same basic set of procedures because they share the same underlying vulnerabilities. Barlow

and colleagues (2004, p. 205) state that the necessary components of treatment of the emotional disorders include "(a) altering antecedent cognitive reappraisals; (b) preventing emotional avoidance; and (c) facilitating action tendencies not associated with the emotion that is dysregulated." These components map well onto the presence of cognitive biases and dysregulated emotion in the anxiety disorders. However, there is still a distance to go in the study of cognition–emotion interactions in the anxiety disorders, and these interactions are not yet that well reflected in anxiety treatments. With the possible exception of some cognitive bias modification procedures (see MacLeod & Clarke, Chapter 29, this volume), most CBTs rely heavily on the engagement of conscious, strategic, and effortful cognitive restructuring procedures to ignite change in unconscious, automatic, and implicit cognitive processes. It is clear that important therapeutic gains can be realized in this way, but it is less clear that this is an efficient way to proceed. Although much implicit learning surely takes place during exposure to feared situations, this is an area scarcely studied and a fertile area for future research.

References

Amir, N., Beard, C., & Bower, E. (2005). Interpretation bias and social anxiety. *Cognitive Therapy and Research, 29*, 433–443.

Amir, N., Beard, C., Burns, M., & Bomyea, J. (2009). Attention modification program in individuals with generalized anxiety disorder. *Journal of Abnormal Psychology, 118*, 28–33.

Amir, N., Beard, C., Taylor, C. T., Klumpp, H., Elias, J., Burns, M., et al. (2009). Attention training in individuals with generalized social phobia: A randomized controlled trial. *Journal of Consulting and Clinical Psychology, 77*, 961–973.

Amir, N., Bomyea, J., & Beard, C. (2010). The effect of single-session interpretation modification on attention bias in socially anxious individuals. *Journal of Anxiety Disorders, 24*, 178–182.

Amir, N., Bower, E., Briks, J., & Freshman, M. (2003). Implicit memory for negative and positive social information in individuals with and without social anxiety. *Cognition and Emotion, 17*, 567–583.

Amir, N., Elias, J., Klumpp, H., & Przeworski, A. (2003). Attentional bias to threat in social phobia: Facilitated processing of threat or difficulty disengaging attention from threat? *Behaviour Research and Therapy, 41*, 1325–1335.

Amir, N., Foa, E. B., & Coles, M. E. (1998). Automatic activation and strategic avoidance of threat-relevant information in social phobia. *Journal of Abnormal Psychology, 107*, 285–290.

Amir, N., Foa, E. B., & Coles, M. E. (2000). Implicit memory bias for threat-relevant information in individuals with generalized social phobia. *Journal of Abnormal Psychology, 109*, 713–720.

Amir, N., McNally, R. J., Riemann, B. C., & Clements, C. (1996). Implicit memory bias for threat in panic disorder: Application of the "white noise" paradigm. *Behaviour Research and Therapy, 34*, 157–162.

Anderson, B., Goldin, P. R., Kurita, K., & Gross, J. J. (2008). Self-representation in social anxiety disorder: Linguistic analysis of autobiographical narratives. *Behaviour Research and Therapy, 46*, 1119–1125.

Arntz, A., Voncken, M., & Goosen, A. C. A. (2007). Responsibility and obsessive–compulsive disorder: An experimental test. *Behaviour Research and Therapy, 45*, 425–435.

Ashbaugh, A. R., & Radomsky, A. S. (2011). Memory for physiological feedback in social anxiety disorder: The role of fear of bodily sensations. *Cognitive Therapy and Research, 35*, 304–316.

Asmundson, G. J. G., Sandler, L. S., Wilson, K. G., & Walker, J. R. (1992). Selective attention toward physical threat in patients with panic disorder. *Journal of Anxiety Disorders, 6*, 295–303.

Asmundson, G. J. G., & Stein, M. B. (1994). Selective processing of social threat in patients with generalized social phobia: Evaluation using a dot-probe paradigm. *Journal of Anxiety Disorders, 8*, 107–117.

Bar-Haim, Y., Lamy, D., Pergamin, L., Bakermans-Kranenburg, M., & van IJzendoorn, M. H. (2007). Threat-related attentional bias in anxious and nonanxious individuals: A meta-analytic study. *Psychological Bulletin, 133*, 1–24.

Barlow, D. H., Allen, L. B., & Choate, M. L. (2004). Towards a unified treatment for emotional disorders. *Behavior Therapy, 35*, 205–230.

Beard, C., & Amir, N. (2010). Negative interpretation bias mediates the effect of social anxiety on state anxiety. *Cognitive Therapy and Research, 34*, 292–296.

Beck, A. T., & Emery, G., & Greenberg, R. L. (1985). *Anxiety disorders and phobias: A cognitive perspective.* New York: Basic Books.

Beck, J. G., Stanley, M. A., Averill, P. M., Baldwin, L. E., & Deagle, E. A. (1992). Attention and memory for threat in panic disorder. *Behaviour Research and Therapy, 30*, 619–629.

Becker, E. S., Roth, W. T., Andrich, M., & Margraf, J. (1999). Explicit memory in anxiety disorders. *Journal of Abnormal Psychology, 108*, 153–163.

Behar, E., Zuellig, A. R., & Borkovec, T. D. (2005). Thought and imaginal activity during worry and trauma recall. *Behavior Therapy, 36*, 157–168.

Berntsen, D. (1996). Involuntary autobiographical memories. *Applied Cognitive Psychology, 10*, 435–454.

Borkovec, T. D., & Inz, J. (1990). The nature of worry in generalized anxiety disorder: A predominance of thought activity. *Behaviour Research and Therapy, 28*, 153–158.

Borkovec, T. D., Alcaine, O. M., & Behar, E. (2004). Avoidance theory of worry. In R. G. Heimberg, C. L. Turk, & D. S. Mennin (Eds.), *Generalized anxiety disorder: Advances in research and practice* (pp. 77–108). New York: Guilford Press.

Bower, G. H. (1981). Mood and memory. *American Psychologist, 36*, 129–148.

Bradley, B. P., Mogg, K., White, J., Groom, C., & de Bono, J. (1999). Attentional bias for emotional faces in generalized anxiety disorder. *British Journal of Clinical Psychology, 38*, 267–278.

Bradley, B. P., Mogg, K., & Williams, R. (1995). Implicit and explicit memory for emotion-congruent information in clinical depression and anxiety. *Behaviour Research and Therapy, 33*, 755–770.

Ceschi, G., Van der Linden, M., Dunker, D., Perroud, A., & Brédart, S. (2003). Further exploration memory bias in compulsive washers. *Behaviour Research and Therapy, 41*, 737–748.

Charash, M., & McKay, D. (2009). Disgust and contamination fear: Attention, memory, and judgment of stimulus situations. *International Journal of Cognitive Therapy, 2,* 53–65.

Cisler, J. M., Bacon, A. K., & Williams, N. L. (2009). Phenomenological characteristics of attentional biases towards threat: A critical review. *Cognitive Therapy and Research, 33,* 221–234.

Cisler, J. M., Olatunji, B., Feldner, M., & Forsyth, J. (2010). Emotion regulation and the anxiety disorders: An integrative review. *Journal of Psychopathology and Behavioral Assessment, 32,* 68–82.

Clark, D. M. (1986). A cognitive approach to panic. *Behaviour Research and Therapy, 24,* 461–470.

Clark, D. M., Salkovskis, P. M., Hackmann, A., Middleton, H., Anastasiades, P., & Gelder, M. (1994). A comparison of cognitive therapy, applied relaxation, and imipramine in the treatment of panic disorder. *British Journal of Psychiatry, 164,* 759–769.

Clark, D. M., Salkovskis, P. M., Öst, L., Breitholtz, E., Koehler, K. A., Westling, B. E., et al. (1997). Misinterpretation of body sensations in panic disorder. *Journal of Consulting and Clinical Psychology, 65,* 203–213.

Cloitre, M., Cancienne, J., Heimberg, R. G., Holt, C. S., & Liebowitz, M. R. (1995). Memory bias does not generalize across anxiety disorders. *Behaviour Research and Therapy, 33,* 305–307.

Cloitre, M., & Liebowitz, M. R. (1991). Memory bias in panic disorder: An investigation of the cognitive avoidance hypothesis. *Cognitive Therapy and Research, 15,* 371–386.

Cloitre, M., Shear, K., Cancienne, J., & Zeitlin, S. (1994). Implicit and explicit memory for catastrophic associations to bodily sensation words in panic disorder. *Cognitive Therapy and Research, 18,* 225–240.

Cody, M. W., & Teachman, B. A. (2010). Post-event processing and memory bias for performance feedback in social anxiety. *Journal of Anxiety Disorders, 24,* 468–479.

Coles, M. E., & Heimberg, R. G. (2002). Memory biases in the anxiety disorders: Current status. *Clinical Psychology Review, 22,* 587–627.

Coles, M. E., & Heimberg, R. G. (2005). Recognition bias for critical faces in social phobia: A replication and extension. *Behaviour Research and Therapy, 43,* 109–120.

Coles, M. E., Turk, C. L., & Heimberg, R. G. (2002). The role of memory perspective in social phobia: Immediate and delayed memories for role-played situations. *Behavioural and Cognitive Psychotherapy, 30,* 415–425.

Coles, M. E., Turk, C. L., & Heimberg, R. G. (2007). Memory bias for threat in generalized anxiety disorder: The potential importance of stimulus relevance. *Cognitive Behaviour Therapy, 36,* 65–73.

Coles, M. E., Turk, C. L., Heimberg, R. G., & Fresco, D. M. (2001). Effects of varying levels of anxiety within social situations: Relationship to memory perspective and attributions in social phobia. *Behaviour Research and Therapy, 39,* 651–665.

Constans, J. I., Foa, E. B., Franklin, M. E., & Mathews, A. (1995). Memory for actual and imagined events in OC checkers. *Behaviour Research and Therapy, 33,* 665–671.

D'Argembeau, A., Van der Linden, M., d'Acremont, M., & Mayers, I. (2006). Phenomenal characteristics of autobiographical memories for social and non-social events in social phobia. *Memory, 14,* 637–647.

Erwin, B. A., Heimberg, R. G., Marx, B. P., & Franklin, M. E. (2006). Traumatic and socially stressful life events among persons with social anxiety disorder. *Journal of Anxiety Disorders, 20,* 896–914.

Eysenck, M. W., MacLeod, C., & Mathews, A. (1987). Cognitive functioning and anxiety. *Psychological Research, 49,* 189–195.

Eysenck, M. W., Mogg, K., May, J., Richards, A., & Mathews, A. (1991). Bias in interpretation of ambiguous sentences related to threat in anxiety. *Journal of Abnormal Psychology, 100,* 144–150.

Foa, E. B., Amir, N., Gershuny, B., Molnar, C., & Kozak, M. J. (1997). Implicit and explicit memory in obsessive–compulsive disorder. *Journal of Anxiety Disorders, 11,* 119–129.

Foa, E. B., Franklin, M. E., Perry, K. J., & Herbert, J. D. (1996). Cognitive biases in generalized social phobia. *Journal of Abnormal Psychology, 105,* 433–439.

Foa, E. B., & McNally, R. J. (1986). Sensitivity to feared stimuli in obsessive-compulsives: A dichotic listening analysis. *Cognitive Therapy and Research, 10,* 477–485.

Fox, E., Russo, R., Bowles, R., & Dutton, K. (2001). Do threatening stimuli draw or hold visual attention in subclinical anxiety? *Journal of Experimental Psychology: General, 130,* 681–700.

Fox, E., Russo, R., & Dutton, K. (2002). Attentional bias for threat: Evidence for delayed disengagement from emotional faces. *Cognition and Emotion, 16*, 355–379.

Freeston, M. H., Dugas, M. J., & Ladouceur, R. (1996). Thoughts, images, worry, and anxiety. *Cognitive Therapy and Research, 20*, 265–273.

Friedman, B. H., Thayer, J. F., & Borkovec, T. D. (2000). Explicit memory bias for threat words in generalized anxiety disorder. *Behavior Therapy, 31*, 745–756.

Gilboa-Schechtman, E., Foa, E. B., & Amir, N. (1999). Attentional biases for facial expressions in social phobia: The face-in-the-crowd paradigm. *Cognition and Emotion, 13*, 305–318.

Goldin, P. R., & Gross, J. J. (2010). Effects of mindfulness-based stress reduction (MBSR) on emotion regulation in social anxiety disorder. *Emotion, 10*, 83–91.

Goldin, P. R., Manber, T., Hakimi, S., Canli, T., & Gross, J. J. (2009). Neural bases of social anxiety disorder: Emotional reactivity and cognitive regulation during social and physical threat. *Archives of General Psychiatry, 66*, 170–180.

Goldin, P. R., Ramel, W., & Gross, J. J. (2009). Mindfulness meditation training and self-referential processing in social anxiety disorder: Behavioral and neural effects. *Journal of Cognitive Psychotherapy, 23*, 242–257.

Gross, J. J. (1998). The emerging field of emotion regulation: An integrative review. *Review of General Psychology, 2*, 271–299.

Hackmann, A., Clark, D. M., & McManus, F. (2000). Recurrent images and early memories in social phobia. *Behaviour Research and Therapy, 38*, 601–610.

Hackmann, A., Surawy, C., & Clark, D. M. (1998). Seeing yourself through others' eyes: A study of spontaneously occurring images in social phobia. *Behavioural and Cognitive Psychotherapy, 26*, 3–12.

Hallion, L. S., & Ruscio, A. M. (2011). A meta-analysis of the effect of cognitive bias modification on anxiety and depression. *Psychological Bulletin, 137*, 940–958.

Harvey, A. G., Clark, D. M., Ehlers, A., & Rapee, R. M. (2000). Social anxiety and self-impression: Cognitive preparation enhances the beneficial effects of video feedback following a stressful social task. *Behaviour Research and Therapy, 38*, 1183–1192.

Harvey, A. G., Watkins, E. R., Mansell, W., & Shafran, R. (2004). *Cognitive behavioural*

processes across psychological disorders: A transdiagnostic approach to research and treatment. New York: Oxford University Press.

Hayes, S., Hirsch, C. R., Krebs, G., & Mathews, A. (2010). The effects of modifying interpretation bias on worry in generalized anxiety disorder. *Behaviour Research and Therapy, 48*, 171–178.

Hazlett-Stevens, H., & Borkovec, T. D. (2004). Interpretive cues and ambiguity in generalized anxiety disorder. *Behaviour Research and Therapy, 42*, 881–892.

Heimberg, R. G., Brozovich, F. A., & Rapee, R. M. (2010). A cognitive-behavioral model of social anxiety disorder: Update and extension. In S. G. Hofmann & P. M. DiBartolo (Eds.), *Social anxiety: Clinical, developmental, and social perspectives* (2nd ed., pp. 395–422). New York: Academic Press.

Hertel, P. T., Brozovich, F. A., Joormann, J., & Gotlib, I. H. (2008). Biases in interpretation and memory in generalized social phobia. *Journal of Abnormal Psychology, 117*, 278–288.

Heuer, K., Lange, W., Isaac, L., Rinck, M., & Becker, E. S. (2010). Morphed emotional faces: Emotion detection and misinterpretation in social anxiety. *Journal of Behavior Therapy and Experimental Psychiatry, 41*, 418–425.

Hirsch, C. R., Clark, D. M., & Mathews, A. (2006). Imagery and interpretations in social phobia: Support for the combined cognitive biases hypothesis. *Behavior Therapy, 37*, 223–236.

Hirsch, C. R., Clark, D. M., Mathews, A., & Williams, R. (2003). Self-images play a causal role in social phobia. *Behaviour Research and Therapy, 41*, 909–921.

Hirsch, C. R., Hayes, S., Mathews, A., Perman, G., & Borkovec, T. (2012). The extent and nature of imagery during worry and positive thinking in generalized anxiety disorder. *Journal of Abnormal Psychology, 121*, 238–243.

Hirsch, C. R., & Mathews, A. (2000). Impaired positive inferential bias in social phobia. *Journal of Abnormal Psychology, 109*, 705–712.

Hirsch, C. R., Mathews, A., & Clark, D. M. (2007). Inducing an interpretation bias changes self-imagery: A preliminary investigation. *Behaviour Research and Therapy, 45*, 2173–2181.

Hirsch, C. R., Mathews, A., Clark, D. M., Williams, R., & Morrison, J. A. (2003). Negative self-imagery blocks inferences. *Behaviour Research and Therapy, 41,* 1383–1396.

Hirsch, C. R., Mathews, A., Clark, D. M., Williams, R., & Morrison, J. A. (2006). The causal role of negative imagery in social anxiety: A test in confident public speakers. *Journal of Behavior Therapy and Experimental Psychiatry, 37,* 159–170.

Hirsch, C. R., Meynen, T., & Clark, D. M. (2004). Negative self-imagery in social anxiety contaminates social interactions. *Memory, 12,* 496–506.

Kabat-Zinn, J. (2003). Mindfulness-based interventions in context: Past, present, and future. *Clinical Psychology: Science and Practice, 10,* 144–156.

Koster, E. H. W., Crombez, G., Verschuere, B., & De Houwer, J. (2006). Attention to threat in anxiety-prone individuals: Mechanisms underlying attentional bias. *Cognitive Therapy and Research, 30,* 635–643.

Koszycki, D., Benger, M., Shlik, J., & Bradwejn, J. (2007). Randomized trial of a meditation-based stress reduction program and cognitive behavior therapy in generalized social anxiety disorder. *Behaviour Research and Therapy, 45,* 2518–2526.

Lipton, M. G., Brewin, C. R., Linke, S., & Halperin, J. (2010). Distinguishing features of intrusive images in obsessive–compulsive disorder. *Journal of Anxiety Disorders, 24,* 816–822.

Llera, S. J., & Newman, M. G. (2010a). Effects of worry on physiological and subjective reactivity to emotional stimuli in generalized anxiety disorder and nonanxious control participants. *Emotion, 10,* 640–650.

Llera, S. J., & Newman, M. G. (2010b, November). *Revisiting emotional avoidance in GAD.* Paper presented at the annual meeting of the Association of Behavioral and Cognitive Therapies, San Francisco, CA.

Lundh, L., Czyzykow, S., & Öst, L. (1997). Explicit and implicit memory bias in panic disorder with agoraphobia. *Behaviour Research and Therapy, 35,* 1003–1014.

Lundh, L., & Öst, L. (1996). Recognition bias for critical faces in social phobics. *Behaviour Research and Therapy, 34,* 787–794.

Lundh, L., & Öst, L. (1997). Explicit and implicit memory bias in social phobia: The role of subdiagnostic type. *Behaviour Research and Therapy, 35,* 305–317.

Lundh, L., Thulin, U., Czyzykow, S., & Öst, L. (1998). Recognition bias for safe faces in panic disorder with agoraphobia. *Behaviour Research and Therapy, 36,* 323–337.

MacLeod, C., Mathews, A., & Tata, P. (1986). Attentional bias in emotional disorders. *Journal of Abnormal Psychology, 95,* 15–20.

MacLeod, C., & McLaughlin, K. (1995). Implicit and explicit memory bias in anxiety: A conceptual replication. *Behaviour Research and Therapy, 33,* 1–14.

MacLeod, C., Rutherford, E., Campbell, L., Ebsworthy, G., & Holker, L. (2002). Selective attention and emotional vulnerability: Assessing the causal basis of their association through the experimental manipulation of attentional bias. *Journal of Abnormal Psychology, 111,* 107–123.

Mathews, A., & MacLeod, C. (1994). Cognitive approaches to emotion and emotional disorders. *Annual Review of Psychology, 45,* 25–50.

Mathews, A., Mogg, K., Kentish, J., & Eysenck, M. (1995). Effect of psychological treatment on cognitive bias in generalized anxiety disorder. *Behaviour Research and Therapy, 33,* 293–303.

Mathews, A., Mogg, K., May, J., & Eysenck, M. (1989). Implicit and explicit memory bias in anxiety. *Journal of Abnormal Psychology, 98,* 236–240.

Mattia, J. I., Heimberg, R. G., & Hope, D. A. (1993). The revised Stroop color-naming task in social phobics. *Behaviour Research and Therapy, 31,* 305–313.

McManus, F., Clark, D. M., & Hackmann, A. (2000). Specificity of cognitive biases in social phobia and their role in recovery. *Behavioural and Cognitive Psychotherapy, 28,* 201–209.

McNally, R. J., & Foa, E. B. (1987). Cognition and agoraphobia: Bias in the interpretation of threat. *Cognitive Therapy and Research, 11,* 567–581.

McNally, R. J., Otto, M. W., & Hornig, C. D. (2001). The voice of emotional memory: Content-filtered speech in panic disorder, social phobia and major depressive disorder. *Behaviour Research and Therapy, 39,* 1329–1337.

McTeague, L. M., Lang, P. J., Laplante, M., Cuthbert, B. N., Strauss, C. C., & Bradley, M. M. (2009). Fearful imagery in social phobia: Generalization, comorbidity, and physiological reactivity. *Biological Psychiatry, 65,* 374–382.

Mennin, D. S., Heimberg, R. G., Turk, C. L., & Fresco, D. M. (2005). Preliminary evidence for an emotion dysregulation model of generalized anxiety disorder. *Behaviour Research and Therapy, 43,* 1281–1310.

Mennin, D. S., Holaway, R. M., Fresco, D. M., Moore, M. T., & Heimberg, R. G. (2007). Delineating components of emotion and its dysregulation in anxiety and mood psychopathology. *Behavior Therapy, 38,* 284–302.

Mennin, D. S., McLaughlin, K. A., & Flanagan, T. J. (2009). Emotion regulation deficits in generalized anxiety disorder, social anxiety disorder, and their co-occurrence. *Journal of Anxiety Disorders, 23,* 866–871.

Mitte, K. (2008). Memory bias for threatening information in anxiety and anxiety disorders: A meta-analytic review. *Psychological Bulletin, 134,* 886–911.

Mogg, K., & Bradley, B. P. (1998). A cognitive-motivational analysis of anxiety. *Behaviour Research and Therapy, 36,* 809–848.

Mogg, K., Bradley, B. P., De Bono, J., & Painter, M. (1997). Time course of attentional bias for threat information in non-clinical anxiety. *Behaviour Research and Therapy, 35,* 297–303.

Mogg, K., Bradley, B. P., Miles, F., & Dixon, R. (2004). Time course of attentional bias for threat scenes: Testing the vigilance–avoidance hypothesis. *Cognition and Emotion, 18,* 689–700.

Mogg, K., Holmes, A., Garner, M., & Bradley, B. P. (2008). Effects of threat cues on attentional shifting, disengagement and response slowing in anxious individuals. *Behaviour Research and Therapy, 46,* 656–667.

Moscovitch, D. A., Gavric, D. L., Merrifield, C., Bielak, T., & Moscovitch, M. (2011). Retrieval properties of negative vs. positive mental images and autobiographical memories in social anxiety: Outcomes with a new measure. *Behaviour Research and Therapy, 49,* 505–517.

Moser, J. S., Hajcak, G., Huppert, J. D., Foa, E. B., & Simons, R. F. (2008). Interpretation bias in social anxiety as detected by event-related brain potentials. *Emotion, 8,* 693–700.

Newman, M. G., & Llera, S. J. (2011). A novel theory of experiential avoidance in generalized anxiety disorder: A review and synthesis of research supporting a contrast avoidance model of worry. *Clinical Psychology Review, 31,* 371–382.

Nunn, J. D., Stevenson, R. J., & Whalan, G. (1984). Selective memory effects in agoraphobic patients. *British Journal of Clinical Psychology, 23,* 195–201.

O'Banion, K., & Arkowitz, H. (1977). Social anxiety and selective memory for affective information about the self. *Social Behavior and Personality, 5,* 321–328.

Obsessive Compulsive Cognitions Working Group. (2003). Psychometric validation of the Obsessive Beliefs Questionnaire and the Interpretation of Intrusions Inventory. *Behaviour Research and Therapy, 41,* 863–878.

Posner, M. I. (1980). Orienting of attention. *Quarterly Journal of Experimental Psychology, 32,* 3–25.

Rachman, S. (1997). A cognitive theory of obsessions. *Behaviour Research and Therapy, 35,* 793–802.

Radomsky, A. S., & Rachman, S. (1999). Memory bias in obsessive–compulsive disorder (OCD). *Behaviour Research and Therapy, 37,* 605–618.

Radomsky, A. S., & Rachman, S. (2004). The importance of importance in OCD memory research. *Journal of Behavior Therapy and Experimental Psychiatry, 35,* 137–151.

Radomsky, A. S., Rachman, S., & Hammond, D. (2001). Memory bias, confidence and responsibility in compulsive checking. *Behaviour Research and Therapy, 39,* 813–822.

Rapee, R. M. (1994). Failure to replicate a memory bias in panic disorder. *Journal of Anxiety Disorders, 8,* 291–300.

Rapee, R. M., & Heimberg, R. G. (1997). A cognitive-behavioral model of anxiety in social phobia. *Behaviour Research and Therapy, 35,* 741–756.

Rapee, R. M., McCallum, S. L., Melville, L. F., Ravenscroft, H., & Rodney, J. M. (1994). Memory bias in social phobia. *Behaviour Research and Therapy, 32,* 89–99.

Rapee, R. M., & Lim, L. (1992). Discrepancy between self- and observer ratings of performance in social phobics. *Journal of Abnormal Psychology, 101,* 728–731.

Rinck, M., & Becker, E. S. (2005). A comparison of attentional biases and memory biases in women with social phobia and major depression. *Journal of Abnormal Psychology, 114,* 62–74.

Rinck, M., Becker, E. S., Kellermann, J., & Roth, W. T. (2003). Selective attention in anxiety: Distraction and enhancement in visual search. *Depression and Anxiety, 18,* 18–28.

Rodebaugh, T. L., Heimberg, R. G., Schultz,

L. T., & Blackmore, M. (2010). The moderated effects of video feedback in the context of social anxiety disorder. *Journal of Anxiety Disorders, 24,* 663–671.

Rodebaugh, T. L., & Rapee, R. M. (2005). Those who think they look worst respond best: Self-observer discrepancy predicts response to video feedback following a speech task. *Cognitive Therapy and Research, 29,* 705–715.

Roemer, L., & Orsillo, S. M. (2008). Efficacy of an acceptance-based behavior therapy for generalized anxiety disorder: Evaluation in a randomized controlled trial. *Journal of Consulting and Clinical Psychology, 76,* 1083–1089.

Rohner, J. (2004). Memory-based attentional biases: Anxiety is linked to threat avoidance. *Cognition and Emotion, 18,* 1027–1054.

Salemink, E., Hertel, P., & Mackintosh, B. (2010). Interpretation training influences memory for prior interpretations. *Emotion, 10,* 903–907.

Salters-Pedneault, K., Roemer, L., Tull, M. T., Rucker, L., & Mennin, D. S. (2006). Evidence of broad deficits in emotion regulation associated with chronic worry and generalized anxiety disorder. *Cognitive Therapy and Research, 30,* 469–480.

Schmidt, N. B., Richey, J. A., Buckner, J. D., & Timpano, K. R. (2009). Attention training for generalized social anxiety disorder. *Journal of Abnormal Psychology, 118,* 5–14.

Smith, T. W., Ingram, R. E., & Brehm, S. S. (1983). Social anxiety, anxious self-preoccupation, and recall of self-relevant information. *Journal of Personality and Social Psychology, 44,* 1276–1283.

Speckens, A. E. M., Hackmann, A., Ehlers, A., & Cuthbert, B. (2007). Intrusive images and memories of earlier adverse events in patients with obsessive compulsive disorder. *Journal of Behavior Therapy and Experimental Psychiatry, 38,* 411–422.

Spokas, M., Luterek, J. A., & Heimberg, R. G. (2009). Social anxiety and emotional suppression: The mediating role of beliefs. *Journal of Behavior Therapy and Experimental Psychiatry, 40,* 283–291.

Stopa, L., & Jenkins, A. (2007). Images of the self in social anxiety: Effects on the retrieval of autobiographical memories. *Journal of Behavior Therapy and Experimental Psychiatry, 38,* 459–473.

Tata, P. R., Liebowitz, J. A., Prunty, M. J., Cameron, M., & Pickering, A. D. (1996). Attentional bias in obsessional compulsive disorder. *Behaviour Research and Therapy, 34,* 53–60.

Teachman, B. A., Marker, C. D., & Clerkin, E. M. (2010). Catastrophic misinterpretations as a predictor of symptom change during treatment for panic disorder. *Journal of Consulting and Clinical Psychology, 78,* 964–973.

Teachman, B. A., Smith-Janik, S., & Saporito, J. (2007). Information processing biases and panic disorder: Relationships among cognitive and symptom measures. *Behaviour Research and Therapy, 45,* 1791–1811.

Tobon, J. I., Ouimet, A. J., & Dozois, D. J. A. (2011). Attentional bias in anxiety disorders following cognitive behavioral treatment. *Journal of Cognitive Psychotherapy, 25,* 114–129.

Tolin, D. F., Abramowitz, J. S., Brigidi, B. D., Amir, N., Street, G. P., & Foa, E. B. (2001). Memory and memory confidence in obsessive-compulsive disorder. *Behaviour Research and Therapy, 39,* 913–927.

Tran, T. B., Hertel, P. T., & Joormann, J. (2011). Cognitive bias modification: Induced interpretive biases affect memory. *Emotion, 11,* 145–152.

Treanor, M., Erisman, S. M., Salters-Pedneault, K., Roemer, L., & Orsillo, S. M. (2011). Acceptance-based behavioral therapy for GAD: Effects on outcomes from three theoretical models. *Depression and Anxiety, 28,* 127–136.

Tuna, Ş., Tekcan, A. İ., & Topçuoğlu, V. (2005). Memory and metamemory in obsessive-compulsive disorder. *Behaviour Research and Therapy, 43,* 15–27.

Turk, C. L., Heimberg, R. G., Luterek, J. A., Mennin, D. S., & Fresco, D. M. (2005). Emotion dysregulation in generalized anxiety disorder: A comparison with social anxiety disorder. *Cognitive Therapy and Research, 29,* 89–106.

Wells, A., Clark, D. M., & Ahmad, S. (1998). How do I look with my mind's eye?: Perspective taking in social phobic imagery. *Behaviour Research and Therapy, 36,* 631–634.

Wenzel, A., & Cochran, C. (2006). Autobiographical memories prompted by automatic thoughts in panic disorder and social phobia. *Cognitive Behaviour Therapy, 35,* 129–137.

Wenzel, A., Jackson, L. C., & Holt, C. S. (2002). Social phobia and the recall of autobiographical memories. *Depression and Anxiety, 15,* 186–189.

Wenzel, A., Werner, M. M., Cochran, C. K., & Holt, C. S. (2004). A differential pattern of autobiographical memory retrieval in social phobic and nonanxious individuals. *Behavioural and Cognitive Psychotherapy, 32*, 1–13.

Werner, K. H., Goldin, P. R., Ball, T. M., Heimberg, R. G., & Gross, J. J. (2011). Assessing emotion regulation in social anxiety disorder: The Emotion Regulation Interview. *Journal of Psychopathology and Behavioral Assessment, 33*, 346–354.

White, L. K., Suway, J. G., Pine, D. S., Bar-Haim, Y., & Fox, N. A. (2011). Cascading effects: The influence of attention bias to threat on the interpretation of ambiguous information. *Behaviour Research and Therapy, 49*, 244–251.

Wild, J., & Clark, D. M. (2011). Imagery rescripting of early traumatic memories in social phobia. *Cognitive and Behavioral Practice, 18*, 433–443.

Wild, J., Hackmann, A., & Clark, D. M. (2007). When the present visits the past: Updating traumatic memories in social phobia. *Journal of Behavior Therapy and Experimental Psychiatry, 38*, 386–401.

Wild, J., Hackmann, A., & Clark, D. M. (2008). Rescripting early memories linked to negative images in social phobia: A pilot study. *Behavior Therapy, 39*, 47–56.

Wilhelm, S., McNally, R. J., Baer, L., & Florin, I. (1996). Directed forgetting in obsessive–compulsive disorder. *Behaviour Research and Therapy, 34*, 633–641.

Williams, J. M. G., Watts, F. N., MacLeod, C., & Mathews, A. (1988). *Cognitive psychology and emotional disorders*. Chichester, UK: Wiley.

CHAPTER 24

Cognition and Depression

Mechanisms Associated with the Onset and Maintenance of Emotional Disorder

Peter C. Clasen, Seth G. Disner, and Christopher G. Beevers

Over the past 40 years, a continually evolving literature has examined the role of cognition in depression. Initially, efforts focused on measuring self-reported negative cognition via questionnaires. This has since transitioned into the use of experimental tasks and paradigms designed to measure how information is attended to, processed, encoded, and recalled. As a result, there is now a substantial body of research evidence that generally supports the idea that depression is characterized by negatively biased cognition and information processing (i.e., attention, memory, and interpretation) (Gotlib & Joormann, 2010). More recent efforts have attempted to integrate these findings with genetic and brain-imaging approaches so that the neurobiology of these cognitive biases can be identified.

This chapter aims to review what we believe to be among the most exciting research in this area. We first review how depression is typically defined and the prevalence and incidence of it. We then provide an overview of the dominant cognitive model of depression. Next, we identify cognitive biases associated with depression vulnerability and the maintenance of depression. We then briefly review attempts to determine whether cognitive biases are causally implicated in depression. We conclude with

a brief review of research that integrates cognitive biases with other levels of analyses (e.g., genetic, neural). By doing so, we hope to provide a comprehensive overview of research examining cognitive factors in depression. We believe this is an exciting time to be conducting research that examines the interface between cognition and depression. We hope that you will feel the same way after reading this chapter.

Description and Epidemiology of Depression

Major depressive disorder (MDD) is a common, recurrent, and impairing condition that predicts future suicide attempts, interpersonal problems, unemployment, substance abuse, and delinquency (Kessler & Walters, 1998). According to the World Health Organization, 121 million people are currently suffering from MDD, and it is a leading cause of disability. The annual economic cost of MDD in the United States alone is also quite large—billions of dollars annually—due to medical expenditures, lost productivity, and other costs (Greenberg, Stiglin, Finkelstein, & Berndt, 1993; Wang, Simon, & Kessler, 2003). Furthermore, MDD accounts for more than two-thirds of the 30,000 reported suicides each year (Beautrais et al., 1996).

To be diagnosed with MDD, a person must experience either depressed mood or anhedonia (a loss of interest or pleasure) for most of the day, nearly every day, for at least a 2-week period. Four additional symptoms (e.g., insomnia, fatigue, hopelessness) are also required to be present (for more detail, see the *Diagnostic and Statistical Manual of Mental Disorders*, 4th edition, text revision [American Psychiatric Association, 2000]). These symptoms must cause significant distress or impairment in important areas of functioning and should not be attributable to substances (e.g., drug abuse, medication changes), medical conditions (e.g., hypothyroidism), or the death of a loved one.

Recent epidemiological research indicates that the 12-month prevalence rate for MDD is 6.6% (95% confidence interval [CI], 5.9–7.3%) among adults residing in the United States. Lifetime prevalence for MDD is 16.2% (95% CI, 15.1–17.3%) (Kessler et al., 2003). Put differently, approximately 13.5 million Americans experienced MDD in the past year, and 34 million adults have experienced MDD at some point in their life. Approximately 51% who experienced MDD in the past year, received health care treatment for it, although treatment was considered adequate in only 21% of the cases (Beautrais et al., 1996). Thus, MDD is a prevalent and pervasive mental health disorder that is unfortunately not treated optimally in the United States.

Obtaining adequate treatment is important, as the course of MDD tends to be relatively prolonged. One of the largest studies of MDD recovery among individuals seeking treatment found that 50% of the sample recovered from MDD within 6 months, 70% within 12 months, and 81% within 24 months. Approximately 17% did not recover within the 5-year follow-up period (Keller et al., 1992). The first 6 months represent a particularly important time period for MDD recovery, as the rate of MDD recovery significantly slows thereafter. Similarly, Kessler and Wang (2009) write that time to recovery from MDD in non-treatment-seeking populations "appears to be highly variable, although epidemiological evidence is slim" (p. 29). One study found that 40% had recovered from MDD by 5 weeks and 90%

had recovered within 12 months (McLeod, Kessler, & Landis, 1992). Another study reported that mean time to recovery was 4 months and that approximately 90% had recovered by 12 months (Kendler, Walters, & Kessler, 1997). Taken together, these data suggest that most participants from a community sample recover from MDD within 12 months.

Given this enormous impact at societal and individual levels, there is a clear need to better understand factors that contribute to the onset of MDD so that efficacious treatments for this disorder can be developed and disseminated. Although a range of theories has been proposed (e.g., Beck, 1967; Ferster, 1973; Joiner & Coyne, 1999; Mayberg, 1997; Schildkraut, 1965), cognitive theories of depression have significant empirical support. We now review the prominent cognitive models of depression in some detail.

Cognitive Theories of Depression

Cognitive models of depression provide a compelling explanation for who is likely to become depressed. For the most part, cognitive models of MDD are diathesis–stress models of psychopathology. These models posit that an underlying vulnerability (diathesis) is necessary and sufficient to produce the disorder if and when the person encounters an activating event (stress). According to cognitive models, cognitive mechanisms play a key role in vulnerability to the onset and maintenance of MDD (e.g., Abramson, Metalsky, & Alloy, 1989; Beck, 1967; Ingram, 1984; Teasdale, 1988).

Perhaps the best known cognitive model of depression was developed by Beck (1967, 1976). Beck's model postulates that individuals who are vulnerable to MDD harbor depressotypic schemas, or internal knowledge structures (e.g., beliefs, attitudes, memories) that influence information-processing operations, such as selective attention and memory search (also see Segal & Shaw, 1986; Williams, Watts, MacLeod, & Mathews, 1997). For example, if an individual holds the belief that he is worthless, he may focus on internal explanations for a negative event (e.g., "It's all my fault that I lost my job—I have nothing to offer this company") instead of examining other possible explanations (e.g., bad economy, poor management). This internal focus includes selective attention to, and recall of, schema-congruent information, which exacerbates negative mood and further reinforces schematic beliefs. Schematic structures associated with MDD are thought to be organized around fears and concerns about self-worth (Beck, 1967, 1976) and evolve from a range of developmental factors, including genetic predisposition, parental factors, and adverse childhood events (e.g., Beck, 2008; Hammen et al., 1995; Hammen, Shih, & Brennan, 2004).

Consistent with diathesis–stress models, depressotypic schemas are not accessible at all times. Instead, access depends on an activating event that directly or indirectly resonates with schematic themes (e.g., threats to self-worth) (see Beck, 1987). Activating events are considered necessary and sufficient to trigger schematic processing. Once activated, schematic processing involves the initiation of negative, self-referent information-processing biases that underlie the onset and maintenance of MDD (Ingram, 1984; Ingram, Miranda, & Segal, 1998; Teasdale, 1988).

Over the past 40 years, a host of evidence has accumulated supporting and refining the central tenants of this model. We review this evidence below, differentiating between mechanisms associated with depression vulnerability and those underlying the prolonged experience of negative emotion. This differentiation is useful for the organization of this review, but the reader will quickly note significant overlap among associated mechanisms. Importantly, the majority of extant research is correlational and predominantly cross-sectional. Thus, the bulk of empirical support for cognitive models of depression is descriptive and does not address the causal role of cognition in the onset and maintenance of MDD. Following our review, we discuss this critical limitation and point to promising areas of research aimed at addressing this gap in the literature.

Cognitive Vulnerability to Depression

Cognitive models explicitly define the circumstances in which schema activation will initiate depressive emotions. These circumstances occur when an activating event directly or indirectly resonates with schematic themes (e.g., Beck, 1987). Therefore, in order to identify mechanisms associated with the initiation of depressive emotions, it is essential to first activate the latent schematic structure. This presents a host of methodological challenges for researchers, including identifying individuals who may harbor a depressotypic schema but who are not currently depressed (i.e., depression vulnerability) and selecting a laboratory procedure that is ethical, valid, and can reliably activate schemas across research participants (Ingram et al., 1998).

Several effective solutions to these challenges have been implemented. Depression-vulnerable samples typically include individuals who are at high risk for developing MDD because they were previously depressed and are currently in remission or because they have a parental history of MDD. Several laboratory procedures have been implemented to putatively activate latent cognitive vulnerabilities among vulnerable individuals, including mood priming, increasing self-awareness, and cognitive load manipulations. Each of these manipulations is thought to facilitate greater access to latent cognitive vulnerabilities to depression.

Mood priming is thought to increase access to negative cognition via spreading activation through associative networks (Ingram, 1984). Increasing attention to or memory for negative stimuli theoretically initiates a cascade of associative processing that involves greater access to negative content and processing biases. Experimentally increasing self-awareness is also thought to trigger this cascade in depression-vulnerable people. By contrast, cognitive load manipulations are thought to increase access to negative cognition by interfering with efforts to control negative thinking. Redirecting limited cognitive resources to some trivial task (e.g., remembering a sequence of digits) theoretically diminishes resources that otherwise would be engaged in managing aversive schema-congruent processing. We review evidence resulting from specific examples of these techniques below. These studies help determine the types of cognitive vulnerabilities that are associated with past and future depression, including biases in attention, memory, attitudes, interpretation, and attributions.

Attentional Bias

Biases in attention have been observed among depression-vulnerable people following a sad mood prime. Sad mood prime manipulations frequently involve inducing a sad mood by having participants listen to sad music, view a sad video, recall a sad memory, or some combination therein. Several studies have demonstrated that mood primes "activate" attentional biases in depression-vulnerable individuals. For instance, never-depressed girls at risk for depression by virtue of a maternal history of depression displayed a stronger attentional bias for sad faces following a sad mood induction than girls without a maternal history of depression (Joormann, Talbot, & Gotlib, 2007). This same bias for sad faces was observed among adults who had remitted from major depression compared to healthy controls (Joormann & Gotlib, 2007; also see Yiend, Barnicot, & Koster, Chapter 6, this volume).

Critically, these attentional biases following a mood prime have been shown to predict the onset of depressive symptoms. Using a short-term longitudinal design, increased attentional bias for negative stimuli following a dysphoric mood induction combined with life stress to predict increases in future dysphoria (Beevers & Carver, 2003). Similarly, soldiers with an attentional bias for sad faces before warzone deployment were more likely to endorse depression if they experienced war zone stress compared to those without an attentional bias for sad stimuli (Beevers, Lee, Wells, Ellis, & Telch, 2011).

Memory Bias

Several studies have also documented memory biases in individuals with remitted depression following a mood prime. Following a mood induction, previously depressed individuals tend to recall more negative information on an incidental recall task than never-depressed individuals (Gilboa & Gotlib, 1997; Teasdale & Dent, 1987; also see Murray, Holland, & Kensinger, Chapter 9, this volume). This bias appears to be specific to sad information, as these groups do not differ in recall of positive or neutral words.

Another study, which used increased self-focus as a prime, also found that formerly depressed individuals recalled more negative words and had fewer incorrectly recalled positive words than never-depressed adults (Hedlund & Rude, 1995). Thus, individuals with remitted depression display biases in attention and memory for negative word stimuli under conditions of sad mood or increased self-awareness.

More work is needed to determine whether these memory biases prospectively predict the onset of depressive symptoms, especially under conditions of stress. However, at least two studies lend preliminary support to this prediction. For example, Bellew and Hill (1991) sampled negative, self-referent memory biases among pregnant women. At baseline, women with these memory biases did not differ from women without these biases on a measure of depressive symptoms. Three months following childbirth, however, women who had demonstrated memory biases at baseline reported higher levels of depressive symptoms. This effect was moderated by the negative impact of intervening life stress on self-esteem. Similar findings have been observed among a group of patients with multiple sclerosis. In this recent study, negative memory biases interacted with intervening life stress to predict higher levels of depressed symptoms at follow-up (Beeney & Arnett, 2008). These findings lend preliminary support to the idea that memory biases prospectively predict the onset of depression under conditions of stress.

Formerly depressed individuals also demonstrate limited access to autobiographical memories. In one study, women who had remitted from depression continued to demonstrate a pattern of reduced specificity when recalling emotional autobiographical memories (e.g., Mackinger, Pachinger, Leibetseder, & Fartacek, 2000). This pattern of overgeneralized autobiographical memory is associated with a more severe course of depression (Brittlebank, Scott, Williams, & Ferrier, 1993) and has been shown to interact with life stress to prospectively predict increases in depression symptoms (Gibbs & Rude, 2004). Below, we further discuss autobiographical memory as a maintaining factor; however, this style of recalling personally relevant events appears to contribute to depression vulnerability, particularly under conditions of stress.

Dysfunctional Attitudes

Besides attention and memory biases, depression-vulnerable individuals also demonstrate dysfunctional attitudes following mood primes. Dysfunctional attitudes are rigid, maladaptive beliefs that typically reflect a person's negative self-schema. Examples of dysfunctional attitudes include "I'm nothing if a person I love doesn't like me" or "If I fail at my work, then I'm a failure as a person" (Weissman & Beck, 1978). People with a past history of depression are more likely to endorse dysfunctional attitudes after a negative mood induction than people with no depression history (Miranda, Gross, Persons, & Hahn, 1998; Miranda & Persons, 1988). Again, the presence of negative mood is critical, as no differences in dysfunctional attitudes are typically observed in the absence of a negative mood (Miranda, Persons, & Byers, 1990; Miranda et al., 1998).

More recently, longitudinal studies have documented that increased dysfunctional thinking before and after a sad mood induction prospectively predicts depressive relapse in previously depressed patients (Segal, Gemar, & Williams, 1999; Segal et al., 2006). In these two important studies, patients with remitted depression were administered the Dysfunctional Attitude Scale (Weissman & Beck, 1978) before and after a negative mood provocation consisting of sad music combined with autobiographical recall of a sad event. In both studies, increases in dysfunctional attitudes following the sad mood provocation predicted depressive relapse during the follow-up period, even when controlling for number of previous depressive episodes (Segal et al., 1999, 2006). In summary, there is considerable evidence that dysfunctional thinking following a sad mood prime is an important marker of vulnerability to depression (Lau, Segal, & Williams, 2004; Scher, Ingram, & Segal, 2005).

Interpretations

Depression vulnerability is also associated with negative interpretations of ambiguous

information under conditions of cognitive load (e.g., Wenzlaff & Bates, 1998). The rationale behind a cognitive load manipulation is that as cognitive resources are depleted, depression-vulnerable individuals are less able to suppress or correct latent cognitive biases. Evidence supports this idea. For example, in one study researchers presented a set of scrambled sentences that could be unscrambled to convey either a positive or negative sentiment (Wenzlaff & Bates, 1998). Currently depressed individuals tend to unscramble significantly more negative sentences compared to nondepressed individuals. Depression-vulnerable individuals (in this case, with remitted depression) do not demonstrate this bias in the absence of a cognitive load. However, in the presence of a cognitive load (e.g., trying to simultaneously remember a six-digit number), the performance of participants with remitted depression mirrors the actively depressed group: They demonstrate a bias toward unscrambling significantly more negative sentences compared to never-depressed people under cognitive load (for similar results with different tasks, see (Wenzlaff & Eisenberg, 2001; Wenzlaff, Rude, Taylor, Stultz, & Sweatt, 2001).

Importantly, this negatively biased interpretation of ambiguous information under cognitive load has been shown to predict the onset of depressive symptoms. For example, Rude, Wenzlaff, Gibbs, Vane, and Whitney (2002) administered the previously described scrambled sentence task in the presence or absence of a cognitive load. Symptoms of depression were then reassessed 4–6 weeks later. Indeed, biases in negative interpretations on the scrambled sentence task when a cognitive load was imposed significantly predicted subsequent increases in depression. This same bias under cognitive load predicted future MDD onset in a later study (Rude, Durham-Fowler, Baum, Rooney, & Maestas, 2009). Thus, biased information processing when cognitive resources are depleted appears to be an important marker of depression vulnerability.

Causal Attributions

Another important cognitive vulnerability involves conditional thinking about the causes of activating events. The hopelessness theory of depression (Abramson et al., 1989) posits that individuals who blame themselves for negative events are more likely to become depressed. Specifically, vulnerable individuals make stable, global, and internal attributions about the causes of negative events but unstable, specific, and external attributions about the causes of positive events. Implicit in this theory is the important role of the activating event. Again, such an event is critical to activate these negative attributions. Moreover, this negative thinking is generally limited to attributions about the self, as depressed individuals do not exhibit global, stable, internal biases when asked to make attributions about negative events that happen to other people (e.g., Schlenker & Britt, 1996; Sweeney, Shaeffer, & Golin, 1982).

In line with the other cognitive biases observed under mood prime, increased self-awareness, and cognitive load, there is consistent evidence that individuals with a negative attributional style are at much higher risk for future MDD. For instance, Alloy and colleagues (2006) reported that high-risk college students (i.e., those with a negative attributional style) were 3.5–6.8 times more likely to experience a first onset of depression and depression recurrence than low-risk college students. Thus, biased attributions about one's role in the causes and consequences of events appear to play an important role in cognitive vulnerability for depression.

Summary

There is now substantial evidence that individuals who are vulnerable for MDD exhibit cognitive biases that increase the likelihood of experiencing future episodes of depression. Such biases are observed in attention, memory, attitudes, interpretations, and attributions. These biases are thought to produce increased generation of negative, self-referent emotions following activating events, thereby increasing risk for the onset (or relapse) of MDD.

Incidentally, the success of laboratory manipulations, such as mood priming, increasing self-focus, and cognitive load, has inspired a better understanding of the properties of "activating" events. Events that increase sad mood, induce greater self-reflection, and/or deplete cognitive resources are expected to trigger schematic information processing associated with depression vulnerability. Cognitive theories posit that activating events are most potent when they resonate with underlying fears about self-worth. Therefore, a more refined perspective on vulnerability must include future efforts to better understand individual differences in reactivity to different classes of events (e.g., social rejection, performance feedback) that are more or less likely to trigger schematic information processing (e.g., Segal, Shaw, Vella, & Katz, 1992).

It is important to note that, so far, our perspective on cognitive vulnerability has focused on mechanisms underlying the onset (or relapse) of depression. The biases reviewed above presumably contribute to the affective symptoms associated with depression, including sadness and/or anhedonia. If these affective symptoms decayed relatively quickly, however, they would not constitute MDD. Indeed, these hallmark symptoms must occur for a period of 2 weeks or longer to warrant a diagnosis of MDD. Therefore, depression is characterized not only by biases associated with the generation of sadness and anhedonia, but also by biases that prolong the experience of these affective symptoms. In the next section, we review cognitive processes associated with the maintenance of depression.

Cognitive Factors That Maintain Negative Emotion[1]

Before reviewing the literature, we briefly remind the reader of relevant aspects of the cognitive model presented earlier in this chapter. According to cognitive theories,

[1]Cognitive models suggest that information-processing biases will only occur when schemas are activated. For currently depressed individuals it is assumed that schemas are already accessible and that information-processing biases are actively maintaining the disorder. Therefore, mood primes are not needed and cognitive functioning of depressed and nondepressed individuals can be compared directly. This methodological convenience may explain why there are far more studies of maintenance than vulnerability factors. Furthermore, it should be noted that researchers frequently use dysphoric individuals (i.e., individuals with elevated depressive symptoms who have not been diagnosed with MDD) within this paradigm.

schema activation influences information-processing systems such as those mediating selective attention and memory search. Schema-induced biases promote preferential processing of schema-congruent information. Thus, attention and memory systems are biased toward negative information and filter out positive information. This preferential processing of negative information results in a self-perpetuating, elaborative cycle that serves to reinforce negative cognitive biases and depressed mood (Beck, 1967). For these reasons, biased elaboration of negative, self-referent material is considered the "engine" that maintains MDD (Ingram, 1984; Teasdale, 1988). Biased elaboration in depression has been observed in many forms, including attention, memory, and rumination. Biased elaboration appears to involve deficits in cognitive control when processing mood-congruent information. These deficits also appear to undermine efforts to regulate negative emotions in MDD, further maintaining the disorder. Finally, biases underlying expectations about the experience of reward may also exacerbate and prolong depressive symptoms. We review evidence supporting this view of depression maintenance below.

Attentional Bias

Early efforts to observe attentional biases in MDD focused on automatic orienting biases toward negative stimuli typically found among individuals with anxiety disorders; however, depressed individuals did not consistently demonstrate this bias (Mogg, Bradley, & Williams, 1995). A subtle change in design, permitting participants to engage with emotional stimuli longer, yielded a more consistent pattern of results. When depressed individuals have extended time to engage with emotional stimuli (i.e., greater than 1,000 milliseconds [ms]), they show reliable evidence of preferential attention for mood-congruent information (e.g., Bradley, Mogg, & Lee, 1997; Gotlib, Krasnoperova, Yue, & Joormann, 2004; also see Yiend, Barnicot, & Koster, Chapter 6, this volume).

Together, these findings led to the hypothesis that depressed individuals do not automatically orient to mood-congruent information, but once it enters their awareness they preferentially elaborate on it (Mogg

& Bradley, 2005). Elaboration involves a deeper level of semantic and associative processing that relies on and produces stronger connections between semantic properties of stimuli and internally stored knowledge (Craik & Tulving, 1975; Klein & Loftus, 1988). In depression, the elaboration hypothesis posits that individuals display elaborative biases for mood-congruent information because they are inclined to engage in deeper-level associative processing between mood-congruent stimuli and internal representations of themselves (e.g., Ingram, 1984; Wisco, 2009).

The elaboration hypothesis is supported by research using gaze registration technology to measure allocation of visual attention to emotional stimuli. Several researchers have reported that depressed participants show biases in the allocation of attention toward mood-congruent information using these paradigms (Eizenman et al., 2003; Caseras, Garner, Bradley, & Mogg, 2007; Kellough, Beevers, Ellis, & Wells, 2008; Leyman, De Raedt, Vaeyens, & Philippaerts, 2011). This includes passive viewing tasks where participants freely decide where to allocate attention across an array of emotional stimuli (e.g., sad, happy, fearful, neutral) for extended periods of time (e.g., 30 seconds) (e.g., Kellough et al., 2008). These findings suggest that in depression, elaboration is generally specific to mood-congruent information, it persists over time, and is resistant to distraction from competing emotional images presented concurrently (also see Siegle, Granholm, Ingram, & Matt, 2001).

These findings support the notion that depressed individuals engage in preferential and sustained attention for sad stimuli. However, it remains unclear whether this is because stimuli are mood-congruent, self-referential, or both (see Wisco, 2009). This distinction is not trivial. Understanding which stimuli are most likely to produce elaboration is critical to improve research methods aimed at elucidating the mechanics of this processing bias. This involves future efforts to identify stimulus properties that most reliably trigger elaborative attention in MDD. In any case, the elaboration hypothesis has gained traction due to converging evidence at other levels of cognitive analysis, including research on memory biases.

Memory Bias

Memory biases for mood-congruent information are perhaps the most reliable cognitive findings in the depression literature (Mathews & MacLeod, 2005; Matt, Vázquez, & Campbell, 1992; Williams et al., 1997; also see Murray, Holland, & Kensinger, Chapter 9, this volume). However, these findings are generally limited to experiments where encoding facilitates elaboration of mood-congruent information (see Watkins, 2002). When depressed individuals have time to process semantic features, such as emotional valence or self-referential properties of emotional stimuli, they are better at recalling mood-congruent information compared to nondepressed individuals. In light of the attentional findings reviewed above, these findings may represent a consequence of encoding and consolidation biases mediated by attention. However, relatively few studies have explored the link between these biases. One recent experiment demonstrated that dysphoric individuals who engage in more elaborative attention allocation for emotional stimuli (measured with gaze registration) also recall these stimuli better (Wells, Beevers, Robison, & Ellis, 2010). More work is needed to explore the relationship between attention and memory biases associated with MDD.

Regardless, preferential recall of mood-congruent information has important implications for the prolonged experience of negative emotions in depression. These biases suggest that depressed individuals have limited access to internal representations of past events and, importantly, representations of themselves (e.g., autobiographical memories). These possibilities are supported by evidence that depressed individuals tend to recall more negative autobiographical memories, enhance the negative features of these memories, and even inaccurately reappraise memories in negative ways (e.g., Ben-Zeev, Young, & Madsen, 2009). Thus, in the same way that depressed individuals selectively elaborate on external stimuli, they demonstrate similar preferences when accessing internal representations (also see Williams, 1996). This limited universe of available self-representations helps reinforce schematic beliefs and perpetuate the elaborative cycle.

Rumination

Biased recall of autobiographical memories is not the only self-reflective process thought to help maintain MDD. Rumination, or the tendency to reflect and brood on the causes and consequences of depressed mood, represents a self-reflective process that is closely associated with MDD (Nolen-Hoeksema, 1991; Nolen-Hoeksema, Wisco, & Lyubomirsky, 2008; also see Watkins, Chapter 21, this volume). Examples of ruminative thoughts include "Why do I always react this way?" and "Why do I have problems other people don't have?" (Nolen-Hoeksema & Morrow, 1991). Similar to the attentional biases reviewed above, rumination is characterized as an elaborative process that is resistant to distraction (Nolen-Hoeksema et al., 2008). Rumination is associated with the prolonged experience of negative mood and diminished efforts (both cognitive and behavioral) to repair negative mood (e.g., (Lyubomirsky & Nolen-Hoeksema, 1993, 1995; Lyubomirsky, Tucker, Caldwell, & Berg, 1999). Therefore, rumination is considered a relatively stable style of elaborative self-reflection that contributes to the maintenance of depression.

More recently, researchers have sought to parse the features of rumination that make it an aversive form of self-reflection. According to this work, rumination is dangerous because it is associated with aversive modes of self-focus. One feature of maladaptive self-focus involves thinking about oneself in an abstract, conceptual, and decontextualized way (Teasdale, 1999). Compared to thinking about oneself in a more concrete and contextualized fashion, this abstract self-focus has been associated with a variety of aversive outcomes associated with MDD, including overgeneral autobiographical memory, reduced social problem solving, and rumination (e.g., Watkins & Baracaia, 2002; Watkins & Teasdale, 2001, 2004). Another feature of maladaptive self-focus involves the tendency to take a more immersed perspective during self-reflection (i.e., reliving events from a first-person perspective rather than recalling events from a third-person perspective) (e.g., Kross, Ayduk, & Mischel, 2005). This immersed self-focus has been linked with a variety of adverse mood-related outcomes and is associated with rumination (Ayduk & Kross, 2008; Kross & Ayduk, 2008, 2009). Thus, a growing body of research suggests that rumination perpetuates depression, in part, because it facilitates maladaptive modes of self-focus.

These findings raise important questions about why people ruminate. Research suggests that individuals ruminate because they hold positive beliefs about the consequences of rumination (e.g., Papageorgiou & Wells, 2001, 2003). More specifically, they believe that rumination helps them gain insight and understanding into the causes of depressed mood, solve complex problems, and prevent future mistakes (Watkins & Baracaia, 2001). These metacognitive beliefs about the utility of ruminative thinking help perpetuate its use, further maintaining depressed mood.

It is important to note that elaboration is not limited to effortful self-reflection. In fact, elaboration of negative emotion in MDD appears to remain "active" even when it is unwanted. Evidence suggests that some depressed individuals engage in thought suppression to limit chronic reexposure to negative information (Wenzlaff & Bates, 1998; Wenzlaff et al., 2001). Evidence also suggests that this strategy not only fails to successfully reduce negative mood, but actually promotes elaborative processes such as rumination (e.g., Wenzlaff & Luxton, 2003; Wenzlaff & Wegner, 2000). Together, these findings indicate that elaborative processes prolong negative emotion even when depressed individuals attempt to actively suppress them.

Cognitive Control of Emotional Information

So far, we have reviewed evidence of biased operations associated with the maintenance of MDD, including selective attention, memory search, and rumination. This work highlights the biased elaborative nature of these operations, but does not identify mechanisms underlying their expression. Cognitive control processes, including the ability to disengage attention and inhibit distracting information, are considered fundamental to operations such as selective attention, memory search, and self-reflection (e.g., Miller & Cohen, 2001; Posner & Rothbart, 1998).

For this reason, researchers have sought to identify cognitive control deficits among individuals with MDD.

Increasingly, researchers are reporting that depressed individuals exhibit deficits in cognitive control when processing mood-congruent information. For example, using an adaptation of Posner's (1980) exogenous cueing task, researchers have demonstrated that depressed and dysphoric individuals have difficulty disengaging attention from mood-congruent information (e.g., Koster, De Raedt, Goeleven, Franck, & Crombez, 2005; Koster, De Raedt, Leyman, & De Lissnyder, 2010). These difficulties are unique to mood-congruent information, as depressed and dysphoric individuals do not show similar deficits for neutral or positive stimuli. Also, these difficulties are unique to conditions involving extended time to engage with emotional stimuli (i.e., 1,500 ms), suggesting that these deficits are a feature of elaborative processing (see De Raedt & Koster, 2010), although it should be noted that there is some controversy about whether these tasks are pure assessments of attention disengagement (e.g., Mogg, Holmes, Garner, & Bradley, 2008).

Similar cognitive control deficits are found in tasks that require inhibition. Inhibitory control prevents distracting environmental information from interfering with goal-directed processing and therefore represents an important tool for regulating emotion (see Joormann & Gotlib, 2010; Nigg, 2000). Joormann and colleagues have developed and adapted several tasks capable of measuring the ability to inhibit distracting mood-congruent information. On these tasks, depressed individuals consistently demonstrate deficits inhibiting mood-congruent information (e.g., Goeleven, De Raedt, Baert, & Koster, 2006; Joormann, 2004). Thus, depressed individuals not only have trouble getting attention off mood-congruent information, they also have trouble inhibiting the intrusion of distracting mood-congruent information.

Deficits in cognitive control for mood-congruent information may underlie elaborative processing biases in MDD. For example, difficulty disengaging attention from sad stimuli may help explain the expression of mood-congruent elaborative attention (reviewed above). Inhibitory deficits have been linked to the pattern of mood-congruent deficits observed in MDD (e.g., Hertel, 1997; Hertel & Rude, 1991). Moreover, biases associated with attentional disengagement and inhibitory control are associated with rumination (Joormann, 2006; Koster, De Lissnyder, Derakshan, & De Raedt, 2011). Thus, an increasing body of research indicates that biases at the level of cognitive control facilitate the expression of elaborative processes putatively associated with the maintenance of MDD. The extent to which these cognitive control biases cause elaborative processing in MDD remains an important avenue for future research.

In addition to facilitating elaborative attention and rumination, cognitive control biases may also help maintain depression via effects on emotion regulation. A well-established literature suggests that adaptive emotion regulation depends on cognitive control processes (e.g., (Gross, 1998; Ochsner & Gross, 2005; also see Suri, Sheppes, & Gross, Chapter 11, this volume). Biases in cognitive control, therefore, theoretically influence depressed peoples' ability to successfully regulate negative emotions. There is some evidence to support this proposition. In one recent study, cognitive control biases in MDD were associated with reduced implementation of adaptive emotion regulation strategies, such as reappraisal, and increased implementation of maladaptive strategies, such as thought suppression and rumination (Joormann & Gotlib, 2010). These findings are exciting because they highlight growing speculation that biased cognitive control deficits in MDD mediate a variety of processes that maintain depression. Nevertheless, future work is needed to continue exploring this hypothesis.

Distorted Expectations and Reduced Sensitivity to Rewards

In addition to difficulty regulating negative emotions, MDD is associated with diminished reactivity to positive emotions, including the experience of reward. This diminished reactivity is thought to exacerbate and prolong depressive symptoms. Cognitive biases may also underlie this putative maintaining factor. For example, depressed individuals tend to distort expected rewards, overestimating the amount of reward they expect to feel for a given outcome (Yuan & Kring, 2009). They tend to set rigid conditional goals, believing that they will feel better only if they can achieve some discrete, usually difficult to attain, reward (Hadley & MacLeod, 2010). At the same time, depressed individuals show evidence of reduced sensitivity to rewarding stimuli (e.g., Epstein et al., 2006; Heller et al., 2009; Pizzagalli et al., 2009). When individuals place a high value on expected rewards but experience little actual reward, they report increased negative affect (e.g., Moberly & Watkins, 2010). Depression, hopelessness, and suicidal ideation are all associated with large discrepancies between idealized and actual outcomes (Cornette, Strauman, Abramson, & Busch, 2009; Higgins, Klein, & Strauman, 1985). Therefore, overestimation of positive outcomes and diminished sensitivity to reward likely contribute to the maintenance of MDD.

Summary

There is now a large body of research supporting the idea that depressed individuals preferentially elaborate on mood-congruent information. Evidence of these biases can be observed across measures of attention, memory, and rumination. Biased elaboration on mood-congruent information is thought to help maintain MDD. Deficits in cognitive control, such as the ability to disengage attention from mood-congruent stimuli, may underlie this style of elaborative processing. Cognitive control biases may also undermine efforts to successfully regulate depressive emotions, further maintaining MDD. Distorted expectations about rewards also represent important cognitive biases underlying the prolonged experience of depression.

Future Directions

Throughout the chapter we have commented on important areas of future research. In the remainder of the chapter we highlight two future directions we consider critical to the development of cognitive models of depression. These include the need to causally manipulate cognitive factors associated with depression and the need to integrate cognitive models with biological models of vulnerability and maintenance of MDD. In each section, we briefly highlight exciting ongoing work addressing these important areas of research.

Causally Manipulating Cognitive Factors That Maintain Depression

Work reviewed to this point identifies several cognitive biases that are associated with depression. However, most of this work is correlational. Therefore, it is unclear which, if any, of these biases are causally implicated in the onset and maintenance of MDD. This remains an important challenge to cognitive theories of depression.

Experiments that manipulate (and subsequently ameliorate) putative cognitive biases and examine subsequent effects on the onset and maintenance of depression are critical for determining causality. So-called cognitive bias modification studies use this paradigm to test causal hypotheses about putative mechanisms underlying the maintenance of MDD (e.g., Mathews & Mackintosh, 2000; Wilson, MacLeod, Mathews, & Rutherford, 2006; also see MacLeod & Clarke, Chapter 29, this volume). We briefly review two lines of research that are representative of this nascent but important literature.

One example of cognitive bias modification is attention training. This form of training involves manipulating stimulus–response contingencies in well-established cognitive tasks (e.g., dot probe, exogenous cueing) to train attention toward, or away from, a desired class of stimuli (e.g., positive, negative). In a randomized controlled design, active training for depression can involve training attention away from negative stimuli or toward positive stimuli. Thus, active training aims to ameliorate the putative attentional bias toward negative stimuli that theoretically prolongs depression. In this design, active training is compared to a placebo manipulation that involves no bias modification.

Using this design, Wells and Beevers (2010) reported that dysphoric individuals trained away from negative stimuli reported significantly fewer depressive symptoms at 2-week follow-up compared to individuals in the control condition. Baert, De Raedt, Schacht, and Koster (2010) reported similar results when training attention toward positive words and away from negative words among individuals with mild depression severity. However, depressed individuals with more severe symptoms demonstrated increased symptoms following attention training. More work is needed to replicate these findings and explore differences in response to attention training at varying levels of depression severity. Nevertheless, these preliminary findings support the notion that attentional biases play a causal role in the experience of depressive symptoms.

Another example of cognitive bias modification is concreteness training. As outlined above, the tendency to think abstractly, generally, and in a decontextualized manner may causally contribute to the maintenance of depression (e.g., Watkins & Moulds, 2005). Prior work has shown that training participants to focus on concrete features of events during self-reflection (i.e., thinking about the details of the event) rather than focusing on abstract implications (i.e., thinking about the causes, meanings, and implications of a negative event) significantly reduced emotional reactivity to a failure (Moberly & Watkins, 2006; Watkins, Moberly, & Moulds, 2008). This training has also been shown to reduce depressive symptoms in dysphoric and depressed individuals (Watkins, Baeyens, & Read, 2009; Watkins et al., 2011). Moreover, a proof-of-principle test indicates that reductions in depressive symptoms may be related to increases in concrete thinking following the training intervention (Watkins et al., 2009). Together, this evidence suggests that a cognitive bias to reflect more abstractly on negative events may, in fact, play a causal role in the maintenance of depression.

Integrating across Levels of Analysis

In this chapter we focused on reviewing evidence of cognitive biases in MDD from a cognitive level of analysis. Obviously, this is only one level of analysis for understanding mechanisms underlying depression. A substantial body of research has focused on identifying biological mechanisms associated with vulnerability and maintenance of MDD. Integrating cognitive and biological models represents an opportunity to develop a more comprehensive understanding of

MDD. Efforts to integrate these models are well underway; we briefly review two important examples below.

One example of integration involves understanding associations between genetic and cognitive vulnerability for depression. A common polymorphism in a gene regulating serotonin transmission (5-HTTLPR) has been associated with increased sensitivity to the adverse effects of stress (see Caspi, Hariri, Holmes, Uher, & Moffitt, 2010, for a review), including increased vulnerability for MDD (Caspi et al., 2003; Karg, Burmeister, Shedden, & Sen, 2011; but see Risch et al., 2009). This diathesis–stress framework is consistent with cognitive models of depression vulnerability. Efforts to integrate these models indicate that individuals with a genetic vulnerability for MDD also display information-processing biases associated with cognitive vulnerability for depression (e.g., Beevers, Ellis, Wells, & McGeary, 2010; Beevers, Gibb, McGeary, & Miller, 2007; Beevers, Marti, et al., 2011; Beevers, Wells, Ellis, & McGeary, 2009). Moreover, several studies now demonstrate that life stress interacts with genetic vulnerability to predict processing biases associated with the onset and maintenance of MDD (e.g., Antypa & Van der Does, 2010; Clasen, Wells, Knopik, McGeary, & Beevers, 2011). Efforts to integrate genetic and cognitive models of depression vulnerability are helping to identify who is most likely to demonstrate cognitive biases associated with MDD. These biases may represent key intermediary phenotypes for the onset of MDD among genetically vulnerable individuals who experience significant life stress.

A second important area of integration involves exploring associations between cognitive biases and the neural systems that putatively instantiate cognition and emotion. Broadly, functional neuroimaging studies indicate that MDD is associated with increased reactivity to negative information in brain regions associated with processing aversive emotions (e.g., amygdala) and inefficient recruitment of regions underlying cognitive control (e.g., dorsolateral prefrontal cortex) (e.g., Mayberg, 1997; Phillips, Drevets, Rauch, & Lane, 2003). Importantly, this pattern is associated with elaborative cognitive biases thought to maintain MDD, including biased attention, memory,

rumination, and cognitive control (e.g., Beevers, Clasen, Stice, & Schnyer, 2010; Berman et al., 2011; Cooney, Joormann, Eugène, Dennis, & Gotlib, 2010; Siegle, Thompson, Carter, Steinhauer, & Thase, 2007). Efforts to integrate cognitive and neural findings in MDD are helping define a circumscribed network of brain regions that, presumably, mediates cognitive biases (see Disner, Beevers, Haigh, & Beck, 2011, for a recent review). Understanding how this network gives rise to cognitive biases associated with depression is an exciting avenue for future research. This research promises to inspire a deeper understanding of cognitive and emotional process generally by elucidating when, how, and why these processes go awry in MDD.

These are just two examples of how cognitive bias research can be integrated with other levels of analysis. Additional work is now needed to examine complex etiological models of depression that link these various mechanisms. By studying factors that maintain depression across levels of analyses (e.g., cognitive, genetic, neural, environmental), we may be able to develop more comprehensive models of depression maintenance. Developing an integrative model is also in line with a central tenet of National Institute of Mental Health's strategic plan to strengthen the public health impact of translational research (Insel, 2009) and, perhaps more importantly, should yield a fuller, more nuanced understanding of this complex and debilitating disorder.

Conclusion

Depression is a common, recurrent, and impairing condition that can have devastating impact on individuals, families, and society in general (Kessler & Walters, 1998). There is clear indication that cognitive factors play an important role in both the onset and maintenance of the disorder. A host of information-processing biases, including biased attention, memory, and interpretation, have been associated with MDD. Cognitive vulnerability research supports the idea that these biases are latent among vulnerable individuals and can be accessed through activating events. Work on maintaining factors suggests that once cognitive biases are activated, sustained elaboration of negative, self-referential material plays a key role in maintaining MDD. Correlational research designs have been essential for identifying information-processing biases associated with depression. Nevertheless, experimental designs are now required to discover which of these biases, if any, play a causal role in the onset and maintenance of MDD. Finally, although it is also important to understand cognitive biases associated with MDD, it is also important to note that these processes do not work in isolation. Thus, we look forward to additional research that attempts to integrate cognitive models with other factors known to contribute to the disorder, including genetics and neurobiology.

References

Abramson, L. Y., Metalsky, G. I., & Alloy, L. B. (1989). Hopelessness depression: A theory-based subtype of depression. *Psychological Review, 96*, 358–372.

Alloy, L. B., Abramson, L. Y., Whitehouse, W. G., Hogan, M. E., Panzarella, C., & Rose, D. T. (2006). Prospective incidence of first onsets and recurrences of depression in individuals at high and low cognitive risk for depression. *Journal of Abnormal Psychology, 115*, 145–156.

American Psychiatric Association. (2000). *Diagnostic and statistical manual of mental disorders* (4th ed., text rev.). Washington, DC: Author.

Antypa, N., & Van der Does, A. J. W. (2010). Serotonin transporter gene, childhood emotional abuse and cognitive vulnerability to depression. *Genes, Brain, and Behavior, 9*, 615–620.

Ayduk, O., & Kross, E. (2008). Enhancing the pace of recovery: Self-distanced analysis of negative experiences reduces blood pressure reactivity. *Psychological Science, 19*, 229–231.

Baert, S., De Raedt, R., Schacht, R., & Koster, E. H. W. (2010). Attentional bias training in depression: Therapeutic effects depend on depression severity. *Journal of Behavior Therapy and Experimental Psychiatry, 41*, 265–274.

Beautrais, A. L., Joyce, P. R., Mulder, R. T., Fergusson, D. M., Deavoll, B. J., & Nightingale, S. K. (1996). Prevalence and comorbidity of mental disorders in persons making serious suicide attempts: A case-control study. *American Journal of Psychiatry, 153*, 1009–1014.

Beck, A. T. (1967). *Depression: clinical, experimental, and theoretical aspects*. New York: Harper & Row.

Beck, A. T. (1976). *Cognitive therapy and the emotional disorders*. Oxford, UK: International Universities Press.

Beck, A. T. (1987). Cognitive models of depression. *Journal of Cognitive Psychotherapy, 1*(1), 5–37.

Beck, A. T. (2008). The evolution of the cognitive model of depression and its neurobiological correlates. *American Journal of Psychiatry, 165*, 969–977.

Beeney, J., & Arnett, P. A. (2008). Stress and memory bias interact to predict depression in multiple sclerosis. *Neuropsychology, 22*, 118–126.

Beevers, C. G., & Carver, C. S. (2003). Attentional bias and mood persistence as prospective predictors of dysphoria. *Cognitive Therapy and Research, 27*, 619–637.

Beevers, C. G., Clasen, P., Stice, E., & Schnyer, D. (2010). Depression symptoms and cognitive control of emotion cues: A functional magnetic resonance imaging study. *Neuroscience, 167*, 97–103.

Beevers, C. G., Ellis, A. J., Wells, T. T., & McGeary, J. E. (2010). Serotonin transporter gene promoter region polymorphism and selective processing of emotional images. *Biological Psychology, 83*, 260–265.

Beevers, C. G., Gibb, B. E., McGeary, J. E., & Miller, I. W. (2007). Serotonin transporter genetic variation and biased attention for emotional word stimuli among psychiatric inpatients. *Journal of Abnormal Psychology, 116*, 208–212.

Beevers, C. G., Lee, H.-J., Wells, T. T., Ellis, A. J., & Telch, M. J. (2011). Association of pre-deployment gaze bias for emotion stimuli with later symptoms of PTSD and depression in soldiers deployed in Iraq. *American Journal of Psychiatry, 168*, 735–741.

Beevers, C. G., Marti, C. N., Lee, H.-J., Stote, D. L., Ferrell, R. E., Hariri, A. R., et al. (2011). Associations between serotonin transporter gene promoter region (*5-HTTLPR*) polymorphism and gaze bias for emotional information. *Journal of Abnormal Psychology, 120*, 187–197.

Beevers, C. G., Wells, T. T., Ellis, A. J., & McGeary, J. E. (2009). Association of the serotonin transporter gene promoter region

(5-HTTLPR) polymorphism with biased attention for emotional stimuli. *Journal of Abnormal Psychology, 118*, 670–681.

Bellew, M., & Hill, A. B. (1991). Schematic processing and the prediction of depression following childbirth. *Personality and Individual Differences, 12*, 943–949.

Ben-Zeev, D., Young, M. A., & Madsen, J. W. (2009). Retrospective recall of affect in clinically depressed individuals and controls. *Cognition and Emotion, 23*, 1021–1040.

Berman, M. G., Nee, D. E., Casement, M., Kim, H. S., Deldin, P., Kross, E., et al. (2011). Neural and behavioral effects of interference resolution in depression and rumination. *Cognitive, Affective, and Behavioral Neuroscience, 11*, 85–96.

Bradley, B. P., Mogg, K., & Lee, S. C. (1997). Attentional biases for negative information in induced and naturally occurring dysphoria. *Behaviour Research and Therapy, 35*, 911–927.

Brittlebank, A. D., Scott, J., Williams, J. M., & Ferrier, I. N. (1993). Autobiographical memory in depression: State or trait marker? *British Journal of Psychiatry, 162*, 118–121.

Caseras, X., Garner, M., Bradley, B. P., & Mogg, K. (2007). Biases in visual orienting to negative and positive scenes in dysphoria: An eye movement study. *Journal of Abnormal Psychology, 116*, 491–497.

Caspi, A., Hariri, A. R., Holmes, A., Uher, R., & Moffitt, T. E. (2010). Genetic sensitivity to the environment: The case of the serotonin transporter gene and its implications for studying complex diseases and traits. *American Journal of Psychiatry, 167*, 509–527.

Caspi, A., Sugden, K., Moffitt, T. E., Taylor, A., Craig, I. W., Harrington, H., et al. (2003). Influence of life stress on depression: Moderation by a polymorphism in the *5-HTT* gene. *Science, 301*, 386–389.

Clasen, P. C., Wells, T. T., Knopik, V. S., McGeary, J. E., & Beevers, C. G. (2011). *5-HTTLPR* and BDNF Val66Met polymorphisms moderate effects of stress on rumination. *Genes, Brain, and Behavior, 10*, 740-746.

Cooney, R. E., Joormann, J., Eugène, F., Dennis, E. L., & Gotlib, I. H. (2010). Neural correlates of rumination in depression. *Cognitive, Affective, and Behavioral Neuroscience, 10*, 470–478.

Cornette, M. M., Strauman, T. J., Abramson, L. Y., & Busch, A. M. (2009). Self-discrepancy and suicidal ideation. *Cognition and Emotion, 23*, 504–527.

Craik, F. I. M., & Tulving, E. (1975). Depth of processing and the retention of words in episodic memory. *Journal of Experimental Psychology: General, 104*, 268–294.

De Raedt, R., & Koster, E. H. W. (2010). Understanding vulnerability for depression from a cognitive neuroscience perspective: A reappraisal of attentional factors and a new conceptual framework. *Cognitive, Affective, and Behavioral Neuroscience, 10*, 50–70.

Disner, S. G., Beevers, C. G., Haigh, E. A. P., & Beck, A. T. (2011). Neural mechanisms of the cognitive model of depression. *Nature Reviews Neuroscience, 12*, 467–477.

Eizenman, M., Yu, L. H., Grupp, L., Eizenman, E., Ellenbogen, M., Gemar, M., et al. (2003). A naturalistic visual scanning approach to assess selective attention in major depressive disorder. *Psychiatry Research, 118*, 117–128.

Epstein, J., Pan, H., Kocsis, J. H., Yang, Y., Butler, T., Chusid, J., et al. (2006). Lack of ventral striatal response to positive stimuli in depressed versus normal subjects. *American Journal of Psychiatry, 163*, 1784–1790.

Ferster, C. B. (1973). A functional anlysis of depression. *American Psychologist, 28*, 857–870.

Gibbs, B. R., & Rude, S. S. (2004). Overgeneral autobiographical memory as depression vulnerability. *Cognitive Therapy and Research, 28*, 511–526.

Gilboa, E., & Gotlib, I. (1997). Cognitive biases and affect persistence in previously dysphoric and never-dysphoric individuals. *Cognition and Emotion, 11*, 517–538.

Goeleven, E., De Raedt, R., Baert, S., & Koster, E. H. W. (2006). Deficient inhibition of emotional information in depression. *Journal of Affective Disorders, 93*, 149–157.

Gotlib, I. H., & Joormann, J. (2010). Cognition and depression: Current status and future directions. *Annual Review of Clinical Psychology, 6*, 285–312.

Gotlib, I. H., Krasnoperova, E., Yue, D. N., & Joormann, J. (2004). Attentional biases for negative interpersonal stimuli in clinical depression. *Journal of Abnormal Psychology, 113*, 121–135.

Greenberg, P. E., Stiglin, L. E., Finkelstein, S. N., & Berndt, E. R. (1993). The economic burden of depression in 1990. *Journal of Clinical Psychiatry, 54*, 405–418.

Gross, J. J. (1998). The emerging field of emotion regulation: An integrative review. *Review of General Psychology, 2*, 271–299.

Hadley, S. A., & MacLeod, A. K. (2010). Conditional goal-setting, personal goals and hopelessness about the future. *Cognition and Emotion, 24*, 1191–1198.

Hammen, C., Burge, D., Daley, S. E., Davila, J., Paley, B., & Rudolph, K. D. (1995). Interpersonal attachment cognitions and prediction of symptomatic responses to interpersonal stress. *Journal of Abnormal Psychology, 104*, 436–443.

Hammen, C., Shih, J. H., & Brennan, P. A. (2004). Intergenerational transmission of depression: Test of an interpersonal stress model in a community sample. *Journal of Consulting and Clinical Psychology, 72*, 511–522.

Hedlund, S., & Rude, S. S. (1995). Evidence of latent depressive schemas in formerly depressed individuals. *Journal of Abnormal Psychology, 104*, 517–525.

Heller, A. S., Johnstone, T., Shackman, A. J., Light, S. N., Peterson, M. J., Kolden, G. G., et al. (2009). Reduced capacity to sustain positive emotion in major depression reflects diminished maintenance of fronto-striatal brain activation. *Proceedings of the National Academy of Sciences, 106*, 22445–22450.

Hertel, P. T. (1997). On the contributions of deficent cognitive control to memory impairments in depression. *Cognition and Emotion, 11*, 569–583.

Hertel, P. T., & Rude, S. S. (1991). Depressive deficits in memory: Focusing attention improves subsequent recall. *Journal of Experimental Psychology: General, 120*, 301–309.

Higgins, E. T., Klein, R., & Strauman, T. (1985). Self-concept discrepancy theory: A psychological model for distinguishing among different aspects of depression and anxiety. *Social Cognition, 3*(1), 51–76.

Ingram, R. E. (1984). Toward an information-processing analysis of depression. *Cognitive Therapy and Research, 8*, 443–477.

Ingram, R. E., Miranda, J., & Segal, Z. V. (1998). *Cognitive vulnerability to depression.* New York: Guilford Press.

Insel, T. R. (2009). Translating scientific opportunity into public health impact: A strategic plan for research on mental illness. *Archives of General Psychiatry, 66*, 128–133.

Joiner, T. E., & Coyne, J. C. (Eds.). (1999). *The interactional nature of depression: Advances in interpersonal approaches.* Washington, DC: American Psychological Association.

Joormann, J. (2004). Attentional bias in dysphoria: The role of inhibitory processes. *Cognition and Emotion, 18*, 125–147.

Joormann, J. (2006). Differential effects of rumination and dysphoria on the inhibition of irrelevant emotional material: Evidence from a negative priming task. *Cognitive Therapy and Research, 30*, 149–160.

Joormann, J., & Gotlib, I. H. (2007). Selective attention to emotional faces following recovery from depression. *Journal of Abnormal Psychology, 116*, 80–85.

Joormann, J., & Gotlib, I. H. (2010). Emotion regulation in depression: Relation to cognitive inhibition. *Cognition and Emotion, 24*, 281–298.

Joormann, J., Talbot, L., & Gotlib, I. H. (2007). Biased processing of emotional information in girls at risk for depression. *Journal of Abnormal Psychology, 116*, 135–143.

Karg, K., Burmeister, M., Shedden, K., & Sen, S. (2011). The serotonin transporter promoter variant *(5-HTTLPR)*, stress, and depression meta-analysis revisited: Evidence of genetic moderation. *Archives of General Psychiatry, 68*, 444–454.

Keller, M. B., Lavori, P. W., Mueller, T. I., Endicott, J., Coryell, W., Hirschfeld, R. M. A., et al. (1992). Time to recovery, chronicity, and levels of psychopathology in major depression: A 5-year prospective follow-up of 431 subjects. *Archives of General Psychiatry, 49*, 809–816.

Kellough, J. L., Beevers, C. G., Ellis, A. J., & Wells, T. T. (2008). Time course of selective attention in clinically depressed young adults: An eye tracking study. *Behaviour Research and Therapy, 46*, 1238–1243.

Kendler, K. S., Walters, E. E., & Kessler, R. C. (1997). The prediction of length of major depressive episodes: Results from an epidemiological sample of female twins. *Psychological Medicine, 27*, 107–117.

Kessler, R. C., Berglund, P., Demler, O., Jin, R., Koretz, D., Merikangas, K. R., et al. (2003). The epidemiology of major depressive disorder results from the National Comorbidity Survey Replication (NCS-R). *Journal of the American Medical Association, 289*, 3095–3105.

Kessler, R. C., & Walters, E. E. (1998). Epidemiology of DSM-III-R major depression and minor depression among adolescents and young adults in the National Comorbidity Survey. *Depression and Anxiety, 7,* 3–14.

Kessler, R. C., & Wang, P. S. (2009). Epidemiology of depression. In I. H, Gotlib & C. L. Hammen (Eds.), *Handbook of depression* (2nd ed., pp. 5–22). New York: Guilford Press.

Klein, S. B., & Loftus, J. (1988). The nature of self-referent encoding: The contributions of elaborative and organizational processes. *Journal of Personality and Social Psychology, 55,* 5–11.

Koster, E. H. W., De Lissnyder, E., Derakshan, N., & De Raedt, R. (2011). Understanding depressive rumination from a cognitive science perspective: The impaired disengagement hypothesis. *Clinical Psychology Review, 31,* 138–145.

Koster, E. H. W., De Raedt, R., Goeleven, E., Franck, E., & Crombez, G. (2005). Mood-congruent attentional bias in dysphoria: Maintained attention to and impaired disengagement from negative information. *Emotion, 5,* 446–455.

Koster, E. H. W., De Raedt, R., Leyman, L., & De Lissnyder, E. (2010). Mood-congruent attention and memory bias in dysphoria: Exploring the coherence among information-processing biases. *Behaviour Research and Therapy, 48,* 219–225.

Kross, E., & Ayduk, O. (2008). Facilitating adaptive emotional analysis: Distinguishing distanced-analysis of depressive experiences from immersed-analysis and distraction. *Personality and Social Psychology Bulletin, 34,* 924–938.

Kross, E., & Ayduk, O. (2009). Boundary conditions and buffering effects: Does depressive symptomology moderate the effectiveness of distanced-analysis for facilitating adaptive self-reflection? *Journal of Research in Personality, 43,* 923–927.

Kross, E., Ayduk, O., & Mischel, W. (2005). When asking "why" does not hurt: Distinguishing rumination from reflective processing of negative emotions. *Psychological Science, 16,* 709–715.

Lau, M. A., Segal, Z. V., & Williams, J. M. G. (2004). Teasdale's differential activation hypothesis: Implications for mechanisms of depressive relapse and suicidal behaviour. *Behaviour Research and Therapy, 42,* 1001–1017.

Leyman, L., De Raedt, R., Vaeyens, R., & Philippaerts, R. M. (2011). Attention for emotional facial expressions in dysphoria: An eye-movement registration study. *Cognition and Emotion, 25,* 111–120.

Lyubomirsky, S., & Nolen-Hoeksema, S. (1993). Self-perpetuating properties of dysphoric rumination. *Journal of Personality and Social Psychology, 65,* 339–349.

Lyubomirsky, S., & Nolen-Hoeksema, S. (1995). Effects of self-focused rumination on negative thinking and interpersonal problem solving. *Journal of Personality and Social Psychology, 69,* 176–190.

Lyubomirsky, S., Tucker, K. L., Caldwell, N. D., & Berg, K. (1999). Why ruminators are poor problem solvers: Clues from the phenomenology of dysphoric rumination. *Journal of Personality and Social Psychology, 77,* 1041–1060.

Mackinger, H. F., Pachinger, M. M., Leibetseder, M. M., & Fartacek, R. R. (2000). Autobiographical memories in women remitted from major depression. *Journal of Abnormal Psychology, 109,* 331–334.

Mathews, A., & Mackintosh, B. (2000). Induced emotional interpretation bias and anxiety. *Journal of Abnormal Psychology, 109,* 602–615.

Mathews, A., & MacLeod, C. (2005). Cognitive vulnerability to emotional disorders. *Annual Review of Clinical Psychology, 1,* 167–195.

Matt, G. E., Vázquez, C., & Campbell, W. K. (1992). Mood-congruent recall of affectively toned stimuli: A meta-analytic review. *Clinical Psychology Review, 12,* 227–255.

Mayberg, H. S. (1997). Limbic–cortical dysregulation: A proposed model of depression. *Journal of Neuropsychiatry and Clinical Neurosciences, 9,* 471–481.

McLeod, J. D., Kessler, R. C., & Landis, K. R. (1992). Speed of recovery from major depressive episodes in a community sample of married men and women. *Journal of Abnormal Psychology, 101,* 277–286.

Miller, E. K., & Cohen, J. D. (2001). An integrative theory of prefrontal cortex function. *Annual Review of Neuroscience, 24,* 167–202.

Miranda, J., Gross, J. J., Persons, J. B., & Hahn, J. (1998). Mood matters: Negative mood induction activates dysfunctional attitudes in women vulnerable to depression. *Cognitive Therapy and Research, 22,* 363–376.

Miranda, J., & Persons, J. B. (1988). Dysfunctional attitudes are mood-state dependent. *Journal of Abnormal Psychology, 97,* 76–79.

Miranda, J., Persons, J. B., & Byers, C. N. (1990). Endorsement of dysfunctional beliefs depends on current mood state. *Journal of Abnormal Psychology, 99,* 237–241.

Moberly, N. J., & Watkins, E. R. (2006). Processing mode influences the relationship between trait rumination and emotional vulnerability. *Behavior Therapy, 37,* 281–291.

Moberly, N. J., & Watkins, E. R. (2010). Negative affect and ruminative self-focus during everyday goal pursuit, *24,* 729–739.

Mogg, K., & Bradley, B. P. (2005). Attentional bias in generalized anxiety disorder versus depressive disorder. *Cognitive Therapy and Research, 29,* 29–45.

Mogg, K., Bradley, B. P., & Williams, R. (1995). Attentional bias in anxiety and depression: The role of awareness. *British Journal of Clinical Psychology, 34*(Pt. 1), 17–36.

Mogg, K., Holmes, A., Garner, M., & Bradley, B. P. (2008). Effects of threat cues on attentional shifting, disengagement and response slowing in anxious individuals. *Behaviour Research and Therapy, 46,* 656–667.

Nigg, J. T. (2000). On inhibition/disinhibition in developmental psychopathology: Views from cognitive and personality psychology and a working inhibition taxonomy. *Psychological Bulletin, 126,* 220–246.

Nolen-Hoeksema, S. (1991). Responses to depression and their effects on the duration of depressive episodes. *Journal of Abnormal Psychology, 100,* 569–582.

Nolen-Hoeksema, S., & Morrow, J. (1991). A prospective study of depression and posttraumatic stress symptoms after a natural disaster: The 1989 Loma Prieta earthquake. *Journal of Personality and Social Psychology, 61,* 115–121.

Nolen-Hoeksema, S., Wisco, B. E., & Lyubomirsky, S. (2008). Rethinking rumination. *Perspectives on Psychological Science, 3,* 400–424.

Ochsner, K. N., & Gross, J. J. (2005). The cognitive control of emotion. *Trends in Cognitive Sciences, 9,* 242–249.

Papageorgiou, C., & Wells, A. (2001). Metacognitive beliefs about rumination in recurrent major depression. *Cognitive and Behavioral Practice, 8,* 160–164.

Papageorgiou, C., & Wells, A. (2003). An empirical test of a clinical metacognitive model of rumination and depression. *Cognitive Therapy and Research, 27,* 261–273.

Phillips, M. L., Drevets, W. C., Rauch, S. L., &

Lane, R. (2003). Neurobiology of emotion perception: II. Implications for major psychiatric disorders. *Biological Psychiatry, 54,* 515–528.

Pizzagalli, D. A., Holmes, A. J., Dillon, D. G., Goetz, E. L., Birk, J. L., Bogdan, R., et al. (2009). Reduced caudate and nucleus accumbens response to rewards in unmedicated individuals with major depressive disorder. *American Journal of Psychiatry, 166,* 702–710.

Posner, M. I. (1980). Orienting of attention. *Quarterly Journal of Experimental Psychology, 32,* 3–25.

Posner, M. I., & Rothbart, M. K. (1998). Attention, self-regulation and consciousness. *Philosophical Transactions of the Royal Society of London. Series B: Biological Sciences, 353,* 1915–1927.

Risch, N., Herrell, R., Lehner, T., Liang, K.-Y., Eaves, L., Hoh, J., et al. (2009). Interaction between the serotonin transporter gene *(5-HTTLPR),* stressful life events, and risk of depression: A meta-analysis. *Journal of the American Medical Association, 301,* 2462–2471.

Rude, S. S., Durham-Fowler, J. A., Baum, E. S., Rooney, S. B., & Maestas, K. L. (2009). Self-report and cognitive processing measures of depressive thinking predict subsequent major depressive disorder. *Cognitive Therapy and Research, 34,* 107–115.

Rude, S. S., Wenzlaff, R., Gibbs, B., Vane, J., & Whitney, T. (2002). Negative processing biases predict subsequent depressive symptoms. *Cognition and Emotion, 16,* 423–440.

Scher, C. D., Ingram, R. E., & Segal, Z. V. (2005). Cognitive reactivity and vulnerability: Empirical evaluation of construct activation and cognitive diatheses in unipolar depression. *Clinical Psychology Review, 25,* 487–510.

Schildkraut, J. J. (1965). The catecholamine hypothesis of affective disorders: A review of supporting evidence. *American Journal of Psychiatry, 122,* 509–522.

Schlenker, B. R., & Britt, T. W. (1996). Depression and the explanation of events that happen to self, close others, and strangers. *Journal of Personality and Social Psychology, 71,* 180–192.

Segal, Z. V., Gemar, M., & Williams, S. (1999). Differential cognitive response to a mood challenge following successful cognitive therapy or pharmacotherapy for unipolar depression. *Journal of Abnormal Psychology, 108,* 3–10.

Segal, Z. V., Kennedy, S., Gemar, M., Hood, K., Pedersen, R., & Buis, T. (2006). Cognitive reactivity to sad mood provocation and the prediction of depressive relapse. *Archives of General Psychiatry, 63,* 749–755.

Segal, Z. V., & Shaw, B. F. (1986). Cognition in depression: A reappraisal of Coyne and Gotlib's critique. *Cognitive Therapy and Research, 10,* 671–693.

Segal, Z. V., Shaw, B. F., Vella, D. D., & Katz, R. (1992). Cognitive and life stress predictors of relapse in remitted unipolar depressed patients: Test of the congruency hypothesis. *Journal of Abnormal Psychology, 101,* 26–36.

Siegle, G. J., Granholm, E., Ingram, R. E., & Matt, G. E. (2001). Pupillary and reaction time measures of sustained processing of negative information in depression. *Biological Psychiatry, 49,* 624–636.

Siegle, G. J., Thompson, W., Carter, C. S., Steinhauer, S. R., & Thase, M. E. (2007). Increased amygdala and decreased dorsolateral prefrontal BOLD responses in unipolar depression: Related and independent features. *Biological Psychiatry, 61,* 198–209.

Sweeney, P. D., Shaeffer, D. E., & Golin, S. (1982). Pleasant events, unpleasant events, and depression. *Journal of Personality and Social Psychology, 43,* 136–144.

Teasdale, J. D. (1988). Cognitive vulnerability to persistent depression. *Cognition and Emotion, 2,* 247–274.

Teasdale, J. D. (1999). Emotional processing, three modes of mind and the prevention of relapse in depression. *Behaviour Research and Therapy, 37*(Suppl. 1), S53–S77.

Teasdale, J. D., & Dent, J. (1987). Cognitive vulnerability to depression: An investigation of two hypotheses. *British Journal of Clinical Psychology, 26*(Pt. 2), 113–126.

Wang, P. S., Simon, G., & Kessler, R. C. (2003). The economic burden of depression and the cost-effectiveness of treatment. *International Journal of Methods in Psychiatric Research, 12,* 22–33.

Watkins, E. R., Baeyens, C. B., & Read, R. (2009). Concreteness training reduces dysphoria: Proof-of-principle for repeated cognitive bias modification in depression. *Journal of Abnormal Psychology, 118,* 55–64.

Watkins, E. R., & Baracaia, S. (2001). Why do people ruminate in dysphoric moods? *Personality and Individual Differences, 30,* 723–734.

Watkins, E. R., & Baracaia, S. (2002). Rumination and social problem-solving in depression.

Behaviour Research and Therapy, 40, 1179–1189.

Watkins, E. R., Moberly, N. J., & Moulds, M. L. (2008). Processing mode causally influences emotional reactivity: Distinct effects of abstract versus concrete construal on emotional response. *Emotion, 8,* 364–378.

Watkins, E. R., & Moulds, M. L. (2005). Distinct modes of ruminative self-focus: Impact of abstract versus concrete rumination on problem solving in depression. *Emotion, 5,* 319–328.

Watkins, E. R., Taylor, R. S., Byng, R., Baeyens, C., Read, R., Pearson, K., et al. (2012). Guided self-help concreteness training as an intervention for major depression in primary care: A Phase II randomized controlled trial. *Psychological Medicine, 42,* 1359–1371.

Watkins, E. R., & Teasdale, J. D. (2001). Rumination and overgeneral memory in depression: Effects of self-focus and analytic thinking. *Journal of Abnormal Psychology, 110,* 353–357.

Watkins, E. R., & Teasdale, J. D. (2004). Adaptive and maladaptive self-focus in depression. *Journal of Affective Disorders, 82,* 1–8.

Watkins, P. (2002). Implicit memory bias in depression. *Cognition and Emotion, 16,* 381–402.

Weissman, A. N., & Beck, A. T. (1978). Development and validation of the Dysfunctional Attitude Scale: A preliminary investigation. In *Proceedings of the annual meeting of the American Educational Research Association.* Toronto, ON.

Wells, T. T., & Beevers, C. G. (2010). Biased attention and dysphoria: Manipulating selective attention reduces subsequent depressive symptoms. *Cognition and Emotion, 24,* 719–728.

Wells, T. T., Beevers, C. G., Robison, A. E., & Ellis, A. J. (2010). Gaze behavior predicts memory bias for angry facial expressions in stable dysphoria. *Emotion, 10,* 894–902.

Wenzlaff, R. M., & Bates, D. E. (1998). Unmasking a cognitive vulnerability to depression: How lapses in mental control reveal depressive thinking. *Journal of Personality and Social Psychology, 75,* 1559–1571.

Wenzlaff, R. M., & Eisenberg, A. R. (2001). Mental control after dysphoria: Evidence of a suppressed, depressive bias. *Behavior Therapy, 32,* 27–45.

Wenzlaff, R. M., & Luxton, D. D. (2003). The role of thought suppression in depressive rumination. *Cognitive Therapy and Research, 27,* 293–308.

Wenzlaff, R. M., Rude, S. S., Taylor, C. J., Stultz, C. H., & Sweatt, R. A. (2001). Beneath the veil of thought suppression: Attentional bias and depression risk. *Cognition and Emotion, 15,* 435–452.

Wenzlaff, R. M., & Wegner, D. M. (2000). Thought suppression. *Annual Review of Psychology, 51,* 59–91.

Williams, J. M. G. (1996). Depression and the specificity of autobiographical memory. In D. Rubin (Ed.), *Remembering our past: Studies in autobiographical memory* (pp. 244–267). Cambridge, UK: Cambridge University Press.

Williams, J. M. G., Watts, F. N., MacLeod, C. M., & Mathews, A. (1997). *Cognitive psychology and emotional disorders* (2nd ed.). New York: Wiley.

Wilson, E. J., MacLeod, C., Mathews, A., & Rutherford, E. M. (2006). The causal role of interpretive bias in anxiety reactivity. *Journal of Abnormal Psychology, 115,* 103–111.

Wisco, B. E. (2009). Depressive cognition: Self-reference and depth of processing. *Clinical Psychology Review, 29,* 382–392.

Yuan, J. W., & Kring, A. M. (2009). Dysphoria and the prediction and experience of emotion. *Cognition and Emotion, 23,* 1221–1232.

CHAPTER 25

Emotional Awareness

Attention Dysregulation in Borderline Personality Disorder

Ryan W. Carpenter, Stephanie Bagby-Stone, and Timothy J. Trull

Borderline personality disorder (BPD) is a severe mental disorder associated with extreme emotional, behavioral, and interpersonal dysfunction. Individuals with BPD have a maladaptive personality style that is present in a variety of contexts, emerges by early adulthood, and leads to distinct patterns of dysfunction in behavior and relationships. BPD affects 1–3% of the general population and is the most common personality disorder in clinical settings, representing 10% of the patients in outpatient settings, 15–20% of the patients in inpatient settings, and 30–60% of patients diagnosed with personality disorders (Lenzenweger, Lane, Loranger, & Kessler, 2007; Trull, Jahng, Tomko, Wood, & Sher, 2010; Widiger & Trull, 1993). BPD is associated with interpersonal and occupational impairment, increased risk for suicide, and higher rates of treatment in both medical and psychiatric settings (Skodol et al., 2002). Finally, BPD is frequently comorbid with other personality disorders and with Axis I disorders, and this comorbidity is associated with poorer outcome (Skodol et al., 2002).

Researchers have typically approached BPD from an emotion-based perspective, focusing primarily, though not exclusively, on the role of emotion dysregulation in the cause and maintenance of the disorder (e.g., Lieb, Zanarini, Schmahl, Linehan, & Bohus, 2004; Linehan, 1993; Trull et al., 2008). Although this line of study has proven fruitful, it has led to a relative neglect of dysregulation on the other, cognitive, side of the equation. This is a potentially costly oversight because cognition can influence emotion, and dysregulation in one domain may interact with and mutually reinforce dysregulation in the other (Matthews & MacLeod, 2005; Ochsner & Gross, 2005). Therefore, there is a need to consider cognition and emotion together in the context of BPD.

We refer to cognition here broadly. Cognitive processes, including executive function, memory, working memory, and attention, have been explored among patients diagnosed with BPD. Several of these studies found support for dysregulated cognition, whereas others did not (Dell'Osso, Berlin, Serati, & Altamura, 2010; Driessen et al., 2000; Haaland, Esperaas, & Landrø, 2009; Kunert, Druecke, Sass, & Herpertz, 2003; Lenzenweger, Clarkin, Fertuck, & Kernberg, 2004). Of these studies, however, many employed batteries of neuropsychological tests covering multiple processes, which may lack precision in measuring relevant cognitive processes and identifying specific neural correlates. Additionally, some of them (e.g., Dell'Osso et al., 2010; Haaland et al., 2009; Lenzenweger et al., 2004) found support for dysfunction in one domain and not in others, and the domains of dysfunction are not consistent across studies. Although suggestive, it is difficult to take away firm conclusions from this body of work.

Cognitive processes can also be considered within the context of associated neural structures that include a number of brain regions, especially the prefrontal cortex, orbitofrontal cortex, hippocampus, and the anterior cingulate cortex (ACC). In this case, the evidence for cognitive dysregulation in BPD is more straightforward. Studies suggest that BPD involves dysfunction of the frontal–limbic network, which consists of the ACC, orbitofrontal and dorsolateral prefrontal cortex, and hippocampus (for reviews, see Dell'Osso et al., 2010; Schmahl & Bremner, 2006). The frontal–limbic network also involves the amygdala, which is important in emotion processing, suggesting a possible interaction of cognitive and emotion dysregulation in BPD.

Parts of the frontal–limbic network— the dorsolateral prefrontal cortex and the ACC—are important components in the anterior attention system, which is involved in the conscious allocation of attentional resources (Posner, 1992; Posner & Dehaene, 1994). Attention, and its dysregulation, may therefore be important for increasing our understanding of BPD and emotion dysregulation. Attentional dysregulation may describe a number of different attention-related problems (for a detailed examination of attention, see Yiend, Barnicot, & Koster, Chapter 6, this volume). In this chapter we focus on two: attentional bias and reduced attentional capacity. Attentional bias refers to a tendency to focus on specific stimuli (e.g., negative events) and reduced attentional capacity to a reduction in the amount of information a person can attend to at one time. We propose that attention dysregulation in these areas is present in BPD and that the two types of dysregulation interact to contribute to the development of the disorder. This proposal follows from Linehan's (1993) biosocial theory of BPD, which hypothesizes that BPD patients possess an attentional bias toward negative emotional

cues and a narrowing of attentional focus that is congruent with their negative mood state.

In this chapter we first compare BPD to a psychological disorder with ties to both BPD and attention dysregulation, attention-deficit/hyperactivity disorder (ADHD), in order to illustrate the potential role of attention dysregulation in BPD. Next, we briefly review the research that has investigated attentional processes in the development and maintenance of BPD. Finally, we examine several domains relevant to BPD and suggest how attention and emotion dysregulation may interact to cause a number of BPD symptoms.

BPD and ADHD

BPD and ADHD share numerous symptoms, including impulsivity and affect dysregulation, as well as other clinical features such as substance abuse, low self-esteem, disturbed interpersonal relationships, and aversive inner tension (Davids & Gastpar, 2005; Philipsen, 2006). Features of BPD broadly overlap with ADHD symptoms, especially regarding impulsivity (Philipsen, 2006). More striking, many of the symptoms associated with adult ADHD (e.g., inattentiveness, hyperactivity, affective lability, hot temper, disorganization, and impulsivity) are commonly found in BPD (Ferrer et al., 2010; Fossati, Novella, Donati, Donini, & Maffei, 2002).

Research on functional brain anatomy also reveals similarities between BPD and ADHD. As mentioned in the introduction, the frontal–limbic network may mediate the expression of most BPD symptoms (Dell'Osso et al., 2010; Schmahl & Bremner, 2006), whereas in ADHD, frontal–striatal dysfunction is thought to mediate the disorder's expression (Philipsen, 2006; Wilens, Faraone, & Biederman, 2004). Neuroimaging data from adults with ADHD and BPD reveal dysfunction in both the prefrontal cortex, corresponding with attention deficits, and the orbitofrontal cortex dysfunction implicated in impulsivity and emotional instability (Philipsen, 2006).

There is a high degree of comorbidity between personality disorders (especially Cluster B disorders) and adult ADHD (Biederman, 2004; Faraone et al., 2000; Philipsen, 2006; Wilens et al., 2004). ADHD in childhood has been shown to be significantly associated with BPD in adulthood (Fossati et al., 2002). Furthermore, studies have estimated that childhood ADHD diagnoses were present in 41.25–59.5% of adult patients with BPD and 16.1% of adult patients with BPD received ADHD diagnoses in adulthood (Fossati et al., 2002; Philipsen et al., 2008).

Multiple studies have attempted to clarify the relationship between BPD and ADHD (Andrulonis, Glueck, Stroebel, & Vogel, 1982; Ferrer et al., 2010; Fossati et al., 2002; Philipsen, 2006; Philipsen et al., 2008). In an early attempt to classify BPD, Andrulonis and colleagues (1982) described how BPD could be viewed either on a continuum with affective disorders and atypical psychoses or with organic brain dysfunction, including episodic dyscontrol syndrome and/or adult minimal brain dysfunction (the diagnostic precursors to intermittent explosive disorder and ADHD, respectively). More recently, the overlap in symptoms has led some to postulate that BPD and ADHD are two dimensions of a single disorder and that the development of BPD may largely depend on exposure to negative childhood experiences (Philipsen, 2006). Others view BPD as a heterogeneous disorder with proposed impulsive, affective, or dissociative subgroups, with ADHD being a risk factor for some but not all of these groups (Davids & Gastpar, 2005). In an attempt to categorize patients with BPD, Ferrer and colleagues (2010) found that those with BPD and ADHD were a more homogeneous impulsive subtype, whereas those without ADHD had more anxious and depressive symptoms. Van Dijk, Lappenschaar, Kan, Verkes, and Buitelaar (2011) explored the role of temperament and personality traits in patients with BPD and ADHD and discovered that the personality trait of novelty seeking was associated with the inattentive symptoms of ADHD. The highest ratings in novelty seeking were found in patients with both disorders, suggesting that this temperament may predispose individuals to co-occurring BPD and ADHD diagnoses. Although interesting, more research is vital to help distinguish clear subgroups of BPD, revise and refine diagnostic criteria, direct therapeutic interventions, and better delineate BPD's relationship to disorders of attention.

The degree of overlap in BPD and ADHD clinical symptoms, as well as neuroimaging findings, would indicate that treatments that are effective for ADHD might also be beneficial for patients with BPD. Regarding psychotherapeutic interventions, patients with ADHD and those with BPD both respond well to a cognitive-behavioral treatment, dialectical behavioral therapy (DBT), which includes components of mindfulness, distress tolerance, emotion modulation, and interpersonal effectiveness (Davids & Gastpar, 2005; Hesslinger et al., 2002; Philipsen, 2006).

In ADHD, stimulant medications (e.g., methylphenidate [MPH] or dextroamphetamine [D-AMPH] enhance dopaminergic activity and are effective in the treatment of attention deficits. Several studies, trials, and case reports have been published looking into the possibility of BPD treatment with such stimulants (e.g., Golubchik, Sever, & Weizman, 2009; Schulz, Cornelius, Schulz, & Soloff, 1988; van Reekum & Links, 1994). In general, published data show a possible benefit; however, the limited number and type of these reports greatly restrict definitive conclusions regarding the long-term efficacy and tolerability of psychostimulant medications in the treatment of BPD. Larger, longer, randomized, placebo-controlled studies are needed to replicate current findings and to further elucidate the exact effects of psychostimulants on specific symptoms and functioning of patients with BPD.

Despite the similarities between BPD and ADHD, there are also noteworthy differences. BPD is more commonly diagnosed in females (3:1; American Psychiatric Association, 2000), at least within clinical samples. In children, ADHD is much more common in males (3:1 in community samples and 10:1 in clinic-referred samples), although the difference reduces to 3:2 in adults (Biederman, 2004). In addition, coping methods for dealing with aversive tension and affect dysregulation in these disorders vary greatly; patients with ADHD are characterized by risk taking and novelty seeking, whereas patients with BPD engage in self-harm and dissociation (Davids & Gastpar, 2005; Philipsen, 2006). Also, the interpersonal and social functioning of these patients differs significantly (Philipsen, 2006).

In summary, BPD and ADHD share a number of suggestive similarities, including symptoms such as impulsivity and affect dysregulation, and are frequently commorbid. Although these similarities may be superficial, it may also be that they are the result of the same underlying mechanisms. Alternatively, there may be a specific subset of individuals with BPD that is characterized by attention dysregulation. Although attention likely does not play the central role in BPD that it plays in ADHD, knowledge about its dysregulation in the latter may still inform both research and treatment of the former.

BPD and Attention

One of the first investigators to make a link between attention dysregulation and BPD was Murray (1979), who proposed, based on clinical experience, that individuals with BPD may have a history of mild brain dysfunction. Among other cognitive difficulties, mild brain dysfunction included attentional deficits in both focusing and sustaining attention, as well as overall capacity. More recent studies have examined attentional deficits empirically and with greater specificity. In a review, LeGris and van Reekum (2006) surveyed 15 studies that examined selective and/or sustained attention deficits in individuals with BPD on tests including the continuous performance test, the attention network test (ANT), the backward masking test, and the Wechsler Adult Intelligence Scale (WAIS) Digital Symbol subtest. Over half of these studies reported some level of impairment.

For example, Posner and colleagues (2002) found evidence for impaired performance in individuals with BPD on the ANT, a computerized behavioral test of three different functions of attention: alerting, orienting, and conflict resolution. Controls were either selected at random or to match individuals with BPD on (high) levels of negative affect and (low) levels of effortful control. Results indicated that there were no differences between groups on alerting or orienting, but that individuals with BPD were significantly worse than normal controls on conflict

resolution. Conflict resolution is measured in terms of the time a participant needs to overcome the interference of an incongruent distracter and correctly respond. This was calculated on the ANT by subtracting the average reaction time on congruent trials from the average reaction time on incongruent trials. Interestingly, matched controls fell between the BPD group and the normal controls and were not significantly different from either. This pattern of findings suggests that high-negative affectivity and low-effortful control may partially explain the slowed responses in the BPD group, though not entirely, given that the matched controls were no different from the normal controls. It is curious that high-negative affectivity was associated with poorer conflict resolution, as the ANT involves no emotional stimuli. However, similar tasks of conflict resolution have been shown to generate emotion-related responses (Hajcak & Foti, 2008). It is possible that individuals high on negative affectivity became more frustrated by the task, leading to problems in conflict resolution. In any case, that individuals with BPD were impaired in conflict resolution on a cognitive task supports the idea that they have impaired executive attention, slowing them on the complicated task of separating goal-related information from irrelevant distracters.

Other studies have found evidence for attentional deficits in the context of emotional stimuli. Several studies have examined performance by individuals with BPD on the emotional Stroop task. The basic Stroop paradigm (Stroop, 1935) is a measure of cognitive inhibition, or the ability to suppress interfering information, a construct related to conflict resolution. Performance on the task is associated with activation in brain regions related to attention, including the parietal lobe (Carter, Mintun, & Cohen, 1995; Peterson et al., 1999; Taylor, Kornblum, Lauber, Minoshima, & Koeppe, 1997), lateral prefrontal cortex (Carter et al., 1995; Taylor et al., 1997), and the ACC (Carter et al., 1995; Peterson et al., 1999). In the typical Stroop task, individuals are presented words displayed in different colors and must ignore the word and name the color. In the emotional Stroop task, the words vary in their emotional significance. In theory, individuals sensitive to emotionally charged stimuli will have more diffi-cultly suppressing their inclination to read the words, slowing their reaction times. This could be due to a hypervigilance for emotion-related cues or an inability to redi-rect attention from emotion-related cues.

Using the emotional Stroop task, Arntz, Appels, and Sieswerda (2000) found that individuals with BPD were slower than controls, but not slower than individuals with Cluster C personality disorder diagno-ses, to name colors on trials with negative emotion words than on trials with neutral words, which they interpreted as evidence that individuals with a Cluster C diagnosis are hypervigilant for emotionally charged stimuli. Later studies (Sieswerda, Arntz, & Kindt, 2007; Sieswerda, Arntz, Mertens, & Vertommen, 2007) found that individuals with BPD were slower than individuals with a Cluster C diagnosis than normal controls at performing the Stroop on both positive-and negative-valenced trials. Other studies, contrarily, failed to find effects for emo-tional stimuli, but did find that individu-als with BPD were slower across all stimuli (Domes et al., 2006; Sprock, Rader, Kend-all, & Yoder, 2000; Wingenfeld, Rullkoet-ter, et al., 2009). This finding, however, is tempered by the fact that Kunert and col-leagues (2003) found that patients with BPD, although nonsignificantly slower than con-trols, were less likely to make errors, raising the possibility of a speed–accuracy tradeoff. Additionally, Wingenfeld, Mensebach, and colleagues (2009) found that deficits on an emotional Stroop using personally relevant stimuli were specifically related to comorbid posttrraumatic stress disorder (PTSD).

An increasing number of studies has used imaging to explore differences in brain structure and functioning in individuals with BPD, some of which suggest atten-tion dysregulation. As mentioned above, Schmahl and Bremner (2006) found evi-dence for reduced activity and/or volume of the structures that make up the frontal–limbic system. This finding suggests a fail-ure of attention-related structures to regu-late the amygdala and supports the idea that BPD may involve a dysregulated interaction between attention and emotion. Addition-ally, Schmahl and colleagues (Schmahl et al., 2003; Schmahl, Vermetten, Elzinga, & Bremner, 2004) found that female patients

with BPD with a history of childhood abuse showed decreased activation in the right ACC in one study and a failure to activate, relative to controls, the ACC in another.

Returning to the emotional Stroop, Wing-enfeld, Rullkoeter, and colleagues (2009) tested whether the responses of individuals with BPD to emotional stimuli correlated with reduced frontal–limbic system activa-tion. They did not find any reaction time differences between individuals with BPD and controls for positive, negative, or neu-tral words, but did find that individuals with BPD were slower overall at responding. More interestingly, on trials with negative, relative to neutral, words, the control group showed an increase in activation in the ACC and frontal lobe areas, whereas the BPD group did not. This effect was particularly strong in controls when the negative stimuli were selected specifically to relate to a stress-ful event participants self-reported before the experiment. The findings supported ACC dysregulation, and therefore attention dysregulation, as interfering in emotion pro-cessing in BPD, although the interpretation of reduced activation is not straightforward. For example, the finding of no increase in the BPD group does not tell us about their aver-age level of activation, only that the change in encountered conflict was smaller for the BPD group than for controls. It may be that the BPD group had a smaller reaction to the negative stimuli, or that they attempted to avoid processing the content of the negative stimuli. Either option could result in the lack of ACC activation.

In summary, both the behavioral and imaging evidence for attentional deficits in BPD are mixed, especially for studies exam-ining impairments related to emotional stimuli. One possible reason for inconsistent results is that most of the studies that have examined attention dysregulation in BPD have used heterogeneous samples, without selecting for the presence of particular BPD symptoms (e.g., affective instability, impul-sivity). This is potentially a problem, as there are a large number of ways to obtain a BPD diagnosis. Thus, without selection crite-ria, two different samples may, by chance, vary systematically on symptom frequency. It may be that particular symptoms are tied to attention dysregulation whereas others are not. It is also possible that attention dysregulation is tied to a specific subgroup of individuals with BPD that have yet to be identified. Lack of appropriate selection criteria may similarly account for at least some of the inconsistent findings in the sections below.

That being said, there are some encouraging results considering that, thus far, relatively little work has been done. There is a need to move beyond finding a presence or absence of deficit and to be driven by theory. A clearer understanding of why a process may be impaired will increase the probability of finding positive and meaningful results. Toward that end, we briefly review several domains relevant to BPD that appear to involve both attention and emotion dysregulation. We hope that by doing so, we may identify some of the ways in which attention dysregulation, along with emotion dysregulation, contributes to BPD, which future research can elucidate further.

Emotion Dysregulation

Although discussed throughout this chapter, in this section we focus specifically on emotion dysregulation and discuss how it, or, more precisely, affective instability, can be caused by, and, in turn, cause attention dysregulation. Affective instability is a symptom of BPD that involves extreme changes in affect over the course of time, often in response to stressful life events such as interpersonal conflict. A large part of regulating affect may depend on whether an individual chooses to attend to or ignore a stimulus; in other words, whether he or she engages in approach or avoidance. Both can have negative consequences when they are the result of attention dysregulation. We briefly review how dysregulated approach and avoidance can differentially lead to emotion dysregulation and how this may contribute to affective instability in BPD.

Approach

Emotion dysregulation may occur when an individual attends to emotionally significant information to a maladaptive degree. Focusing on negative events can lead to increased arousal and negative thinking, which, in turn, leads to a greater focus and expectancy

of negative events, creating a feedback loop. This is the process of rumination (Nolen-Hoeksema, Wisco, & Lyubomirsky, 2008; see Watkins, Chapter 21, this volume), which has been shown to increase negative affect, despite the fact that it is generally engaged in for the opposite purpose. Rumination can be conceptualized as a failure to shift attention away from negative content or affect. BPD has been found to be associated with rumination (Baer & Sauer, 2011; Selby, Anestis, Bender, & Joiner, 2009), perhaps indicating a reduced ability to shift attentional resources in the context of emotional stimuli.

Avoidance

Avoiding information with negative emotional significance can have consequences as well. Philippot, Baeyens, and Douilliez (2006) found that closely attending to information with emotional significance can leave individuals less emotionally affected by it, despite the fact that most people believe the opposite to be true and instinctively avoid thinking deeply about events associated with negative emotions, such as anxiety. Although Philippot et al. used undergraduates and patients with anxiety disorders as participants, it is easy to see how their research might apply to BPD. Individuals with BPD have been shown to be hypervigilant to negative stimuli in their environment (Arntz, Appels, & Sieswerda, 2000; Sieswerda, Arntz, & Kindt, 2007; Sieswerda, Arntz, Mertens, & Vertommen, 2007). However, although they may be very good at detecting such stimuli, individuals with BPD may shy away from processing them. As Philippot and colleagues show, this avoidance could have opposite the intended result: Although attention is shifted away from the distressing stimuli, emotion dysregulation increases.

It is important to note that the interaction of attention and emotion need not always have negative effects. Garland and colleagues (2010), working from the broaden-and-build theory of positive emotions (Fredrickson, 1998, 2003, 2009), differentiate the ways positive and negative emotion can direct attention. Whereas negative emotions, as discussed, may lead to a narrowing of attention onto negative stimuli and through processes such as rumination (also see Schmitz, De Rosa, & Anderson, 2009; Talarico, LaBar, & Rubin, 2004), positive emotions can potentially have the reverse effect, broadening attention and leading to greater awareness of context (Johnson, Waugh, & Fredrickson, 2010; Waugh & Fredrickson, 2006). This, in turn, can further broaden attention, creating an "upward," rather than "downward" spiral or feedback loop (Garland et al., 2010). Broadening attention can have a number of positive effects, including relief of psychopathological symptoms. Garland and colleagues propose that intentionally generated positive emotions can be used as a therapeutic intervention, as a means to interrupt and reverse negative feedback loops. It is important to note, however, that it may be too simplistic to assume that the experience of negative affect narrows attention and the experience of positive affect broadens attention. Rather, it may be the motivational intensity of affect that leads to a broad versus narrow focus of attention (Gable & Harmon-Jones, 2010; Harmon-Jones, Gable, & Price, 2011). Individuals with BPD may have a propensity to experience high-motivation negative emotions (e.g., anger), while seldom experiencing low-motivation positive emotions.

One current therapeutic intervention that may work by broadening attention and generating positive emotions is mindfulness meditation. Mindfulness involves present-focused self-regulation in a moment-to-moment manner. Emphasis is placed on monitoring internal and external stimuli in a nonjudgmental way (Garland, 2007; Lutz, Slagter, Dunne, & Davidson, 2008) and involves training one's attention to operate at a broad, open-ended level that has been shown to improve attentional processes (Jha, Krompinger, & Baime, 2007; Slagter, Lutz, Greischar, Nieuwenhuis, & Davidson, 2009). Mindfulness meditation differs from other forms of meditation in that it does not prescribe focusing on one stimulus or object (e.g., a candle flame) but rather involves allowing one's attention to shift from one stimulus or object to the next as experiences change throughout the day. One is not mindful of any one thing, but is mindful of both internal sensations/processes and external stimuli as they present themselves.

In this way, mindfulness training is believed to broaden one's attentional capacity.

Garland and colleagues (2010) propose that this training may trigger positive emotions in an individual. In other words, not only can positive emotions lead to broadened attention, but broadened attention may lead to the experience of positive emotions (Fredrickson & Joiner, 2002). There is some support for this claim: Studies have found that mindfulness led to increases in positive emotions in a sample of healthy adults (Nyklíček & Kuijpers, 2008) and a sample of patients with comorbid rheumatoid arthritis and depression (Zautra et al., 2008). Additionally, Lynch, Chapman, Rosenthal, Kuo, and Linehan (2006) proposed that mindfulness may promote change by fostering an internal state that leads individuals to create new, more positive associations with stimuli previously viewed as negative. These new associations would possibly lead to more positive emotions. Although it remains to be determined whether this increase in positive emotions mediates improvement in symptoms, the interaction between emotion and attention again appears to be mutually reciprocating. As already stated, however, it may not be positive affect per se that is responsible for the broadening of attention that is believed to result from mindfulness training but instead the low-approach motivation nature of the positive affect (experiencing, but not doing or seeking) that is responsible for this effect.

Mindfulness is an important component of DBT, which has been shown empirically to be effective in the treatment of individuals with BPD (Lynch, Trost, Salsman, & Linehan, 2007). It would be interesting to see if there is an increase in positive emotions in patients with BPD in DBT similar to that found in the above studies and, if so, whether this positive interaction of attention and emotion might, in part, explain the effects of DBT.

Impulsivity

Impulsivity is one of the core symptoms of BPD (Lieb et al., 2004; Trull, Tomko, Brown, & Scheiderer, 2010). Individuals with BPD have high rates of alcohol and drug use and disorders (Skodol, Oldham, & Gallaher, 1999; Trull, Sher, Minks-Brown, Durbin, & Burr, 2000), and a tendency to engage in maladaptive behaviors, including aggressive outbursts, bingeing, and sexual promiscuity. They have consistently higher levels of self-reported impulsivity than controls (e.g., Domes et al., 2006; Ferraz et al., 2009; Jacob et al., 2010; Kunert et al., 2003). Although much attention has been paid to the assessment of impulsivity and its consequences in BPD, there has been less emphasis on understanding why individuals with BPD are impulsive, although Linehan (1993) linked impulsivity to negative affect. It should be no surprise that we propose that impulsivity in BPD is the result of an interaction of emotion and attention dysregulation.

Such an interaction has been previously outlined by Selby, Anestis, and Joiner (2008) in their emotional cascade model. This model, validated in undergraduates, builds from the idea of dysregulated approach behavior, detailed earlier, stating that a small amount of negative affect due to a negative stimulus may be increased exponentially through rumination, catastrophizing, or other similar cognitive processes, resulting in a feedback loop. When negative affect becomes great enough, the model predicts that individuals engage in behavior that disrupts the feedback loop, acting as a sort of safety valve and reducing emotion dysregulation. This behavior tends to be impulsive and maladaptive, especially when the negative affect is intense. This may be because, as attention is increasingly focused on the emotional stimulus, individuals do not have sufficient capacity to carefully think through how to best regulate their emotions. Selby and colleagues (2008) associated these types of impulsive behaviors with Whiteside and Lynam's (2001) urgency subtype of impulsivity, which has been separately linked to BPD (Whiteside, Lynam, Miller, & Reynolds, 2005).

The emotional cascade model thus offers a means of conceptualizing impulsivity in BPD and how cognition, emotion, and attention all might intersect in the disorder to produce dysregulated behavior (also see Selby et al., 2009). Individuals with BPD may overfocus on negative stimuli, leading to an increase in negative affect, which in turn leads to an increase in ineffective cognitive strategies to reduce that affect (e.g., rumination), leading to a greater attentional focus on the negative stimulus (or other, new negative stimuli), and so on, until the cycle is broken by impulsive behavior.

In this way, impulsivity can be characterized as the behavioral consequence of attention dysregulation. That is, impulsive behavior results from some failure to take into account important internal or external information when making a decision. Of course, although attention dysregulation may be a necessary condition of impulsivity, it is not sufficient; emotion dysregulation also plays a key role. A major question that needs to be addressed, then, is whether emotion or attention is more important in causing impulsive behavior in individuals with BPD: that is, whether BPD is better characterized by strong affective impulses (emotion dysregulation) overriding normal controls (normal attention) or by moderate affective impulses (normal emotion) breaking through weak controls (attention dysregulation). There is more evidence available supporting the case for emotion dysregulation, but, as already discussed, studies have found attention dysregulation in the absence of emotion stimuli. It is also important to note that these explanations are not mutually exclusive. Impulsivity in BPD likely involves dysregulation in both areas. The exact interaction of the two remains to be determined.

However, the emotional cascade model would seem to suggest that individuals with BPD should engage in impulsive behaviors only when they are emotionally dysregulated. That is, emotion dysregulation would be a necessary condition of impulsive behavior. One way to test this hypothesis is to assess individuals with BPD for impulsivity in an experimental setting, where emotional content can be controlled. This can be accomplished with tests of behavioral response inhibition, a common way to behaviorally operationalize impulsivity. Tasks of behavioral inhibition (e.g., a go/no-go task) typically involve the establishment of a response, usually at the detection of a particular stimulus, which participants must periodically, but unpredictably, withhold or inhibit at the detection of a second type of stimulus. Their ability to do so is their measure of behavioral inhibition, which is calculated based on reaction time or the number of errors made.

Studies comparing individuals with BPD and controls on behavioral inhibition, however, are inconsistent, with some (Dinn et al. 2004; Ferraz et al., 2009; Jacob et al., 2010; Kunert et al., 2003; Lampe et al., 2007) finding no difference, whereas others find less inhibition in individuals with BPD (Coffey, Schumacher, Baschnagel, Hawk, & Holloman, 2011; Leyton et al., 2001; McCloskey et al., 2009; Nigg, Silk, Stavro, & Miller, 2005; Rentrop et al., 2008). Despite the inconsistency in the literature, the existence of some findings of impaired behavioral inhibition in the absence of emotional stimuli would seem to suggest that emotion dysregulation is not a necessary precursor for impulsive behavior in individuals with BPD, although it may be sufficient. In order to determine the relationship between emotion dysregulation and impulsivity in individuals with BPD, future studies of BPD and behavioral response inhibition should manipulate emotional content as another variable.

Emotion Recognition

A number of studies have explored the association between BPD and the detection and recognition of emotion in others, particularly via facial cues (for a review, see Domes, Schulze, & Herpertz, 2009). Individuals with BPD might be expected to be adept at the detection of emotions in others, as emotion dysregulation suggests sensitivity to emotion-related cues in the environment (Linehan, 1993). Such sensitivity could result from early learning—a result of, for example, early childhood abuse followed by years of reinforcing experience.

There is some support for this hypothesis. Scott, Levy, Adams, and Stevenson (2011) found that undergraduates high on BPD traits were better at identifying negative emotions from pictures of eye regions than students low on BPD traits, but no different at identifying positive or neutral emotions. However, the high-BPD group also showed a greater tendency to associate negative emo-

tions with all stimuli types. Using computer morphing techniques to ensure strong experimental control, Lynch, Rosenthal, and colleagues (2006) showed participants with and without BPD images of faces that transitioned from neutral expressions to ones of sadness, happiness, surprise, anger, fear, or disgust. Participants had to identify the correct emotion as quickly as possible. The BPD group was able to identify all emotions more quickly than controls, thus using less information to make identifications. This effect could not be explained by a speed–accuracy tradeoff. In a replication, however, Domes and colleagues (2008) failed to find differences between groups, although the BPD group did show a reduction in reaction time over the course of the experiment. The authors suggested that, over time, the faces became familiar to participants and, thus, that individuals with BPD may show increased sensitivity, but only for familiar faces.

Other studies, however, have reported contrary results, finding individuals with BPD to be no different from, or worse than, controls at detecting emotions in others. For example, although Wagner and Linehan (1999) found that individuals with BPD were more accurate than controls and participants with a history of childhood sexual abuse at the detection of fear, participants also had a bias to report fear across all trials. Domes and colleagues (2008) found a similar bias, only for anger instead of fear. Minzenberg, Poole, and Vinogradov (2006) found that individuals with BPD were no different from controls at identifying emotions based on facial or prosodic cues in isolation, but were less accurate when the two cue types were combined. Several other studies found that individuals with BPD were significantly worse than controls at recognizing emotions, especially negative ones (Bland, Williams, Scharer, & Manning, 2004; Levine, Marziali, & Hood, 1997). Dyck and colleagues (2009) found a recognition deficit in individuals with BPD when under time pressure, but not when given unlimited time to respond.

The amygdala has been found to be important in recognizing negative emotions, and, suggestively, is smaller in volume and more active in individuals with BPD (Hall,

Olabi, Lawrie, & McIntosh, 2010; Nunes et al., 2009; Schmahl & Bremner, 2006). However, it is not clear whether these structural and functional differences would lead to more accurate detection or to a propensity to interpret ambiguous cues negatively (possibilities that both find support in the literature). Two studies have used functional imaging in the context of emotion recognition with facial cues in individuals with BPD, both of which found abnormalities in prefrontal and amygdala areas (Donegan et al., 2003; Minzenberg, Fan, New, Tang, & Siever, 2007).

Regardless of whether individuals with BPD are more or less accurate at detecting emotions in others, they do appear to pay increased attention to them. Although an ability to detect emotions more quickly or more accurately would be adaptive in certain situations, it could more often have negative consequences. Facial cues, after all, are not perfect indicators of emotions, nor of their intensity. Being more aware of facial cues, whether the interpretation of them is accurate or not, may leave individuals more likely to overreact to them. Sometimes, for the sake of our relationships, it is better to overlook the emotions we generate in others, especially when they are momentary and quickly controlled. Individuals who are less able to do this are likely to have more interpersonal conflict, as is seen with individuals with BPD. A similar case could be made for individuals who tend to be inaccurate or biased at detecting emotions.

Thus, individuals with BPD appear to have a propensity to attend to and detect facial cues, accurately or otherwise, and, possibly, to associate them with negative emotions. The detection of negative emotions may serve as distressing emotional stimuli to individuals with BPD, increasing their physiological arousal, creating emotion dysregulation, and decreasing their attentional capacity. This reduction in capacity may render them less able to thoroughly process additional facial cues. Given their already established bias, they would be prone to continue to associate these cues with negative emotions, which, in turn, would lead to further increased arousal and reduced capacity, creating a feedback loop similar to that discussed previously. Future studies could test whether the accuracy of individuals with BPD in emotion recognition decreases as a function of detection of negative emotions, regardless of whether those detections are correct or not.

Alternatively, however, individuals with BPD, upon detecting negative affectivity, may engage in attentional avoidance, similar to the effect described by Philippot and colleagues (2006). This, too, could conceivably lead to reduced accuracy in emotion recognition, as attention is refocused elsewhere, while increasing emotional distress. Although not directly examining BPD, Berenson and colleagues (2009) found that individuals high in rejection sensitivity performed worse than individuals with low rejection sensitivity on two attention-related tasks using social threat cues. The first, an emotional Stroop task, incorporated rejection-related words. Individuals high on rejection sensitivity were slower. The second, a visual probe task, used faces with threatening or pleasant expressions. Individuals high on rejection sensitivity showed a bias to avoid the threatening stimuli. Furthermore, participants who took the visual probe task were assessed for borderline features, and borderline features predicted avoidance of threatening faces. These findings suggest a different mechanism for abnormal emotion recognition in individuals with BPD: They avoid processing emotions upon recognizing them, potentially leading to both reduced recognition and emotion dysregulation.

Similar to emotion dysregulation more generally, then, abnormal emotion recognition in BPD may involve both approach- and avoidance-related processes. Whether individuals with BPD engage primarily in one or the other likely depends on the individual and the situation. It is possible that emotion recognition in BPD depends on the current mood state of the individual, with the result of frequent flipping back and forth between approach and avoidance. For example, an individual with BPD might initially attend very closely to a loved one's facial expressions, angrily looking for signs of rejection, only to shift away, suddenly afraid of actually detecting them. Then he or she might resume processing a few moments later, when the loved one makes what seems to be a suspicious comment.

Self-Injury and Pain

Individuals with BPD have a paradoxical relationship with pain. In experimental settings using induced pain methodology (e.g., heat stimuli, electric shock, the cold pressor task), they show consistently greater tolerance to pain and report less pain overall compared to controls (Niedtfeld et al., 2010; Russ et al., 1992), an effect that is even stronger under conditions of distress (Bohus et al., 2000; Ludäscher et al., 2007). This high tolerance occurs despite their low distress tolerance (Gratz, Rosenthal, Tull, Lejeuz, & Gunderson, 2006) and high prevalence in chronic headache and pain populations (Saper & Lake, 2002; Tragesser, Bruns, & Disorbio, 2010). This paradox may be partly due to the effects of emotion dysregulation, which has been shown to inhibit pain sensitivity (Rhudy & Meagher, 2003). That is, individuals with BPD may primarily experience greater pain tolerance when in a state of emotional distress. However, emotion dysregulation cannot account entirely for their higher pain tolerance, as they were found to differ from controls in studies that did not manipulate distress.

Related to pain tolerance, a majority of individuals with BPD engage in self-injurious behavior (SIB) over their lifetime—that is, behavior that intentionally damages the body but lacks lethal intent (Dulit, Fyer, Leon, Brodsky, & Frances, 1994; Zanarini et al., 2008). There are multiple explanations for why BPD individuals engage in SIB (Nock, 2010), but one of the chief reasons that individuals with BPD report is to relieve distress or to regulate affect (Chapman, Gratz & Brown, 2006; Nock, 2010).

The perception of pain can be divided into two broad areas, affective motivation and sensation discrimination, each of which has its own network in the brain (Treede, Kenshalo, Gracely, & Jones, 1999). Affective motivation involves higher-level processing of, and responding to, pain and involves brain regions important to both emotion (e.g., the amygdala) and attention processing (e.g., the ACC). In this way, SIB may be a means of emotion regulation via a refocusing of attention. As already discussed in connection with the emotional cascade model,

when caught in a feedback loop that they are unable to free themselves from, individuals with BPD may engage in maladaptive behavior in order to reduce their distress. In the case of SIB, individuals with BPD may break the loop by activating the brain's pain response, which requires attentional resources. The importance of attentional processes to the experience of pain, and vice versa, might explain, at least in part, the high prevalence of SIB in individuals with BPD (Selby et al., 2009).

Some support for this idea has been found. Schmahl and colleagues (2006) found that individuals with BPD reported less pain in response to heat stimulation and showed reduced neural activation relative to controls. After adjusting for subjective pain level, individuals with BPD showed greater activity in the left dorsolateral prefrontal cortex and reduced activity in the parietal cortex. In support of the hypothesis that individuals with BPD may engage in SIB to refocus attentional processes, individuals with BPD also showed deactivation in the perigenual ACC and the right amygdala, whereas controls did not. Deactivation in the perigenual ACC may be related to processes intended to concentrate cognitive and emotional resources toward goal-focused behavior (Gusnard & Raichle, 2001) or handling emotional states (Simpson, Drevets, Snyder, Gusnard, & Raichle, 2001). Deactivation in the perigenual ACC may, therefore, have been directly responsible for the deactivation found in the right amygdala. If accurate, this would provide a mechanism for attentional processes to interrupt and exert control over emotion dysregulation.

However, amygdala deactivation may not be specific to BPD. Kraus and colleagues (2009) compared individuals with BPD with and without co-occurring PTSD on a pain induction task. There was no difference in pain sensitivity across groups, but individuals in the comorbid group showed greater amygdala deactivation, suggesting that amygdala deactivation is not the central antinociceptive mechanism in individuals with BPD. The association between BPD and pain response may involve more than dysregulation in attention and emotion processes. For example, BPD has been linked to dysregulation of the endogenous opioid system, which is heavily involved in the experience of pain (Bandelow, Schmahl, Falkai, & Wedekind, 2010; Stanley & Siever, 2010). Ultimately, evidence has shown consistently that there is something important about how individuals with BPD experience and process pain, although we are still working to fully understand the biological mechanisms involved.

Conclusion

We have briefly reviewed the available literature on attention and BPD and described how attention and emotion processes may interact to yield many of the symptoms associated with BPD, including affective instability, impulsivity, interpersonal deficits, and SIB. We also reviewed the similarities between BPD and ADHD, a disorder with strong ties to attention dysregulation.

There is evidence in the literature that BPD involves dysregulation of attention, perhaps specific to the context of emotional stimuli. Attention dysregulation may lead to emotion dysregulation in BPD, creating a distressing feedback loop and resulting in maladaptive and impulsive or SIB. It may also lead to rejection sensitivity and social hypersensitivity, as well as a number of other negative consequences. Emotion dysregulation can also lead to attentional problems, especially narrowing of attention. It is important to realize that neither one exists in isolation, but that there is strong evidence that each contributes to the other.

There are several limitations in the current work on attention and BPD. Chief among these is the inconsistency of findings. As mentioned previously, one of the reasons for the inconsistency of results may be the failure of researchers to ensure the selection of participants with relevant symptoms, such as impulsivity and affective instability. Interestingly, the most consistent set of results we reviewed dealt with pain and self-injury in BPD, of which most, if not all, of the studies included only participants with a clear history of SIB. This is an important point, and future studies should be conducted following a careful consideration of selection criteria. That is, given the heterogeneity of BPD, we believe that researchers interested

in studying particular criteria (e.g., affective instability, impulsivity) should take steps to ensure that all participants in their studies possess those criteria. Despite the inconsistency, however, we believe there is a great deal to gain from researchers investigating attention dysregulation in BPD, especially in the context of emotion dysregulation. The results obtained thus far are promising, but much remains to be understood.

References

American Psychiatric Association. (2000). *Diagnostic and statistical manual of mental disorders* (4th ed., text rev.). Washington, DC: Author.

Andrulonis P. A., Glueck B. C., Stroebel C. F., & Vogel N. G. (1982). Borderline personality subcategories. *Journal of Nervous and Mental Disease, 170*, 670–679.

Arntz, A., Appels, C., & Sieswerda, S. (2000). Hypervigilance in borderline disorder: A test with the emotional Stroop paradigm. *Journal of Personality Disorders, 14*, 366–373.

Baer, R. A., & Sauer, S. E. (2011). Relationships between depressive rumination, anger rumination, and borderline personality features. *Personality Disorders: Theory, Research, and Treatment, 2*, 142–150.

Bandelow, B., Schmahl, C., Falkai, P., & Wedekind, D. (2010). Borderline personality disorder: A dysregulation of the endogenous opioid system? *Psychological Review, 117*, 623–636.

Berenson, K. R., Gyurak, A., Ayduk, O., Downey, G., Garner, M. J., Mogg, K., et al. (2009). Rejection sensitivity and disruption of attention by social threat cues. *Journal of Research in Personality, 43*, 1064–1072.

Biederman, J. (2004). Impact of comorbidity in adults with attention-deficit/hyperactivity disorder. *Journal of Clinical Psychiatry, 65*(Suppl. 3), 3–7.

Bland, A. R., Williams, C. A., Scharer, K., & Manning, S. (2004). Emotion processing in borderline personality disorders. *Issues in Mental Health Nursing, 25*, 655–672.

Bohus, M., Limberger, M., Ebner, U., Glocker, F. X., Schwarz, B., Wernz, M., et al. (2000). Pain perception during self-reported distress and calmness in patients with borderline personality disorder and self-mutilating behavior. *Psychiatry Research, 95*, 251–260.

Carter, C. S., Mintun, M., & Cohen, J. D. (1995). Interference and facilitation effects during selective attention: An H215O PET study of Stroop task performance. *NeuroImage, 2,* 264–272.

Chapman, A. L., Gratz, K. L., & Brown, M. Z. (2006). Solving the puzzle of deliberate self-harm: The experiential avoidance model. *Behaviour Research and Therapy, 44,* 371–394.

Coffey, S. F., Schumacher, J. A., Baschnagel, J. S., Hawk, L. W., & Holloman, G. (2011). Impulsivity and risk-taking in borderline personality disorder with and without substance use disorders. *Personality Disorders: Theory, Research, and Treatment, 2,* 128–141.

Davids, E. & Gastpar, M. (2005). Attention deficit hyperactivity disorder and borderline personality disorder. *Progress in Neuro-Psychopharmacology and Biological Psychiatry, 29,* 865–877.

Dell'Osso B., Berlin H. A., Serati M., & Altamura, A. C. (2010). Neuropsychobiological aspects, comorbidity patterns and dimensional models in borderline personality disorder. *Neuropsychobiology, 61,* 169–179.

Dinn, W. M., Harris, C. L., Aycicegi, A., Greene, P. B., Kirkley, S. M., & Reilly, C. (2004). Neurocognitive function in borderline personality disorder. *Progress in Neuro-Psychopharmacology and Biological Psychiatry, 28,* 329–341.

Domes, G., Czieschnek, D., Weidler, F., Berger, C., Fast, K., & Herpertz, S. C. (2008). Recognition of facial affect in borderline personality disorder. *Journal of Personality Disorders, 22,* 135–147.

Domes, G., Schulze, L., & Herpertz, S. C. (2009). Emotion recognition in borderline personality disorder: A review of the literature. *Journal of Personality Disorders, 23,* 6–19.

Domes, G., Winter, B., Schnell, K., Vohs, K., Fast, K., & Herpertz, S. C. (2006). The influence of emotions on inhibitory functioning in borderline personality disorder. *Psychological Medicine, 36,* 1163–1172.

Donegan, N., Sanislow, C. A., Blumberg, H. P., Fulbright, R. K., Lacadie, C., Skudlarski, P., et al. (2003). Amygdala hyperreactivity in borderline personality disorder: Implications for emotional dysregulation. *Biological Psychiatry, 54,* 1284–1293.

Driessen, M., Herrmann, J., Stahl, K., Zwaan, M., Meier, S., Hill, A., et al. (2000). Magnetic resonance imaging volumes of the hippocampus and the amygdala in women with borderline personality disorder and early traumatization. *Archives of General Psychiatry, 57,* 1115–1122.

Dulit, R. A., Fyer, M. R., Leon, A. C., Brodsky, B. S., & Frances, A. J. (1994). Clinical correlates of self-mutilation in borderline personality disorder. *American Journal of Psychiatry, 151,* 1305.

Dyck, M., Habel, U., Slodczyk, J., Schlummer, J., Backes, V., Schneider, F., et al. (2009). Negative bias in fast emotion discrimination in borderline personality disorder. *Psychological Medicine, 39,* 855–864.

Faraone, S. V., Biederman, J., Spencer, T., Wilens, T., Seidman, L. J., Mick, E., et al. (2000). Attention-deficit/hyperactivity disorder in adults: An overview. *Biological Psychiatry, 48,* 9–20.

Ferraz, L., Vallez, M., Navarro, J., Gelabert, E., Martinsantos, R., & Subira, S. (2009). Dimensional assessment of personality and impulsiveness in borderline personality disorder. *Personality and Individual Differences, 46,* 140–146.

Ferrer, M., Andion, O., Matali, J., Valero, S., Navarro, J. A., Ramos-Quiroga, J. A., et al. (2010). Comorbid attention-deficit/hyperactivity disorder in borderline patients defines an impulsive subtype of borderline personality disorder. *Journal of Personality Disorders, 24,* 812–822.

Fossati, A., Novella, L., Donati, D., Donini, M., & Maffei, C. (2002). History of childhood attention deficit/hyperactivity disorder symptoms and borderline personality disorder: A controlled study. *Comprehensive Psychiatry, 43,* 369–377.

Fredrickson, B. L. (1998). What good are positive emotions? *Review of General Psychology, 2,* 300–319.

Fredrickson, B. L. (2003). The value of positive emotions: The emerging science of positive psychology is coming to understand why it's good to feel good. *American Scientist, 91,* 330–335.

Fredrickson, B. L. (2009). *Positivity: Groundbreaking research reveals how to embrace the hidden strength of positive emotions, overcome negativity, and thrive.* New York: Crown.

Fredrickson, B. L., & Joiner, T. (2002). Positive emotions trigger upward spirals toward emotional well-being. *Psychological Science, 13,* 172–175.

Gable, P., & Harmon-Jones, E. (2010). The motivational dimensional model of affect: Implications for breadth of attention, memory, and cognitive categorisation. *Cognition and Emotion, 24*, 322–337.

Garland, E. L. (2007). The meaning of mindfulness: A second-order cybernetics of stress, metacognition, and coping. *Complementary Health Practice Review, 12*, 15–30.

Garland, E. L., Fredrickson, B., Kring, A. M., Johnson, D. P., Meyer, P. S., & Penn, D. L. (2010). Upward spirals of positive emotions counter downward spirals of negativity: Insights from the broaden-and-build theory and affective neuroscience on the treatment of emotion dysfunctions and deficits in psychopathology. *Clinical Psychology Review, 30*, 849–864.

Golubchik, P., Sever, J., & Weizman, A. (2009). Influence of methylphenidate treatment on smoking behavior in adolescent girls with attention-deficit/hyperactivity and borderline personality disorders. *Clinical Neuropharmacology, 32*, 239–242.

Gratz, K. L., Rosenthal, M. Z., Tull, M. T., Lejuez, C. W., & Gunderson, J. G. (2006). An experimental investigation of emotion dysregulation in borderline personality disorder. *Journal of Abnormal Psychology, 115*, 850–855.

Gusnard, D. A., Raichle, M. E. (2001). Searching for a baseline: Functional imaging and the resting human brain. *National Review of Neuroscience, 33*, 685–694.

Haaland, V. Ø., Esperaas, L., & Landrø, N. I. (2009). Selective deficit in executive functioning among patients with borderline personality disorder. *Psychological Medicine, 39*, 1733–1743.

Hajcak, G., & Foti, D. (2008). Errors are aversive: Defensive motivation and the error-related negativity. *Psychological Science, 19*, 103–108.

Hall, J., Olabi, B., Lawrie, S. M., & McIntosh, A. M. (2010). Hippocampal and amygdala volumes in borderline personality disorder: A meta-analysis of magnetic resonance imaging studies. *Personality and Mental Health, 4*, 172–179.

Harmon-Jones, E., Gable, P. A., & Price, T. F. (2011). Toward an understanding of the influence of affective states on attentional tuning: Comment on Friedman and Förster (2010). *Psychological Bulletin, 137*, 508–512.

Hesslinger, B., Tebartz van Elst, L., Nyberg, E., Dykierek, P., Richter, H., et al. (2002). Psychotherapy of attention deficit hyperactivity disorder in adults: A pilot study using a structured skills training program. *European Archives of Psychiatry and Clinical Neuroscience, 252*, 177–184.

Jacob, G. A., Gutz, L., Bader, K., Lieb, K., Tüscher, O., & Stahl, C. (2010). Impulsivity in borderline personality disorder: Impairment in self-report measures, but not behavioral inhibition. *Psychopathology, 43*, 180–188.

Jha, A., Krompinger, J., & Baime, M. (2007). Mindfulness training modifies subsystems of attention. *Cognitive, Affective, and Behavioral Neuroscience, 7*, 109–119.

Johnson, K., Waugh, C., & Fredrickson, B. (2010). Smile to see the forest: Facially expressed positive emotions broaden cognition. *Cognition and Emotion, 24*, 299–321.

Kraus, A., Esposito, F., Seifritz, E., Di Salle, F., Ruf, M., Valerius, G., et al. (2009). Amygdala deactivation as a neural correlate of pain processing in patients with borderline personality disorder and co-occurrent posttraumatic stress disorder. *Biological Psychiatry, 65*, 819–822.

Kunert, H. J., Druecke, H. W., Sass, H., & Herpertz, S. C. (2003). Frontal lobe dysfunctions in borderline personality disorder?: Neuropsychological findings. *Journal of Personality Disorders, 17*, 497–509.

Lampe, K., Konrad, K., Kroener, S., Fast, K., Kunert, H. J., & Herpertz, S. C. (2007). Neuropsychological and behavioural disinhibition in adult ADHD compared to borderline personality disorder. *Psychological Medicine, 37*, 1717–1729.

LeGris, J., & van Reekum, R. (2006). The neuropsychological correlates of borderline personality disorder and suicidal behaviour. *Canadian Journal of Psychiatry, 51*, 131–142.

Lenzenweger, M. F., Clarkin, J. F., Fertuck, E. A., & Kernberg, O. F. (2004). Executive neurocognitive functioning and neurobehavioral systems indicators in borderline personality disorder: A preliminary study. *Journal of Personality Disorders, 18*, 421–438.

Lenzenweger, M. F., Lane, M. C., Loranger, A. W., & Kessler, R. C. (2007). DSM-IV personality disorders in the National Comorbidity Survey Replication. *Biological Psychiatry, 62*, 553–564.

Levine, D., Marziali, E., & Hood, J. (1997). Emotion processing in borderline personality disorders. *Journal of Nervous and Mental Disease, 185*, 240–246.

Leyton, M., Okazawa, H., Diksic, M., Paris, J., Rosa, P., Mzengeza, S., et al. (2001). Brain regional α-[^{11}C]methyl-L-tryptophan trapping in impulsive subjects with borderline personalitydisorder. *American Journal of Psychiatry, 158*, 775–782.

Lieb, K., Zanarini, M. C., Schmahl, C., Linehan, M. M., & Bohus, M. (2004). Borderline personality disorder. *Lancet, 364*, 453–461.

Linehan, M. M. (1993). *Cognitive-behavioral treatment of borderline personality disorder.* New York: Guilford Press.

Ludäscher, P., Bohus, M., Lieb, K., Philipsen, A., Jochims, A., & Schmahl, C. (2007). Elevated pain thresholds correlate with dissociation and aversive arousal in patients with borderline personality disorder. *Psychiatry Research, 149*, 291–296.

Lutz, A., Slagter, H. A., Dunne, J. D., & Davidson, R. J. (2008). Attention regulation and monitoring in meditation. *Trends in Cognitive Sciences, 12*, 163–169.

Lynch, T. R., Chapman, A. L., Rosenthal, M. Z., Kuo, J. R., & Linehan, M. M. (2006). Mechanisms of change in dialectical behavior therapy: Theoretical and empirical observations. *Journal of Clinical Psychology, 62*, 459–480.

Lynch, T. R., Rosenthal, M. Z., Kosson, D. S., Cheavens, J. S., Lejuez, C. W., & Blair, R. J. R. (2006). Heightened sensitivity to facial expressions of emotion in borderline personality disorder. *Emotion, 6*, 647–655.

Lynch, T. R., Trost, W. T., Salsman, N., & Linehan, M. M. (2007). Dialectical behavior therapy for borderline personality disorder. *Annual Review of Clinical Psychology, 3*, 181–205.

Mathews, A., & MacLeod, C. (2005). Cognitive vulnerability to emotional disorders. *Annual Review of Clinical Psychology, 1*, 167–195.

McCloskey, M. S., New, A. S., Siever, L. J., Goodman, M., Koenigsberg, H. W., Flory, J. D., et al. (2009). Evaluation of behavioral impulsivity and aggression tasks as endophenotypes for borderline personality disorder. *Journal of Psychiatric Research, 43*, 1036–1048.

Minzenberg, M. J., Fan, J., New, A. S., Tang, C. Y., & Siever, L. J. (2007). Fronto-limbic dysfunction in response to facial emotion in borderline personality disorder: An event-related fMRI study. *Psychiatry Research, 155*, 231–243.

Minzenberg, M. J., Poole, J. H., & Vinogradov, S. (2006). Social-emotion recognition in borderline personality disorder. *Comprehensive Psychiatry, 47*, 468–474.

Murray, M. E. (1979). Minimal brain dysfunction and borderline personality adjustment. *American Journal of Psychotherapy, 33*, 391–403.

Niedtfeld, I., Schulze, L., Kirsch, P., Herpertz, S. C., Bohus, M., & Schmahl, C. (2010). Affect regulation and pain in borderline personality disorder: A possible link to the understanding of self-injury. *Biological Psychiatry, 68*, 383–391.

Nigg, J. T., Silk, K. R., Stavro, G., & Miller, T. (2005). Disinhibition and borderline personality disorder. *Development and Psychopathology, 17*, 1129–1149.

Nock, M. K. (2010). Self-injury. *Annual Review of Clinical Psychology, 6*, 339–363.

Nolen-Hoeksema, S., Wisco, B. E., & Lyubomirsky, S. (2008). Rethinking rumination. *Perspectives on Psychological Science, 3*, 400–424.

Nunes, P. M., Wenzel, A., Borges, K. T., Porto, C. R., Caminha, R. M., & de Oliveira, I. R. (2009). Volumes of the hippocampus and amygdala in patients with borderline personality disorder: A meta-analysis. *Journal of Personality Disorders, 23*, 333–345.

Nyklíček, I., & Kuijpers, K. F. (2008). Effects of mindfulness-based stress reduction intervention on psychological well-being and quality of life: Is increased mindfulness indeed the mechanism? *Annals of Behavioral Medicine, 35*, 331–340.

Ochsner, K. N., & Gross, J. J. (2005). The cognitive control of emotion. *Trends in Cognitive Sciences, 9*, 242–249.

Peterson, B. S., Skudlarski, P., Gatenby, J. C., Zhang, H., Anderson, A. W., & Gore, J. C. (1999). An fMRI study of Stroop word–color interference: Evidence for cingulate subregions subserving multiple distributed attentional systems. *Biological Psychiatry, 45*, 1237–1258.

Philippot, P., Baeyens, C., & Douilliez, C. (2006). Specifying emotional information: Regulation of emotional intensity via executive processes. *Emotion, 6*, 560–571.

Philipsen, A. (2006). Differential diagnosis and comorbidity of attention-deficit/hyperactivity disorder (ADHD) and borderline personality disorder (BPD) in adults. *European Archives* of Psychiatry and Clinical Neuroscience, 256(Suppl. 1), 42–46.

Philipsen, A., Limberger, M. F., Lieb, K., Feige, B., Kleindienst, N., Ebner-Priemer, U., et al. (2008). Attention-deficit hyperactivity disorder as a potentially aggravating factor in borderline personality disorder. British Journal of Psychiatry, 192, 118–123.

Posner, M. I. (1992). Attention as a cognitive and neural system. Current Directions in Psychological Science, 1, 11–14.

Posner, M. I., & Dehaene, S. (1994). Attentional networks. Trends in Neurosciences, 17, 75–79.

Posner, M. I., Rothbart, M. K., Vizueta, N., Levy, K. N., Evans, D. E., Thomas, K. M., et al. (2002). Attentional mechanisms of borderline personality disorder. Proceedings of the National Academy of Sciences of the United States of America, 99, 16366–16370.

Rentrop, M., Backenstrass, M., Jaentsch, B., Kaiser, S., Roth, A., Unger, J., et al. (2008). Response inhibition in borderline personality disorder: Performance in a go/no-go task. Psychopathology, 41, 50–57.

Rhudy, J. L., & Meagher, M. W. (2003). Negative affect: Effects on an evaluative measure of human pain. Pain, 104, 617–626.

Russ, M. J., Roth, S. D., Lerman, A., Kakuma, T., Harrison, K., Shindledecker, R. D., et al. (1992). Pain perception in self-injurious patients with borderline personality disorder. Biological Psychiatry, 32, 501–511.

Saper, J. R., & Lake, A. E. (2002). Borderline personality disorder and the chronic headache patient: Review and management recommendations. Headache, 42, 663–674.

Schmahl, C. G., Bohus, M., Esposito, F., Treede, R.-D., Di Salle, F., Greffrath, W., et al. (2006). Neural correlates of antinociception in borderline personality disorder. Archives of General Psychiatry, 63, 659–667.

Schmahl, C. G., & Bremner, J. D. (2006). Neuroimaging in borderline personality disorder. Journal of Psychiatric Research, 40, 419–427.

Schmahl, C. G., Elzinga, B. M., Vermetten, E., Sanislow, C., Mcglashan, T. H., & Bremner, J. D. (2003). Neural correlates of memories of abandonment in women with and without borderline personality disorder. Biological Psychiatry, 3223, 142–151.

Schmahl, C. G., Vermetten, E., Elzinga, B. M.,

& Bremner, J. D. (2004). A positron emission tomography study of memories of childhood abuse in borderline personality disorder. Biological Psychiatry, 55, 759–765.

Schmitz, T. W., De Rosa, E., & Anderson, A. K. (2009). Opposing influences of affective state valence on visual cortical encoding. Journal of Neuroscience, 29, 7199–7207.

Schulz, S. C., Cornelius, J., Schulz, P. M., & Soloff, P. H. (1988). The amphetamine challenge test in patients with borderline disorder. American Journal of Psychiatry, 145, 809–814.

Scott, L. N., Levy, K. N., Adams, R. B., & Stevenson, M. T. (2011). Mental state decoding abilities in young adults with borderline personality disorder traits. Personality Disorders: Theory, Research, and Treatment, 2, 98–112.

Selby, E. A., Anestis, M. D., Bender, T. W., & Joiner, T. E., Jr. (2009). An exploration of the emotional cascade model in borderline personality disorder. Journal of Abnormal Psychology, 118, 375–387.

Selby, E. A., Anestis, M. D., & Joiner, T. E. (2008). Understanding the relationship between emotional and behavioral dysregulation: Emotional cascades. Behaviour Research and Therapy, 46, 593–611.

Sieswerda, S., Arntz, A., & Kindt, M. (2007). Successful psychotherapy reduces hypervigilance in borderline personality disorder. Behavioural and Cognitive Psychotherapy, 35, 387–402.

Sieswerda, S., Arntz, A., Mertens, I., & Vertommen, S. (2007). Hypervigilance in patients with borderline personality disorder: Specificity, automaticity, and predictors. Behaviour Research and Therapy, 45, 1011–1024.

Simpson, J. R. Jr., Drevets, W. C., Snyder, A. Z., Gusnard, D. A., Raichle, M. E. (2001). Emotion induced changes in human medial prefrontal cortex: II. During anticipatory anxiety. Proceedings of the National Academy of Science of the United States of America, 98, 688–693.

Skodol, A. E., Gunderson, J. G., Pfohl, B., Widiger, T. A., Livesley, W. J., & Siever, L. J. (2002). The borderline diagnosis: I. Psychopathology, comorbidity, and personality structure. Biological Psychiatry, 51, 936–950.

Skodol, A. E., Oldham, J. M., & Gallaher, P. E. (1999). Axis II comorbidity of substance use disorders among patients referred for treatment of personality disorders. *American Journal of Psychiatry, 156,* 733.

Slagter, H. A., Lutz, A., Greischar, L. L., Nieuwenhuis, S., & Davidson, R. J. (2009). Theta phase synchrony and conscious target perception: Impact of intensive mental training. *Journal of Cognitive Neuroscience, 21,* 1536–1549.

Sprock, J., Rader, T. J., Kendall, J. P., & Yoder, C. Y. (2000). Neuropsychological functioning in patients with borderline personality disorder. *Journal of Clinical Psychology, 56,* 1587–1600.

Stanley, B., & Siever, L. J. (2010). The interpersonal dimension of borderline personality disorder: Toward a neuropeptide model. *American Journal of Psychiatry, 167,* 24–39.

Stroop, J. R. (1935). Studies of interference in serial verbal reactions. *Journal of Experimental Psychology: General, 18,* 643–662.

Talarico, J. M., LaBar, K. S., & Rubin, D. C. (2004). Emotional intensity predicts autobiographical memory experience. *Memory and Cognition, 32,* 1118–1132.

Taylor, S. F., Kornblum, S., Lauber, E. J., Minoshima, S., & Koeppe, R. A. (1997). Isolation of specific interference processing in the Stroop task: PET activation studies. *NeuroImage, 6,* 81–92.

Tragesser, S. L., Bruns, D., & Disorbio, J. M. (2010). Borderline personality disorder features and pain: The mediating role of negative affect in a pain patient sample. *Clinical Journal of Pain, 26,* 348–353.

Treede, R. D., Kenshalo, D. R., Gracely, R. H., & Jones, A. K. P. (1999). The cortical representation of pain. *Pain, 79,* 105–111.

Trull, T. J., Jahng, S., Tomko, R. L., Wood, P. K., & Sher, K. J. (2010). Revised NESARC personality disorder diagnoses: Gender, prevalence, and comorbidity with substance dependence disorders. *Journal of Personality Disorders, 24,* 412–426.

Trull, T. J., Sher, K. J., Minks-Brown, C., Durbin, J., & Burr, R. (2000). Borderline personality disorder and substance use disorders: A review and integration. *Clinical Psychology Review, 20,* 235–53.

Trull, T. J., Solhan M. B., Tragesser S. L., Jahng S., Wood P. K., Piasecki T. M., et al. (2008). Affective instability: Measuring a core feature of borderline personality disorder with ecological momentary assessment. *Journal Abnormal Psychology, 117,* 647–661.

Trull, T. J., Tomko, R., Brown, W., & Scheiderer, E. (2010). Borderline personality disorder in 3-D: Dimensions, symptoms, and measurement challenges. *Social and Personality Psychology Compass, 11,* 1057–1069.

van Dijk, F. E., Lappenschaar, M., Kan, C. C., Verkes, R. J., & Buitelaar, J. K. (2011). Symptomatic overlap between attention-deficit/hyperactivity disorder and borderline personality disorder in women: The role of temperament and character traits. *Comprehensive Psychiatry, 53,* 39–47.

van Reekum, R. & Links, P. S. (1994). N of 1 study: Methylphenidate in a patient with borderline personality disorder and attention deficit hyperactivity disorder. *Canadian Journal of Psychiatry, 39,* 186–187.

Wagner, A. W., & Linehan, M. M. (1999). Facial expression recognition ability among women with borderline personality disorder: Implications for emotion regulation? *Journal of Personality Disorders, 13,* 329–344.

Waugh, C. E., & Fredrickson, B. (2006). Nice to know you: Positive emotions, self–other overlap, and complex understanding in the formation of a new relationship. *Journal of Positive Psychology, 1,* 93–106.

Whiteside, S. P., & Lynam, D. R. (2001). The five-factor model and impulsivity: Using a structural model of personality to understand impulsivity. *Personality and Individual Differences, 30,* 669–689.

Whiteside, S. P., Lynam, D. R., Miller, J. D., & Reynolds, S. K. (2005). Validation of the UPPS impulsive behavior scale: A four-factor model of impulsivity. *European Journal of Personality, 19,* 559–574.

Widiger, T. A., & Trull, T. J. (1993). Borderline and narcissistic personality disorders. In H. Adams & P. Sutker (Eds.), *Comprehensive handbook of psychopathology* (2nd ed., pp. 371–394). New York: Plenum Press.

Wilens, T. E., Faraone, S. V., & Biederman, J. (2004). Attention-deficit/hyperactivity disorder in adults. *Journal of the American Medical Association, 292,* 619–623.

Wingenfeld, K., Mensebach, C., Rullkoetter, N., Schlosser, N., Schaffrath, C., Woermann, F. G., et al. (2009). Relevant words in borderline personality disorder is strongly related to comorbid posttraumatic personality disorder. *Journal of Personality, 23,* 141–155.

Wingenfeld, K., Rullkoetter, N., Mensebach,

C., Beblo, T., Mertens, M., Kreisel, S., et al. (2009). Neural correlates of the individual emotional Stroop in borderline personality disorder. *Psychoneuroendocrinology, 34,* 571–586.

Zanarini, M. C., Frankenburg, F. R., Reich, D. B., Fitzmaurice, G., Weinberg, I., & Gunderson, J. G. (2008). The 10-year course of physically self-destructive acts reported by borderline patients and Axis II comparison subjects. *Acta Psychiatrica Scandinavica, 117,* 177–184.

Zautra, A. J., Davis, M. C., Reich, J. W., Nicassio, P., Tennen, H., Finan, P., et al. (2008). Comparison of cognitive behavior and mindfulness meditation interventions on adaptation to rheumatoid arthritis for patients with and without history of recurrent depression. *Journal of Clinical and Consulting Psychology, 76,* 408–421.

CHAPTER 26

Emotion, Motivation, and Cognition in Bipolar Spectrum Disorders

A Behavioral Approach System Perspective

Lauren B. Alloy, Ashleigh R. Molz, Olga V. Obraztsova,
Benjamin G. Shapero, Abigail L. Jenkins, Shimrit K. Black,
Kim E. Goldstein, Denise R. LaBelle, Elaine M. Boland,
and Lyn Y. Abramson

Bipolar disorder is a disorder of mood dysregulation involving extreme contrasts in mood, motivation, cognition, and behavior that occur within the same individual. At times, individuals with bipolar disorder exhibit hypomania or mania involving euphoric mood, excessive goal striving, supercharged energy, racing thoughts, decreased need for sleep, and overconfident cognition. However, at other times, they become depressed and feel sad, unmotivated, lethargic, hopeless, and have low self-esteem. Within the bipolar category, a group of disorders appears to form a spectrum of severity (see Figure 26.1) from the milder cyclothymic disorder, to bipolar II disorder, to full-blown bipolar I disorder at the most severe end of the continuum (e.g., Akiskal, Djenderedjian, Rosenthal, & Khani, 1977; Alloy, Urosevic, et al., 2012; Birmaher et al., 2009; Cassano et al., 1999; Goodwin & Jamison, 2007). Moreover, milder forms of bipolar disorder sometimes progress to the more severe forms (e.g., Akiskal et al., 1977; Alloy, Urosevic, et al., 2012; Birmaher et al., 2009; Kochman et al., 2005). Approximately 4.4% of the U.S. population exhibits a disorder in the bipolar spectrum (Merikangas et al., 2007), and these disorders are often associated with severe personal, social, and economic costs. For example, individuals with bipolar spectrum disorders experience divorce, substance abuse, suicide, and impairment in academic and occupational functioning at high rates (e.g., Angst, Stassen, Clayton, & Angst, 2002; Conway, Compton, Stinson, & Grant, 2006; Judd et al., 2008; Nusslock, Alloy, Abramson, Harmon-Jones, & Hogan, 2008). On the other hand, some individuals with bipolar spectrum disorders experience a more benign course and are high achievers (Johnson, 2005).

In this chapter, we attempt to understand bipolar spectrum disorders from the perspective of a behavioral approach system (BAS) hypersensitivity model. First, we present the BAS hypersensitivity model of bipolar disorder and consider its role in the onset and course of bipolar spectrum disorders. Then, in the sections that follow, we review findings on the cognitive and motivational styles of individuals with bipolar disorders; the role of life events in triggering bipolar symptoms and mood episodes; emotion pro-

SEVERITY

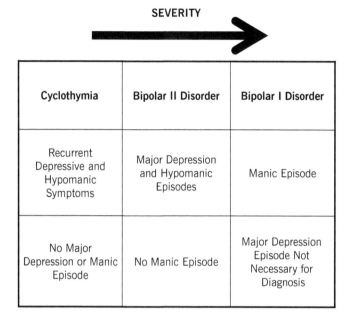

Cyclothymia	Bipolar II Disorder	Bipolar I Disorder
Recurrent Depressive and Hypomanic Symptoms	Major Depression and Hypomanic Episodes	Manic Episode
No Major Depression or Manic Episode	No Manic Episode	Major Depression Episode Not Necessary for Diagnosis

FIGURE 26.1. Spectrum of bipolar disorders. The disorders in the spectrum are more severe as one moves from left to right.

cessing and emotion regulation strategies associated with bipolar disorders; the neurobiological substrates of the cognitive, motivational, and emotional dysregulation in bipolar disorders; and cognitive-behavioral treatment approaches for these disorders. In each of these sections we integrate the findings with the BAS hypersensitivity model of bipolar spectrum disorders.

BAS Hypersensitivity Model of Bipolar Spectrum Disorders

What explains the highs and lows of mood, confidence, energy, and motivation observed in individuals with bipolar disorders? A BAS hypersensitivity model of bipolar spectrum disorders may provide an overarching, explanatory model for integrating cognitive, emotional, motivational, stress, and neural processes involved in the onset and course of bipolar spectrum disorders. As described in greater detail in Chapter 18 of this volume (Harmon-Jones, Price, Peterson, Gable, & Harmon-Jones), the BAS is a biobehavioral system that regulates approach motivation and goal-directed behavior to attain rewards and actively avoid punishments

(e.g., Gray, 1994). It is activated by goal- or reward-relevant stimuli, which can be either internal (expectancies of goal attainment) or external (presence of a desired goal). BAS activation has been associated with increased incentive motivation, reward sensitivity, motor behavior, and positive goal-striving emotions such as hope and happiness (e.g., Depue & Collins, 1999; Gray, 1994), as well as with anger when goal striving is frustrated or blocked (Carver, 2004; Harmon-Jones & Allen, 1998; Harmon-Jones & Sigelman, 2001). The BAS has also been linked with a reward-sensitive neural network involving dopaminergic neurons that project between several emotion- and reward-relevant brain structures in the limbic and frontal cortical systems (Depue & Iacono, 1989).

Depue and colleagues (Depue & Iacono, 1989; Depue, Krauss, & Spoont, 1987) proposed a BAS hypersensitivity model of bipolar spectrum disorders that has been expanded and updated recently (Alloy & Abramson, 2010; Alloy, Abramson, Urosevic, Bender, & Wagner, 2009; Johnson, 2005; Urosevic, Abramson, Harmon-Jones, & Alloy, 2008). This model provides a single theme—approach motivation/reward sensitivity—within which to organize a diverse array of symptoms and account for both poles of bipolar disorder. According to this model, an overly sensitive BAS that is hyperreactive to goal- and reward-relevant cues is the vulnerability for bipolar spectrum disorders (see Figure 26.2). BAS hypersensitivity can lead to excessive BAS activation in response to events involving rewards or goal striving and attainment. In turn, this excessive activation is hypothesized to lead to (hypo)manic symptoms, such as excessive goal-directed behavior, increased energy, decreased need for sleep, optimism, grandiosity, and euphoria (or irritability if the BAS activation-triggering event involves goal frustrations or obstacles). BAS hypersensitivity can also lead to excessive BAS deactivation or shutdown of behavioral approach/ engagement in response to events involving definite failures, losses, or nonattainment of goals. In turn, this excessive deactivation

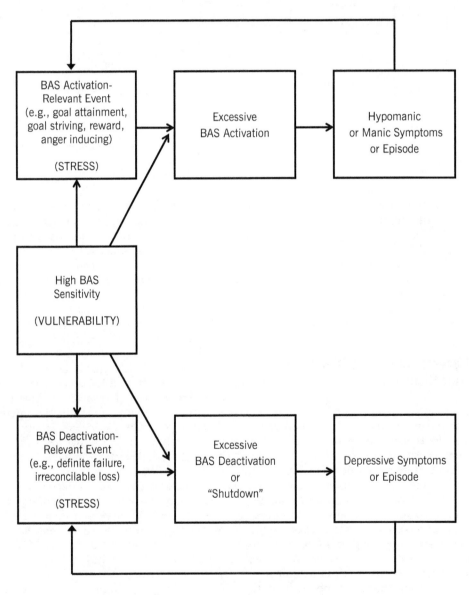

FIGURE 26.2. BAS hypersensitivity model of bipolar disorder.

is hypothesized to lead to depressive symptoms, such as decreased goal-directed activity, decreased energy, loss of interest and anhedonia, hopelessness, and sadness.

In sum, according to the BAS hypersensitivity model, individuals with or vulnerable to bipolar spectrum disorders have a single vulnerability, a hypersensitive BAS, but polarity-specific BAS-relevant triggers for (hypo)manic and depressive episodes (e.g., Alloy, Abramson, Urosevic, et al., 2009; Urosevic et al., 2008). Moreover, among bipolar spectrum individuals, those with the highest BAS/reward sensitivity may be most likely to develop a bipolar disorder at the severe end of the spectrum (e.g., bipolar I), as found by Alloy, Urosevic, and colleagues (2012). Little is known about the exact nature of the dysregulation associated with BAS hypersensitivity, but Urosevic and colleagues (2008) hypothesized that BAS hypersensitivity may lead to a greater reactivity to BAS-relevant events, a faster rise in BAS activation or deactivation in response to BAS-relevant events, and a slower recovery of BAS activation or deactivation back to baseline. And, indeed, Wright, Lam, and Brown (2008) reported that a greater number of previous mood episodes predicted a slower time to recover BAS activity back to baseline from rewards or frustrations in euthymic bipolar I patients compared to controls.

It is important to emphasize that the hypothesized vulnerability to bipolar disorders in this model is a tendency (i.e., a propensity) toward excessive BAS activation and deactivation, not the actual activation or deactivation itself, which is considered the more proximal precursor of mood symptoms and episodes. This overly sensitive BAS (vulnerability) may combine with the experience of BAS-activating or BAS-deactivating life events (the stress) to lead to excessive activation or deactivation of approach motivation, respectively, and, in turn, (hypo)manic or depressive symptoms or episodes. Consequently, high BAS sensitivity is hypothesized to provide vulnerability both to initial onset and to a more severe course of bipolar spectrum disorders, as well as to recurrences of mood symptoms and episodes.

A growing body of evidence supports the BAS hypersensitivity model of bipolar spectrum disorders. Individuals with disorders in the bipolar spectrum or at risk for bipolar disorder by virtue of exhibiting a hypomanic personality exhibit significantly higher levels of self-reported BAS sensitivity, as well as greater responsiveness to rewards on behavioral tasks, than do individuals without mood disorders or hypomanic personality, even controlling for concurrent (hypo)manic and depressive symptoms (Alloy et al., 2008; Carver & Johnson, 2009; Hayden et al., 2008; Meyer, Johnson, & Carver, 1999; Meyer, Johnson, & Winters, 2001; Salavert et al., 2007). Studies of individuals with bipolar disorder in remitted or euthymic states are of special interest because they assess BAS sensitivity or reward responsiveness independent of any mood state-related biases. Euthymic patients with bipolar I disorder exhibit higher self-reported BAS sensitivity (Salavert et al., 2007) and greater reward responsiveness on a behavioral task (Hayden et al., 2008) than healthy controls. In addition, BAS sensitivity remains stable across fluctuations in clinical symptoms (Meyer et al., 2001). Finally, Alloy and colleagues (2006) selected 18- to 24-year-old participants with high versus moderate levels of BAS sensitivity on two different self-report measures (Carver & White, 1994; Torrubia, Avila, Molto, & Caseras, 2001) and compared the two groups on lifetime history of mood disorders, current symptoms, and personality, blind to their BAS scores. Individuals with high BAS sensitivity were 6 times more likely to meet diagnostic criteria for a lifetime bipolar spectrum disorder (50%) than those with moderate BAS sensitivity (8.3%), and they also scored higher on measures of hypomanic symptoms and personality. Of course, the causal direction of the association between high BAS sensitivity and increased lifetime bipolar disorders in this retrospective study is unclear.

BAS Sensitivity and the Onset and Course of Bipolar Spectrum Disorders

Several longitudinal studies have examined whether BAS sensitivity and associated traits such as goal striving and reward responsiveness predict the onset and course of bipolar spectrum disorders, as hypothesized by the BAS hypersensitivity model. We review these findings next.

Initial Onset of Bipolar Spectrum Disorders

Although there has been increased recognition of bipolar disorders in prepubertal children (see Youngstrom, Birmaher, & Findling, 2008, for a review), the initial onset of the adult form of bipolar disorder usually occurs in adolescence, between ages 15–19 (for a review, see Alloy, Bender, et al., 2012). Employing a prospective version of the behavioral high-risk design, Alloy, Bender, and colleagues (2012) selected 14- to 19-year-old adolescents with high versus moderate levels of BAS sensitivity, based on two self-report measures (Carver & White, 1994; Torrubia et al., 2001), who had no prior history of a bipolar spectrum disorder, and followed them prospectively. Participants also completed measures of ambitious goal striving (Johnson & Carver, 2006) and behavioral reward responsiveness (Al-Adawi, Powell, & Greenwood, 1998) at baseline. Controlling for length of follow-up, initial (hypo)manic and depressive symptoms, and family history of bipolar disorder, Alloy, Bender, and colleagues found that the high-BAS sensitivity group was significantly more likely, and had a shorter time, to develop a first onset of a bipolar spectrum disorder than the moderate BAS sensitivity group. In addition, higher reward responsiveness on a behavioral task and more ambitious goal striving for popular fame and financial success also predicted a shorter time to first onset of a bipolar spectrum disorder, with ambitious goal setting partially mediating the BAS risk group effect.

Course of Bipolar Spectrum Disorders

Prodromes

Prodromes are the early signs and symptoms that precede the acute clinical phase of an illness and represent the earliest course of a disorder. Studies indicate that the most frequently reported prodromal signs of an impending manic episode are decreased sleep and increased goal-directed activity (Lam & Wong, 1997; Lam, Wong, & Sham, 2001; Lam et al., 2003; Wong & Lam, 1999), and individuals who respond to a manic prodrome by actively decreasing their goal-directed activity are less likely to have a manic relapse than those who do not cope in this way (Lam et al., 2001, 2003). Conversely, decreased goal-directed activity, decreased energy, and decreased pleasure are some of the most commonly reported prodromal symptoms of an impending bipolar depressive episode (e.g., Lam & Wong, 1997; Molnar, Feeney, & Fava, 1988; Smith & Tarrier, 1992; Wong & Lam, 1999), and individuals who respond to a depressive prodrome by increasing their goal-directed activity are less likely to experience depressive relapses over follow-up (Lam et al., 2001). The finding that increased and decreased goal-directed activity are immediate harbingers of manic and depressive episodes, respectively, is consistent with the BAS hypersensitivity model of bipolar disorders.

Relapse, Recurrence, and Progression along the Bipolar Spectrum

Several longitudinal studies have examined BAS sensitivity as a predictor of relapses or recurrences of mood episodes in individuals with bipolar spectrum disorders. Meyer and colleagues (2001) found that bipolar I patients' self-reported BAS sensitivity at recovery predicted greater manic symptoms over follow-up. Similarly, controlling for initial manic and depressive symptoms, Salavert and colleagues (2007) reported that over 18 months of follow-up, bipolar I patients who relapsed with a hypomanic or manic episode had higher, and those who relapsed with a depressive episode had lower, BAS sensitivity at baseline than patients who remained asymptomatic. Similarly, controlling for baseline hypomanic and depressive symptoms, Alloy and colleagues (2008) found that over a 3-year follow-up, higher baseline self-reported BAS sensitivity predicted a shorter time to relapse with hypomanic or manic episodes among individuals with bipolar II disorder or cyclothymia. In addition, higher self-reported reward responsiveness showed a trend to predict shorter time to relapse with a major depressive episode.

Milder disorders in the bipolar spectrum sometimes worsen and progress to more severe diagnoses over time. Alloy, Urosevic, and colleagues (2012) found that controlling for length of follow-up, initial hypomanic and depressive symptoms, and treatment seeking, higher baseline BAS sensitivity (particularly the Fun-Seeking subscale) predicted a greater likelihood of conversion to bipolar II disorder among individuals with initial cyclothymia or bipolar disorder not otherwise specified (BiNOS), and a greater likelihood of conversion to bipolar I disorder among individuals with initial bipolar II disorder, cyclothymia, or BiNOS.

Impairment versus Success

Paradoxically, bipolar disorder has been associated both with academic/occupational impairment and substance abuse as well as with high levels of achievement and accomplishment (Johnson, 2005). Theoretically, high BAS sensitivity is associated both with excessive reward seeking that could lead to substance abuse and engagement in risky activities that may result in impairment, as well as with high goal striving that could lead to achievement. Thus, other factors may combine with high BAS sensitivity to determine whether impairment or accomplishment predominates in the course of an individual's bipolar disorder.

Impulsivity, defined as rash, unplanned behavior without reflection, is elevated in bipolar disorder and stable across mood episodes (Swann, Dougherty, Pazzaglia, Pham, & Moeller, 2004) and may be relevant to predicting impairment versus success in individuals with bipolar disorders. In factor analyses, measures of rash impulsivity load on a separate factor from measures of BAS and reward sensitivity, although the two factors are correlated (see Alloy, Bender, et al., 2009, for a review). High impulsivity and high BAS sensitivity both predicted conversion to bipolar I disorder among participants with bipolar II, cyclothymia, or BiNOS in the Alloy, Urosevic, and colleagues (2012) study. In addition, Alloy, Bender, and colleagues (2009) found that both high BAS sensitivity and high impulsivity predicted substance abuse problems over longitudinal follow-up in individuals with bipolar spectrum disorders, and impulsivity completely mediated the comorbidity between bipolar disorder and prospective substance abuse in the sample. In a study of academic achieve-

ment, Nusslock and colleagues (2008) found that, overall, undergraduates with bipolar spectrum disorders had worse grade point averages (GPAs), more dropped classes, and were more likely to withdraw from college than healthy controls. However, those bipolar participants who were high in BAS sensitivity but low in impulsivity had significantly higher GPAs than those with high BAS sensitivity and high impulsivity or those with low BAS sensitivity, regardless of impulsivity levels. In other words, when combined with low impulsivity, high BAS sensitivity was associated with higher academic achievement. Thus, high BAS sensitivity may be more likely to lead to a negative course of bipolar disorder when it is combined with high impulsivity.

BAS-Relevant Cognitive and Motivational Styles and Bipolar Spectrum Disorders

Given the empirical support for BAS hypersensitivity as a predictor of symptoms and mood episodes, initial onset, and course of bipolar spectrum disorders, it becomes relevant to better understand the cognitive and motivational characteristics of individuals with bipolar disorders and/or high BAS sensitivity. According to the BAS theory, certain types of cognitive and motivational styles may be associated with high BAS sensitivity. For instance, from a BAS perspective, individuals with bipolar spectrum disorders should exhibit cognitive styles related to the themes of high drive/incentive motivation and goal attainment that are associated with BAS hypersensitivity. Cognitive styles involving high incentive motivation would include ambitious goal-setting, perfectionism (e.g., "a person should do well at everything") and self-criticism when high goals are not met. Moreover, Alloy, Abramson, Walshaw, and colleagues (2009) demonstrated that these BAS-relevant cognitive styles did, in fact, correlate with high BAS sensitivity.

Consistent with this hypothesis, individuals with and at risk for bipolar spectrum disorders specifically have been found to exhibit such BAS-relevant cognitive styles. For example, individuals with bipolar disorder have cognitive styles focused on performance evaluation (Rosenfarb, Becker, Khan, & Mintz, 1988; Scott, Stanton, Garland, &

Ferrier, 2000). This concern with performance has generally been studied by examining an individual's tendency to be self-critical and perfectionistic. Perfectionism is characterized by a predisposition toward flawlessness or an idealized goal and people who have high levels of perfectionism tend to have high expectations for themselves. Self-criticism is closely related to perfectionism; if perfectionistic individuals fail to meet their own expectations, they are more likely to evaluate themselves harshly. Research suggests that individuals with bipolar spectrum disorders exhibit more perfectionism and a higher need to achieve compared to healthy controls (Alloy, Abramson, Walshaw, et al., 2009; Goldberg, Gerstein, Wenze, Welker, & Beck, 2008; Lam, Wright, & Smith, 2004; Scott et al., 2000). In addition, studies have found higher levels of self-criticism in individuals with bipolar spectrum disorders compared to healthy controls (Alloy, Abramson, Walshaw, et al., 2009; Rosenfarb et al., 1988) and that self-critical styles prospectively predict a greater likelihood of a (hypo)manic episode (Alloy, Abramson, Walshaw, et al., 2009). Moreover, cognitive styles characterized by perfectionism and self-criticism have been found to be significantly associated with high self-reported BAS sensitivity (Alloy, Abramson, Walshaw, et al., 2009). Consequently, in a study that examined individuals vulnerable to developing bipolar spectrum disorders by virtue of their BAS hypersensitivity, individuals with high BAS sensitivity also had significantly higher levels of perfectionism and self-criticism (Stange et al., 2013) than those with moderate BAS sensitivity, indicating that these BAS-related cognitive styles may contribute to the development of a bipolar disorder.

In addition, individuals with bipolar spectrum disorders have been observed to exhibit styles of overly ambitious goal striving and excessive sensitivity to rewards compared with controls, consistent with the BAS hypersensitivity model and Johnson's (2005) related goal dysregulation theory (Alloy, Abramson, Walshaw, et al., 2009; Carver & Johnson, 2009; Eisner, Johnson, & Carver, 2008; Gruber & Johnson, 2009; Johnson & Carver, 2006; Johnson & Jones, 2009; Johnson, Ruggero, & Carver, 2005; Meyer

& Krumm-Merabet, 2003). For example, individuals with or vulnerable to bipolar disorder set goals of fame, wealth, and power for themselves that are very difficult to attain (e.g., having a major role in a movie, earning $20 million, or becoming president of the United States; Carver & Johnson, 2009; Gruber & Johnson, 2009; Johnson & Carver, 2006; Johnson, Eisner, & Carver, 2009). They also have high expectations for long-term academic and occupational success (Meyer & Krumm-Merabet, 2003). Individuals with bipolar disorders are also less likely than controls to decrease their goal-striving efforts after unexpectedly high progress toward a goal (Fulford, Johnson, Llabre, & Carver, 2010). Such cognitive–motivational styles have been related to prospective increases in manic symptoms among individuals with bipolar disorder. Lozano and Johnson (2001) reported that high achievement-striving styles predicted increases in manic symptoms in bipolar I patients over a 6-month follow-up. Theoretically, BAS hypersensitivity should lead to such ambitious goal striving, and consistent with this view, Alloy, Bender, and colleagues (2012) found that ambitious goal-setting mediated the prospective relationship between high BAS sensitivity and first onset of bipolar spectrum disorder.

Even after achieving a success, individuals with bipolar disorders exhibit greater emotional and cognitive responsiveness to rewards than controls (Eisner et al., 2008; Hayden et al., 2008; Johnson et al., 2005). That is, they exhibit greater positive emotion, confidence, and further increases in goal striving following small initial successes, and they overgeneralize from a particular success to broader aspects of their lives (Eisner et al., 2008). They are also more likely to endorse overly optimistic views of the future when something positive happens in their lives (Johnson & Jones, 2009; also Stange et al., 2013). In addition, positive overgeneralization from success has been found to be associated with risk for mania (Eisner et al., 2008).

In sum, BAS sensitivity has been significantly associated with several BAS-relevant cognitive–motivational styles in individuals with bipolar disorders (Alloy, Abramson, Walshaw, et al., 2009) and those at risk for bipolar disorder (Stange et al., 2013). Importantly, because BAS hypersensitivity has been shown to be a specific risk factor for bipolar disorder, it would be expected that individuals with bipolar spectrum disorders would not show differences in non-BAS-relevant cognitive styles. Consistent with this hypothesis, research supports the specificity of BAS-relevant cognitive styles to bipolar disorder and has shown that individuals with bipolar disorder do not differ from healthy controls on other types of maladaptive cognitive styles (e.g., approval seeking, dependency) characteristic of unipolar depression (Alloy, Abramson, Walshaw, et al., 2009).

BAS-Relevant Life Events and Bipolar Spectrum Disorders

Evidence suggests that environmental factors also play an important role in the onset and course of bipolar disorder, triggering bipolar mood episodes and symptoms (Alloy et al., 2005). More specifically, recent reviews (e.g., Alloy et al., 2005; Johnson, 2005) indicate that both negative and positive life events trigger (hypo)mania in bipolar spectrum individuals, whereas only negative life events precipitate bipolar depression. Several prospective studies of bipolar spectrum samples have examined the association between life events and bipolar mood episodes. Findings from these studies support a relationship between increased stress/negative life events and higher relapse rates across 6-month (Hammen & Gitlin, 1997) and 2-year follow-ups (Ellicott, Hammen, Gitlin, Brown & Jamison, 1990). Hunt, Bruce-Jones, and Silverstone (1992) found similar evidence for increased relapse rates in bipolar spectrum individuals following a month in which a severe life event took place. In addition, one prospective study found that when bipolar spectrum individuals experience negative life events concurrent with a mood episode, episode duration is significantly prolonged (Johnson & Miller, 1997). Of note, there have been a few studies that have not supported the predictive relationship between negative or positive life events and bipolar mood episode relapse (e.g., McPherson, Herbinson, & Romans, 1993; Pardoen et al., 1996).

According to the BAS hypersensitivity model of bipolar disorder, specific types of life events are hypothesized to trigger the onset of initial and recurring bipolar mood episodes and symptoms. In response to BAS activation-relevant events such as goal striving/attainment events and anger provocation events (e.g., goal obstacles or insults), individuals with a hypersensitive BAS are thought to respond with (hypo)manic symptoms and/or episodes. In comparison, the BAS model postulates that bipolar depressive episodes are precipitated by BAS-deactivating events such as irreconcilable failures and losses (Depue & Iacono, 1989; Urosevic et al., 2008).

Consistent with the BAS hypersensitivity model, several studies have found that the occurrence of goal striving/attainment events predict an increase in (hypo)manic symptoms and episodes over a range of follow-ups (e.g., Johnson, Cueller, et al., 2008; Nusslock, Abramson, Harmon-Jones, Alloy, & Hogan, 2007). For example, in their two relevant studies, Johnson and colleagues (2000; Johnson, Cueller, et al., 2008) found that goal attainment events predicted increases in manic, but not depressive, symptoms in a sample of individuals with bipolar I disorder. They reported that this relationship did not hold true for positive life events in general, but was specific to the BAS activation events. Similarly, Nusslock and colleagues (2007) found that students with bipolar II disorder or cyclothymia who were engaged in a goal-striving event (studying for and taking final exams) were significantly more likely to develop a new hypomanic episode (42%), but not depression, compared to other bipolar students who did not take final exams (4%). Alloy, Abramson, Urosevic, and colleagues (2009) reported that in individuals in the bipolar spectrum, BAS activation events prospectively predicted increases in hypomanic symptoms, whereas BAS deactivation events predicted depressive symptoms over a 1-year follow-up. Finally, BAS-activating anger-inducing events also have been linked to increased hypomanic symptoms (Carver, 2004; Harmon-Jones et al., 2002); however, prospective longitudinal studies have yet to examine the relationship between anger-provoking events and (hypo)manic episodes in bipolar spectrum individuals.

BAS-Relevant Cognitive Vulnerability–Stress Interaction

As previously discussed, several BAS-relevant cognitive styles, such as perfectionism, high goal striving, and high self-criticism, have been identified as vulnerabilities for bipolar mood episodes. More recently, researchers have examined how these BAS-relevant cognitive styles may interact with the occurrence of life events to predict the onset of bipolar mood episodes. Specifically, controlling for initial symptoms and the total number of events experienced, Francis-Raniere, Alloy, and Abramson (2006) found that among individuals with bipolar spectrum disorders, BAS-relevant cognitive styles such as self-criticism and perfectionism interacted with positive and negative life events congruent with those styles to prospectively predict increases in hypomanic and depressive symptoms, respectively.

Stress Generation in Bipolar Spectrum Disorders

An important component of the BAS hypersensitivity model of bipolar disorders, as elucidated by Urosevic and colleagues (2008), and in line with Hammen's (1991) stress generation model, is the transactional, bidirectional influences between BAS-related life events and bipolar mood symptoms. In one study, Urosevic and colleagues (2010) found that in comparison to healthy controls, individuals with bipolar spectrum disorders reported significantly higher rates of BAS-activating and -deactivating life events over follow-up. Given that the rates of BAS-activating and -deactivating events were significantly correlated with each other in the sample, the same bipolar individuals were experiencing high rates of both types of BAS-relevant events. These findings suggest that individuals with bipolar spectrum disorders may actually experience more BAS-activating and -deactivating events through processes of stress generation, which, in turn, can trigger onsets of additional (hypo) manic and depressive symptoms and episodes. Thus, bipolar individuals may both generate, and react more strongly to, BAS-relevant events in a "two-hit" model of vulnerability to bipolar mood dysregulation.

Emotional Dysfunction and Mood Regulation Strategies in Bipolar Spectrum Disorders

Emotion and Reward Processing in Bipolar Disorder

Many lines of research have revealed impairments in various emotional skills in bipolar disorder. For example, several studies of facial emotion recognition have indicated that individuals with bipolar disorder tend to have difficulty identifying and categorizing images of emotional facial expressions (Bozikas, Tonia, Fokas, Karavatos, & Kosmidis, 2006; Getz, Shear, Strakowski, 2003; Summers, Papadopoulou, Bruno, Cipolotti, & Ron, 2006). Other studies have found that individuals with bipolar disorder have difficulty recalling negative memories and a poorer ability to process negative interpersonal cues during positive mood states (Eich, Macaulay, & Lam, 1997; Lembke & Ketter, 2002). Furthermore, research suggests that compared to low-risk individuals, those at increased risk for bipolar disorder display more robust startle eyeblink attenuation and heightened cardiac vagal tone (both correlates of positive emotion) in response to positively valenced stimuli (Gruber, Johnson, Oveis, & Keltner, 2008; Sutton & Johnson, 2002).

Of particular relevance to the BAS hypersensitivity model of bipolar disorder, several studies have revealed impairments in emotional reward processing in bipolar disorder (see Suri, Sheppes, & Gross, Chapter 11, this volume, for a discussion of emotion regulation and cognition). For example, Johnson and colleagues (2005) showed that individuals at risk for mania show higher positive affect and self-confidence in response to false success feedback in comparison to controls. In addition, Hayden and colleagues (2008) reported that euthymic individuals with bipolar disorder exhibit greater responsiveness to rewards on a behavioral task involving monetary incentives than do healthy controls. Pizzagalli, Goetz, Ostacher, Iosifescu, and Perlis (2008) found that individuals with bipolar disorder, even when euthymic, exhibited dysfunctional reward learning in a probabilistic reward task requiring integration of reward information over time, because they showed hypersensitivity to single rewards on the task.

Bipolar disorder is unique from other forms of psychopathology in that euphoric mania is the only psychopathological state characterized by a positively valenced, high-arousal emotional state. Inasmuch as positive emotions are generally associated with positive outcomes (e.g., Fredrickson, 1998), the role of positive emotion in psychopathology is less understood. Previous studies suggest that abnormalities in positive emotion may be associated with an increased risk for mania (Carver & Johnson, 2009). Converging research suggests that individuals with bipolar disorder display elevated levels of positive emotion not only in the context of reward (Meyer et al., 2001; Johnson et al., 2005), but across a wide range of contexts and emotional stimuli (Hofmann & Meyer, 2006). Interestingly, and consistent with the BAS hypersensitivity model of bipolar disorder, individuals at high risk for mania show elevated levels of positive emotions typically associated with reward and achievement, such as joy and happiness, but not other non-BAS-related positive emotions (Gruber et al., 2008; Gruber & Johnson, 2009).

Mood Regulation Strategies in Bipolar Disorder

The strategies that individuals use to attempt to regulate their mood states may play a role in aberrant emotional processes in bipolar disorder. One emotion regulation strategy that may contribute to these difficulties with emotional processing is rumination on both positive and negative affect. Rumination can be defined as perseverative attention on an affective state (see Watkins, Chapter 21, this volume, for detailed analysis of rumination). Research in this area emerged from Nolen-Hoeksema's response styles theory (1991), which suggests that individuals use a variety of functional and dysfunctional strategies to regulate their emotions, especially feelings of sadness. A ruminative response style to sad mood is characterized by passive thinking about the causes and consequences of one's depressive symptoms (Nolen-Hoeksema, 1991). Rumination on negative affect is a central feature of unipolar depression, and given that a significant proportion of individuals with bipolar disorder also experience depressive episodes, it is not surprising that heightened levels of rumination on sad affect are also prevalent in bipolar disorder (Alloy, Abramson, Flynn, et al., 2009; Knowles, Tai, Christensen, & Bentall, 2005; Thomas & Bentall, 2002). Moreover, rumination predicted the subsequent onset of depressive episodes among individuals with bipolar spectrum disorders (Alloy, Abramson, Flynn, et al., 2009).

A unique feature of bipolar disorder is that in addition to heightened levels of rumination on negative affect, bipolar individuals also exhibit elevated levels of rumination on positive affect in comparison to controls or people with major depressive disorder (Johnson, McKenzie, & McMurrich, 2008). In addition, individuals vulnerable to mania by virtue of exhibiting a hypomanic personality (Feldman, Joormann, & Johnson, 2008) or by virtue of exhibiting high BAS sensitivity (Stange et al., 2013) also show higher rumination on positive affect than individuals lower in hypomanic personality or BAS sensitivity. Furthermore, it has been shown that the use of positive rumination is associated with a more severe course of bipolar disorder characterized by more frequent manic episodes (Gruber, Eidelman, Johnson, Smith, & Harvey, 2012). Individuals may be especially prone to use positive rumination as an emotion regulation strategy in order to bolster self-esteem and confidence when approaching new challenges. Positive rumination may serve to increase positive affect by focusing attention on one's positive self-qualities, positive affective experience, and favorable life circumstances (Feldman et al., 2008; Martin & Tesser, 1996).

Another emotion regulation strategy associated with positive affect in individuals with bipolar disorder is dampening. Unlike rumination on positive affect, which seeks to increase or maintain positive mood, the goal of dampening is to decrease the duration or intensity of positive affect (Feldman et al., 2008). Levels of dampening in response to positive affect are higher in individuals both at risk for, and with a history of, manic episodes (Feldman et al., 2008; Gruber et al., 2012; Johnson & Jones, 2009). Although it may appear counterintuitive that bipolar individuals would want to both increase and decrease their positive affect, it has been suggested that individuals may be capable of engaging in either strategy in response to positive mood, and it is likely that they choose their response based on their interpretation of the event (Mansell, Morrison, Reid, Lowens, & Tai, 2007). Individuals also may choose to dampen their positive affect as a way to maintain control of their mood and attempt to prevent a full-blown manic episode, as discussed in the section on prodromes of bipolar disorder, above (Lam et al., 2001).

The reviewed literature suggests that individuals with bipolar disorder engage in a variety of emotion regulation strategies. An unanswered question remains as to whether this variety is due to some underlying emotion regulation deficit in bipolar disorder or because bipolar individuals are forced to broaden their repertoire of emotion regulation strategies in order to deal with the array of intense mood states associated with the disorder.

Neurobiological Substrates of BAS Dysregulation in Bipolar Spectrum Disorders

Electroencephalogram and Neuroimaging Findings

There are several brain regions involved in a reward-sensitive neural network that are thought to be associated with BAS dysregulation. Specifically, research suggests that extreme fluctuations in the activation and deactivation of the BAS in individuals with bipolar disorder may be linked with abnormalities of frontal cortical areas, including dorsolateral prefrontal cortex (DLPFC), anterior cingulate cortex (ACC), orbitofrontal cortex (OFC), and dorsomedial prefrontal cortex (Depue & Iacono, 1989). Furthermore, it has been proposed that other brain regions involved in the reward system may also play a role in BAS dysregulation (e.g., ventral tegmental area, amygdala, nucleus accumbens, ventral pallidum, septum, and hippocampus; Urosevic et al., 2008). Nonetheless, most of the literature relates left frontal activity to BAS activation and, as such, implicates abnormal functioning of left frontal regions in BAS dysregulation

problems experienced by individuals with bipolar disorder.

For example, much research in humans has focused on left frontal cortical activity as a neurobiological index of the BAS (Coan & Allen, 2004; Urosevic et al., 2008). Studies have observed an association between greater left frontal cortical activity, as measured by electroencephalogram (EEG), and high scores on self-report measures of BAS sensitivity (Harmon-Jones & Allen, 1997; Sutton & Davidson, 1997), as well as with experimentally manipulated reward motivational states (Miller & Tomarken, 2001; Sobotka, Davidson, & Senulis, 1992; see also Coan & Allen, 2004; Urosevic et al., 2008). A separate EEG study reported a relationship between greater activity within the left DLPFC and the medial OFC and a stronger response bias to reward-related cues (Pizzagalli, Sherwood, Henriques, & Davidson, 2005). With regard to neurobiological mechanisms underlying BAS dysregulation in bipolar disorder, EEG research has shown that individuals with bipolar spectrum disorders display greater relative left frontal cortical activation compared with healthy controls in preparation for solving difficult anagrams when they have the opportunity to obtain rewards (i.e., win money; Harmon-Jones et al., 2008). Similarly, in response to an anger-evoking event, Harmon-Jones and colleagues (2002) found that proneness to (hypo)mania was related to increased left frontal cortical activity, whereas proneness to depression was related to decreased left frontal cortical activity. This finding suggests that the tendency to respond to anger provocation with BAS activation and approach (proneness to hypomania) rather than with BAS deactivation and withdrawal (proneness to depression) is associated with greater relative left frontal cortical activity. Kano, Nakamura, Matsuoka, Iida, and Nakajima (1992) also reported greater relative left frontal EEG activity in individuals in a manic episode and greater relative right frontal activity in individuals in a major depressive episode. Importantly, Nusslock, Harmon-Jones, and colleagues (2012) found that greater left frontal cortical activity predicted a worse course of bipolar disorder. Individuals with cyclothymia or bipolar II disorder who progressed to developing bipolar I disorder over follow-up exhibited initially greater (relative) left frontal activation at rest than did individuals in the bipolar spectrum who did not progress to bipolar I.

Functional magnetic resonance imaging (fMRI) work conducted in individuals with bipolar disorder also implicates the left prefrontal cortex in BAS dysregulation. A recent study examining patients with mania on a monetary incentive delay task found stronger responses in the left lateral OFC during expectation of increasing gain and weaker responses in this region to increasing loss cues, as compared with controls (Bermpohl et al., 2010). Furthermore, a study investigating performance of patients with mania on a reward-based decision-making task found that the patients showed a task-related increase in activation of the left dorsal ACC but decreased activation in the frontal pole relative to controls (Rubinsztein et al., 2001). Controls, on the other hand, demonstrated significantly more task-related activation in the inferior frontal gyrus, compared with the patients with mania. Finally, in an fMRI study involving a card-guessing game for monetary wins and losses, Nusslock, Almeida, and colleagues (2012) found that relative to healthy controls, individuals with bipolar I disorder in a euthymic state showed elevated activity in brain regions implicated in the processing of rewards (ventral striatum and OFC) during anticipation of rewards, but not during anticipation of losses.

Some studies have identified that individuals with bipolar disorders demonstrate structural abnormalities of these same brain regions implicated in BAS dysregulation. For example, research reports volume reductions in the OFC (Lyoo, Hwang, Sim, Dunn, & Renshaw, 2006; Nugent et al., 2006), the DLPFC (Dickstein et al., 2005; Haznedar et al., 2005) and the anterior cingulate (Chiu et al., 2007). Although lateralization effects are more prominent in functional studies of the frontal cortex in bipolar disorder, some structural studies also have shown abnormalities restricted to the left hemisphere (Fountoulakis, Giannakopoulos, Kövari, & Bouras, 2008; Houenou et al., 2011). Moreover, lesions of brain structures implicated in the reward system (OFC, thalamus, caudate) in the right hemisphere have been associated with occurrence of secondary mania (Robinson, Boston, Starkstein, & Price, 1988),

presumably because of increased left frontal activation unregulated by the right hemisphere due to the lesions. Likewise, lesions of the left hemisphere near the frontal pole are associated with depressive symptoms (Narushima, Kosler, & Robinson, 2003; Robinson et al., 1988).

Dopaminergic Functioning

Dopamine (DA) has been implicated as a critical neurotransmitter in the underlying neuropathology of dysregulated reward systems and bipolar disorder. Amphetamine abuse, which increases dopamine availability within the synapse, is phenotypically similar to mania, in that it is characterized by higher levels of impulsive and risk-taking behavior, increased sexual activity and interest, faster speech and thinking, reduced need for sleep, expansivity, grandiosity, and euphoria (Cousins, Butts, & Young, 2009; Verhoeff et al., 2000). In contrast, experimental reduction in DA availability via artificial suppression of molecular precursors to DA also precipitates a depression-like state, in which the individual exhibits lowered mood, anhedonia, slowed thinking, and lethargy (Nutt et al., 2007). Additionally, pharmacotherapies for bipolar disorder have been shown to act on DA circuitry, and lithium, an indirect DA antagonist that has been used widely as a mood stabilizer in bipolar disorder, has also been shown to treat manic presentations of amphetamine abuse (Naranjo, Tremblay, Lescia, & Busto, 2001; Nutt, 2006).

Apart from evidence from pharmacotherapies and artificial behavioral analogues, there is also genetic and molecular evidence linking the altered cognitive and affective functioning observed in bipolar disorder to alterations in DA synthesis. Catechol-o-methyltransferase (COMT) is an enzyme responsible for the degradation of DA within synapses in the prefrontal cortex, and a genetic polymorphism in the allele responsible for its transcription has been associated with alterations in cognitive performance, affective responsivity, and also risk for developing bipolar disorder (Smolka et al., 2005). Similarly, polymorphisms in the DA transporter genes have also been found in individuals with alterations in reward sensitivity and bipolar disorders (Camara et al., 2010;

Missale, Nash, Robinson, Jaber, & Caron, 1998). Finally, a manic mood state has been associated with elevated levels of DA metabolites in cerebrospinal fluid, suggesting an excess of DA release within the brain during mania. This evidence supports a pharmacological model of mania and depression with DA as a central mediator.

Generally, evidence has shown that individuals with bipolar disorder evidence deficits in attention, memory, and some tasks of executive functioning mediated by DA. Individuals with bipolar disorder also perform more poorly on tasks that are highly complex or involve time constraints, such as tasks of verbal learning or fluency and processing speed (Bearden, Hoffman, & Cannon, 2001; Goodwin, Martinez-Aran, Glahn, & Vieta, 2008). Rather than a specific cognitive deficit, individuals with bipolar disorder may have a lowered "ceiling" of cognitive functioning, and thus, they will evidence impairments on tasks with higher cognitive loads regardless of their domain. Dopamine has been implicated in these processes in that it is one of the primary neurotransmitters (along with norepinephrine) responsible for the functioning of the DLPFC, a region that subserves these executive functions. Dopamine's ability to appropriately mediate cognitive function has an inverted U-shaped influence, in that too much or too little impairs cognition, whereas moderate amounts are necessary for optimal functioning (Gamo & Arnsten, 2011). The lowered threshold for maximum cognitive capability thus is consistent with a model of bipolar disorder in which DA responding is generally sensitized to stimulation, particularly reward. Further supporting the role of DA in the cognitive and affective presentation of bipolar disorder is the consistent finding of impaired attention in individuals with bipolar disorder (Goodwin et al., 2008). The regulation of attention is an executive function that is closely associated with DA function, and impoverished sustained and selective attention has been associated with hypodopaminergic activity. It is not surprising, then, that attention-deficit/hyperactivity disorder (ADHD) has been consistently associated with bipolar disorder, with some studies suggesting that ADHD in children may be a risk factor for bipolar disorder in adulthood, and others finding a high comorbidity between the two disorders in both children and adults (Bearden et al., 2001).

Alterations in DA-mediated reward pathways in bipolar disorder have also been noted, suggesting that DA dysfunction may be influential in the BAS hypersensitivity model of bipolar disorder (Abler, Greenhouse, Ongur, Walter, & Heckers, 2008; Berk et al., 2007). Consistent with the high rates of comorbidity with substance use disorders, individuals with bipolar disorder have evidenced decreased tonic and phasic DA signaling in reward pathways, much like those with sensation seeking and drug/alcohol abuse (Abler et al., 2008). This finding could be consistent with a BAS hypersensitivity model in which the individual at risk for bipolar disorder does not get the appropriate level of arousal and adaptive feedback to cease or modulate maladaptive goal-striving behaviors. A recent study of variations in the D2 dopamine receptors and COMT revealed that the interaction of the genotypes was associated with the Drive, Fun-Seeking, and total scores from Carver and White's measure of BAS sensitivity. Higher BAS scores were also associated with significantly lower prolactin levels, a known endocrine marker for elevated DA activity (Reuter, Schmitz, Corr, & Hennig, 2006). Alterations in DA functioning and the associated changes in cognition and emotion could thus represent a molecular correlate of the personality characteristics described by the BAS hypersensitivity model of bipolar disorder.

Cognitive-Behavioral Therapy for Bipolar Spectrum Disorders

Cognitive-behavioral therapy (CBT) is a well-documented and empirically supported treatment for unipolar depression (see Deckersbach, Gershuny, & Otto, 2000, for a thorough review) that has been extended to bipolar spectrum disorders as well. CBT centers on the overarching hypothesis that maladaptive cognitive patterns provide cognitive vulnerability to depression, which is then triggered by stressful life events. CBT targets these maladaptive thinking patterns in an effort to generate a less depressogenic information-processing scheme (Hollon, 2006; Nusslock, Abramson, Harmon-Jones, Alloy, & Coan, 2009). Recent research has suggested that maladaptive cognitive styles are also at work in bipolar spectrum disorders (Alloy et al., 2005). However, as discussed in the section on cognitive styles, above, among individuals with bipolar spectrum disorders, some unique cognitive patterns have been documented that fall directly in line with the high drive/incentive motivation associated with high BAS sensitivity.

Nusslock and colleagues (2009) conducted a thorough review of the implications of research on the cognitive profiles of individuals with bipolar disorder in line with the BAS hypersensitivity theory for the usefulness of CBT for bipolar disorder. The authors note that whereas traditional CBT for bipolar disorder typically targets state-dependent negative automatic thoughts and underlying state-independent dysfunctional schemas, there is a growing body of research suggesting that targeting the cognitive prodrome of bipolar disorder may be a more proactive strategy than merely addressing the automatic thoughts expressed during affective episodes (Lam et al., 2003). This approach would take advantage of the fact that the individual's coping strategies may not yet be overwhelmed by affective symptoms, thus allowing for the possibility of relapse prevention (Smith & Tarrier, 1992). As reviewed in the above section on prodromes, research has shown that the cognitive prodromes of manic episodes are characterized by the type of goal striving and heightened expectations of success that are consistent with the BAS hypersensitivity model (Nusslock et al., 2009). Research has also shown that increased goal-directed activity is one of the most common behavioral prodromes of mania and is a predictor of increased rates of manic episodes (Lam et al., 2001). CBT from a BAS model perspective would invite the individual to examine his or her ambitious goal striving and surge of self-confidence and reframe them as early warning signs of mania, rather than as thoughts to be considered independently of their disorder (Nusslock et al., 2009). With this technique, the individual would be better equipped to identify a manic prodrome from a mere good mood.

This same prodrome-focused approach can be directed to the red flags of low self-esteem and decreased goal striving that can occur following an achievement failure in the BAS hypersensitivity model (Johnson et al., 2005; Lam et al., 2000). Urosevic and colleagues (2008) suggest that low-efficacy expectancy, resulting from a failure in an achievement domain, can result in BAS deactivation. In this light, low self-esteem, feelings of low self-efficacy, and decreased goal-directed activity can be treated as depressive prodromes and focused on in much the same way as negative automatic thoughts or schemas. Focusing on acquainting the individual with his or her own personal BAS-relevant prodromes may aid in the prevention of depressive relapse. Moreover, behavioral activation strategies such as exercise, goal striving, and other pleasurable activities may help target BAS deactivation (Nusslock et al., 2009).

Conclusion

In this chapter we presented a BAS hypersensitivity model of bipolar disorder and reviewed evidence indicating that the model shows much promise in predicting the onset and course of bipolar spectrum disorders. In addition, our review suggested that individuals with bipolar spectrum disorders are characterized specifically by BAS-relevant cognitive and motivational styles involving perfectionism, self-criticism, overly ambitious goal striving, reward sensitivity, and positive overgeneralization from success. They also exhibit emotional processing dysfunctions, are emotionally hyperresponsive to rewards, and tend to engage in rumination on both positive and negative moods, prolonging and intensifying these mood states. Life events that are BAS-relevant specifically appear to trigger mood episodes and symptoms in individuals with bipolar spectrum disorders, consistent with the BAS hypersensitivity theory, and cognitive-behavioral therapeutic strategies that target dysregulated goal-directed behavior during prodromes of mood episodes may be efficacious in preventing relapse and a severe course of bipolar disorder. Finally, individuals with bipolar spectrum disorders appear to exhibit relatively greater left frontal cortical activation, a neurobiological index of BAS activity. They differ from controls on structural and functional imaging of brain areas involved in neural reward pathways, and they exhibit abnormalities in dopaminergic functioning, a neurotransmitter system also implicated in reward processing.

In sum, considerable evidence suggests that dysregulation of approach motivation and reward processing is central to an understanding of the psychopathology of bipolar spectrum disorders. Future research on the BAS hypersensitivity model of bipolar disorders should address some of the current limitations of the model and prior research designed to test it. For example, most studies that have tested whether BAS or reward hypersensitivity predicts the onset and course of bipolar spectrum disorders primarily have used self-report measures of BAS sensitivity. Future studies may benefit from using additional behavioral and neurobiological (e.g., fMRI) assessments of reward sensitivity. Second, the existing self-report measures of BAS sensitivity do a better job of assessing dysregulation of the BAS in an upward (activation) direction than in the downward (deactivation) direction. Thus, further instrument development is needed to more powerfully test the BAS hypersensitivity model of bipolar disorders. Finally, most prior studies assess the propensity for the BAS to become overactivated (dysregulated), but not the dysregulation itself. Thus, future research would benefit from a focus on developing a better understanding of the nature of emotional, cognitive, motivational, and neurobiological BAS dysregulation in bipolar disorders and the underlying causes of such dysregulation.

Acknowledgment

Preparation of this chapter was supported by National Institute of Mental Health Grant No. MH 77908 to Lauren B. Alloy.

References

Abler, B., Greenhouse, I., Ongur, D., Walter, H., & Heckers, S. (2008). Abnormal reward system activation in mania. *Neuropsychopharmacology, 33*, 2217–2227.

Akiskal, H. S., Djenderedjian, A. H., Rosenthal, R. H., & Khani, M. K. (1977). Cyclothymic disorder: Validating criteria for inclusion in the bipolar affective group. *American Journal of Psychiatry, 134*, 1227–1233.

Al-Adawi, S., Powell, J. H., & Greenwood, R. J. (1998). Motivational deficits after brain injury: A neuropsychological approach using new assessment techniques. *Neuropsychology, 12*, 115–124.

Alloy, L. B., & Abramson, L. Y. (2010). The role of the behavioral approach system (BAS) in bipolar spectrum disorders. *Current Directions in Psychological Science, 19*, 189–194.

Alloy, L. B., Abramson, L. Y., Flynn, M., Liu, R. T., Grant, D. A., Jager-Hyman, S., et al. (2009). Self-focused cognitive styles and bipolar spectrum disorders: Concurrent and prospective associations. *International Journal of Cognitive Therapy, 2*, 354–372.

Alloy, L. B., Abramson, L. Y., Urosevic, S., Bender, R. E., & Wagner, C. A. (2009). Longitudinal predictors of bipolar spectrum disorders: A behavioral approach system (BAS) perspective. *Clinical Psychology: Science and Practice, 16*, 206–226.

Alloy, L. B., Abramson, L. Y., Urosevic, S., Walshaw, P. D., Nusslock, R., & Neeren, A. M. (2005). The psychosocial context of bipolar disorder: Environmental, cognitive, and developmental risk factors. *Clinical Psychology Review, 25*, 1043–1075.

Alloy, L. B., Abramson, L. Y., Walshaw, P. D., Cogswell, A., Grandin, L. D., Hughes, M. E., et al. (2008). Behavioral approach system and behavioral inhibition system sensitivities: Prospective prediction of bipolar mood episodes. *Bipolar Disorders, 10*, 310–322.

Alloy, L. B., Abramson, L. Y., Walshaw, P. D., Cogswell, A., Smith, J., Hughes, M., et al. (2006). Behavioral approach system (BAS) sensitivity and bipolar spectrum disorders: A retrospective and concurrent behavioral high-risk design. *Motivation and Emotion, 30*, 143–155.

Alloy, L. B., Abramson, L. Y., Walshaw, P. D., Gerstein, R. K., Keyser, J. D., Whitehouse, W. G., et al. (2009). Behavioral approach system (BAS): Relevant cognitive styles and bipolar spectrum disorders—concurrent and prospective associations. *Journal of Abnormal Psychology, 118*, 459–471.

Alloy, L. B., Bender, R. E., Wagner, C. A., Whitehouse, W. G., Abramson, L. Y., Hogan, M. E., et al. (2009). Bipolar spectrum: Substance use co-occurrence—behavioral approach system

(BAS) sensitivity and impulsiveness as shared personality vulnerabilities. *Journal of Personality and Social Psychology, 97*, 549–565.

Alloy, L. B., Bender, R. E., Whitehouse, W. G., Wagner, C. A., Liu, R. T., Grant, D. A., et al. (2012). High behavioral approach system (BAS) sensitivity, reward responsiveness, and goal-striving predict first onset of bipolar spectrum disorders: A prospective behavioral high-risk design. *Journal of Abnormal Psychology, 121*, 339–351.

Alloy, L. B., Urosevic, S., Abramson, L. Y., Jager-Hyman, S., Nusslock, R., Whitehouse, W. G., et al. (2012). Progression along the bipolar spectrum: A longitudinal study of predictors of conversion from bipolar spectrum conditions to bipolar I and II disorders. *Journal of Abnormal Psychology, 121*, 16–27.

Angst, F., Stassen, H. H., Clayton, P. J., & Angst, J. (2002). Mortality of patients with mood disorders: Follow-up over 34–38 years. *Journal of Affective Disorders, 68*, 167–181.

Bearden, C. E., Hoffman, K. M., & Cannon, T. D. (2001). The neuropsychology and neuroanatomy of bipolar affective disorder: A critical review. *Bipolar Disorders, 3*, 106–150.

Berk, M., Dodd, S., Kauer-Sant-anna, M., Malhi, G. S., Bourin, M, Kapczinski, F., et al. (2007). Dopamine dysregulation syndrome: Implications for a dopamine hypothesis of bipolar disorder. *Acta Psychiatrica Scandinavica: Supplementum, 116*, 41–49.

Bermpohl, F., Kahnt, T., Dalanay, U., Hägele, C., Sajonz, B., Wegner, T., et al. (2010). Altered representation of expected value in the orbitofrontal cortex in mania. *Human Brain Mapping, 31*, 958–969.

Birmaher, B., Axelson, D., Goldstein, B., Strober, M., Gill, M. K., Hunt, J., et al. (2009). Four-year longitudinal course of children and adolescents with bipolar spectrum disorders: The Course and Outcome of Bipolar Youth (COBY) study. *American Journal of Psychiatry, 166*, 795–804.

Bozikas, V. P., Tonia, T., Fokas, K., Karavatos, A., & Kosmidis, M. H. (2006). Impaired emotion processing in remitted patients with bipolar disorder. *Journal of Affective Disorders, 91*, 53–56.

Camara, E., Kra, U. M., Cunillera, T., Marcopallare, J., Cucurell, D., Nager, W., et al. (2010). The effects of COMT (Val108/158Met) and DRD4 (SNP 2521) dopamine genotypes on brain activations related to valence and magnitude of rewards. *Cerebral Cortex, 4*, 1985–1996.

Carver, C. S. (2004). Negative affect deriving from the behavioral approach system. *Emotion, 4*, 3–22.

Carver, C. S., & Johnson, S. (2009). Tendencies toward mania and tendencies toward depression have distinct motivational, affective, and cognitive correlates. *Cognitive Therapy and Research, 33*, 552–569.

Carver, C. S., & White, T. L. (1994). Behavioral inhibition, behavioral activation, and affective responses to impending reward and punishment: The BIS/BAS scales. *Journal of Personality and Social Psychology, 67*, 319–333.

Cassano, G. B., Dell'Osso, L., Frank, E., Miniati, M., Fagiolini, A., Shear, K., et al. (1999). The bipolar spectrum: A clinical reality in search of diagnostic criteria and an assessment methodology. *Journal of Affective Disorders, 54*, 319–328.

Chiu, S., Widjaja, F., Bates, M. E., Voelbel, G. T., Pandina, G., Marble, J., et al. (2007). Anterior cingulate volume in pediatric bipolar disorder and autism. *Journal of Affective Disorders, 105*, 93–99.

Coan, J. A., & Allen, J. J. B. (2004). Frontal EEG asymmetry as a moderator and mediator of emotion. *Biological Psychology, 67*, 7–49.

Conway, K. P., Compton, W., Stinson, F. S., & Grant, B. F. (2006). Lifetime comorbidity of DSM-IV mood and anxiety disorders and specific drug use disorders: Results from the National Epidemiologic Survey on Alcohol and related conditions. *Journal of Clinical Psychiatry, 67*, 247–257.

Cousins, D. A., Butts, K., & Young, A. H. (2009). The role of dopamine in bipolar disorder. *Bipolar Disorders, 11*, 787–806.

Deckersbach, T., Gershuny, B. S., & Otto, M. W. (2000). Cognitive-behavioral therapy for depression: Applications and outcome. *Psychiatric Clinics of North America, 23*, 795–809.

Depue, R. A., & Collins, P. F. (1999). Neurobiology of the structure of personality: Dopamine, facilitation of incentive motivation, and extraversion. *Behavioral and Brain Sciences, 22*, 491–517.

Depue, R. A., & Iacono, W. G. (1989). Neurobehavioral aspects of affective disorders. *Annual Reviews in Psychology, 40*, 457–492.

Depue, R. A., Krauss, S., & Spoont, M. R. (1987). A two-dimensional threshold model of seasonal bipolar affective disorder. In D. Magnusson & A. Ohman (Eds.), *Psychopathology: An interactional perspective* (pp. 95–123). New York: Academic Press.

Dickstein, D. P., Milham, M. P., Nugent, A. C., Drevets, W. C., Charney, D. S., Pine, D. S., et al. (2005). Frontotemporal alterations in pediatric bipolar disorder: Results of a voxel-based morphometry study. *Archives of General Psychiatry, 62,* 734–741.

Eich E., Macaulay, D., & Lam R. W. (1997). Mania, depression, and mood dependent memory. *Cognition and Emotion, 11,* 607–618.

Eisner, L., Johnson, S. L., & Carver, C. S. (2008). Cognitive responses to failure and success relate uniquely to bipolar depression versus mania. *Journal of Abnormal Psychology, 117,* 154–163.

Ellicott, A., Hammen, C., Gitlin, M., Brown, G., & Jamison, K. (1990). Life events and the course of bipolar disorder. *American Journal of Psychiatry, 147,* 1194–1198.

Feldman, G., Joormann, J., & Johnson, S. (2008). Responses to positive affect: A self-report measure of rumination and dampening. *Cognitive Therapy and Research, 32,* 507–525.

Fountoulakis, K. N., Giannakopoulos, P., Kövari, E., & Bouras, C. (2008). Assessing the role of cingulate cortex in bipolar disorder: Neuropathological, structural, and functional imaging data. *Brain Research Reviews, 59,* 9–21.

Francis-Raniere, E., Alloy, L. B., & Abramson, L. Y. (2006). Depressive personality styles and bipolar spectrum disorders: Prospective tests of the event congruency hypothesis. *Bipolar Disorders, 8,* 382–399.

Fredrickson, B. L. (1998). What good are positive emotions? *Review of General Psychology, 2,* 300–319.

Fulford, D., Johnson, S. L., Llabre, M. M., & Carver, C. S. (2010). Pushing and coasting in dynamic goal pursuit: Coasting is attenuated in bipolar disorder. *Psychological Science, 21,* 1021–1027.

Gamo, N. J., & Arnsten, A. F. T. (2011). Molecular modulation of prefrontal cortex: Rational development of treatments for psychiatric disorders. *Behavioral Neuroscience, 125,* 282–296.

Getz, G. E., Shear, P. K., & Strakowski, S. M. (2003). Facial affect recognition deficits in bipolar disorder. *Journal of the International Neuropsychological Society, 9,* 623–632.

Goldberg, J. F., Gerstein, R. K., Wenze, S. J., Welker, T. M., & Beck, A. T. (2008). Dysfunctional attitudes and cognitive schemas in bipolar manic and unipolar depressed outpatients: Implications for cognitively based psychotherapeutics. *Journal of Nervous and Mental Disease, 196,* 207–210.

Goodwin, F. K., & Jamison, K. R. (2007). *Manic–depressive illness* (2nd ed.). New York: Oxford University Press.

Goodwin, G. M., Martinez-Aran, A., Glahn, D. C., & Vieta, E. (2008). Cognitive impairment in bipolar disorder: Neurodevelopment or neurodegeneration? An ECNP expert meeting report. *European Neuropsychopharmacology, 18,* 787–793.

Gray, J. A. (1994). Three fundamental emotion systems. In P. Eckman & R. J. Davidson (Eds.), *The nature of emotion: Fundamental questions* (pp. 243–247). New York: Oxford University Press.

Gruber, J., Eidelman, P., Johnson, S. L., Smith, B., & Harvey, A. G. (2012). Hooked on a feeling: Rumination about positive and negative emotion in inter-episode bipolar disorder. *Journal of Abnormal Psychology, 120,* 956–961.

Gruber, J., & Johnson, S. L. (2009). Positive emotional traits and ambitious goals among people at risk for bipolar disorder: The need for specificity. *International Journal of Cognitive Therapy, 2*(2), 176–187.

Gruber, J., Johnson, S. L., Oveis, C., & Keltner, D. (2008). Risk for mania and positive emotional responding: Too much of a good thing? *Emotion, 8,* 23–33.

Hammen, C. (1991). Generation of stress in the course of unipolar depression. *Journal of Abnormal Psychology, 100,* 555–561.

Hammen, C., & Gitlin, M. (1997). Stress reactivity in bipolar patients and its relation to prior history of depression. *American Journal of Psychiatry, 154,* 856–857.

Harmon-Jones, E., Abramson, L. Y., Nusslock, R., Sigelman, J. D., Urosevic, S., Turonie, L. D., et al. (2008). Effect of bipolar disorder on left frontal cortical responses to goals differing in valence and task difficulty. *Biological Psychiatry, 63,* 693–698.

Harmon-Jones, E., Abramson, L. Y., Sigelman, J. D., Bohlig, A., Hogan, M. E., & Harmon-Jones, C. (2002). Proneness to hypomania/mania symptoms or depression symptoms and asymmetrical frontal cortical responses to an anger evoking event. *Journal of Personality and Social Psychology, 82,* 610–618.

Harmon-Jones, E., & Allen, J. J. B. (1998). Anger and prefrontal brain activity: EEG asymmetry consistent with approach motivation despite negative affect valence. *Journal of Personality and Social Psychology, 74,* 1310–1316.

Harmon-Jones, E., & Allen, J. J. B. (1997). Behavioral activation sensitivity and resting frontal EEG asymmetry: Covariation of putative indicators related to risk for mood disorders. *Journal of Abnormal Psychology, 106,* 159–163.

Harmon-Jones, E., & Sigelman, J. D. (2001). State anger and prefrontal brain activity: Evidence that insult-related relative left prefrontal activity is associated with experienced anger and aggression. *Journal of Personality and Social Psychology, 80,* 797–803.

Hayden, E. P., Bodkins, M., Brenner, C., Shekhar, A., Nurnberger, J. I., O'Donnell, B. F., et al. (2008). A multimethod investigation of the behavioral activation system in bipolar disorder. *Journal of Abnormal Psychology, 117,* 164–170.

Haznedar, M. M., Roversi, F., Pallanti, S., Baldini-Rossi, N., Schnur, D. B., Licalzi, E. M., et al. (2005). Fronto-thalamo-striatal gray and white matter volumes and anisotropy of their connections in bipolar spectrum illnesses. *Biological Psychiatry, 57,* 733–742.

Hofmann, B. U., & Meyer, T. D. (2006). Mood fluctuations in people putatively at risk for bipolar disorders. *British Journal of Clinical Psychology, 45,* 105–110.

Hollon, S. D. (2006). Cognitive therapy in the treatment and prevention of depression. In T. E. Joiner, J. S. Brown, & J. Kistner (Eds.), *The interpersonal, cognitive, and social nature of depression* (pp. 131–151). Mahwah, NJ: Erlbaum.

Houenou, J., Frommberger, J., Carde, S., Glasbrenner, M., Diener, C., Leboyer, M., et al. (2011). Neuroimaging-based markers of bipolar disorder: Evidence from two meta-analyses. *Journal of Affective Disorders, 132,* 344–355.

Hunt, N., Bruce-Jones, W., & Silverstone, T. (1992). Life events and relapse in bipolar affective disorder. *Journal of Affective Disorders, 25,* 13–20.

Johnson, S. L. (2005). Mania and dysregulation in goal pursuit: A review. *Clinical Psychology Review, 25,* 241–262.

Johnson, S. L., & Carver, C. S. (2006). Extreme goal setting and vulnerability to mania among undiagnosed young adults. *Cognitive Therapy and Research, 30,* 377–395.

Johnson, S. L., Cueller, A. K., Ruggero, C., Winett-Perlman, C., Goodnick, P., White, R., et al. (2008). Life events as predictors of mania and depression in bipolar I disorder. *Journal of Abnormal Psychology, 117,* 268–277.

Johnson, S. L., Eisner, L., & Carver, C. S. (2009). Elevated expectancies among persons diagnosed with bipolar disorder. *British Journal of Clinical Psychology, 48,* 217–222.

Johnson, S. L., & Jones, S. (2009). Cognitive correlates of mania risk: Are responses to success, positive moods, and manic symptoms distinct or overlapping? *Journal of Clinical Psychology, 65,* 891–905.

Johnson, S. L., McKenzie, G., & McMurrich, S. (2008). Ruminative responses to negative and positive affect among students diagnosed with bipolar disorder and major depressive disorder. *Cognitive Therapy and Research, 32,* 702–713.

Johnson, S. L., Meyer, B., Winett, C., & Small, J. (2000). Social support and self-esteem predict changes in bipolar depression but not mania. *Journal of Affective Disorders, 58,* 79–86.

Johnson, S. L., & Miller, I. (1997). Negative life events and time to recovery from episodes of bipolar disorder. *Journal of Abnormal Psychology, 106,* 449–457.

Johnson, S. L., Ruggero, C. J., & Carver, C. S. (2005). Cognitive, behavioral, and affective responses to reward: Links with hypomanic symptoms. *Journal of Social and Clinical Psychology, 24,* 894–906.

Johnson, S. L., Sandrow, D., Meyer, B., Winters, R., Miller, I., Solomon, D., et al. (2000). Increases in manic symptoms after life events involving goal attainment. *Journal of Abnormal Psychology, 109,* 721–727.

Judd, L. L., Schettler, P. J., Solomon, D. A., Maser, J. D., Coryell, W., Endicott, J., et al. (2008). Psychosocial disability and work role function compared across the long-term course of bipolar I, bipolar II, and unipolar major depressive disorders. *Journal of Affective Disorders, 108,* 49–58.

Kano, K., Nakamura, M., Matsuoka, T., Iida, H., & Nakajima, T. (1992). The topographical features of EEGs in patients with affective disorders. *Electroencephalography and Clinical Neurophysiology, 83,* 124–129.

Knowles, R., Tai, S., Christensen, I., & Bentall, R. (2005). Coping with depression and vulnerability to mania: A factor analytic study of the Nolen-Hoeksema (1991) response style questionnaire. *British Journal of Clinical Psychology, 44,* 99–112.

Kochman, F. J., Hantouche, E. G., Ferrari, P., Lancrenon, S., Bayart, D., & Akiskal, H. S. (2005). Cyclothymic temperament as a prospective predictor of bipolarity and suicidality in children and adolescents with major depressive disorder. *Journal of Affective Disorders, 85,* 181–189.

Lam, D. H., Bright, J., Jones, S., Hayward, P., Schuck, N., Chisholm, D., et al. (2000). Cognitive therapy for bipolar illness: A pilot study of relapse prevention. *Cognitive Therapy and Research, 24,* 503–520.

Lam, D. H., Watkins, E. R., Hayward, P., Bright, J., Wright, K., Kerr, N., et al. (2003). A randomized controlled study of cognitive therapy for relapse prevention for bipolar affective disorder: Outcome of the first year. *Archives of General Psychiatry, 60,* 145–152.

Lam, D. H., & Wong, G. (1997). Prodromes, coping strategies, insight and social functioning in bipolar affective disorders. *Psychological Medicine, 27,* 1091–1100.

Lam, D. H., Wong, G., & Sham, P. (2001). Prodromes, coping strategies and the course of illness in bipolar affective disorder: A naturalistic study. *Psychological Medicine, 31,* 1397–1402.

Lam, D. H., Wright, K., & Sham, P. (2005). Sense of hyper-positive self and response to cognitive therapy in bipolar disorder. *Psychological Medicine, 35,* 69–77.

Lam, D. H., Wright, K., & Smith, N. (2004). Dysfunctional assumptions in bipolar disorder. *Journal of Affective Disorders, 79,* 193–199.

Lembke, A., & Ketter, T. A. (2002). Impaired recognition of facial emotion in mania. *American Journal of Psychiatry, 159,* 302–304.

Lozano, B. E., & Johnson, S. L. (2001). Can personality traits predict increases in manic and depressive symptoms? *Journal of Affective Disorders, 63,* 103–111.

Lyoo, I. K., Hwang, J., Sim, M., Dunn, B. J., & Renshaw, P. F. (2006). Advances in magnetic resonance imaging methods for the evaluation of bipolar disorder. *CNS Spectrums, 11,* 269–280.

Mansell, W., Morrison, A. P., Reid, G., Lowens, I., & Tai, S. (2007). The interpretation of, and responses to, changes in internal states: An integrative cognitive model of mood swings and bipolar disorders. *Behavioural and Cognitive Psychotherapy, 35,* 515–539.

Martin, L. T., & Tesser, A. (1996). Some ruminative thoughts. In R. S. Wyer, Jr. (Ed.), *Ruminative thoughts* (pp. 1–47). Hillsdale, NJ: Erlbaum.

McPherson, H., Herbinson, P., & Romans, S. (1993). Life events and relapse in established bipolar affective disorder. *British Journal of Psychiatry, 163,* 381–385.

Merikangas, K. R., Akiskal, H. S., Angst, J., Greenberg, P. E., Hirschfeld, R. M. A., Petukhova, M., et al. (2007). Lifetime and 12–month prevalence of bipolar spectrum disorder in the National Comorbidity Survey Replication. *Archives of General Psychiatry, 64,* 543–552.

Meyer, B., Johnson, S. L., & Carver, C. S. (1999). Exploring behavioral activation and inhibition sensitivities among college students at risk for bipolar spectrum symptomatology. *Journal of Psychopathology and Behavioral Assessment, 21,* 275–292.

Meyer, B., Johnson, S. L., & Winters, R. (2001). Responsiveness to threat and incentive in bipolar disorder: Relations of the BIS/BAS scales with symptoms. *Journal of Psychopathology and Behavioral Assessment, 23,* 133–143.

Meyer, T. D., & Krumm-Merabet, C. (2003). Academic performance and expectations for the future in relation to a vulnerability marker for bipolar disorders: The hypomanic temperament. *Personality and Individual Differences, 35,* 785–796.

Miller, A., & Tomarken, A. J. (2001). Task-dependent changes in frontal brain asymmetry: Effects of incentive cues, outcome expectancies, and motor responses. *Psychophysiology, 38,* 500–511.

Missale, C., Nash, S. R., Robinson, S. W., Jaber, M., & Caron, M. G. (1998). Dopamine receptors: From structure to function. *Physiological Reviews, 78,* 189–225.

Molnar, G. J., Feeney, M. G., & Fava, G. A. (1988). Duration and symptoms of bipolar prodromes. *American Journal of Psychiatry, 145,* 1576–1578.

Naranjo, C. A., Tremblay, L. K., Lescia, K., & Busto, U. E. (2001). The role of the brain reward system in depression. *Progress in Neuro-Psychopharmacology and Biological Psychiatry, 25,* 781–823.

Narushima, K., Kosler, J. T., & Robinson, R. G. (2003). A reappraisal of poststroke depression, intra- and inter-hemispheric lesion location using meta-analysis. *Journal of Neuropsychiatry and Clinical Neuroscience, 15,* 422–430.

Nolen-Hoeksema, S. (1991). Responses to

depression and their effects on the duration of depressive episodes. *Journal of Abnormal Psychology, 100,* 569–582.

Nugent, A. C., Milham, M. P., Bain, E. E., Mah, L., Cannon, D. M., Marrett, S., et al. (2006). Cortical abnormalities in bipolar disorder investigated with MRI and voxel-based morphometry. *NeuroImage, 30,* 485–497.

Nusslock, R., Abramson, L. Y., Harmon-Jones, E., Alloy, L. B., & Coan, J. (2009). Psychosocial interventions for bipolar disorder: Perspective from the behavioral approach system (BAS) dysregulation theory. *Clinical Psychology: Science and Practice, 16,* 449–469.

Nusslock, R., Abramson, L. Y., Harmon-Jones, E., Alloy, L. B., & Hogan, M. E. (2007). A goal-striving life event and the onset of bipolar episodes: Perspective from the behavioral approach system (BAS) dysregulation theory. *Journal of Abnormal Psychology, 116,* 105–115.

Nusslock, R., Alloy, L. B., Abramson, L. Y., Harmon-Jones, E., & Hogan, M. E. (2008). Impairment in the achievement domain in bipolar spectrum disorders: Role of behavioral approach system (BAS) hypersensitivity and impulsivity. *Minerva Pediatrica, 60,* 41–50.

Nusslock, R., Almeida, J. R. C., Forbes, E. E., Versace, A., LaBarbara, E. J., Klein, C. R., et al. (2012). Waiting to win: Elevated striatal and orbitofrontal cortical activity during reward anticipation in euthymic bipolar adults. *Bipolar Disorders, 14,* 249–260.

Nusslock, R., Harmon-Jones, E., Alloy, L. B., Urosevic, S., Goldstein, K., & Abramson, L. Y. (2012). Elevated left mid-frontal cortical activity prospectively predicts conversion to bipolar I disorder. *Journal of Abnormal Psychology, 121,* 592–601.

Nutt, D. J. (2006). The role of dopamine and norepinephrine in depression and antidepressant treatment. *Journal of Clinical Psychiatry, 67(S6),* 3–8.

Nutt, D. J., Demyttenaere, K., Janka, Z., Aarre, T., Bourin, M., Canonico, P. L., et al. (2007). The other face of depression, reduced positive affect: The role of catecholamines in causation and cure. *Journal of Psychopharmacology, 21,* 461–471.

Pardoen, D., Bauwens, F., Dramaix, M., Tracy, A., Genevrois, C., Staner, L., et al. (1996). Life events and primary affective disorders: A one year prospective study. *British Journal of Psychiatry, 169,* 160–166.

Pizzagalli, D. A., Goetz, E., Ostacher, M., Iosifescu, D. V., & Perlis, R. H. (2008). Euthymic patients with bipolar disorder show decreased reward learning in a probabilistic reward task. *Biological Psychiatry, 64,* 162–168.

Pizzagalli, D. A., Sherwood, R. J., Henriques, J. B., & Davidson, R. J. (2005). Frontal brain asymmetry and reward responsiveness: A source-localization study. *Psychological Science, 16,* 805–813.

Reuter, M., Schmitz, A., Corr, P., & Hennig, J. (2006). Molecular genetics support Gray's personality theory: The interaction of COMT and DRD2 polymorphisms predicts the behavioural approach system. *International Journal of Neuropsychopharmacology, 9,* 155–66.

Robinson, R. G., Boston, J. D., Starkstein, S. E., & Price, T. R. (1988). Comparison of mania and depression after brain injury: Causal factors. *American Journal of Psychiatry, 145,* 172–178.

Rosenfarb, I. S., Becker, J., Khan, A., & Mintz, J. (1988). Dependency and self-criticism in bipolar and unipolar depressed women. *British Journal of Clinical Psychology, 37,* 409–414.

Rubinsztein, J. S., Fletcher, P. C., Rogers, R. D., Ho, L. W., Aigbirhio, F. I., Paykel, E. S., et al. (2001). Decision-making in mania: A PET study. *Brain, 124,* 2550–2563.

Salavert, J., Caseras, X., Torrubia, R., Furest, S., Arranz, B., Duenas, R., et al. (2007). The functioning of the behavioral activation and inhibition systems in bipolar I euthymic patients and its influence in subsequent episodes over an 18-month period. *Personality and Individual Differences, 42,* 1323–1331.

Scott, J., Stanton, B., Garland, A., & Ferrier, I. N. (2000). Cognitive vulnerability in patients with bipolar disorder. *Psychological Medicine, 30,* 467–472.

Smith, J., & Tarrier, N. (1992). Prodromal symptoms in manic depressive psychosis. *Social Psychiatry and Psychiatric Epidemiology, 27,* 245–248.

Smolka, M. N., Schumann, G., Wrase, J., Grusser, S. M., Flor, H., Mann, K., et al. (2005). Catechol-O-methyltransferase val158met genotype affects processing of emotional stimuli in the amygdala and prefrontal cortex. *Journal of Neuroscience, 25,* 836–842.

Sobotka, S. S., Davidson, R. J., & Senulis, J. A. (1992). Anterior brain asymmetries in response to reward and punishment. *Electro-*

encephalography and Clinical Neurophysiology, 83, 236–247.

Stange, J. P., Shapero, B. G., Jager-Hyman, S. G., Grant, D. A., Abramson, L. Y., & Alloy, L. B. (2013). Behavioral approach system (BAS)–relevant cognitive styles in individuals with high versus moderate BAS sensitivity: A behavioral high-risk design. *Cognitive Therapy and Research, 37*, 139–149.

Summers, M., Papadopoulou, K., Bruno, S., Cipolotti, L., & Ron, M. A. (2006). Bipolar I and bipolar II disorder: Cognition and emotion processing. *Psychological Medicine, 36*, 1799–1809.

Sutton, S. K., & Davidson, R. J. (1997). Prefrontal brain asymmetry: A biological substrate of the behavioral approach and inhibition systems. *Psychological Science, 8*, 204–210.

Sutton, S. K., & Johnson, S. L. (2002). Hypomanic tendencies predict lower startle magnitudes during pleasant pictures. *Psychophysiology, 39*(Suppl.), S80.

Swann, A. C., Dougherty, D. M., Pazzaglia, P., Pham, M., & Moeller, F. G. (2004). Impulsivity: A link between bipolar disorder and substance abuse. *Bipolar Disorders, 6*, 204–212.

Thomas, J., & Bentall, R. P. (2002). Hypomanic traits and response styles to depression. *British Journal of Clinical Psychology, 41*, 309–313.

Torrubia, R., Avila, C., Molto, J., & Caseras, X. (2001). The Sensitivity to Punishment and Sensitivty to Reward Questionnaire (SPSRQ) as a measure of Gray's anxiety and impulsivity dimensions. *Personality and Individual Differences, 31*, 837–862.

Urosevic, S., Abramson, L. Y., Alloy, L. B., Nusslock, R., Harmon-Jones, E., Bender, R. E., et al. (2010). Increased rates of events that activate or deactivate the behavioral approach system, but not events related to goal attainment, in bipolar spectrum disorders. *Journal of Abnormal Psychology, 119*, 610–615.

Urosevic, S., Abramson, L. Y., Harmon-Jones, E., & Alloy, L. B. (2008). Dysregulation of the behavioral approach system (BAS) in bipolar spectrum disorders: Review of theory and evidence. *Clinical Psychology Review, 28*, 1188–1205.

Verhoeff, P., Seneca, N., Zoghbi, S. S., Seibyl, J. P., Charney, D. S., & Innis, R. B. (2000). Brain SPECT imaging of amphetamine-induced dopamine release in euthymic bipolar disorder patients. *American Journal of Psychiatry, 157*, 1108–1114.

Wong, G., & Lam, D. (1999). The development and validation of the coping inventory for prodromes of mania. *Journal of Affective Disorders, 53*, 57–65.

Wright, K. A., Lam, D., & Brown, R. G. (2008). Dysregulation of the behavioral activation system in remitted bipolar I disorder. *Journal of Abnormal Psychology, 117*, 838–848.

Youngstrom, E. A., Birmaher, B., & Findling, R. L. (2008). Pediatric bipolar disorder: Validity, phenomenology, and recommendations for diagnosis. *Bipolar Disorders, 10*, 194–214.

Differentiating the Cognition–Emotion Interactions That Characterize Psychopathy versus Externalizing

Arielle R. Baskin-Sommers and Joseph P. Newman

Disinhibitory psychopathology encompasses a broad range of traits and behaviors that is epitomized by psychopathy and externalizing (Gorenstein & Newman, 1980; Krueger, Markon, Patrick, & Iacono, 2005; Patrick & Zempolich, 1998; Patrick, Zempolich, & Levenston, 1997; Poythress & Hall, 2011; Zuckerman, 1978). Psychopathic individuals are characterized by difficulty establishing genuine relationships, minimal and superficial affective experience, an impulsive behavioral style, and a chronic antisocial lifestyle that entails great costs to society as well as for affected individuals (e.g., incarceration). Alternatively, externalizing individuals often display excessive reward seeking, intense hostility and reactive aggression, and poor impulse control (Buckholtz et al., 2010; Gorenstein & Newman, 1980; Krueger et al., 2005; Pridmore, Chambers, & McArthur, 2005; Newman & Lorenz, 2003). Although both psychopathy and externalizing are characterized by antisociality, impulsivity, irresponsibility, and aggression, these syndromes are commonly measured and expressed in distinct manners.

Psychopathy is a severe psychopathological disorder affecting approximately 1% of the general population and 25% of incar-

cerated male offenders (Hare, 2006; Neumann & Hare, 2008). The gold standard measure of psychopathy, particularly with incarcerated samples, is Hare's Psychopathy Checklist—Revised (PCL-R; 2003). The PCL-R, an interview-based measure, identifies individuals displaying a combination of disinhibited traits (i.e., impulsivity, irresponsibility), a chronic antisocial lifestyle, and a variety of interpersonal and affective symptoms (i.e., callousness, glibness, superficial charm, shallow emotions). Because the impulsivity and antisocial lifestyle symptoms apply to most disinhibitory psychopathology, it is the callous–unemotional traits that distinguish psychopathy from externalizing disorders (i.e., antisocial personality disorder, substance abuse/dependence) and externalizing personality traits (e.g., low constraint).

In contrast to psychopathy, the externalizing spectrum encompasses a heterogeneous mixture of disorders, including conduct disorder, substance use disorders, and antisocial personality disorder. In prison populations, externalizing disorders are much more prominent than psychopathy (e.g., the prevalence of antisocial personality disorder [50–80%] is more than double the prevalence of psychopathy in male prisoners). By definition, the externalizing construct is not intended to identify a specific disorder or set of symptoms. Rather, it is intended to identify a heritable predisposition (i.e., latent variable) to diverse forms of disinhibitory psychopathology (Gorenstein & Newman, 1980; Iacono, Malone, & McGue, 2008). In some cases, this latent variable is identified by extracting the common variance associated with conduct disorder, adult antisocial behavior, and symptoms of a substance use disorder (Iacono et al., 2008). In other cases, externalizing is identified using measures of personality/temperament that include low constraint, impulsivity, negative emotionality, high extraversion, and high neuroticism. When defined in this way, investigators identify externalizing using broad-spectrum measures of personality, such as the Multidimensional Personality Questionnaire (MPQ; Patrick, Curtin, Tellegen, 2002) or, more recently, questionnaires designed to assess the array of predisposing traits more directly (e.g., Externalizing Spectrum Inventory; Krueger, Markon, Patrick, Benning, & Kramer, 2007).

The distinction between psychopathy and externalizing is complicated by virtue of their overlapping behavior problems. Nearly all incarcerated individuals with psychopathy qualify for conduct disorder and antisocial personality disorder, and most also qualify for one or more substance use disorders (Smith & Newman, 1990). Thus, if using these behavioral symptoms alone, it would be extremely difficult to distinguish between psychopathy and externalizing. However, as already noted, the callous–unemotional traits serve to differentiate psychopathy from the more emotionally reactive style (e.g., high reward seeking and negative emotionality) associated with externalizing. Moreover, although laboratory-based characterizations of psychopathy and externalizing commonly emphasize etiologically relevant attentional, executive system, and emotion-related dysfunction (Gorenstein & Newman, 1980; Newman, 1997; Patrick, 2007), close inspection of the specific pattern of process-level results associated with psychopathy and externalizing reveal that they are remarkably different. As a result of the differences in assessment and process-level functioning, we believe that progress

in understanding the serious behavior problems associated with psychopathy and externalizing depends on disentangling the divergent etiological pathways associated with their disinhibitory psychopathology.

The primary goal of this chapter is to distinguish between the cognitive–affective processes contributing to psychopathy and externalizing. Toward this end, we (1) review key findings in psychopathy and externalizing for the purpose of identifying their respective attentional, executive functioning, and affective abnormalities; (2) introduce an integrative model of cognitive–affective interactions as a framework for specifying and distinguishing the dysfunctional interactions operating in psychopathy and externalizing; and (3) based on the proposed model, discuss treatment implications for these syndromes. Before continuing, it is important to note that the scope of the studies reviewed in this chapter is not all-inclusive. We specifically examine reports that help us characterize and distinguish the dysfunctional cognition–emotion interactions operating in psychopathy and externalizing. In our view, failure to distinguish the dysfunctional cognitive–affective interactions associated with psychopathy and externalizing is a primary factor impeding etiological understanding as well as the development of more successful treatment strategies in both domains.

Attention

To understand the proposed roles for attention in the etiology of psychopathy and externalizing, it is important to first clarify the processes that may be operating in them. Models of selective attention suggest that there is a continuum of early and late influences. Early selective attention may act as a "fixed bottleneck" that, once established, blocks the processing of secondary information that is not goal relevant (Driver, 2001). Such selection is presumed to involve the serial processing of incoming information. Alternatively, selective attention may operate at a later stage (e.g., Luck & Hillyard, 1999). In traditional models of late selection, information is initially encoded in parallel, and then selection occurs after stimulus identification or semantic encoding (Corbetta, Miezin, Dobmeyer, Shulman, & Petersen, 1991; Duncan, 1980) as a function of memory and response selection processes that bias attention in a manner consistent with an individual's top-down, goal-directed focus (Driver, 2001). Of particular relevance, the distinction between these stages highlights the extent to which selective attention reflects a relatively automatic gating (early) out of distracting stimuli, as opposed to the influence of higher-order regulatory processes (late) that sustain a goal-relevant focus of attention. The following review suggests that individuals with psychopathy are uniquely associated with an early attention bottleneck, whereas externalizing individuals are primarily associated with dysfunction at a later stage of attention.

According to Newman and colleagues (e.g., Newman & Baskin-Sommers, 2011), an early attention bottleneck plays a crucial role in moderating the behavior and decision-making deficits associated with psychopathy. Psychopaths are oblivious to potentially meaningful peripheral information because they fail to reallocate attention while engaged in goal-directed behavior (MacCoon, Wallace, & Newman, 2004; Newman, 1998; Patterson & Newman, 1993). This difficulty balancing simultaneous demands to process goal-directed and peripheral information creates a bias whereby psychopaths are unresponsive to information unless it is a central aspect of their goal-directed focus of attention (Jutai & Hare, 1983; Kiehl, Hare, McDonald, & Brink, 1999).

An important implication of the attention bottleneck is that the emotion deficits commonly associated with psychopathy may vary as a function of attentional focus. A recent experiment by Newman and colleagues (2010) involving fear-potentiated startle (FPS) provides striking support for this hypothesis. Of note, existing evidence suggests that FPS is generated via the amygdala (Grillon, Ameli, Goddard, Woods, & Davis, 1994). The task used in this study required participants to view and categorize letter stimuli that could also be used to predict the administration of electric shocks. Instructions engaged either a goal-directed focus on threat-relevant information (i.e., the color that predicted electric shocks) or an alternative, threat-irrelevant dimension

of the letter stimuli (i.e., in a low-load condition, participants responded to indicate letter case; in a high-load condition, participants responded to indicate whether or not a letter stimulus matched one that occurred two back). The results provided no evidence of a psychopathy-related deficit in FPS under conditions that focused attention on the threat-relevant dimension. However, PCL-R psychopathy scores were significantly and inversely related to FPS under conditions that required participants to focus on an alternative, threat-irrelevant dimension of stimuli (i.e., when threat cues were peripheral) (Figure 27.1A).

Although the results from Newman and colleagues (2010) provided some of the strongest evidence to date that the fear deficit of individuals high on psychopathy is moderated by attention, the study did not specify the attentional mechanism underlying this effect. Baskin-Sommers, Curtin, and Newman (2011) specified this attentionally mediated abnormality in a new sample of offenders by measuring FPS in four conditions that crossed attentional focus (threat vs. alternative focus) with early versus late presentation of goal-relevant cues. First, the authors replicated the key findings reported by Newman and colleagues (2010): The deficit in FPS in individuals high on psychopathy was virtually nonexistent under conditions that focused attention on the threat-relevant dimension of the experimental stimuli (i.e., threat-focus conditions), but was pronounced when threat-relevant cues were peripheral to their primary focus of attention (i.e., alternative-focus conditions). More specifically, the psychopathic deficit in FPS was apparent only in the early alternative-focus condition, in which threat cues were presented after the alternative goal-directed focus was already established (Figure 27.1B). This finding implicates an early attention bottleneck as a proximal mechanism for deficient response modulation in psychopathy (see Newman & Baskin-Sommers, 2011). Additionally, Larson and colleagues (2012) have recently completed an imaging study using this paradigm with an independent sample of inmates. Preliminary results suggest that individuals with psychopathy as compared to those without it display significantly lower activation in the right-dorsal amygdala in the early alternative-focus con-

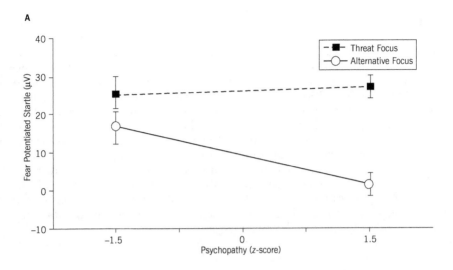

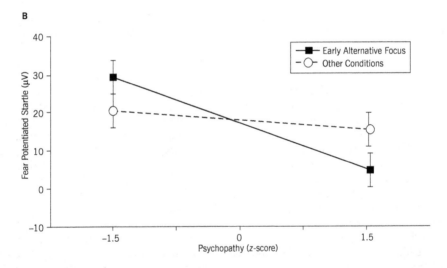

FIGURE 27.1. Fear-potentiated startle (FPS) as a function of PCL-R psychopathy (± 1.5 *SD* from the mean) and condition. (A) As reported by Newman et al. (2010), prisoners high on psychopathy displayed significantly lower FPS than prisoners low on psychopathy in the alternative-focus conditions. High- and low-psychopathic prisoners displayed comparable FPS in the threat-focus condition. (B) As reported by Baskin-Sommers et al. (2011a), prisoners high on psychopathy, compared to those low on psychopathy, displayed significantly lower FPS in the early alternative-focus condition, but comparable FPS in the other three conditions.

dition, but there was no difference in amygdala activation between the two groups (psychopathic vs. nonpsychopathic) in the early threat-focus condition. These results corroborate the idea that attention moderates the fearlessness of individuals with psychopathy, as evidenced by the appearance and disappearance of deficits in FPS and amygdala activation as a function of focus of attention.

There is equally clear evidence that the core inhibitory deficit in psychopathy is moderated by attention. Using a go/no-go learning task, Newman and Kosson (1986) examined passive avoidance (i.e., inhibition of punished responses) learning under reward-and-punishment versus punishment-only conditions. When participants were focused on avoiding punishment (punishment-only), there were no group differences in passive avoidance. However, when punishment was peripheral to the primary focus of earning rewards (reward-and-punishment), those with psychopathy committed significantly more passive avoidance errors than controls. Thus, the deficit in passive avoidance learning of individuals with psychopathy, like their FPS deficits, is moderated by their focus of attention (see also Arnett, Smith & Newman, 1997; Newman, Patterson, Howland, & Nichols, 1990). Individuals with psychopathy also display deficits in reversal learning (Budhani, Richell, & Blair, 2006; Hornak et al., 2004) and in gambling tasks (Bechara, Damasio, Tranel, & Damasio, 1997; Mitchell, Colledge, Leonard, & Blair, 2002; Newman, Patterson, & Kosson, 1987; cf. Lösel & Schmucker, 2004; Schmitt, Brinkley, & Newman, 1999), which also require participants to reallocate goal-directed attention.

Despite strong evidence for the role of an attention bottleneck in moderating affective reactivity in psychopathy, the evidence reviewed to this point does not preclude the possibility that a fundamental deficit in emotion processing undermines the motivation or capacity of these individuals to redirect attention (Blair & Mitchell, 2009; Lykken, 1995). However, there is now substantial evidence demonstrating that individuals with psychopathy display similar attentional abnormalities on laboratory tasks involving motivationally neutral peripheral information.

In standard versions of the color–word and number Stroop tasks, participants first perceive the conflicting elements and must then reprioritize attention to the appropriate element of the display (i.e., late selective attention; MacLeod, 1998). Thus, the quality of response depends on the participant's ability to resolve the conflict prior to making a response using executive functions, such as cognitive control (Botvinick, Braver, Barch, Carter, & Cohen, 2001). Under such conditions, individuals with psychopathy and those without it show comparable levels of interference (Blair et al., 2006; Hiatt, Schmitt, & Newman, 2004; Smith, Arnett, & Newman, 1992). Conversely, on Stroop-like tasks that facilitate early selection of goal-relevant information by spatially or temporally separating the incongruent elements of the display, individuals with psychopathy display significantly less interference than nonpsychopathic individuals, who still show significant interference under these conditions (Hiatt et al., 2004; Mitchell, Richell, Leonard, & Blair, 2006; Newman, Schmitt, & Voss, 1997; Vitale, Brinkley, Hiatt, & Newman, 2007). Such findings suggest that for individuals with psychopathy, an early attention bottleneck effectively blocks the processing of conflicting information, reducing the salience of the conflict and obviating the need to use executive functions to inhibit the distracting/conflicting information. Therefore, in certain contexts, individuals with psychopathy are effectively oblivious to distraction and remain focused on their goal, whereas nonpsychopathic individuals answer the automatic call for processing and are influenced by the conflict regardless of experimental context (Patterson & Newman, 1993).

Corroborating this attention-bottleneck-based interpretation of the Stroop data, Zeier, Maxwell, and Newman (2009) used a modified Erikson flanker task with an attentional cueing manipulation to examine whether an early attention bottleneck is a crucial factor differentiating sensitivity to response conflict in individuals with psychopathy. On some trials, pretrial cueing was used so that participants could orient attention to the location of the task-relevant target before the target and distracting flanker stimuli were presented (i.e., early selection). On other trials, the pretrial cues directed attention to both the target and distracter locations (i.e., late selection). Whereas participants with psychopathy displayed significantly less interference than controls in the former condition, they displayed nonsignificantly more interference in the latter condition.

Similarly, Wolf and colleagues (2011) evaluated the early attention bottleneck hypothesis using a more traditional assessment of attention, the attentional blink (AB) task. In the AB paradigm, participants identify targets in a rapid serial visual presentation (RSVP). Because distracters are presented almost immediately after targets, they elicit a response conflict between attending to the target and attending to the distracters. The magnitude of the AB appears to reflect the consequences of prioritizing attention to the first target (T1) over competing demands to reallocate attention in order to process all stimuli in the RSVP; the greater the conflict and resulting prioritizing of T1, the greater the AB. As predicted by the attention bottleneck hypothesis, offenders high on psychopathy displayed a significantly smaller AB (i.e., less conflict and fewer missed targets) than offenders low on psychopathy and this difference was apparent from the earliest possible postconflict lag time (i.e., lag 2, the second stimulus presented after T1). Such evidence is consistent with the idea that once they focus attention on goal-relevant information, individuals with psychopathy are essentially oblivious to goal-irrelevant information that elicits conflict in others.

Combined, these studies show that participants with psychopathy are significantly less sensitive to information if it is peripheral to a preestablished focus of goal-directed behavior. Moreover, the fact that this abnormality applies to affectively neutral as well as to affectively significant peripheral information implicates an early attention bottleneck that undermines the processing of goal-incongruent cues regardless of affective significance (Hiatt et al., 2004; Jutai & Hare, 1983; Mitchell et al., 2006; Vitale et al., 2007).

The attentional abnormality in externalizing individuals tends to be quite different. Not only do they perform differently than individuals with psychopathy on the Baskin-Sommers, Curtin, and Newman (2011) fear-conditioning paradigm and other tasks, such as AB, but they appear to display a different set of attention-related problems. Research on externalizing-specific performance implicates strong attentional orienting to salient and/or motivationally significant cues (Derryberry & Reed, 1994; Tiffany & Conklin, 2000) and a tendency to overallocate attentional resources to events of motivational significance (Ávila & Parcet, 2001; Baskin-Sommers, Wallace, MacCoon, Curtin, & Newman, 2010; Wallace & Newman, 1997). Thus, once a stimulus is identified as intrinsically important, engagement of higher-order cognitive processes is required to regulate a response. This later stage of attentional selection, which links up with executive functions to sustain a goal-relevant focus, appears dysfunctional in externalizing individuals.

Using the Baskin-Sommers, Curtin, and Newman (2011) instructed fear paradigm, a pattern distinct from the psychopathy effect emerged among externalizing individuals. When threat information was the primary focus of attention and presented first, trait externalizing (i.e., high-negative affect and low constraint) was significantly associated with greater FPS. Conversely, under conditions that instructed participants to focus on threat-relevant information but presented an irrelevant letter prior to the threat-relevant cues, externalizing was associated with nonsignificantly smaller FPS (Baskin-Sommers et al., 2012). One interpretation of these findings is that externalizing individuals have an intrinsic bias that primes them to orient attention toward motivationally significant information more strongly than other individuals. This recruitment of attention that prioritizes the goal-relevant processing of threat information, in turn, impairs other executive control processes and results in emotional hyperreactivity. Conversely, when a stimulus occurs that is at odds with this goal, such as an irrelevant distracting letter, it is necessary to alter the focus of attention and employ executive functions to facilitate goal-directed behavior. In externalizing this reallocation of attention and effort appears to disrupt fluent processing, resulting in an attenuated threat response. Such findings suggest that attentional processes, and their interaction with executive control processes, are at the root of the externalizing-related dysfunction. Moreover, in light of the fact that the externalizing effect was specific to the early threat-focus condition, whereas the psychopathy effect was specific to the early alternative-focus condition, the results indicate that the abnormal attentional responses associated with psychopathy and externalizing are clearly distinct.

Similarly, externalizing-related performance on the AB paradigm is easily differentiated from psychopathy-related performance and consistent with the purported externalizing-based attentional bias. Individuals with high externalizing (as measured by MPQ-based Impulsive Antisociality; Benning, Patrick, Blonigen, Hicks, & Iacono, 2005, or antisocial personality disorder) displayed a significantly greater AB (i.e., less accurate T2 identification) than individuals with low externalizing scores. Thus, externalizing individuals appear to overallocate attention to salient information (i.e., T1), and this attentional response temporarily (AB lasts for approximately 300–400 milliseconds [ms]) impairs information processing, resulting in an inability to update expectations concerning the present situation. This study further clarifies the attentional dysfunction operating in externalizing and, moreover, distinguishes it from the abnormalities associated with psychopathy.

Adaptive self-regulation requires a balance of attention to goal-relevant and peripheral information (MacCoon et al., 2004). On the one hand, adaptive behavior requires "that we respond to objects that are outside the current focus of attention, i.e., those that do not match current settings for selecting stimuli and responses" (Corbetta, Patel & Shulman, 2008, p. 306). On the other hand, effective goal-directed behavior requires not becoming overly distracted by stimuli outside the current goal-directed focus or overallocating attentional resources to particularly salient information. The former appears especially relevant for psychopathy. The early attention bottleneck facilitates the selection of goal-relevant information at the expense of overlooking information that might otherwise modulate the goal-directed behavior of individuals with psychopathy. Externalizing individuals do not show this type of deficit. Rather, they are characterized by a tendency to overcommit attentional resources to salient environmental events at the expense of processing other goal-relevant information (i.e., the latter requirement for adaptive self-regulation). In other words, both psychopathy and externalizing are associated with disordered attentional processing, but the characteristic attentional dysfunction in psychopathy involves an early attention bottleneck that interferes with information intake, whereas externalizing is associated with a later selective attention dysfunction that interferes with executive control.

Executive Function

Morgan and Lilienfeld (2000) define executive functioning as an "umbrella term that refers to the cognitive processes that allow for future, goal-oriented behavior" (p. 114).

More specifically, executive functions are a constellation of higher-order cognitive processes that facilitate the planning, initiation, and regulation of behavior (Giancola & Tarter, 1999).

When studying externalizing, it is hard to ignore the substantial behavioral, imaging, and event-related potential (ERP) evidence that such individuals have impaired executive functioning (Iacono et al., 2008). First, using behavioral tasks, executive functions such as working memory (e.g., measured by go/no-go discrimination tasks) and cognitive control (e.g., measured by Stroop interference) have been shown to be particularly deficient in externalizing individuals (Dolan, Bechara, & Nathan, 2008; Endres et al., 2011; Morgan & Lilienfeld, 2000). Second, neuroimaging studies involving externalizing individuals (e.g., antisocial personality disorder; Raine, Lencz, Bihrle, LaCasse, & Colletti, 2000) detect both structural and functional abnormalities in regions of the frontal cortex that have been associated with executive functions (e.g., anterior cingulate cortex [ACC]; Davidson, Pizzagalli, Nitschke, & Kalin, 2003; Raine et al., 2000; orbitofrontal cortex [OFC]; Seguin, 2004). Lastly, ERP studies consistently report inverse relationships between increased levels of externalizing and the amplitude and latency of the P300 and error related negativity (ERN).

Externalizing is regularly associated with deficits in P300 during oddball paradigms (i.e., participants respond to target stimuli that occur infrequently and unpredictably within a series of target-frequent stimuli) and task-relevant stimuli in non-oddball tasks (Bernat, Nelson, Steele, Gehring & Patrick, 2011; Costa et al., 2000; Patrick et al., 2006; Polich, Pollock, & Bloom, 1994). A deficiency in this component suggests disruptions in the updating of working memory and integrating information into existing networks (Bernat et al., 2011). Correspondingly, even though posterior brain regions typically generate the P300, the externalizing-related P300 amplitude reduction is often largest at frontocentral sites, suggesting that this P300 indexes the executive functioning deficit typically associated with anterior brain regions (e.g., ACC; Nelson, Patrick, & Bernat, 2011). Additionally, reports of significant externalizing-related reductions in ERN suggest inefficient executive function processing related to conflict monitoring and error detection (Hall, Bernat, & Patrick, 2007). Neurally, the ERN is primarily linked to the ACC (Dehaene, Posner, & Tucker, 1994) and supplementary motor area, with other structures, including the PFC, playing a supporting role (Gehring & Knight, 2000). Thus, a deficit in ERN is thought to reflect a deficit in the ACC's executive processes.

Overall, individuals with executive functioning deficits are less able to override maladaptive response inclinations in order to maintain more appropriate and personally beneficial behavior. Consequently, they are at higher risk for persistent rule breaking and committing acts of violence. Thus, deficits in executive functioning may underlie the emotional dysregulation, lack of conscience, and decision-making deficits that have been found to characterize antisocial, externalizing behavior.

Despite the general association between antisocial syndromes/externalizing and executive function deficits (Morgan & Lilienfeld, 2000; see also Blair, 2001), individuals with psychopathy generally do not display deficits on the executive functioning tasks (Blair et al., 2006; Brinkley, Schmitt, & Newman, 2005; Dvorak-Bertsch, Sadeh, Glass, Thornton, & Newman, 2007; Hart, Forth, & Hare, 1990; Hiatt et al., 2004; Munro et al., 2007; Smith et al., 1992; Sutker, Moan, & Allain, 1983). Thus, despite the high level of antisocial behavior displayed by individuals with psychopathy, they do not appear to manifest primary deficits in executive functioning, and in some cases display superior performance on tasks that measure executive functioning (see Stroop discussion above; Hiatt et al., 2004).

Further evidence that executive functioning deficits may be less strongly associated with psychopathy than with externalizing relates to differences in the ERP findings. In the handful of ERP studies on psychopathy that focus on P300 (Jutai, Hare, & Connolly, 1987; Kiehl, Hare, McDonald, & Brink, 1999; Kiehl, Smith, Hare, & Liddle, 2000; Raine & Venables, 1988), the results are more equivocal than those for externalizing. Jutai and colleagues (1987) found no significant difference between individuals

with psychopathy and those without it in the amplitude or latency of the P300. Raine and Venables (1988) reported increased amplitude of parietal P300 in individuals high versus low on psychopathy to visual target stimuli elicited during a continuous performance task (see also Raine, Venable, & Williams, 1990, for faster P300 latency effects in predicting psychopathic behavior). And still other studies show significantly smaller P300 responses in individuals high versus low on psychopathy during visual and auditory oddball tasks (Kiehl et al., 1999). The evidence linking psychopathy and ERN activity is equally mixed. Some evidence suggests that individuals with psychopathy show comparable ERN activity to individuals without it in nonaffective tasks (Brazil et al., 2009; Munro et al., 2007), whereas other evidence reveals attenuated ERN activity, particularly in tasks that have an affective component (Munro et al., 2007). Unfortunately, the results of these studies allow few firm conclusions owing, in large part, to the heterogeneity of the participants and the variety of tasks employed (e.g., oddball, S1–S2 motor response, and aversive differential conditioning tasks).

Conventional wisdom highlights the importance of a person's ability to focus on goal-directed behavior and to screen out salient distracters (i.e., executive functioning) in order to regulate the expression of violent behavior, inappropriate drug use, harmful antisocial behavior, and short-sighted reward seeking (Banfield, Wyland, Macrae, Munte, & Heatherton, 2004; MacCoon et al., 2004; Rueda, Posner, & Rothbart, 2005). In light of the existing evidence with externalizing individuals, there is reason to believe that this mechanism contributes to their behavior problems. However, another group with marked disinhibition, psychopathic individuals do not appear to be deficient in this regard. To the contrary, once their attention is engaged in goal-directed behavior, individuals with psychopathy are abnormally resistant to the influence by peripheral information that routinely modulates the goal-directed behavior of others. As described above, psychopathy appears to reflect abnormalities at an earlier stage of selective attention that moderate executive functioning. Early selection of goal-relevant stimuli diminishes the need for executive functioning to screen out distracting stimuli. Additionally, the psychopathic individual's obliviousness to peripheral information may interfere with recognizing the importance of engaging executive functions to regulate maladaptive responses. Thus, despite what appears to be a normal capacity for executive functioning, psychopathy may often appear to display both superior executive functioning (when early selection obviates the need for utilizing executive functions) and executive functioning deficits (when the need to employ executive functions has not been registered). Paralleling our review of attentional abnormalities, the literature on executive functioning highlights important distinctions between psychopathy and externalizing.

Emotion

Emotion is central to the variety of human experiences. It exerts a powerful influence on behavior, decision making, and reasoning. Here too, however, there is reason to believe that the contributions of emotion to the disinhibited behavior of psychopathic and externalizing individuals are different.

The disinhibited behavior of individuals with psychopathy has most often been understood in the context of the low-fear model (Lykken, 1957). In line with this view, individuals with psychopathy display poor fear conditioning (Lykken, 1957), minimal autonomic arousal (i.e., electrodermal response) in anticipation of aversive events (e.g., loud noises, electric shocks; Hare, 1978), and problems learning to inhibit punished responses (Newman & Kosson, 1986). Additionally, and arguably the most cited evidence of psychopathy-related affective deficits, is the fact that individuals with psychopathy display emotion-modulated startle deficits in picture-viewing paradigms (Patrick, Bradley, & Lang, 1993). In contrast to controls, who display greater startle responses to noise probes while viewing unpleasant versus neutral pictures, this startle potentiation appears to be lacking in participants with psychopathy (see Patrick, 1994). However, this deficit appears to be time-limited. Specifically, those with psychopathy display

startle potentiation deficits when probes are presented shortly after picture onset (e.g., 1.5 seconds), but they display normal emotion-modulated startle when probes are presented later in the picture-viewing interval (e.g., 4 seconds; Levenston, Patrick, Bradley, & Lang, 2000). The restricted nature of the emotion-modulated startle deficit may suggest that a fundamental deficit in the defensive response is not completely accurate and that the processes governing picture viewing in individuals with psychopathy are more complex (see Newman & Baskin-Sommers, 2011, for an attention-related explanation of this finding).

Consistent with the emotion-modulated startle deficit, there is also preliminary evidence that those with psychopathy display less amygdala activation than controls in several domains: aversive conditioning, moral decision making, social cooperation, and memory for emotionally salient words (Birbaumer et al., 2005; Glenn, Raine, & Schug, 2009; Kiehl et al., 2001; Rilling et al., 2007). However, other studies indicate that the amygdala is hyperreactive when individuals with psychopathy view certain emotionally salient information (Muller et al., 2003).

In contrast to the typically hyporeactive affective style in psychopathy, externalizing is more often associated with hyperreactivity to affective cues. In approach/motivation contexts, such as reward or drug seeking, externalizing individuals are characterized by reward hypersensitivity (Buckholtz et al., 2010; Endres, Rickert, Bogg, Lucas & Finn, 2011; Martin & Potts, 2004; Volkow & Li, 2004). For example, impulsive individuals choose immediate rewards over larger delayed rewards (Martin & Potts, 2004). Substance-dependent individuals perform poorly on the Iowa Gambling Task, preferring larger immediate payoffs despite their association with periodic costly punishments that ultimately result in a net loss (Bechara, 2001). Consistent with the assumption that drug cues are rewarding to substance-dependent individuals, they also show increased heart rate and sweat-gland activity in response to drug-related cues in cue reactivity paradigms (Carter & Tiffany, 1999).

In the presence of reward incentives, neurotic extraverts (traits associated with externalizing) commit more passive avoidance errors than introverts do (Newman, Widom, & Nathan, 1985) and fail to pause following punished errors (Nichols & Newman, 1986). On the surface this seems similar to the findings reported above for offenders with psychopathy; however, research suggests that the passive avoidance deficit in neurotic extraverts is mediated by reward sensitivity, whereas the psychopathy effect is not (Newman et al., 1990; Patterson et al., 1987). These findings suggest that externalizing traits may be associated with a fundamental hypersensitivity to rewards.

Importantly, externalizing-related hyperreactivity is not limited to reward contexts. Evidence also shows increased skin conductance and heart rate in response to stressful events (Taylor, Carlson, Iacono, Lykken, & McGue, 1999; Verona, Patrick, & Lang, 2002). These findings suggest that the emotional hyperactivity displayed by externalizing individuals may not be specific to reward, but rather a more general hypersensitivity to motivationally significant information.

A very clear difference in affective response styles between psychopathic and externalizing individuals becomes apparent. Simply put, psychopathic individuals are hyporeactive to emotion information, whereas externalizing individuals are hyperreactive. However, this simple statement can be criticized for being both too specific and not specific enough. For example, as noted above, evidence suggests that the psychopathy-related affective deficit is moderated by attention. In externalizing, there is evidence that both attentional and executive function processes influence affective responding. Thus, focusing on a single deficit (i.e., just emotion, just attention, just executive function) cannot fully capture the process-level dysfunctions that result in behavioral disinhibition.

Integrative Model: The Importance of Cognition–Emotion Interactions

The above review highlights many important research findings related to psychopathy and externalizing. In both syndromes there is evidence that dysfunction at the level of attention, executive function, and/or affect contribute to disinhibition. Moreover,

it appears that psychopathy and externalizing are related to divergent patterns of dysfunction. However, within the research on both syndromes, there is a tendency to focus on one specific process. Of course, though, these processes do not operate in a vacuum. There is a wealth of existing research suggesting that attention, executive function, and affect are interrelated processes. Dysfunction associated with any one component may disrupt processing associated with any other component. Understanding how these processes affect each other is too important to ignore, and ultimately it is the relationships (i.e., interactions) among these processes that determine the specific behavior problems related to these distinct syndromes. To the extent that we can distinguish the predisposing cognition–emotion interactions associated with these syndromes and conceptualize their impact on behavior, we are poised to unravel the problem of disinhibitory psychopathology.

Toward this end, we outline an integrative model (Figure 27.2) to illustrate how attention, executive functioning, and affect are interrelated and how the consequences of dysfunction at one process level may affect function at another process level. We believe that this model has a number of advantages. First, it moves away from the typical unitary focus and emphasizes the need for considering multiple processes when attempting to understand disinhibition. Second, it provides a framework for identifying a controlling variable that may initiate the cascade of process-level dysfunction that ultimately results in behavioral disinhibition. The notion of a controlling variable may seem ironic as we propose a movement away from the unitary process approach. However, identifying a controlling variable does not mean that it is the only process needed to understand a person's disinhibitory psychopathology. Rather, this approach provides an opportunity to clarify the impact of interrelated processes on disinhibition. For each syndrome, the model helps us elucidate the multiple interacting influences and specify the divergent pathways that culminate in disinhibited behavior.

As described above, psychopathy is associated with emotional hyporeactivity, an early attention bottleneck, and nonspecific anomalies in executive functions. We propose that the attention bottleneck is the distinctive controlling variable in psychopathy-related disinhibition (Figure 27.2). This is not to deny that psychopathy is often associated with executive function and emotion processing anomalies. However, these anomalies may be usefully understood as a consequence of an early attention bottleneck. Once the bottleneck is established, it blocks the processing of secondary information that is not goal-relevant. Thus, individuals with psychopathy are oblivious to a variety of potentially important stimuli unless they are a central aspect of their prepotent focus of attention. To the extent that the bottleneck filters information at an early

stage of attention, executive functioning is essentially circumvented, as there are fewer perceived conflicts and thus fewer demands for executive control. Of note, we have found that the psychopathy-related deficits in passive avoidance learning, conflict monitoring, electrodermal activity, FPS, and amygdala activation may all be made to appear and disappear in laboratory contexts as a function of experimental manipulations that control the focus of attention. The central role of attention in influencing psychopathic responses across experimental contexts highlights its role as a controlling variable in psychopathy. This understanding of the cognition–emotion interactions

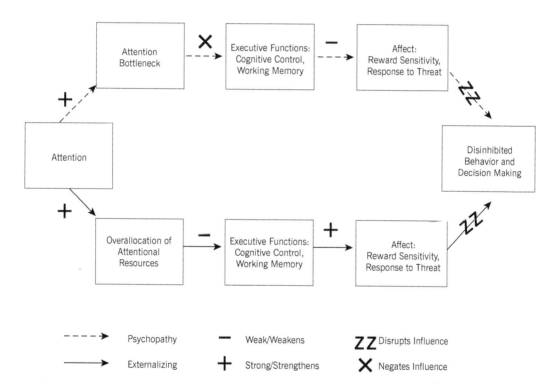

FIGURE 27.2. Integrative model of cognition–emotion interactions in psychopathy and externalizing. First, externalizing (solid line) involves an overallocation of attentional resources, which in turn impairs executive functions that normally moderate responding, including inhibition, shifting, and control, and results in dysregulated affective responses and behavioral disinhibition. Second, psychopathy (dashed line) is best characterized by an early attention bottleneck that disrupts the processing of information, particularly when it is peripheral to the primary goal. To the extent that the bottleneck filters information at an early stage of attention, executive functioning is essentially circumvented, as there are fewer conflicts or cognitive demands. Nevertheless, strong executive functioning reinforces the early attention bottleneck (Baskin-Sommers, Curtin, & Newman, 2011). Moreover, to the extent that affective information is not the main focus of attention, it receives little or no attention and has minimal impact on behavior. This disrupted influence on behavior and decision making ultimately results in the disinhibited expression of prepotent or dominant responses.

characterizing psychopathy not only provides an integrative context for understanding laboratory-based findings, but may also provide a better context for conceptualizing the often cold-hearted behavior of individuals with psychopathy.

The behavior of psychopathic individuals is highly paradoxical. Their behavior is often deliberate, yet, at times they can be quite impulsive and have little perspective on how their behavior affects themselves and others. This is evident in the strong association between psychopathy and instrumental aggression (i.e., aggression that is deliberate and goal-directed; Blair, 2001) and premeditated murder (i.e. Woodworth & Porter, 2002). Although an attention bottleneck may allow individuals with psychopathy to be more effective at filtering out distraction and focusing narrowly on personal goals (i.e., deliberateness of behavior), it may also leave them vulnerable to overallocating attention to goal-relevant cues at the expense of processing other context-relevant information (i.e., impulsivity of behavior). This inflexible focus on personal goals may also underlie the self-centered, callous traits associated with psychopathy. More generally, a deficit in the ability to process multiple aspects of a situation may leave individuals with psychopathy oblivious to the potentially devastating consequences (i.e., the distress response of others) of their behavior. Given this attentional perspective, it is interesting to speculate that the harmful behavior of individuals with psychopathy (e.g., instrumental aggression, fraud) may not reflect innate callousness. Rather, they are callously oblivious to information that is not directly and immediately related to their goal. That is, psychopathic individuals' abnormal cognition–emotion interaction, guided by an abnormal attention bottleneck, may effectively preclude response inhibition, conflict monitoring, affective processing, and self-regulation.

In contrast to psychopathy, the process-level dysfunctions in externalizing appear best characterized by an overallocation of attentional resources (i.e., late selective attention), deficits in executive functions, and hyperemotionality. At this time, determining which of these processes is the controlling variable in externalizing-related disinhibition is less clear-cut than it is for psychopathy. Relatively few studies have systematically attempted to disambiguate whether it is emotional hyperreactivity, attention, or executive function that is the controlling variable in externalizing disinhibition. However, one scenario that seems to be associated with many of the externalizing findings may be that the overallocation of limited capacity processing resources to salient stimuli exacerbates emotional reactions and consequently decreases cognitive resources available for processing subsequent stimuli (Figure 27.2). That is, when expecting motivationally significant/salient information, externalizing individuals overallocate attentional resources, which in turn may also impair executive functions that normally moderate responding, including inhibition, shifting, and control. Ultimately, the impact of information on behavior will depend on the application of resources associated with executive function, but the proposed model suggests that these downstream executive function effects in the dysfunctional cascade begin with an overallocation of resources at the attentional stage. Although novel and speculative at this time, this proposal is consistent with the strong attentional orienting to salient cues, dysfunction in identifying T2 stimuli in the attentional blink task, difficulty classifying rare or unexpected stimuli in the oddball task, and problems shifting focus to inhibit drug craving and violent responses of externalizing individuals. Moreover, much like in psychopathy, this unique understanding of the interactions between cognition and emotion in externalizing may provide a more nuanced understanding for why individuals with this behavioral disinhibition behave the way they do.

Externalizing individuals are reactive in their behavior and tend to let emotions get the best of them. As such, these individuals are prone to excessive reward (e.g., monetary) seeking, reactive aggression (i.e., aggression often in response to frustration or threat), and other strong urges (e.g., drug cravings) that overwhelm their inhibitory controls (i.e., executive functions). Describing individuals with such problems, Skeem and colleagues (2004) note that they are "anxious, emotionally volatile, hostile, and impulsive, and they are heavy substance abusers" (p. 399). Thus, unlike psychopathic individuals, externalizing individuals, do not engage in disinhibited behavior (i.e., gambling, substance use reactive aggression) because of intentional premeditated goals or obliviousness to the drawbacks associated with these behaviors. Rather, they may be disinhibited because of an inability to engage in cognitive control under affectively charged circumstances, stemming from an overcommitment of attentional resources to motivationally salient information (e.g., a drug, a threat), resulting in affective hyper-reactivity (e.g., substance use, aggression). Although more research needs to be done to support this point of view, ultimately, the behavior of externalizing individuals is clearly a function of abnormal cognition–emotion interactions, rather than a deficit in a single process that hampers effective self-regulation.

The purpose of outlining an integrative model for characterizing crucial cognition–emotion interactions in psychopathy and externalizing is to specify the dysfunctional processes that contribute to each syndrome and understand how these processes form a network that culminates in distinct patterns of disinhibition. In addition to confirming that they are different syndromes, the unique empirical and behavioral correlates of psychopathy and externalizing highlight their distinct and complex cognitive–affective deficits. Moreover, the specification of these distinct interactions may aid in the development of targeted intervention and treatment programs to address the dysfunctional processes.

Treatment

To date, many of the canonical behavioral and cognitive treatments for disinhibitory psychopathology have proven ineffective, particularly in cases of psychopathy. Individuals with externalizing disorders are usually perceived as resistant to treatment, especially psychotherapy. Moreover, individuals with alcohol dependence and antisocial features have significantly worse outcomes in treatment than those without these features (Compton, Cottler, Jacobs, Ben-Abdallah, & Spitznagel, 2003). For those with psychopathy, it has been proposed that "popular prison treatment and socialization

programs may actually make psychopaths worse than they were before. . . . Group therapy and insight-oriented programs help psychopaths develop better ways of manipulating, deceiving and using people but do little to help them understand themselves" (Hare, 2006, p. 717). Supporting this notion, not only are individuals with psychopathy more likely to reoffend, but after treatment they reoffend at a higher rate and more violently than nontreated individuals with psychopathy (Hughes, Hughes, Hollin, & Champion, 1997; Ogloff, Wong, & Greenwood, 1990; O'Neil, Lidz, & Heilbrun, 2003; Rice, Harris, & Cormier, 1992). Nonetheless, with advancing knowledge regarding cognition–emotion interactions that undermine the ability of psychopathic and externalizing individuals to self-regulate, new treatment options are on the horizon (Hare & Neumann; 2009; Skeem, Poythress, Edens, Lilienfeld, & Cale, 2003; Wallace & Newman, 2004; Wallace, Schmitt, Vitale, & Newman, 2000; Wallace, Vitale, & Newman, 1999).

Among those treatment possibilities being explored currently is that of cognitive remediation. *Cognitive remediation* refers to an approach that trains the individual in particular cognitive skills, such as paying attention to contextual cues, applying working memory, and sustaining attention (Klingberg, 2010; Wykes & Van der Gaag, 2001). In healthy adults, Klingberg and colleagues have shown that working memory training not only improves overall working memory capacity, but also changes the functioning of dopamine neurotransmission and brain plasticity (McNab et al., 2009). Research on disorders with known cognitive abnormalities, such as attention-deficit/hyperactivity disorder and schizophrenia, has begun to assess the efficacy of cognitive remediation as a treatment strategy (Stevenson, Whitmont, Bornholt, Livesey, & Stevenson, 2002; Wykes et al., 2003). For example, the application of working memory training has demonstrated durable improvement in memory (Wykes et al., 2007).

Given the dysfunctional cognition–emotion interactions associated with externalizing and psychopathy, it may be possible to develop cognitive remediation treatments that target the specific deficits of these individuals. Thus, as seen in McNab and colleagues (2009), with explicit practice and skill building in attentional selection, executive functioning, and reactivity to affective information, improvement in these functions may be reflected in brain-related measures and ultimately behavior.

Externalizing individuals are overreactive to affective and motivationally salient information and have poor executive function capabilities. For example, a training task that focuses on exposure to distressing cues and requires executive functions to regulate responses and emotional reactivity might be quite effective. Along this line, distress tolerance tasks, such as the paced auditory serial addition test (PASAT), provide a means to measure performance and, over time, improvement on difficult or frustrating cognitive tasks (Zvolensky, Vujanovic, Bernstein, & Leyro, 2010). Preliminary evidence suggests that the latency of task engagement on the PASAT predicts the ability to maintain substance use abstinence (Daughters et al., 2005).

Individuals with psychopathy are oblivious to affective, inhibitory, and punishment cues (Newman & Kosson, 1986) that contraindicate ongoing goal-directed behavior (i.e., mismatch information; Baskin-Sommers et al., 2010; Hiatt et al., 2004; Newman et al., 2010). Although the possibility has yet to be directly investigated, it is plausible that tasks that emphasize balancing attention between primary and peripheral information (i.e., affective and neutral) and paying attention to rule changes may induce changes in specific attentional pathways that are associated with attention to contextual information—and thereby reduce the disinhibited behavior of individuals with psychopathy. Corroborating this idea is evidence from work with the card perseveration task (Newman et al., 1987). Under typical conditions, individuals with psychopathy selected significantly more cards at the expense of losing more money. However, in another condition, in which participants were forced to pause 5 seconds before selecting the next card, individuals with psychopathy did not display a disinhibited response style and performed like nonpsychopathic individuals. Thus, when individuals with psychopathy were forced to stop and reflect, there was a change in the quality of their decision making.

In fact, Newman and collaborators have designed cognitive–affective interventions that are believed to target the specific cognitive, affective, decision-making, and self-regulation deficits associated with externalizing and psychopathy, respectively. The potential advantage of such treatment is that it is based on an etiological theory that targets the unique deficits associated with externalizing and psychopathy.

Closing Remarks

The concept of equifinality is used in relation to syndromes involving similar phenotypic expressions (e.g., violence, impulsivity, substance abuse), but which appear to reflect different etiological/developmental pathways. In this regard, it is noteworthy that cognitive–affective accounts of externalizing and psychopathy appear to be relatively distinct. Based on existing evidence, externalizing-related disinhibition involves affective hyperreactivity, a tendency to overallocate attention toward motivationally salient information (e.g., threat, rewards, drug cues), and a deficit in executive functions (e.g., cognitive control, inhibition, working memory). Ultimately, the cascade of events results in behavioral as well as emotional dysregulation. Alternatively, for psychopathy, we propose that this form of disinhibition stems from an early attention bottleneck that precludes the processing of peripheral information, including affective information, resulting in a myopic perspective on goal-directed behavior and poor decision making.

Externalizing and psychopathy are behaviorally similar disorders associated with etiologically distinct pathways. Although the general processes associated with these pathways may be discussed using similar terms (e.g., *attention, executive function*, and *affective dysfunction*), it is clear that they function differently in each and combine to produce two relatively distinct syndromes. It is important for future research to keep these multifaceted relationships (i.e., cognition–emotion interactions) in mind and work toward a specified understanding of the diverse pathways to disinhibition. Moreover, with regard to disinhibitory psychopathology more generally, understanding these cognition–emotion interactions will aid in working toward specified treatment and prevention programs.

References

Arnett, P. A., Smith, S. S., & Newman, J. P. (1997). Approach and avoidance motivation in incarcerated psychopaths during passive avoidance. *Journal of Personality and Social Psychology, 72*, 1413–1428.

Ávila, C., & Parcet, M. A. (2001). Personality and inhibitory deficits in the stop-signal task: The mediating role of Gray's anxiety and impulsivity. *Personality and Individual Differences, 29*, 975–986.

Banfield, J., Wyland, C. L., Macrae, C. N., Munte, T. F., & Heatherton, T. F. (2004). The cognitive neuroscience of self-regulation. In R. F. Baumeister & K. D. Vohs (Eds.), *The handbook of self-regulation* (pp. 62–83.) New York: Guilford Press.

Baskin-Sommers, A. R., Curtin, J. J., & Newman, J. P. (2011). Specifying the attentional selection that moderates the fearlessness of psychopathic offenders. *Psychological Science, 22*, 226–234.

Baskin-Sommers, A. R., Curtin, J. J, Larson, C. L., Stout, D, Kiehl, K., & Newman, J. P. (2012). Characterizing the anomalous cognition-emotion interactions in externalizing. *Biological Psychology, 911*, 48–58.

Baskin-Sommers, A. R., Wallace, J., MacCoon, D., Curtin, J., & Newman, J. (2010). Clarifying the factors that undermine behavioral inhibition system functioning in psychopathy. *Personality Disorders: Theory, Research, and Treatment, 1*, 203–217.

Bechara, A. (2001). Neurobiology of decision making: Risk and reward. *Seminars in Clinical Neuropsychiatry 6*, 205–216.

Bechara, A., Damasio, H., Tranel, D., & Damasio, A. R. (1997). Deciding advantageously before knowing the advantageous strategy. *Science, 275*, 1293–1295.

Benning, S. D., Patrick, C. J., Blonigen, D. M., Hicks, B. M., & Iacono, W. G. (2005). Estimating facets of psychopathy from normal personality traits: A step toward community-epidemiological investigations. *Assessment, 12*, 3–18.

Bernat, E. M., Nelson, L. D., Steele, V., Gehrig, W. J., & Patrick, C. J. (2011). Externalizing psychopathology and gain/loss feedback in

a simulated gambling task: Dissociable components of brain response revealed by time–frequency analysis. *Journal of Abnormal Psychology, 120*, 352–364.

Birbaumer, N., Veit, R., Lotze, M., Erb, M., Christiane, H., Grodd, W., et al. (2005). Fear conditioning in psychopathy: A functional magnetic resonance imaging study. *Archives of General Psychiatry, 62*, 799–805.

Blair, K. S., Newman, C. C., Mitchell, D. G. V., Richell, R. A., Leonard, A., Morton, J., et al. (2006). Differentiating among prefrontal substrates in psychopathy: Neuropsychological test findings. *Neuropsychology, 20*, 153–165.

Blair, R. J. R. (2001). Neuro-cognitive models of aggression, the antisocial personality disorders, and psychopathy. *Journal of Neurology, Neurosurgery, and Psychiatry, 71*, 727–731.

Blair, R. J. R., & Mitchell, D. V. G. (2009). Psychopathy, attention, and emotion. *Psychological Medicine, 39*, 543–555.

Botvinick, M., Braver, T., Barch, D., Carter, C., & Cohen, J. (2001). Conflict monitoring and cognitive control. *Psychological Review, 108*, 624–652.

Botvinick, M. M., Cohen, J. D., Carter, C. S. (2004). Conflict monitoring and anterior cingulate cortex: An update. *Trends in Cognitive Science, 8*, 539–546.

Brazil, I. A., de Bruijn, E. R. A., Bulten, B. H., von Borries, A. K. L., van Lankveld, J. J. M., Buitelaar, J. K., et al. (2009). Early and late components of error-monitoring in violent offenders with psychopathy. *Biological Psychiatry, 65*, 137–143.

Brinkley, C. A., Schmitt, W. A., & Newman, J. P. (2005). Semantic processing in psychopathic offenders. *Personality and Individual Differences, 38*, 1047–1056.

Buckholtz, J. W., Treadway, M. T., Cowan, R. L., Woodward, N. D., Li, R., Ansari, M. S. (2010). Dopaminergic network differences in human impulsivity. *Science, 329*, 532.

Budhani, S., Richell, R. A., & Blair, R. J. (2006). Impaired reversal but intact acquisition: Probabilistic response reversal deficits in adult individuals with psychopathy. *Journal of Abnormal Psycholology, 115*, 552–558.

Carter, B. L., & Tiffany, S. T. (1999). Meta-analysis of cue reactivity in addiction research. *Addiction, 94*, 327–340.

Compton, W. M., III, Cottler, L. B., Jacobs, J. L., Ben-Abdallah, A., & Spitznagel, E. L. (2003). The role of psychiatric disorders in predicting drug dependence treatment outcomes. *American Journal of Psychiatry, 60,* 890–895.

Corbetta, M., Miezin, F. M., Dobmeyer, S., Shulman, G. L., & Petersen, S. E. (1991). Selective and divided attention during visual discriminations of shape, color, and speed: Functional anatomy by positron emission tomography. *Journal of Neuroscience, 11,* 2383–2402.

Corbetta, M., Patel, G., & Shulman, G. L. (2008). The reorienting system of the human brain: From environment to theory of mind. *Neuron, 58,* 306–324.

Costa, L., Bauer, L., Kuperman, S., Porjesz, B., O'Connor, S., Hesselbrock, V., et al. (2000). Frontal P300 decrements, alcohol dependence, and antisocial personality disorder. *Biological Psychiatry, 47,* 1064–1071.

Daughters, S. B., Lejuez, C. W., Bornovalova, M. A., Kahler, C. W., Strong, D. R., & Brown, R. A. (2005). Distress tolerance as a predictor of early treatment dropout in a residential substance abuse treatment facility. *Journal of Abnormal Psychology, 114,* 729–734.

Davidson, R. J., Pizzagalli, D., Nitschke, J. B., & Kalin, N. H. (2003). Parsing the subcomponents of emotion and disorders of emotion: Perspectives from affective neuroscience. In R. J. Davidson, K. R. Scherer, & H. H. Goldsmith (Eds.), *Handbook of affective sciences* (pp. 8–24). New York: Oxford University Press.

Dehaene, S., Posner, M. I., & Tucker, D. M. (1994). Localization of a neural system for error detection and compensation. *Psychological Science, 5,* 303–305.

Derryberry, D., & Reed, M. A. (1994). Temperament and attention: Orienting toward and away from positive and negative signals. *Journal of Personality and Social Psychology, 66,* 1128–1139.

Deveney, C. M., & Pizzagalli, D. A. (2008). The cognitive consequences of emotion regulation: An ERP investigation. *Psychophysiology, 45,* 435–444.

Dolan, S. L., Bechara, A., & Nathan, P. E. (2008). Executive dysfunction as a risk marker for substance abuse: The role of impulsive personality traits. *Behavioral Sciences and the Law, 26,* 799–822.

Driver, J. (2001). A selective review of selective attention research from the past century. *British Journal of Psychology, 92,* 53–78.

Duncan, J. (1980). The locus of interference in the perception of simultaneous stimuli. *Psychological Review, 87,* 272–300.

Dvorak-Bertsch, J. D., Sadeh, N., Glass, S. J., Thornton, D., & Newman, J. P. (2007). Stroop tasks associated with differential activation of anterior cingulate do not differentiate psychopathic and non-psychopathic offenders. *Personality and Individual Differences, 42,* 585–595.

Endres, M. J., Rickert, M. E., Bogg, T., Lucas, J., & Finn, P. R. (2011). Externalizing psychopathology and behavioral disinhibition: Working memory mediates signal discriminability and reinforcement moderates response bias in approach–avoidance learning. *Journal of Abnormal Psychology, 120,* 336–351.

Gao, Y., & Raine, A. (2009). P3 event-related potential impairments in anti-social and psychopathic individuals: A meta-analysis. *Biological Psychology, 82,* 199–210.

Gehring, W. J., & Knight, R. T. (2000). Prefrontal–cingulate interactions in action monitoring. *Nature Neuroscience, 3,* 516–520.

Giancola, P. R., & Tarter, R. E. (1999). Executive cognitive functioning and risk for substance abuse. *Psychological Science, 10,* 203–205.

Glenn, A. L., Raine, A., & Schug, R. A. (2009). The neural correlates of moral decision-making in psychopathy. *Molecular Psychiatry, 14,* 5–6.

Gorenstein, E. E., & Newman, J. P. (1980). Disinhibitory psychopathology: A new perspective and a model for research. *Psychological Review, 87,* 301–315.

Grillon, C., Ameli, R., Goddard, A., Woods, S. W., & Davis, M. (1994). Baseline and fear-potentiated startle in panic disorder patients. *Biological Psychiatry 35,* 431–439.

Hall, R. J., Bernat, E. M., & Patrick, C. J. (2007). Externalizing psychopathology and the error-related negativity. *Psychological Science, 18,* 326–333

Hare, R. D. (1978). Electrodermal and cardiovascular correlates of psychopathy. In R. D. Hare & D. Schalling (Eds.), *Psychopathic behavior: Approaches to research* (pp. 107–143). Chichester, UK: Wiley.

Hare, R. D. (2003). *Manual for the Hare Psychopathy Checklist—Revised* (2nd ed.). Toronto: Multi-Health Systems.

Hare, R. D. (2006). Psychopathy: A clinical and forensic overview. *Psychiatric Clinics of North America, 29,* 709–724.

Hare, R. D., & Neumann, C. S. (2009). Psychopathy: Assessment and forensic implications. *Canadian Journal of Psychiatry, 54,* 791–802.

Hart, S. D., Forth, A. H., & Hare, R. D. (1990). Performance of criminal psychopaths on selected neuropsychological tests. *Journal of Abnormal Psychology, 99,* 374–379.

Hiatt, K. D., Schmitt, W. A., & Newman, J. P. (2004). Stroop tasks reveal abnormal selective attention among psychopathic offenders. *Neuropsychology, 18,* 50–59.

Hornak, J., O'Doherty, J., Bramham, J., Rolls, E. T., Morris, R. G., Bullock, P. R., et al. (2004). Reward-related reversal learning after surgical excisions in orbito-frontal or dorsolateral prefrontal cortex in humans. *Journal of Cognitive Neuroscience, 16,* 463–478.

Hughes, G., Hughes, T., Hollin, C., & Champion, H. (1997). First-stage evaluation of a treatment programme for personality disordered offenders. *Journal of Forensic Psychiatry, 8,* 515–527.

Iacono, W. G., Malone, S. M., & McGue, M. (2008). Behavioral disinhibition and the development of early-onset addiction: Common and specific influences. *Annual Review of Clinical Psychology, 4,* 325–348.

Jutai, J. W., & Hare, R. D. (1983). Psychopathy and selective attention during performance of a complex perceptual-motor task. *Psychophysiology, 20,* 146–151.

Jutai, J. W., Hare, R. D., & Connolly, J. F. (1987). Psychopathy and event-related brain potentials (ERPs) associated with attention to speech stimuli. *Personality and Individual Differences, 8,* 175–184.

Keil, A., Bradley, M. M., Junghöfer, M., Russmann, T., Lowenthal, W., & Lang, P. J. (2007). Cross-modal attention capture by affective stimuli: Evidence from event-related potentials. *Cognitive, Affective, and Behavioral Neuroscience, 7,* 18–24.

Kiehl, K. A., Hare, R. D., McDonald, J. J., & Brink, J. (1999). Semantic and affective processing in psychopaths: An event-related potential (ERP) study. *Psychophysiology, 36,* 765–774.

Kiehl, K. A., Smith, A. M., Hare, R. D., & Liddle, P. F. (2000). An event-related potential investigation of response inhibition in schizophrenia and psychopathy. *Biological Psychiatry, 48,* 210–221.

Kiehl, K. A., Smith, A. M., Hare, R. D., Mendrek, A., Forster, B. B., Brink, J., et al. (2001). Limbic abnormalities in affective processing by criminal psychopaths as revealed by functional magnetic resonance imaging. *Biological Psychiatry, 50,* 677–684.

Klingberg, T. (2010). Training and plasticity of working memory. *Trends in Cognitive Science, 14,* 317–324.

Krueger, R. F., Hicks, B. M., Patrick, C. J., Carlson, S. R., Iacono, W. G., & McGue, M. (2002). Etiologic connections among substance dependence, antisocial behavior, and personality: Modeling the externalizing spectrum. *Journal of Abnormal Psychology, 111,* 411–424.

Krueger, R. F., Markon, K. E., Patrick, C. J., Benning, S. D., & Kramer, M. D. (2007). Linking antisocial behavior, substance use, and personality: An integrative quantitative model of the adult externalizing spectrum. *Journal of Abnormal Psychology, 116*(4), 645–666.

Krueger, R. F., Markon, K. E., Patrick, C. J., & Iacono, W. G. (2005). Externalizing psychopathology in adulthood: A dimensional–spectrum conceptualization and its implications for DSM-V. *Journal of Abnormal Psychology, 114,* 537–550.

Larson, C. L., Baskin-Sommers, A. R., Stout, D. M., Balderson, N. L., Curtin, J. J., Schultz, D. H., et al. (2012). *The interplay of attention and emotion: Top-down attention modulates amygdala activation in psychopathy.* Manuscript submitted for publication.

Levenston, G. K., Patrick, C. J., Bradley, M. M., & Lang, P. J. (2000). The psychopath as observer: Emotion and attention in picture processing. *Journal of Abnormal Psychology, 109,* 373–385.

Lösel, F., & Schmucker, M. (2004). Psychopathy, risk taking, and attention: A differentiated test of the somatic marker hypothesis. *Journal of Abnormal Psychology, 113,* 522–529.

Luck, S. J., & Hillyard, S. A. (1999). The operation of selective attention at multiple stages of processing: Evidence from human and monkey electrophysiology. In M. S. Gazzaniga (Ed.), *The new cognitive neurosciences* (2nd ed., pp. 687–700). Cambridge, MA: MIT Press.

Lykken, D. T. (1957). A study of anxiety in the sociopathic personality. *Journal of Abnormal and Social Psychology, 55,* 6–10.

Lykken, D. T. (1995). *The antisocial personalities.* Hilldale, NJ: Erlbaum.

MacCoon, D. G., Wallace, J. F., & Newman, J. P. (2004). Self-regulation: Context-appropriate balanced attention. In R. F. Baumeister & K. D. Vohs (Eds.), *Handbook of self-regulation: Research, theory, and applications* (pp. 422–444). New York: Guilford Press.

MacLeod, C. M. (1998). Training on integrated

versus separated Stroop tasks: The progression of interference and facilitation. *Memory and Cognition, 26,* 201–211.

Martin, L. E., & Potts, G. F. (2004). Reward sensitivity in impulsivity. *NeuroReport, 15*(9), 1519–1522.

McNab, F., Varrone, A., Farde, L., Jucaite, A., Bystritsky, P., Forssberg, H., et al. (2009). Changes in cortical dopamine D1 receptor binding associated with cognitive training. *Science, 323,* 800–802.

Mitchell, D. G., Colledge, E., Leonard, A., & Blair, R. J. (2002). Risky decisions and response reversal: Is there evidence of orbitofrontal cortex dysfunction in psychopathic individuals? *Neuropsychologia, 40,* 2013–2022.

Mitchell, D. G., Richell, R. A., Leonard, A., & Blair, R. J. R. (2006). Emotion at the expense of cognition: Psychopathic individuals outperform controls on an operant response task. *Journal of Abnormal Psychology, 115,* 559–566.

Morgan, A. B., & Lilienfeld, S. O. (2000). A meta-analytic review of the relation between antisocial behavior and neuropsychological measures of executive function. *Clinical Psychology Review, 20,* 113–136.

Muller, J. L., Sommer, M., Wagner, V., Lange, K., Taschler, H., Roder, C. H., et al. (2003). Abnormalities in emotion processing within cortical and subcortical regions in criminal psychopaths: Evidence from a functional magnetic resonance imaging study using pictures with emotional content. *Biological Psychiatry, 54,* 152–162.

Munro, G. E., Dywan, J., Harris, G. T., McKee, S., Unsal, A., & Segalowitz, S. J. (2007). ERN varies with degree of psychopathy in an emotion discrimination task. *Biological Psychology, 76,* 31–42.

Nelson, L. D., Patrick, C. J., & Bernat, E. M. (2011). Indexing externalizing psychopathology as a multivariate psychophysiological phenotype. *Psychophysiology, 48,* 64–73.

Neumann, C. S., & Hare, R. D. (2008). Psychopathic traits in a large community sample: Links to violence, alcohol use, and intelligence. *Journal of Consulting and Clinical Psychology, 76,* 893–899.

Newman, J. P. (1997). Conceptual models of the nervous system: Implications for antisocial behavior. In D. M. Stoff, J. Breiling, & J. D. Maser (Eds.), *Handbook of antisocial behavior* (pp. 324–335). New York: Wiley.

Newman, J. P. (1998). Psychopathic behavior: An information processing perspective. In D. J. Cooke, R. D. Hare, & A. Forth (Eds.), *Psychopathy: Theory, research and implications for society* (pp. 81–104). Amsterdam: Kluwer.

Newman, J. P., & Baskin-Sommers, A. R. (2011). Early selective attention abnormalities in psychopathy: Implications for self-regulation. In M. I. Posner (Ed.), *Cognitive neuroscience of attention* (2nd ed., pp. 421–440). New York: Guilford Press.

Newman, J. P., Curtin, J. J., Bertsch, J. D., & Baskin-Sommers, A. R. (2010). Attention moderates the fearlessness of psychopathic offenders. *Biological Psychiatry, 67,* 66–70.

Newman, J. P., & Kosson, D. S. (1986). Passive avoidance learning in psychopathic and nonpsychopathic offenders. *Journal of Abnormal Psychology, 95,* 257–263.

Newman, J. P., & Lorenz, A. R. (2003). Response modulation and emotion processing: Implications for psychopathy and other dysregulatory psychopathology. In R. J. Davidson, K. Scherer, & H. H. Goldsmith (Eds.), *Handbook of affective sciences* (pp. 1043–1067). New York: Oxford University Press.

Newman, J. P., Patterson, C. M., Howland, E. W., & Nichols, S. L. (1990). Passive avoidance in psychopaths: The effects of reward. *Personality and Individual Differences, 11,* 1101–1114.

Newman, J. P., Patterson, C. M., & Kosson, D. S. (1987). Response perseveration in psychopaths. *Journal of Abnormal Psychology, 96,* 145–148.

Newman, J. P., Schmitt, W. A., & Voss, W. (1997). The impact of motivationally neutral cues on psychopathic individuals: Assessing the generality of the response modulation hypothesis. *Journal of Abnormal Psychology, 106,* 563–575.

Newman, J. P., Widom, C. S., & Nathan, S. (1985). Passive-avoidance in syndromes of disinhibition: Psychopathy and extraversion. *Journal of Personality and Social Psychology, 48,* 1316–1327.

Nichols, S., & Newman, J. P. (1986). Effects of punishment on response latency in extraverts. *Journal of Personality and Social Psychology, 50,* 624–630.

Ogloff, J., Wong, S., & Greenwood, A. (1990). Treating criminal psychopaths in a therapeutic community program. *Behavioral Sciences and the Law, 8,* 181–190.

O'Neil, M., Lidz, V., & Heilbrun, K. (2003). Adolescents with psychopathic characteristics in a substance abusing cohort: Treatment process and outcomes. *Law and Human Behavior, 27*, 299–313.

Patrick, C. J. (1994). Emotion and psychopathy: Startling new insights. *Psychophysiology, 31*, 319–330.

Patrick, C. J. (2007). Getting to the heart of psychopathy. In H. Herve & J. C. Yuille (Eds.), *The psychopath: Theory, research, and social implications* (pp. 207–252). Hillsdale, NJ: Erlbaum.

Patrick, C. J., Bernat, E., Malone, S. M., Iacono, W. G., Krueger, R. F., & McGue, M. K. (2006). P300 amplitude as an indicator of externalizing in adolescent males. *Psychophysiology, 43*, 84–92.

Patrick, C. J., Bradley, M. M., & Lang, P. J. (1993). Emotion in the criminal psychopath: Startle reflex modulation. *Journal of Abnormal Psychology, 102*, 82–92.

Patrick, C. J., Curtin, J. J., & Tellegen, A. (2002). Development and validation of a brief form of the Multidimensional Personality Questionnaire. *Psychological Assessment, 14*, 150–163.

Patrick, C. J., & Zempolich, K. A. (1998). Emotion and aggression in the psychopathic personality. *Aggression and Violent Behavior, 3*, 303–338.

Patrick, C. J., Zempolich, K. A., & Levenston, G. K. (1997). Emotionality and violent behavior in psychopaths: A biosocial analysis. In A. Raine, D. Farrington, P. Brennan, & S. A. Mednick (Eds.), *The biosocial bases of violence* (pp. 145–161). New York: Plenum Press.

Patterson, C. M., Kosson, D. S., & Newman, J. P. (1987). Reaction to punishment, reflectivity, and passive avoidance learning in extraverts. *Journal of Personality and Social Psychology, 52*, 565–576.

Patterson, C. M., & Newman, J. P. (1993). Reflectivity and learning from aversive events: Toward a psychological mechanism for the syndromes of disinhibition. *Psychological Review, 100*, 716–736.

Polich, J., Pollock, V. E., & Bloom, F. E. (1994). Meta-analysis of P300 amplitude from males at risk for alcoholism. *Psychological Bulletin, 115*, 55–73.

Poythress, N. G., & Hall, J. (2011). Psychopathy and impulsivity reconsidered. *Aggression and Violent Behavior, 16*, 120–134.

Pridmore, S., Chambers, A., & McArthur, M. (2005). Neuroimaging in psychopathy. *Australian and New Zealand Journal of Psychiatry, 39*, 856–865.

Raine, A., Lencz, T., Bihrle, S., LaCasse, L., & Colletti, P. (2000). Reduced prefrontal gray matter volume and reduced autonomic activity in antisocial personality disorder. *Archives of General Psychiatry, 57*, 119–127.

Raine, A., & Venables, P. H. (1988). Enhanced P3 evoked potentials and longer P3 recovery times in psychopaths. *Psychophysiology, 25*, 30–38.

Raine, A., Venable, P. H., & Williams, M. (1990). Relationships between N1, P300, and contingent negative variation recorded at age 15 and criminal behavior at age 24. *Psychophysiology, 27*, 567–74.

Rice, M., Harris, G., & Cormier, C. (1992). An evaluation of a maximum security therapeutic community for psychopaths and other mentally disordered offenders. *Law and Human Behavior, 16*, 399–412.

Rilling, J. K., Glenn, A. L., Jairam, M. R., Pagnoni, G., Goldsmith, D. R., Elfenbein, H. A., et al. (2007). Neural correlates of social cooperation and non-cooperation as a function of psychopathy. *Biological Psychiatry, 61*, 1260–1271.

Rueda, M. R., Posner, M. I., & Rothbart, M. K. (2005). The development of executive attention: Contributions to the emergence of self-regulation. *Developmental Neuropsychology, 28*, 573–594.

Schmitt, W. A., Brinkley, C. A., & Newman, J. P. (1999). Testing Damasio's somatic marker hypothesis with psychopathic individuals: Risk takers or risk averse? *Journal of Abnormal Psychology, 108*, 538–543.

Seguin, J. R. (2004). Neurocognitive elements of antisocial behavior: Relevance of an orbitofrontal cortex account. *Brain and Cognition, 55*, 185–197.

Skeem, J. L., Mulvey, E. P., Appelbaum, P., Banks, S., Grisso, T., Silver, E., et al. (2004). Identifying subtypes of civil psychiatric patients at high risk for violence. *Criminal Justice and Behavior, 31*, 392–437.

Skeem, J. L., Poythress, N., Edens, J. F., Lilienfled, S. O., & Cale, E. M. (2003). Psychopathic personality or personalities?: Exploring potential variants of psychopathy and their implications for risk assessment. *Aggression and Violent Behavior, 8*, 513–546.

Smith, S. S., Arnett, P. A., & Newman, J. P. (1992). Neuropsychological differentiation of psychopathic and nonpsychopathic criminal offenders. *Personality and Individual Differences, 13,* 1233–1245.

Smith, S. S., & Newman, J. P. (1990). Alcohol and drug abuse/dependence in psychopathic and nonpsychopathic criminal offenders. *Journal of Abnormal Psychology, 99,* 430–439.

Stevenson, C. S., Whitmont, S., Bornholt, L., Livesey, D., & Stevenson, R. J. (2002). A cognitive remediation programme for adults with attention deficit hyperactivity disorder. *Australian and New Zealand Journal of Psychiatry, 36,* 610–616.

Sutker, P. B., Moan, C. E., & Allain, A. N. (1983). Assessment of cognitive control in psychopathic and normal prisoners. *Journal of Behavioral Assessment, 5,* 275–287.

Taylor, J., Carlson, S. R., Iacono, W. G., Lykken, D. T., & McGue, M. (1999). Individual differences in electrodermal responsivity to predictable aversive stimuli and substance dependence. *Psychophysiology, 36,* 193–198.

Tiffany, S. T., & Conklin, C. A. (2000). A cognitive processing model of alcohol craving and compulsive alcohol use. *Addiction, 95,* 145–153.

Verona, E., Patrick, C. J., & Lang, A. R. (2002). A direct assessment of the role of state and trait negative emotion in aggressive behavior, *Journal of Abnormal Psychology, 111,* 249–258.

Vitale, J. E., Brinkley, C. A., Hiatt, K. D., & Newman, J. P. (2007). Abnormal selective attention in psychopathic female offenders. *Neuropsychology, 21,* 301–312.

Volkow, N. D., & Li, T. K. (2004). Drug addiction: The neurobiology of behavior gone awry. *Nature Reviews Neuroscience, 5,* 963–970.

Wallace, J. F., & Newman, J. P. (1997). Neuroticism and the attentional mediation of dysregulatory psychopathology. *Cognitive Therapy and Research, 21,* 135–156.

Wallace, J. F., & Newman, J. P. (2004). A theory-based treatment model for psychopathy. *Cognitive and Behavioral Practice, 11,* 178–189.

Wallace, J. R., Schmitt, W. A., Vitale, J. E., & Newman, J. P. (2000). Information processing deficiencies and psychopathy: Implications for diagnosis and treatment. In C. Gacono (Ed.),

The clinical and forensic assessment of psychopathy: A practitioner's guide (pp. 87–109). Mahwah, NJ: Erlbaum.

Wallace, J. F., Vitale, J. E., & Newman, J. P. (1999). Response modulation deficits: Implications for the diagnosis and treatment of psychopathy. *Journal of Cognitive Psychotherapy, 13,* 55–70.

Wolf, R. C., Carpenter, R. W., Warren, C. M., Zeier, J., Baskin-Sommers, A. R., & Newman, J. P. (2011). Reduced susceptibility to the attentional blink deficit in psychopathic offenders: Implications for the attentional bottleneck hypothesis. *Neuropsychology, 26,* 102–109.

Woodworth, M., & Porter, S. (2002). In cold blood: Characteristics of criminal homicides as a function of psychopathy. *Journal of Abnormal Psychology, 111,* 436–445.

Wykes, T., Reeder, C., Landau, S., Everitt, B., Knapp, M., Patel, A., et al. (2007). Cognitive remediation therapy in schizophrenia: Randomised controlled trial. *British Journal of Psychiatry, 190,* 421–427.

Wykes, T., Reeder, C., Williams, C., Corner, J., Rice, C., & Everitt, B. (2003). Are the effects of cognitive remediation therapy (CRT) durable?: Results from an exploratory trial in schizophrenia. *Schizophrenia Research, 61,* 163–174.

Wykes, T., & Van der Gaag, M. (2001). Is it time to develop a new cognitive therapy for psychosis?: Cognitive remediation therapy. *Clinical Psychological Review, 21,* 1227–1238.

Zeier, J. D., Maxwell, J. S., & Newman, J. P. (2009). Attention moderates the processing of inhibitory information in primary psychopathy. *Journal of Abnormal Psychology, 118,* 554–563.

Zuckerman, M. (1978). Sensation seeking and psychopathy. In R. D. Hare & D. Schalling (Eds.), *Psychopathic behavior: Approaches to research* (pp. 165–185). New York: Wiley.

Zvolensky, M. J., Vujanovic, A. A., Bernstein, A., & Leyro, T. (2010). Distress tolerance: Theory, measurement, and relations to psychopathology. *Current Directions in Psychological Science, 19,* 406–410.

CHAPTER 28

Cognition, Emotion, and the Construction of Meaning in Psychotherapy

Leslie S. Greenberg

Significant advances have taken place in understanding the role of emotion and cognition in psychotherapy since our first major presentation on the role of emotion in psychotherapy over two decades ago (Greenberg & Safran, 1987, 1989). Ever since the original debate between Zajonc (1980) and Lazarus (1982) on the primacy of affect, there has been an evolving recognition of the importance of emotion in psychological functioning. This is due in large part to compelling findings in the affective and cognitive neurosciences in the past two decades (e.g., Damasio, 1994, 2003; LeDoux, 1996, 2002) establishing that emotions are not secondary to cognition but a basic component of human functioning in their own right. This chapter reviews both the evolving understanding of the role of emotion and its relationship to cognition in human functioning and the evidence for the role of emotion in therapeutic change.

Emotions as an Adaptive Resource

Over the last decade the tide against the important role of emotions has clearly shifted and it has become clear that they are a fundamentally adaptive resource as opposed to something that needs to be got rid of via catharsis (Freud, 1895) or corrected by reason (Beck, 1976). Emotions involve an embodied meaning system that inform people of the significance of events to their well-being and that organize people for rapid adaptive action (Frijda, 1986; Izard, 1991; Oatley & Jenkins, 1992; Tomkins, 1963). Most theorists of human emotion today agree that emotions are an evolutionary-based adaptive meaning system that helps individuals to survive and function healthily (Ekman, 2003; Frijda, 1986; Izard, 1977; Oatley, Keltner, & Jenkins, 2006; Plutchik, 1980, 2000; Scherer, 2000). From birth on, emotion also is a primary signaling system that communicates intentions and regulates interaction (Sroufe, 1996). Emotion thus regulates self and other and gives life much of its meaning. With the advent of a view of emotion as an adaptive resource, the understanding of its relationship with cognition and its role in human functioning and psychotherapy has changed. This "new look" has begun to set a new agenda for psychological research: to determine under what conditions emotions play a determining role in human experience and how this occurs. The question of whether emotion precedes cognition, or vice versa, has been superseded by one asking under which conditions do emotions influence thought, or vice versa. It also is clear that the emotion versus cognition dichotomy is a false one because emotion is fused with cognition. The more relevant question, especially to psychotherapy, is, how does bodily felt emotional experience influence conscious thought in language?

Neurological Evidence on Affective Primacy

Research emerging from the arena of affective neuroscience supports the conceptualization of emotion and cognition as separate but interacting mental functions mediated by separate but interacting brain systems (LeDoux, 1996). LeDoux (1996) cites research demonstrating that it is possible for our brains to register the emotional meaning of a stimulus before that stimulus has been fully processed by the perceptual system. He also presents research findings that depict the relational interdependence of emotion and cognition in multiple connections between limbic cortices and the neocortex.

In relation to the debate on affective primacy, this work and other studies (Davis, 1989; LeDoux, 1990; Panksepp, Sacks, Crepeau, & Abbott, 1991; Thompson, 1986) suggest that the initial emotional processing of simple sensory features occurs extremely early in the processing sequence, subcortically out of awareness (LeDoux, 1996). This processing occurs prior to the synthesis in consciousness of objects and events from simple sensory perceptions. Learned fear responses therefore do not appear to depend on a complex analysis of the cue stimulus (appraisal) (Lang, 1994).

However, LeDoux's discovery that the amygdala, as well as being activated automatically also receives inputs from the cortex, suggests the operation of a second level of emotional processing. This level allows conscious processing of emotion and involves complex perceptions and concepts received from the cortex. This operation occurs only after a more immediate "intuitive" appraisal of the initial input by the emotional brain. LeDoux (1996) thus suggests that there are two different paths for producing emotion: what he terms the "low road," when the amygdala registers danger and broadcasts an emergency distress signal to brain and body, and the slower "high road," in which the same information is carried through the thalamus to the neocortex. Because the shorter amygdala pathway transmits signals more than twice as fast as the neocortex route, the thinking brain often can't intervene in time to stop emotional responses. Thus the automatic emotional response has already occurred before one can stop it, be it jumping back from a snake, snapping at an inconsiderate spouse, or yelling at a disobedient child.

As LeDoux (1996) emphasized, the initial "precognitive," perceptual, emotional processing of the low road is highly adaptive because it allows people to respond quickly to important events before complex and time-consuming processing has taken place. Lane, Fink, Chua, and Dolan (1997), in investigating the pattern of neural activation associated with attending to one's own emotional experience, found a neural site of emotional awareness that provides a neurological basis for the process of emotion awareness and establishes emotion awareness as a phenomenon in its own right. This finding has important implications for psychotherapy because it suggests that working with emotions directly is necessary if we are to change emotional responding

Neuroscience thus offers a picture of emotion as an independent system that is itself complex, repeatedly interacting within itself and influenced by other systems. Emotion and cognition clearly interact in the brain to produce behavior and experience. Emotions clearly arise from people's perceptions of their circumstances—current, imagined, or recalled (Scherer, 1984, 2000; Moors & Scherer, Chapter 8, this volume). Emotions can be viewed as relatively brief episodes of coordinated changes in several components in response to external or internal events of major significance to the organism (Scherer, 1984, 2000, 2005). These components include (1) *cognitive* components, involved in evaluating the eliciting events and the regulation of ongoing emotion processes; (2) *neurophysiological* components, such as changes in the neuroendocrinological system and the autonomic nervous system; (3) *motivational* components, such as action tendencies; (4) *motor expression*, such as vocal and facial expression; and (5) some sort of *subjective feeling*, the personal experience of an emotion. Each of these components has been proposed to form the definitional core of an emotion. This has been, however, a source of much controversial debate, as these components are only loosely coordinated and do not always occur together (Frijda, 2008).

In summary, findings from the fast-growing field of affective neuroscience demonstrate that the common earlier view that emotion follows cognition is evidently inadequate. Emotion can and often does precede cognition; in fact, emotion is an important regulator of higher cognitive processes and makes an integral contribution to emotional information processing in its own right. One important clinical implication of the neuroscientific research is that because much of the processing involved in the generation of emotional experience occurs independently of, and prior to, conscious, deliberate cognitive operations, therapeutic work on a purely conceptual level of processing is unlikely to produce enduring emotional change. Therapeutic intentions therefore need to target the emotion memory structures that automatically generate emotional responses. Recent experimental research on the memory of fear revealed that changing the emotion schematic structures most likely occurs through the process of memory reconsolidation.

Memory reconsolidation is the process whereby previously consolidated memories are recalled and actively reconfigured (Nader, Schafe, & LeDoux, 2000; Tronson & Taylor, 2007). It is a specific process that serves to maintain, strengthen, and modify memories that are already stored in the long-term memory. The traditional view of memory suggested that once memories undergo the process of consolidation and become part of long-term memory, they are more or less permanent. However, every time a memory is retrieved, the underlying memory trace is once again labile and fragile—requiring another consolidation period, called *reconsolidation*. This reconsolidation period provides another opportunity to disrupt the memory. Abundant evidence in animals indicates that blockade of the reconsolidation process following memory reactivation produces amnesia for the original learning (Nader et al., 2000). Recently, the study of reconsolidation blockade of emotional memory progressed from animals to humans (Brunet et al., 2008; Kindt, Soeter, & Vervliet, 2009; Soeter & Kindt, 2010). The possibility of disrupting a previously acquired emotion memory by blocking reconsolidation has important implications for psychotherapy. Because memory reconsolidation only occurs once a memory is activated, it follows that emotional memories have to be activated in therapy in order to be able to change them.

Psychological Processes in Emotion Generation

Association, appraisal, and degree of goal attainment have all been proposed as important psychological processes in understanding how emotion is generated—which again points to the fusion of emotion and cognitive processes in emotion. Bower's (1981) original associative network theory of emotion is a good example of association as the most fundamental process. Association helps explains some of both the noncognitive and automatic aspects of emotional experience. People thus may become angry or sad by means of associative processes without knowing how situational stimuli are affecting them (Oatley & Johnson-Laird, 1987). However, not all emotions are produced associatively.

Appraisal theory proposes that some form of cognitive evaluation is fundamental. Appraisals are not conscious thoughts, but rather automatic, nonlinguistic evaluations along survival-oriented dimensions that include goal relevance, uncertainty, novelty, danger, pleasure, and ability to cope with a situation (Frijda, 1986; Lazarus, 1991; Scherer, 1984). According to a number of emotion theories, a fundamental source of emotion is an individual's implicit appraisal of situations pertaining to needs, goals, or concerns (Frijda, 1986; Oatley & Jenkins, 1992; Scherer, 1984; Moors & Scherer, Chapter 8, this volume). Emotions are elicited and differentiated on the basis of a person's subjective evaluation or appraisal of the personal significance of a situation. In this view anger is generated only with appraisals of unfairness and blame, and sadness only with appraisals of loss. However, appraisals have been found to account for only about 40% of emotions (Frijda, Kuipers, & ter Schur, 1989), suggesting that there is more to emotion generation than appraisal.

A third type of theory emphasizes desires to maintain or attain a certain desired state or goal. Here, goal frustration is seen as leading to anger without any attribution of wrongdoing or appraisal of blame. Rather the anger is motivated by a desire to change undesirable situations, reinstate goals, or protect boundaries (e.g., Carver & Harmon-Jones, 2009). This process involves a different form of evaluation: a match–mismatch with a desired end state. From this perspective emotions inform us that an important need, value, or goal may be advanced or harmed by a particular situation. Emotions are seen as involved in setting goal priorities (Oatley & Jenkins, 1992) and as providing biologically based action tendencies with which to meet these goals, needs, and concerns (Frijda, 1986). Therefore, dysfunction in the ability to access and process emotions robs people of the information inherent in this highly adaptive orientation and meaning production system (Greenberg & Safran, 1987; Izard, 1977).

In summary, emotions function associatively, appraise situations, inform us, and organize our responses to attain goals and meet needs. They are central to human functioning and therefore to psychotherapy. It becomes crucial to determine under what conditions emotion is and is not governed by cognitive processes; this remains a central task for psychological research, which would then guide therapeutic intervention.

Emotion regulation is another important aspect of emotion process. Even though substantial psychological research has focused on how emotions are regulated by cognitive and other processes (Gross, 2002), there is growing recognition that emotions can also regulate cognitive and behavioral processes, and may be an integral part of how dynamic systems maintain stability across environmental change (Bonanno, 2001; Cole, Martin, & Dennis, 2004; Greenberg & Vander-Kerkhove, 2008; Mennin, 2006). In fact, it has been shown that far more projections lead *away* from the amygdala to other areas of the brain, including the prefrontal cortex, than vice versa (Amaral, Price, Pitkanen, & Carmicheal, 1992). This finding implies that emotional responses have more influence on higher cognitive processes than those cognitive processes have on our emotional responses.

Generally speaking, it is our emotional system that sets a primary mode of processing and subsequently guides more cognitive processing, orienting consciousness to differentially analyze situations occurring in our lives. It thus seems that emotion identifies problems for reason to solve (Greenberg, 2002, 2010; Greenberg & Pascual-Leone, 2001). Evidence supports the role of emotion as a regulator of cognitive processes—for example, by directing of attention and perception, strengthening memory, as well as facilitating judgment and decision making, particularly when information is ambiguous or conveys risk (Bargh & Williams, 2007; Bechara, 2004; Bechara & Damasio, 2005; Damasio, 1994; Forgas & Koch, Chapter 13, this volume; Koenigs et al., 2007; Tucker et al., 2003). Thus, initial emotional responses to an object, a person, or an event can shape subsequent interpretations of that stimulus (e.g., using past emotional reactions in similar experiences to make rapid decisions in an uncertain situation), tagging it as novel, dangerous, or pleasurable and signaling ability to cope (or not) with a situation (Frijda, 1986; Lazarus, 1991; Scherer, 1984). It is these initial emotional responses that need to be the target of therapeutic intervention if we are to help people change the way they see themselves and the world.

In addition to the views of emotion processing described above, more encompassing, multilevel theories that attempt to integrate a variety of different emotion generation processes have arisen to deal with the complexity of human emotion. Leventhal (1984) was the first to suggest that sensory–motor, schematic, and conceptual levels are all involved in generating emotions. This approach was adopted by Greenberg and Safran (1987) to explain the role of emotion in therapeutic change. Teasdale (1993) suggested a nine-level model, starting at a sensory level and moving to a tacit implicational level of processing at the top of the hierarchy, with a conscious propositional level one lower. Power and Dalgleish (2008) have proposed a three-level model similar to Leventhal's, with associative, schematic, and propositional levels. A dynamic rather than a hierarchical model of emotion construction by synthesis has also been proposed by Greenberg and Pascual Leone (1995, 2001) to explain how change occurs.

The type of functioning suggested in these models, in which separate but interacting mental functions are mediated by separate but interacting brain systems, appears to be crucial in understanding a variety of areas of functioning. For example, two types of memory (one factual, the other emotional; van der Kolk, McFarlane, & Weisath, 1996) have been demonstrated as well as two kinds of learning (one a more conceptual, logical form of learning, and the other, a more perceptual and emotionally associative one; Pascual-Leone, 1987, 1990). These views help explain the difference between two ways of knowing: one more conceptual and the other more experiential. More conscious, conceptual forms of processing involve facts and reasoning and are produced by the cortex, whereas more automatic associative forms of processing involve immediate experience and perception and are produced with the aid of the emotional brain. These two systems allow for knowledge by description (conceptual knowing) and knowledge by acquaintance (experiential knowing).

The importance of this distinction in understanding human functioning and therapeutic change has been noted by a number of writers (Bohart & Wugalter, 1991; Buck, 1988; Epstein, 1994; Greenberg, Rice, & Elliott, 1993). These two systems have also been termed *explanation* and *experiencing* (Guidano, 1993). The first is a more conscious declarative process of explaining experience, whereas the second is a more tacit, procedural means of generating affective experience. In this view how individuals consciously make sense of their experience is an important, therapeutic, meaning-construction process, but there also is an independent source of affective experience that has to be organized by conscious meaning construction (cf. Freeman, 2000). In this view meaning results from the dialectical synthesis of emotion and reason. Emotion moves and reason guides. Without emotion there is no action, but without conscious organization there is no coherence. The depth, range, and complexity of emotion cannot develop beyond its instinctual origins without conscious articulation.

An important consequence of this method of functioning is that people can respond emotionally without thought. Damasio (1994, 2000) explains that the tacit experiential level of functioning involves the development of systematic connections between categories of objects and situations and primary emotions. As certain images are stored in memory, they are marked with "somatic information." As these images are stored (an argument with a boss, a moment of tenderness with a spouse), the feelings experienced in those moments also are stored. These emotions then are restored when the image is recalled, producing an emotional experience without an actual train of thought—that is, an embodied process. Memories are thus marked to set off the emotional responses originally set off by the event. The next time a particular memory is recalled, the person will feel the same way unless the emotion schematic of the memory and associations linked to it are revised. This revision can be facilitated therapeutically by attending to bodily felt experience and reexperiencing the emotion-laden memory, thereby making it amenable to new input.

Emotion as a Process

In spite of affect's demonstrated independence of conscious thought, most theorists of human emotion agree that emotion in adult human beings is best understood as a process involving many components. This process often involves some form of stimulus appraisal, physiological arousal, expressive behavior, impulse toward instrumental behavior, and some sort of subjective feeling. With development, however, interpretation, subjective feeling, and visceral and motor responses soon cease to be primary indivisible elements. Rather they are all processes that unfold over time (Ellsworth, 1994). Attention or very simple perceptual appraisals often act as entry points into the realm of emotions (Frijda, 1986; Scherer, 1984), especially in the context of interactions with the environment. As soon as the organism's attention is aroused by some change in the environment or in its stream of consciousness, neural circuits in the brain are activated (LeDoux, 1990; Posner & Rothbart, 1992). The person's heart may speed up, the head may turn, breathing may change. The person now may begin to feel different. Once the organism senses that the stimulus is attractive or aversive, the feelings and all the bodily responses change again. As each succeeding appraisal is made, mind, body, and feeling change yet again. When all the requisite appraisals have been made, quickly or slowly, the person may be able to report being in a state corresponding to one of the known discrete emotions. Paying attention to moment-by-moment bodily experience then becomes important in helping people to symbolize their feelings.

The process of experiencing an emotion clearly involves construction (Greenberg, 2002). Debates about the primacy of cognition, bodily responses, or affect thus make little sense when experience is considered as a process of construction. What is needed, rather, is an integrative view in which human beings are seen as actively constructing their sense of reality, acting as dynamic, self-organizing systems that synthesize many types and levels of information to create their experience (Greenberg & van Balen, 1998). Emotional expression is itself clearly an elaborate cognitive processing task in which data are integrated from many sources in the brain (often in milliseconds), often, in the main, outside awareness. The conscious narrative flow of evaluations, interpretations, and explanations of experience—the reported story of the emotion—only comes afterward. The narrative account is significant as a record in memory of experience, but often is only peripherally related to the process of generating ongoing emotion. In psychotherapy and personality research, thinking about how the cognitive and affective systems work together and how each is blended with the other appears far more profitable than ascertaining which comes first. What is clear is that the simple linear sequence of cognition leads to emotion—one of the early cornerstones of the classical cognitive therapy view of emotion (Beck, 1976)—is oversimplified and misleading in attempting to understand the complex interactions of emotion, cognition, motivation, and behavior.

The question of whether emotional reactions precede or follow their phenomenological "appraisal" should therefore be put to rest. It is only if the definition of cognition is arbitrarily restricted to rational conscious thought in language that it can be placed in opposition to emotion. As we have seen, the question becomes when and under what

conditions emotion is governed by cognitive processes, and vice versa, and under what conditions both are governed by other processes. In addition, it is clear that emotion grows out of biological processes but is also shaped by personal experience and by learning and culture. The reciprocal influence on each other of more biologically based emotional experience and more culturally based explanatory narratives that help people make sense of their experience also needs to be further investigated.

Convergence in Psychotherapeutic Views

All therapeutic approaches appear to be converging on a shared view of emotion as a rapid-action, adaptive, control system that orients people to the relevance of events in their environment to their well-being. All agree that emotion produces tendencies to act in specific ways in response to those events; that emotion plays an independent role in functioning and can impact cognition. There is also consensus that emotion and cognition are automatically and intimately connected in higher-order meaning making and that people are constantly explaining their experience to themselves. How they make sense of their experience influences that very experience.

A striking point of agreement appears to be the shared view that at an automatic or unconscious level, emotional and cognitive structures are highly integrated and that these affective–cognitive (or cognitive–affective) structures are the important targets of treatment. For example, in Beck's updated formulation (1996) this level is called a *mode* and involves conceptual, affective, behavioral, physiological, and motivational components. This is highly similar to Greenberg and colleagues' (1993) definition of emotion schemes in experiential therapy as cognitive, affective, motivational, and behavioral networks that produce emotional experience and meaning in relation to what is significant to people's well-being. These networks bear close similarity to ideas in psychodynamic therapy about internal working models (Bowlby, 1969) and to self–other role relationship models (Horowitz, 1991) in which emotion is viewed as the connective tissue between representations of self and other. Another striking point of agreement is the importance of the meaning construction process: All views are converging on an understanding that there are foundational emotional cues but that how people make sense of their unique emotional experience is crucial to what they experience.

Cumulatively, the above developments in psychotherapy theory combined with the recent understanding of the role of emotion in the brain and in emotion theory to suggest that central to embodied human functioning is a set of cognitive–affective units—what could be called *emotion schemes* to distinguish them from purely cognitive schemas. These cognitive–affective units, or emotion schemes, are based on a variety of levels of processing: in part on affects, desires, and goals; in part on encodings, expectancies, and beliefs; and in part on self-regulatory plans and strategies (Mischel & Shoda, 1995; Oatley, 1992). Early on Lang (1994) suggested that a memory of an emotional episode could be seen as an information network that includes units representing emotional stimuli, somatic or visceral responses, and related semantic (interpretive) knowledge. The memory is activated by input that matches some of its representations, and those elements in the network that are connected are also automatically engaged. Because the circuit is associative, any of the units might initiate or subsequently contribute to the activation process. Lang suggested that these units are likely to be multiply connected and are potentially parts of different overlapping knowledge structures.

Emotions produced by these structures provide a higher-order type of emotional experience (Damasio, 1994)—a level higher than the original biologically based emotion response. These emotional responses have been informed by experience and have benefited from learning. Much automatic adult emotional experience is of this higher order, generated by learned, idiosyncratic schemes that serve to help the individual anticipate future outcomes and to influence decision making (Bechera, Tranel, & Damasio, 2000). These memory-based emotion schemes are triggered automatically and in turn signal the amygdala and anterior cingulate, leading to changes in the viscera and skeletal muscles; the endocrine, neuropeptide, and neurotransmitter systems; and possibly other motor areas of the brain. These changes, together with the often-implicit meaning represented in the prefrontal cortex, generate human beings' complex, synthesized, and embodied sense of self in the world (cf. Teasdale & Barnard, 1996). This sense then is symbolized in conscious awareness and formed into narrative explanations of self, other, and world.

An example of this second, higher-level, more cognitively complex type of emotion would be the pit in one's stomach that one might experience upon unexpectedly encountering an ex-spouse. The trigger is clearly acquired, but the process is still automatic. Regardless of whether or not the experience *can subsequently* be fully articulated (i.e., as to exactly what and why one feels the way one does), the experience nonetheless is tacitly generated. Perhaps most importantly, these memory-based emotion schemes guide appraisals, bias decisions, and serve as blueprints for physiological arousal and action. They act as crucial guides, to which we often need to refer, to enhance reason and decision making. These cognitive–affective emotion schemes are thus a crucial focus of therapeutic attention, and when maladaptive, are important targets of therapeutic change (Greenberg & Paivio, 1997).

Clinically Relevant Research on Emotion

Empirical research on the role of emotion and its interaction with cognition in therapy is growing. A number of authors have found a clear association between in-session emotional activation and expression or arousal and therapy outcome (e.g., Borkovec & Stiles, 1979; Greenberg & Malcolm, 2002; Jaycox et al., 1998; Lang, Melamed, & Hart, 1970; Missirlian, Toukmanian, Warwar, & Greenberg, 2005; Warwar & Greenberg, 1999), whereas others have found that arousal predicted outcome only when specific conditions were met. Iwakabe, Rogan, and Stalikas (2000), for instance, found that high in-session arousal predicted outcome only when the working alliance was good. In a recent study on the relationships between the therapeutic alliance, frequency of aroused emotional expression, and outcome in experiential therapy for the treatment of depression, Carryer and Greenberg (2010) found that a frequency of 25% of emotion episodes, coded as having moderately to highly aroused emotional expression, was found to predict outcome over and above the working alliance. Deviations from this optimal level toward higher or lower frequencies predicted poorer outcome.

Emotional arousal and expression alone, however, appear to be inadequate for therapeutic change. The empirical evidence at hand suggests that emotional processing might be mediated by arousal. For effective emotional processing to occur, the distressing affective experience must be activated and viscerally experienced by the client, but although arousal appears to be essential, it is not necessarily sufficient for therapeutic progress (Greenberg, 2010).The conclusion that client emotional arousal seems to be necessary but not sufficient for positive therapeutic change to occur is consistent with most current emotional processing theories, as they suggest that optimal emotional processing involves emotion activation plus some form of cognitive processing of the activated emotional experience (e.g., Foa & Kozak, 1986; Greenberg, 2002; Greenberg & Safran, 1987; Teasdale, 1999). Authors from the experiential/humanistic paradigm posit that optimal emotional processing involves the integration of cognition and affect and that once contact with emotional experience is achieved, clients must also cognitively orient to that experience as information by exploring, reflecting on, and making sense of it (Greenberg, 2002, 2010; Greenberg & Pascual-Leone, 1995).

As Greenberg and colleagues (Angus & Greenberg 2011; Greenberg, 2010, Greenberg & Angus, 2004; Greenberg & Pascual-Leone, 1997, 2006) point out, symbolizing emotion in awareness promotes reflection on experience to create new meaning, which helps clients develop new narratives to explain their experience. Through language, individuals are able to organize, structure, and ultimately assimilate both their emotional experiences and the events that may have provoked the emotions. In addition, once emotions are expressed in words, people are able to reflect on what they are feeling, create new meanings, evaluate their own emotional experience, and share their experience with others. Evidence for the beneficial effect of putting words to distress-

ing experience and trying to make sense of it comes from the area of expressive writing tasks, an intervention in which individuals write about emotionally stressful material. It has been shown in numerous studies that writing about stressful emotional material has a positive impact on autonomic nervous system activity, immune functioning, and physical and psychological health, and emotional processing has been proposed as the underlying mechanism for theses beneficial effects (Pennebaker, 1997; Pennebaker & Seagal, 1999). In addition to this field of research, a number of other studies provide evidence for the importance of reflecting on aroused emotional experience in therapy (Mergenthaler, 1996; Stalikas & Fitzpatrick, 1995; Watson, 1996). The implication is that emotional processing is best facilitated by the progressive increase and then fading away of expressed emotional arousal over the course of a session. Part of the process involves helping clients to reflect on and make meaning of their emotional experiences as they emerge in the session.

Exploring further the combined effects of emotional arousal and processing, Missirlian and colleagues (2005) used expressed emotional arousal and client perceptual processing, along with working alliance, as predictors of therapeutic outcome in experiential therapy for depression. The levels of client perceptual processing approach (LCPP: Toukmanian, 1996) involves rating particular categories of mental operation. Automated or nonreflective modes of processing, such as recognition and elaboration, are captured in lower level categories, whereas deliberate or controlled and reflective manners of processing, such as reevaluation and integration, are captured in higher-level categories. Missirlian and colleagues found that emotional arousal in conjunction with perceptual processing during midtherapy predicted reductions in depressive and general symptomatology better than either of these variables alone. In a similar project Warwar (2005) studied the extent to which intensity of expressed emotional arousal and depth of experiencing can be used as predictors of therapy outcome, using both peak and modal measures of expressed emotional arousal. She also found expressed emotional arousal at midtherapy to be a significant predictor of the symptom-based measures of outcome, with correlations ranging from .48 to .61 and the combined factors (experiencing and arousal) predicting 58% of the variance in these measures (Beck Depression Inventory [BDI] and Symptom Checklist–90 [SCL-90]). Pascual-Leone and Greenberg (2007), in testing a model of emotional processing derived from task analyses, demonstrated that distress reduction involved moving from states of high arousal and low meaning to low arousal and high meaning. These empirical findings suggest that when emotions are regulated sufficiently to be processed further, it is the combination of their arousal and a more cognitive reflection on their meaning that produces the deepest therapeutic change (Greenberg & Pascual-Leone, 2006; Whelton, 2001).

Another line of research that supports the notion that optimal emotional processing involves helping people to experience and accept their emotions and make sense of them once they are activated comes from extensive research on the concept of depth of experiencing, employing the Experiencing Scale (Klein, Mathieu-Coughlan, & Kiesler, 1986). These scales measure seven levels of depth of experiencing ranging at the low end from abstract and external, to focusing on internal subjective experience in the middle range, to a fluid process of attending to feelings to create meaning and solve problems at the high end. An important assumption underlying the Experiencing Scales is that how people talk about or symbolize experience in language both has an impact on the experiences they have and is a valid index of the quality of their experiencing.

A robust and consistent finding of the research on experiencing is that depth of experiencing is positively related to outcome (Orlinsky, Grawe, & Parks, 1994). Goldman, Greenberg, and Pos (2005) demonstrated that experiencing in relation to "core themes" predicted outcome in emotion-focused therapy (EFT) for depression. Pos, Greenberg, Korman, and Goldman (2003) found that early and late experiencing on emotion episodes predicted reduction of depressive symptoms in a sample of 34 clients who received EFT for depression. They also found that clients' depth of experiencing, as measured by the Experiencing Scale, increased over the course of therapy. These results indicate that early emotional process-

ing skills, even though likely an advantage, do not seem to be as important as the ability to obtain and/or increase depth of emotional processing during therapy.

Watson and Bedard (2006), in studying experiencing in EFT and cognitive-behavioral therapy (CBT), found that clients in the good-outcome group, regardless of treatment group, showed higher experiencing levels than clients in the poor-outcome group, and that clients in the EFT group displayed higher experiencing levels than clients in the CBT group. In addition, they found that clients' experiencing levels significantly increased from early to midtherapy. In a more recent study Pos, Greenberg, and Warwar (2009) measured emotional processing (also operationalized by the Experiencing Scale) and the working alliance across three phases of therapy (beginning, working, and termination) for 74 clients who each received brief experiential psychotherapy for depression. Using path analysis, a model of relationships between these two processes across phases of therapy was proposed and tested, including how these processes relate to predict improvement in the domains of depressive and general symptoms, self-esteem, and interpersonal problems after experiential treatment. Both therapy processes increased significantly across phases of therapy. Controlling for both client processes at the beginning of therapy, working phase emotional processing was found to directly and best predict reductions in depressive and general symptoms, and could directly predict gains in self-esteem. Within working and termination phases of therapy, the alliance significantly contributed to emotional processing and indirectly contributed to outcome. These findings indicate that attending to emotional experiencing— exploring, symbolizing, reflecting upon it, and creating meaning from it—as operationalized and measured by the Experiencing Scale—is important to the successful emotional processing that facilitates positive change in therapy. In addition, in the light of these empirical findings, it seems necessary to extend measurement of optimal processing beyond general measures of mere expression and arousal of emotion because optimal emotional processing appears to involve cognitive reflection on aroused (activated) emotion as an essential ingredient.

Greenberg, Auszra, and Herrmann (2007) developed the concept of emotional productivity and the Emotional Productivity Scale to measure it. They proposed three dimensions of productive emotional processing by clients in therapy: (1) emotion activation, (2) emotion type, and (3) manner of processing. A client is defined as being in a therapeutically productive emotional process when an emotional meaning structure is activated (*emotion activation*) in the session and the person experiences a core primary emotion (*emotion type*) in a mindfully aware manner (*manner of processing*), without either getting stuck in it or becoming a passive victim of the emotion. More specifically, emotional productivity was defined as possessing the following six emotion-related components and one theme-related component: (1) the emotion expressed is primary; (2) the emotion is experienced in the present; (3) the emotion is experienced in an aware manner, which involves (4) the client's experience of him- or herself as an agent rather than a victim of the feeling; (5) the emotion is not overwhelming; (6) the emotional process is fluid rather than blocked; and (7) the emotion is associated with a therapeutically relevant theme.

In an intensive analysis of four good and four poor outcome cases who received EFT for depression, Greenberg and colleagues (2007) found no differences between clients with good or poor outcomes in regard to degree of expressed emotional arousal. They found that good-outcome clients significantly expressed more productive emotions in general as well as significantly more productive highly aroused emotion than did poor-outcome clients. These findings suggest that it may be the productivity of expressed emotion in general, as well as the productivity of more highly aroused emotion, rather than the frequency of highly aroused emotion that is important in facilitating therapeutic change.

Research on depth of experiencing has been shown consistently to relate to outcome across orientations (Klein et al., 1986; Orlinsky & Howard, 1978). For example, Goldman and colleagues (2005), in a study of the experiential therapy of depression, related changes across therapy in clients' depth of experiencing on core themes to outcome. In this study, initial level of client experiencing predicted outcome, and change in experiencing from early to late in therapy accounted for outcome variance over and above early experiencing and the working alliance. Depth of experiencing also has been shown to predict reduction of depressive symptoms in CBT (Castonguay, Goldfried, & Hayes, 1996). These findings suggest that processing one's bodily felt experience and its deepening over time in therapy may well be a core ingredient of change in psychotherapy regardless of approach.

A number of studies have also shown that successful psychodynamic therapies involve a focus on emotion. The more successful therapies have been shown to include more verbalization of emotion and the use of more emotion-focused words by the therapist (Anderson, Bein, Pinnell, & Strupp, 1999; Holzer, Pokorny, Horst, & Luborsky, 1997) and greater emotional activation and reflection by the client (Mergenthaler, 1996). A clear focus on fundamental repetitive and maladaptive emotion structures (Dahl & Teller, 1994; Holzer & Dahl, 1996) has also been shown to be therapeutically productive.

Studies of the behavioral treatment of anxiety disorders has long demonstrated that clients who profited most from systematic desensitization (Borkovec & Stiles, 1979; Lang et al., 1970) and flooding (Watson & Marks, 1971) exhibited higher levels of physiological arousal during exposure. These and other findings suggest that the arousal of the fear-activated phobic memory structures is important for change. Foa and Kozak (1986) have argued that the two conditions necessary for the reduction of pathological fear are the activation of the fear structure and the introduction of new information that is incompatible with the phobic structure. Foa and Jaycox (1998) have demonstrated that emotional processing of trauma facilitates recovery. How people make sense of their emotional experience is proving to be important in predicting both onset and recovery from phobias and trauma (Clarke, 1996).

Clinical research has thus attested to emotion as an important mediator of thought and behavior. The evidence from psychotherapy research indicates that certain types of therapeutically facilitated emotional awareness and arousal, when expressed in supportive relational contexts, in conjunction with some sort of conscious cognitive processing of the emotional experience, are important for therapeutic change in certain classes of people and problems (Greenberg, 2010). Emotion also has been shown to be both adaptive and maladaptive. In therapy, emotions thus at times need to be accessed and used as guides and at other times regulated and modified. The role of the cognitive processing of emotion in therapy has been found to be twofold: either to help make sense of the emotion or to help regulate it.

Principles of Emotional Change

Emotional processing and the emergent meaning-making process are central mechanisms of change in psychotherapy. Emotional change occurs by making sense of one's emotions through awareness, expression, regulation, reflection, and transformation of the emotions in the context of an empathically attuned relationship that facilitates these processes. The principles of emotional change are described below.

Awareness

Awareness of emotion is the most fundamental principle. Once people can identify what they are feeling, they can reconnect to the needs that are signalled by their emotions and are motivated to meet their needs. Becoming aware of and symbolizing core emotional experience in words provides access to both the adaptive information and to the action tendency inherent in the emotion. It is important to note that emotional awareness is not a matter of thinking about feeling, rather it involves *feeling the feeling in awareness*. Only once emotion is felt does its articulation in language become an important component of its awareness. Acceptance of emotional experience, as opposed to its avoidance, is the first step in awareness work. Having accepted the emotion rather than avoided it, the therapist then helps the client utilize the emotion. Clients are helped to make sense of what their emotion is telling them and to identify the goal/ need/concern that it is organizing them to

attain. Emotion is thus used both to inform and to move.

Expression

Expressing emotion in therapy does not involve venting but rather overcoming avoidance to allow a strong experience and expression of previously constricted emotions (Foa & Kozak, 1986; Greenberg & Safran, 1987). Expressive coping may help one attend to and clarify central concerns and serve to promote pursuit of goals. There is a strong human tendency to avoid painful emotions. Normal cognitive processes often distort adaptive unpleasant emotions such as sadness and anger into dysfunctional behavior designed to avoid feeling. First clients must approach emotion by attending to their own emotional experience. This often involves changing the cognitions governing their emotion avoidance (e.g., "It's bad to be angry"). Then clients must allow and tolerate being in live contact with their emotions. These two steps are consistent with notions of exposure. There is a long line of evidence on the effectiveness of exposure to previously avoided feelings (e.g., Foa & Jaycox, 1998).

Regulation

The third principle of emotional processing involves the regulation of emotion. Facilitating the ability to tolerate and regulate having emotional experience is another important change process. Any benefits believed to accrue from the intense expression of emotion are generally predicated on the client's avoidance, overregulation (overcontrol), or suppression of emotion, but it is apparent that for some individuals, psychological disorders, and situations, emotions are under- or dysregulated (Linehan, 1993). Important issues in any treatment, then, are to determine which emotions need to be regulated and how could that regulation be best achieved. Underregulated emotions that require downregulation generally are secondary emotions, such as despair and hopelessness, or primary maladaptive emotions such as the shame of feeling worthless and the anxiety or panic of basic insecurity.

Emotion regulation skills involve a variety of processes: identifying and labeling emotions, allowing and tolerating emotions, gaining perspective, increasing positive emotions, reducing vulnerability to negative emotions, self-soothing, regulatory breathing, and distraction. In short, regulation of emotion involves getting some distance from overwhelming despair and hopeless and/or developing self-soothing capacities to calm and comfort core anxieties. Positive experience and support as well as forms of meditative practice and self-acceptance often are most helpful in achieving a working distance from overwhelming core emotions.

Another important aspect of regulation is developing clients' abilities to tolerate emotion and to self-soothe. Physiological soothing involves activation of the parasympathetic nervous system to regulate heart rate, breathing, and other sympathetic functions that speed up under stress. At the more deliberate behavioral and cognitive levels, promoting clients' abilities to receive and be compassionate toward their emerging painful emotional experience is the first step toward tolerating emotion and self-soothing. It appears that simply acknowledging, allowing, and tolerating emotion also is an important aspect of helping regulate it. This soothing of emotion can be provided by individuals themselves or interpersonally in the form of empathic attunement, acceptance, and validation by another person. Being able to soothe the self develops initially by internalization of the soothing functions of the protective other (Sroufe, 1996; Stern, 1985).

Reflection

In addition to recognizing emotions and symbolizing them in words, promoting further reflection on emotions helps people make sense of their experience and promotes assimilation of that experience into their ongoing self-narratives. What we make of our emotional experience makes us who we are. Reflection helps to create new meaning and develop new *narratives to explain experience* (Angus & Greenberg, 2011; Goldman et al., 2005; Greenberg & Angus, 2004; Greenberg & Pascual-Leone, 1997; Pennebaker, 1995). Through language, individuals are able to organize, structure, and ultimately assimilate both their emotional experiences and the events that may have elicited the emotions. This metalevel clearly involves conscious conceptual processes.

Transformation

The final and probably most important way of dealing with emotion in therapy involves the transformation of emotion by emotion, particularly of maladaptive ones such as fear and shame (Greenberg, 2002). This principle of emotional change suggests that a maladaptive emotional state can be transformed best by activating another, more adaptive emotional state. Spinoza (1677/1967) was the first to note that emotion is needed to change emotion. He proposed that "an emotion cannot be restrained nor removed unless by an opposed and stronger emotion" (p. 195). Reason is seldom sufficient to change automatic emergency-based emotional responses. Darwin (1987), on jumping back from the strike of a snake that was behind glass, noted that, having approached it with the determination *not* to jump back, his will and reason were powerless against the reflexive sense of a danger that he had never personally experienced. Rather than attempting to reason one's way out of a troublesome emotion, one can transform one emotion with another. In time, the coactivation of the more adaptive emotion along with, or in response to, the maladaptive emotion helps transform the maladaptive emotion. While thinking usually changes thoughts, only feeling can change emotions. An important therapeutic goal is thus to arrive at previously unacknowledged maladaptive emotion, not for its good information and motivation, but in order to make it accessible to transformation.

It is important to note that the process of changing emotion via emotion goes beyond catharsis/completion, letting go, exposure, extinction, or habituation in that the maladaptive feeling is not purged, nor does it involve attenuation of emotion by the person feeling it. Rather, another feeling is accessed to transform or undo it, such as accessing anger to change fear. Although exposure to emotion at times may be helpful to overcome affect phobia, in many situations in therapy, change also occurs because one emotion is transformed by another emotion rather than simply attenuating. Emotional change occurs by the activation of an incompatible, more adaptive experience that replaces or transforms the old response. For example, Fredrickson (2001) has shown that a positive emotion may loosen the hold that a negative emotion has on a person's mind by broadening a person's momentary thought–action repertoire. The experience of joy and contentment were found to produce faster cardiovascular recovery from negative emotions than a neutral experience. Frederickson, Mancuso, Branigan, and Tugade (2000) found that resilient individuals cope by recruiting positive emotions to undo negative emotional experiences. In grief, laughter has been found to be a predictor of time to recovery. Thus being able to remember the happy times, to experience joy helps as an antidote to sadness (Keltner & Bonanno, 1997). In depression, a protest-filled, submissive sense of worthlessness can be transformed therapeutically by guiding people to the desire that drives their protest—a desire to be free of their "cages" and to access their feelings of joy and excitement for life. Isen (1999) hypothesized that at least some of the positive effect of happy feelings depends on the effects of the neurotransmitters involved in the emotion of joy on specific parts of the brain that influence purposive thinking.

These studies together indicate that positive emotion can be used to change negative emotion. Davidson (2000) also suggests that the right-hemispheric withdrawal-related negative affect system can be transformed by activation of the approach system in the left prefrontal cortex. This principle applies not only to positive emotions changing negative ones but to changing maladaptive emotions by activating dialectically opposing adaptive emotions (Greenberg, 2002). Thus, in therapy, maladaptive fear or shame, once aroused, can be transformed into security by the activation of more boundary-establishing emotions of adaptive anger or disgust, or by evoking the softer feelings of compassion or forgiveness (Harmon-Jones et al., 2004). The withdrawal tendencies in fear and shame can be transformed by the thrusting forward tendency in newly accessed anger at violation. Once the alternate emotion has been accessed, it transforms or undoes the original state and a new state is forged.

How Does the Therapist Access New Emotions?

The therapist attends to subdominant emotions that are currently being expressed "on the periphery" of a client's awareness and helps the client attend to and experience the more adaptive primary emotions and needs that provide inner resilience. Other methods of accessing new emotion involve using enactment and imagery, remembering a time an emotion was felt, changing how the client views things, or even expressing an emotion for the client (Greenberg, 2002). Once accessed, these new emotional resources begin to undo the psychoaffective motor program previously determining the person's mode of processing. This shift enables the person to challenge the validity of perceptions regarding self and other connected to maladaptive emotion, thereby weakening its hold on them.

There also is growing evidence that some forms of positive affect enhance flexibility, problem solving, and sociability (Isen, 2000). Frederickson (1998) has demonstrated how positive emotions lead to "broaden-and-build" strategies that enhance problem solving. Positive emotions such as joy, interest, pride, and love often expand peoples' momentary thought–action repertoires, and this expansion in turn serves to enhance their resources to cope with life. In addition, research on mood-congruent judgment has shown that moods affect thinking (Mayer & Hanson, 1995). Shifts in mood lead to shifts in thinking. Good moods lead to optimism, bad moods to pessimism. Shifts in mood have clearly been shown to lead to different kinds of reasoning (Palfia & Salovey, 1993).

In a different line of research on the effect of motor expression on experience, Berkowitz (2000) reports a study on the effect of muscular action on mood. Subjects who had talked about an angering incident while making a tightly clenched fist reported having stronger angry feelings, whereas fist clenching led to a reduction in sadness when talking about a sad incident. This finding indicates the effects of motor expression on intensifying congruent emotions but on dampening other emotions. Thus it appears that even the muscular expression of one emotion can change another emotion.

Conclusion

The emotion/motivation, cognitive, and behavioral systems are all important in therapeutic work. Privileging one system for therapeutic attention over the others leads to a narrowing of perspective. Understanding the conditions under which it is optimal to intervene therapeutically with which system is crucial. In this chapter principles for working with emotion have been suggested in order to promote the inclusion of emotion-focused work in an empirically based affective cognitive-behavioral therapy for the new millennium.

In this affective cognitive-behavioral therapy, problems that stem from the low road of emotion, in which automatically activated amygdala-mediated emotion is primary, need to be dealt with in a different manner from emotional problems that come from the high road that involves more deliberate prefrontal cortex processing. Low-road processing is automatic and holistic. When functioning well, it is a source of adaptive intelligence that needs to be in awareness. When dysfunctional, this low-road processing is a source of distress and needs to be regulated and modified using affective change principles. When overregulated, amygdala-mediated emotional reactions would benefit from an approach that facilitates increased awareness, acceptance, expression, identification of discrete emotions, understanding of the basic messages of these emotions, attending to adaptive action tendencies.

High-road processing, on the other hand, is far more culturally derived and is influenced by higher-level goals and plans. Reason is involved in both its generation and alteration. Dysfunction in this system is based on cognitive error, and change involves cognitive change principles. Those problems based on deliberate habitual processes such as faulty thinking or skill deficits are more likely to benefit from psychoeducational and rational methods. These forms of intervention are aimed at changing clients' thinking and behavior and at promoting the practice of new skills. An emotion-focused treatment, however, is most appropriate for people in whom the low road is governing functioning. Here cognition is "hot," and the person lacks the ability to regulate affect storms with will or reason. Here where reason cannot penetrate, cognitive and psychoeducative methods that appeal only to reason and deliberate processing will not work, and emotional change processes will be needed. Change in this domain involves becoming aware of the cues that trigger the amygdala-based affective reactions, as well as purposefully activating the problematic emotions and exposing them to new affective input from a new type of relational experience. Here emotion awareness is necessary, self-soothing will have to be developed, and emotion will be needed to transform emotion.

References

Amaral, D. G., Price, D. L., Pitkanen, A., & Carmichael, S. T. (1992). Anatomical organization of the primate amygdaloid complex. In D. Aggleton (Ed.), *The amygdala* (pp. 1–66). New York: Wiley-Liss.

Anderson, T., Bein, E., Pinnell, B. J., & Strupp, H. H. (1999). Linguistic analysis of affective speech in psychotherapy: A case grammar approach. *Psychotherapy Research, 9,* 88–99.

Angus, L., & Greenberg, L. (2011). *Working with narrative in emotion-focused therapy: Changing stories, healing lives.* Washington, DC: American Psychological Association Press.

Bargh, J. A., & Williams, L. E. (2007). The nonconscious regulation of emotion. In J. J. Gross (Ed.), *Handbook of emotion regulation* (pp. 429–445). New York: Guilford Press.

Beck, A. T. (1976). *Cognitive therapy and emotional disorders.* New York: International Universities Press.

Beck, A. T. (1996). Beyond belief: A theory of modes, personality, and psychopathology. In P. M. Salkovskis (Ed.), *Frontiers of cognitive therapy: The state of the art and beyond* (pp. 1–25). New York: Guilford Press.

Bechara, A. (2004). The role of emotion in decision-making: Evidence from neurological patients with orbitofrontal damage. *Brain and Cognition, 55,* 30–40.

Bechara, A., & Damasio, A. R. (2005). The somatic marker hypothesis: A neural theory of economic decision. *Games and Economic Behavior, 52,* 336–372.

Bechara, A., Tranel, D., & Damasio, H. (2000). Characterization of the decision-making impairment of patients with bilateral lesions of the ventromedial prefrontal cortex. *Brain, 123*, 2189–2202.

Berkowitz, L. (2000). *Causes and consequences of feelings*. Cambridge, UK: Cambridge University Press.

Bohart, A., & Wugalter, S. (1991). Changes in experiential knowing as a common dimension in psychotherapy. *Journal of Integrative and Eclectic Psychotherapy, 10*, 14–37.

Bonanno, G. A. (2001). Emotion self-regulation. In T. J. Mayne & G. A. Bonanno (Eds.), *Emotions: Current issues and future directions* (pp. 251–285). New York: Guilford Press.

Borkovec, T. D., & Stiles, J. (1979). The contribution of relaxation and expectance to fear reduction via graded imaginal exposure to feared stimuli. *Behaviour Research and Therapy, 17*, 529540.

Bower, G. H. (1981). Mood and memory. *American Psychologist, 36*, 129–148.

Bowlby, J. (1969). *Attachment and loss: Volume 1. Attachment*. New York: Basic Books.

Brunet, A., Orr, S. P., Tremblay, J., Robertson, K., Nader, K., & Pitman, R. K. (2008). Effect of post-retrieval propranolol on psychophysiologic responding during subsequent script-driven traumatic imagery in post-traumatic stress disorder. *Journal of Psychiatric Research, 42*, 503–506.

Buck, R. (1988). *Human motivation and emotion*. New York: Wiley.

Carryer, J., & Greenberg, L. (2010). Optimal levels of emotional arousal in experiential therapy of depression. *Journal of Consulting and Clinical Psychology, 78*, 190–199.

Carver, C. S., & Harmon-Jones, E. (2009). Anger is an approach-related affect: Evidence and implications. *Psychological Bulletin, 135*, 183–204.

Castonguay, L. G., Goldfried, M. R., & Hayes, A. M. (1996). Predicting the effect of cognitive therapy for depression: A study of unique and common factors. *Journal of Consulting and Clinical Psychology, 64*, 497–504.

Clarke, D. M. (1996). Panic disorder: From theory to therapy. In P. M. Salkovskis (Ed.), *Frontiers of cognitive therapy: The state of the art and beyond* (pp. 318–344). New York: Guilford Press.

Cole, P., Martin, S., & Dennis, T. (2004). Emotion regulation as a scientific construct: Methodological challenges and directions for child development research. *Child Development, 75*, 317–333.

Dahl, H., & Teller, V. (1994). The characteristics, identification, and applications of frames. *Psychotherapy Research, 4*, 253–276.

Damasio, A. R. (1994). *Descartes' error: Emotion, reason, and the human brain*. New York: Putnam.

Damasio, A. R. (2000). *The feeling of what happens: Body and emotion in the making of consciousness*. New York: Harcourt, Brace.

Damasio, A. (2003). *Looking for Spinoza: Joy, sorrow and the feeling brain*. New York: Harcourt, Brace.

Darwin, C. (1987). *The correspondence of Darwin: 1844–1846* (Vol. 2) (F. Burkhardt & S. Smith, Eds.). Cambridge, UK: Cambridge University Press.

Davidson, R. (2000). Affective style, mood and anxiety disorders: An affective neuroscience approach. In R Davidson (Ed.), *Anxiety, depression and emotion* (pp. 281–297). Oxford, UK: Oxford University Press.

Davis, M. (1989). Neural systems involved in fear-potentiated startle. *Annals of the New York Academy of Sciences, 563*, 165–183.

Ekman, P. (2003). *Emotions revealed*. New York: Holt.

Ellsworth, P. C. (1994). William James and emotion: Is a century of fame worth a century of misunderstanding? *Psychological Review, 101*, 222–229.

Epstein, S. (1994). Integration of the cognitive and psychodynamic unconscious. *American Psychologist, 49*, 709–724.

Foa, E. B., & Jaycox, L. H. (1998). Cognitive-behavioral treatment of posttraumatic stress disorder. In D, Spiegel (Ed.), *Psychotherapeutic frontiers: New principles and practices* (pp. 156–182). Washington, DC: American Psychiatric Association.

Foa, E. B., & Kozak, M. J. (1986). Emotional processing of fear: Exposure to corrective information. *Psychological Bulletin, 99*, 2035.

Fredrickson, B. L. (1998). What good are positive emotions? *Review of General Psychology, 2*, 300–319.

Fredrickson, B L. (2001). The role of positive emotions in positive psychology: The broaden-and-build theory of positive emotions. *American Psychologist, 56*, 218–226.

Fredrickson, B. L., Mancuso, R., Branigan, C., & Tugade, M. (2000). The undoing effect of positive emotions. *Motivation and Emotion, 24*, 237–258.

Freeman, W. J. (2000). Emotion is essential in all intentional behaviors. In M. D. Lewis &

I. Granie (Eds.), *Emotion, development and self-organization dynamic system approaches to emotional development* (pp 209–235). Cambridge, UK: Cambridge University Press.

Freud, S. (1895). *Studies on hysteria. Standard edition of the complete psychological works (1953–74)* (J. Strachey, Ed.). London: Hogarth Press.

Frijda, N. H. (1986). *The emotions.* Cambridge, UK: Cambridge University Press.

Frijda, N. H. (2008). The psychologists' point of view. In M. Lewis, J. M. Haviland-Jones, & L. Feldman Barrett (Eds.), *Handbook of emotions* (3rd ed., pp. 68–87). New York: Guilford Press.

Frijda, N. H., Kuipers, P., & ter Schure, E. (1989). Relations among emotion, appraisal, and emotional action readiness. *Journal of Personality and Social Psychology, 57*(2), 212–228.

Goldman, R. N., Greenberg, L. S., & Pos, A. (2005). Depth of emotional experience and outcome. *Psychotherapy Research, 15,* 248–260.

Greenberg, L. S. (2002). *Emotion-focused therapy: Coaching clients to work through feelings.* Washington, DC: American Psychological Association.

Greenberg, L. S. (2010). *Emotion-focused therapy: Theory, research, and practice.* Washington, DC: American Psychological Association.

Greenberg, L. S., & Angus, L. (2004). The contributions of emotion process to narrative change in psychotherapy: A dialectical constructivist perspective. In L. Angus & J. Mc Leod (Eds.), *The handbook of narrative and psychotherapy* (pp. 331–350). Thousand Oaks, CA: Sage.

Greenberg, L. S., Auszra, L., & Herrmann, I. R. (2007). The relationship among emotional productivity, emotional arousal, and outcome in experiential therapy of depression. *Psychotherapy Research, 17*(4), 482–493.

Greenberg, L. S., & Malcolm, W. (2002). Relating process to outcome. *Journal of Consulting and Clinical Psychology, 70,* 406–416.

Greenberg, L. S., & Paivio, S. C. (1997). *Working with the emotions in psychotherapy.* New York: Guilford Press.

Greenberg, L. S., & Pascual-Leone, A. (2006). Emotion in psychotherapy: A practice-friendly research review. *Journal of Clinical Psychology: In Session, 62,* 611–630.

Greenberg, L. S., & Pascual-Leone, J. (1995). A dialectical constructivist approach to experiential change. In R. A. Neimeyer & M. J. Mahoney (Eds.), *Constructivism in psycho-*

therapy (pp. 169–191). Washington, DC: American Psychological Association.

Greenberg, L. S., & Pascual-Leone, J. (1997). Emotion in the creation of personal meaning. In M. P. Power & C. Brewer (Eds.), *Transformation of meaning in psychological therapies: Integrating theory and practice* (pp. 157–174). New York: Wiley.

Greenberg, L. S., & Pascual-Leone, J. (2001). A dialectical constructivist view of the creation of personal meaning. *Journal of Constructivist Psychology, 14,* 165–186.

Greenberg, L. S., Rice, L. N., & Elliot, R. (1993). *Facilitating emotional change: The moment by moment process.* New York: Guilford Press.

Greenberg, L. S., & Safran, J. D. (1987). *Emotion in psychotherapy.* New York: Guilford Press.

Greenberg, L. S., & Safran, J. D. (1989). Emotion in psychotherapy. *American Psychologist, 44,* 19–29.

Greenberg, L. S., & Van Balen, R. (1998). The theory of experience-centered therapies. In L. S. Greenberg, J. C. Watson, & G. O. Lietaer (Eds.), *Handbook of experiential psychotherapy: Foundations and differential treatment* (pp. 28–57). New York. Guilford Press.

Greenberg, L. S., & Vander-Kerkhove, M. (2008). Emotional experience, expression, and regulation in the psychotherapeutic process. In M. Vander-Kerkhove, C. von Scheve, S. Ismer, S. Jung, & S. Kronast (Eds.), *Regulating emotions: Culture, social necessity, and biological inheritance* (pp. 132–148). Malden, MA: Blackwell.

Gross, J. J. (2002). Emotion regulation: Affective, cognitive, and social consequences. *Psychophysiology, 39,* 281–291.

Guidano, V. (1993). La terapia cognitiva desde una perspectiva evolutio-constructivista. [Cognitive therapy from an evolutionary constructivist perspective]. *Revista de Psicoterapia, 4,* 89–112.

Harmon-Jones, E., Vaughn-Scott, K., Mohr, S., Sigelman, J., & Harmon-Jones, C. (2004). The effect of manipulated sympathy and anger on left and right frontal cortical activity. *Emotion, 4,* 95–101.

Hayes, A. M., & Strauss, J. L. (1998). Dynamic systems theory as a paradigm for the study of change in psychotherapy: An application to cognitive therapy for depression. *Journal of Consulting and Clinical Psychology, 66,* 939–947.

Hayes, S., Strosahl, K. D., & Wilson, K. G.

(1999). *Acceptance and commitment therapy.* New York, Guilford Press.

Holzer, M., & Dahl, H. (1996). How to find frames. *Psychotherapy Research, 6,* 177–197.

Holzer, M., Pokorny, D., Horst, K., & Luborsky, L. (1997). The verbalization of emotions in the therapeutic dialogue: A correlate to treatment outcome? *Psychotherapy Research, 7,* 261–274.

Horowitz, M. (1991). States, schemas and control: General theories for psychotherapy integration. *Journal of Psychotherapy Integration, 1,* 85–102.

Isen, A. M. (1999). Positive affect. In T. Dalgleish & M. Power (Eds.), *The handbook of cognition and emotion* (pp. 521–539). New York: Wiley.

Isen, A. M. (2000). Positive affect and decision making, In M. Lewis & J. M. Haviland-Jones (Eds.), *Handbook of emotions* (2nd ed., pp. 417–435). New York: Guilford Press.

Iwakabe, S., Rogan, K., & Stalikas, A. (2000). The relationship between client emotional expressions, therapist interventions, and the working alliance: An exploration of eight emotional expression events. *Journal of Psychotherapy Integration, 10,* 375–401.

Izard, C. E. (1977). *Human emotions,* New York: Plenum Press.

Izard, C. E. (1991). *The psychology of emotions.* New York: Plenum Press.

Jaycox, L., Foa, E., & Morral, A. (1998). Influence of emotional engagement and habituation on exposure therapy for PTSD. *Journal of Consulting and Clinical Psychology, 66,* 185–192.

Keltner, D., & Bonanno, G. A. (1997). A study of laughter and dissociation: The distinct correlates of laughter and smiling during bereavement. *Journal of Personality and Social Psychology, 73,* 687–702.

Kindt, M., Soeter, M., & Vervliet, B. (2009). Beyond extinction: Erasing human fear responses and preventing the return of fear. *Nature Neuroscience, 12,* 256–258.

Klein, M. H., Mathieu-Couglan, P., & Kiesler, D. J. (1986). The Experiencing Scales. In L. S. Greenberg & W. M. Pinsof (Eds.), *The psychotherapeutic process: A research handbook* (pp. 21–71). New York: Guilford Press.

Koenigs, M., Young, L., Adolphs, R., Tranel, D., Cushman, F., Hauser, M., et al. (2007). Damage to the prefrontal cortex increases utilitarian moral judgements. *Nature, 446,* 908–911.

Lane, R. D., Fink, G. R., Chua, P. M. L., & Dolan, R. J. (1997). Neural activation during selective attention to subjective emotional responses. *NeuroReport, 8,* 3969–3972.

Lang, P. J. (1994). The varieties of emotional experience: A meditation on James–Lange theory. *Psychological Review, 101,* 211–221.

Lang, P. J., Melamed, B. G., & Hart, J. (1970). A psychophysiological analysis of fear modification using an automated desensitization procedure. *Journal of Abnormal Psychology, 76,* 220–234.

Lazarus, R. S. (1982). Thoughts on the relations between emotion and cognition. *American Psychologist, 37,* 1019–1024.

Lazarus, R. S. (1991). *Emotion and adaptation.* New York: Oxford University Press.

LeDoux, J. E. (1990). Information flow from sensation to emotion: Plasticity in the neural computation of stimulus value. In M. Gabriel & J. Moore (Eds.), *Learning and computational neuroscience: Foundations of adaptive networks* (pp. 3–51). Cambridge, MA: MIT Press.

LeDoux, J. E. (1996). *The emotional brain: The mysterious underpinnings of emotional life.* New York: Simon & Schuster.

LeDoux, J. E. (2002). Emotion, memory, and the brain. *Scientific American, 12,* 62–71.

Leventhal, H. (1984). A perceptual motor theory of emotion. In K. R. Scherer & P. Ekman (Eds.), *Approaches to emotion* (pp. 271–291). Hillsdale, NJ: Erlbaum.

Linehan, M. M. (1993). *Cognitive-behavioral treatment of borderline personality disorder.* New York: Guilford Press.

Mayer, J. D., & Hanson, E. (1995). Mood-congruent judgment over time. *Personality and Social Psychology Bulletin, 21,* 237–244.

Mennin, D. S. (2006). Emotion regulation therapy: An integrative approach to treatment resistant anxiety disorders. *Journal of Contemporary Psychotherapy, 36,* 95–105.

Mergenthaler, E. (1996). Emotion-abstraction patterns in verbatim protocols: A new way of describing psychotherapeutic processes. *Journal of Consulting and Clinical Psychology, 64,* 1306–1315.

Mischel, W., & Shoda, Y. (1995). A cognitive-affective system theory of personality: Reconceptualizing situations, dispositions, dynamics, and invariance in personality structure. *Psychological Review, 1102,* 2246–2268.

Missirlian, T., Toukmanian, S., Warwar, S., &. Greenberg, L. S. (2005). Emotional arousal, client perceptual processing, and the working alliance in experiential psychotherapy for depression. *Journal of Consulting and Clinical Psychology, 73,* 861–871.

Nader, K., Schafe, G., & LeDoux, J. E. (2000). Fear memories require protein synthesis in the amygdala for reconsolidation after retrieval. *Nature, 406,* 722–726.

Oatley, K. (1992). *Best laid schemes.* Cambridge, UK: Cambridge University Press.

Oatley, K., & Jenkins, J. (1992). Human emotions: Function and dysfunction. *Annual Review of Psychology, 43,* 55–85.

Oatley, K., & Johnson-Laird, P. N. (1987). Towards a cogntive theory of emotions. *Cognition and Emotion, 1,* 29–50.

Oatley, K., Keltner, D., & Jenkins, J. (2006). *Understanding emotions.* Malden, MA: Wiley–Blackwell.

Ohman, A., & Soares, J. J. F. (1994). Unconscious anxiety: Phobic responses to masked stimuli. *Journal of Abnormal Psychology, 103,* 231–240.

Orlinsky, D. E., Grawe, K., & Parks, B. K. (1994). Process and outcome in psychotherapy: *Noch einmal.* In A. E. Bergin & S. L. Garfield (Eds.), *Handbook of psychotherapy and behavior change* (4th ed, pp. 270–376). New York: Wiley.

Orlinsky, D. E., & Howard, K. I. (1978). The relation of process to outcome in psychotherapy. In S. L. Garfield & A. E. Bergin (Eds.), *Handbook of psychotherapy and behavior change: An empirical analysis* (2nd ed.). New York: Wiley.

Palfia, T., & Salovey, P. (1993). The influence of depressed and elated mood on deductive and inductive reasoning. *Imagination, Cognition, and Personality, 13,* 57–71.

Panksepp, J., Sacks, D. S., Cerepeau, L. J., & Abbot, S. (1991). The psycho- and neurobiology of fear systems in the brain. In M. R. Denny (Ed.), *Fear, avoidance, and phobias: A fundamental analysis* (pp. 7–59). Hillsdale, NJ: Erlbaum.

Pascual-Leone, A., & Greenberg, L. S. (2007). Emotional processing in experiential therapy: Why "the only way out is through." *Journal of Consulting and Clinical Psychology, 75,* 875–887.

Pascual-Leone, J. (1987). Organismic processes for neo-Piagetian theories: A dialectical causal account of cognitive development. *International Journal of Psychology, 22,* 531–570.

Also in A. Demetriou (Ed.), *The neo-Piagetian theories of cognitive development: Towards an integration* (pp. 531–569). Amsterdam: North-Holland.

Pascual-Leone, J. (1990). Emotions, development and psychotherapy: A dialectical–constructivist perspective. In J. D. Safran & L. S. Greenberg (Eds.), *Emotion, psychotherapy, and change* (pp. 302–335). New York: Guilford Press.

Pennebaker, J. W. (1995). *Emotion, disclosure, and health.* Washington, DC: American Psychological Association.

Pennebaker, J. W. (1997). *Opening up: The healing power of expressing emotions.* New York: Guilford Press.

Pennebaker, J., & Seagal, J. (1999). Forming a story: The health benefits of narrative. *Journal of Clinical Psychology, 55,* 1243–1254.

Plutchik, R. (1980). A general psychoevolutionary theory of emotion. In R. Plutchik & H. Kellerman (Eds.), *Emotion: Theory, research, and experience: Vol. 1. Theories of emotion* (pp. 3–33). New York: Academic.

Plutchik, R. (2000). *Emotions in the practice of psychotherapy: Clinical implications of affect theories.* Washington, DC: American Psychological Association.

Pos, A. E., Greenberg, L. S., Korman, L. M., & Goldman, R. N. (2003). Emotional processing during experiential treatment of depression. *Journal of Consulting and Clinical Psychology, 71*(6), 1007–1016.

Pos, A. E., Greenberg, L. S., & Warwar, S. (2009). Testing a model of change in the experiential treatment of depression. *Journal of Consulting and Clinical Psychology, 77,* 1055–1066.

Posner, M. I., & Rothbart, M. K. (1992). Attentional mechanisms and conscious experience. In A. D. Milner & M. D. Rugg (Eds.), *The neuropsychology of consciousness* (pp. 93–111). San Diego, CA: Academic Press.

Power, M., & Dalgleish, T. (2008). *Cognition and emotion: From order to disorder.* New York: Psychology Press.

Scherer, K. R. (1984). Emotion as a multicomponent process: A model and some cross-cultural data. In P. Shaver (Ed.), *Review of personality and social psychology* (Vol. 5, pp. 36–63). Beverly Hills, CA: Sage.

Scherer, K. R. (2000). Emotions as episodes of subsystem synchronization driven by nonlinear appraisal processes. In M. D. Lewis

& I. Granic (Eds.), *Emotion, development, and self-organization: Dynamic systems approaches to emotional development* (pp. 70–99). New York: Cambridge University Press.

Scherer, K. R. (2005). What are emotions? And how can they be measured? *Social Science Information, 44,* 693–727.

Soeter, M., & Kindt, M. (2010). Dissociation response systems: Erasing fear from memory. *Neurobiology of Learning and Memory, 94,* 30–41.

Spinoza, B. (1967). *Ethics* (Part IV). New York: Hafner. (Original work published 1677)

Sroufe, L. A. (1996). *Emotional development: The organization of emotional life in the early years.* New York: Cambridge University Press.

Stalikas, A., & Fitzpatrick, M. (1995). Client good moments: An intensive analysis of a single session. *Canadian Journal of Counselling, 29,* 160–175.

Stern, D. (1985). *The interpersonal world of the infant.* New York: Basic Books.

Teasdale, J. D. (1993). Emotion and two kinds of meaning: Cognitive therapy and applied cognitive science. *Behaviour Research and Therapy, 31,* 339–354.

Teasdale, J. D. (1999). Emotional processing: Three modes of mind and the prevention of relapse in depression. *Behaviour Research and Therapy, 37,* 53–77.

Teasdale, J. D., & Barnard, P. J. (1996). Clinically relevant theory: Integrating clinical insight with cognitive science. In P. M. Salkovskis (Ed.), *Frontiers of cognition therapy* (pp. 26–47). New York: Guilford Press.

Thompson, R. F. (1986). The neurobiology of learning and memory. *Science, 233,* 941–947.

Tomkins, S. (1963). *Affect, imagery and consciousness: The negative affects* (Vol. 1). New York: Springer.

Toukmanian, S. G. (1996). Clients' perceptual processing: An integration of research and practice. In W. Dryden (Ed.), *Research in counselling and psychotherapy: Practical applications* (pp. 184–210). London: Sage.

Tronson, N. C., & Taylor, J. R. (2007). Molecular mechanisms of memory reconsolidation. *Nature Reviews, 8,* 262–275.

Tucker, D., Luu, P., Desmond, R., Jr., Hartrey-Speiser, A., Davey, C., & Flaisch, T. (2003). Corticolimbic mechanisms in emotional decisions. *Emotion, 3,* 127–149.

van der Kolk, B. A., McFarlane, A. C., & Weisath, L. (1996). *Traumatic stress: The effects of overwhelming experience on mind, body, and society.* New York: Guilford Press.

Warwar, S. (2005). Relating emotional processing to outcome in experiential psychotherapy of depression. *Dissertation Abstracts International: Section B: Sciences and Engineering, 66,* 581.

Warwar, S., & Greenberg, L. S. (1999, June). *Emotional processing and therapeutic change.* Paper presented at the annual meeting of the International Society for Psychotherapy Research, Braga, Portugal.

Watson, D., & Clarke, L. A. (1992). Affects separable and inseparable: On the hierarchical arrangement of the negative affects. *Journal of Personality and Social Psychology, 62,* 489–505.

Watson, J. C. (1996). The relationship between vivid description, emotional arousal, and in-session resolution of problematic reactions. *Journal of Consulting and Clinical Psychology, 64,* 459–464.

Watson, J. C., & Bedard, D. (2006). Clients' emotional processing in psychotherapy: A comparison between cognitive-behavioral and process-experienctial psychotherapy. *Journal of Consulting and Clinical Psychology, 74,* 152–159.

Watson, J. P., & Marks, I. M. (1971). Relevant and irrelevant fear in flooding?: A crossover study of phobic patients. *Behavior Therapy, 2,* 275–293.

Whelton, W. (2001). Emotional processes in psychotherapy: Evidence across therapeutic modalities. *Clinical Psychology and Psychotherapy, 11,* 58–71.

Zajonc, R. B. (1980). Feeling and thinking: Preferences need no inferences. *American Psychologist, 35,* 151–175.

CHAPTER 29

Cognitive Bias Modification

A New Frontier in Cognition and Emotion Research

Colin MacLeod and Patrick J. F. Clarke

It is now generally accepted that heightened vulnerability to negative emotions such as anxiety and depression and to clinical disorders involving emotional pathology is characterized by cognitive biases that favor the processing of negative information. For example, it is well established that for individuals who display such vulnerability or pathology, attention is selectively drawn to negative information, interpretation operates to selectively impose negative resolutions on ambiguity, and negative past events may be recalled with disproportionate ease. Such observations have given rise to cognitive theories of emotional dysfunction, according to which these low-level biases in selective information processing make a direct causal contribution to the etiology of dysfunction pathology (e.g., Beck & Clark, 1997; Eysenck, Derakshan, Santos, & Calvo, 2007; Williams, Watts, MacLeod, & Mathews, 1997).

However, despite the pervasive influence of these accounts, the finding that cognitive biases are *characteristic* of emotional dysfunction does not permit the conclusion that these patterns of processing selectivity functionally contribute to such dysfunction. This theoretical position could be adequately tested only if it were possible to directly modify the cognitive bias of inter-

est, in order to test the prediction generated by this causal hypothesis: that emotional vulnerability and the symptoms of emotional pathology will be influenced by this cognitive bias modification. Such a finding not only would confirm that the processing bias in question does causally contribute to emotional dysfunction, but it would raise the exciting possibility that emotional vulnerability might be reduced, and the symptoms of emotional pathology therapeutically attenuated, through clinical interventions that directly modified this type of selective information processing.

The theoretical and applied importance of these potential outcomes helps explain the considerable interest in recently developed techniques designed to modify the low-level cognitive biases implicated in models of emotional vulnerability and dysfunction (cf. Bar-Haim, 2010; Hakamata et al., 2010; Hallion & Ruscio, 2012; Hertel & Mathews, 2011; MacLeod, 2012; MacLeod & Mathews, 2012; Mathews, 2012). Cognitive bias modification (CBM) research is still a young field, as evidenced by the observation that over 70% of CBM publications has appeared within only the past 3 or 4 years (MacLeod & Mathews, 2012). Most of the work to date has sought only to modify attentional or interpretive bias, though new techniques are emerging that promise to extend the range of processing biases that can be targeted using the CBM approach. The present chapter provides an overview of this rapidly developing new field of clinical research. We begin by introducing the general principles that have been employed to transform tasks, previously used to assess cognitive bias, into training procedures designed instead to modify such bias. We then describe the CBM procedures that have been most widely used to induce change in interpretive and attentional bias. Thereafter we review experimental work that has examined the impact of interpretive and attentional bias modification on normal emotional experience, on subclinical manifestations of emotional dysfunction, and on the symptoms of emotional pathology. In the latter half of the chapter we review some of the emerging new directions in CBM research that are likely to prove increasingly influential in future work, including the extension of the bias modification approach to alternative forms of processing selectivity and other clinical conditions, and the use of CBM as a therapeutic tool in real-world clinical settings.

CBM Techniques: Transforming Bias Assessment Procedures into Bias Modification Procedures

As already noted, cognitive theories of emotional vulnerability implicate low-level information processing biases in the development and maintenance of emotional dysfunction. Because these biases commonly are inaccessible through introspection, they do not readily lend themselves to assessment via self-report. Consequently, a variety of cognitive-experimental methodologies have been developed to assess such patterns of processing selectivity. These assessment procedures have, in turn, been amended to transform them into techniques capable of systematically modifying the patterns of selective information processing they were initially designed to assess. This transformation has been accomplished by introducing specific contingencies into these tasks, designed such that they become easier to

perform if the participant adopts a target pattern of processing selectivity. It is anticipated that repeated practice of the tasks configured in this manner will foster a change in cognitive bias to favor the type of selectivity encouraged by the training contingency.

Two features are common to the majority of CBM methodologies (Koster, Fox, & MacLeod, 2009). First, the cognitive bias targeted for change represents a pattern of selective information processing that is known to characterize psychopathology. Second, this cognitive bias is altered in a manner that does not involve instructing the participant to intentionally change such information-processing selectivity. Rather, change in the cognitive bias is induced by introducing into tasks previously used to assess this processing selectivity a contingency designed such that successful task performance will be enhanced by adoption of a new pattern of selectivity. In the following sections we illustrate how these principles have been implemented, focusing first on interpretive bias modification procedures, then on procedures developed to modify attentional bias.

Emotionally Linked Interpretive Bias and Its Modification

Interpretive bias refers to the tendency to selectively impose negative resolutions on ambiguous information. This information-processing bias has a well-established association with clinical psychopathology, being evident in patients diagnosed with depressive and anxiety disorders, and also in individuals with subclinical levels of anxiety and depression (Mathews, 2012). A number of different tasks have been used to assess interpretive bias. Commonly, how the presentation of initial ambiguous prime information impacts on the processing of subsequent targets that are related to alternative negative or non-negative meanings of this preceding ambiguity has been examined. An interpretive bias is revealed by a processing advantage for target stimuli associated with one particular valence of the ambiguous prime. In one variant of this approach participants perform lexical decisions on target words following the presentation of homograph primes that permit negative and non-negative interpretation (e.g., *arms*). These target words can be associated with either the negative meaning (e.g., *weapons*) or the non-negative meaning (e.g., *hands*) of the initial homograph (Richards & French, 1992). Other interpretive bias assessment tasks instead employ descriptions of ambiguous scenarios as the initial primes, then measure speed to process target stimuli related to either the negative or non-negative meanings of these scenarios (Hirsch & Mathews, 1997).

Transforming this interpretive bias assessment approach to yield interpretive bias modification procedures has involved introducing a contingency between the ambiguous prime material and the subsequent target, such that successful task performance will benefit from imposing resolutions on the ambiguous information that favors a single valence. Thus, whereas the interpretive bias assessment task involves presenting targets that are associated equally often with the negative and the non-negative meanings of the initial ambiguous prime, the interpretive bias training task involves consistently presenting targets associated with those meanings of the ambiguous material that share one particular emotional valence. Optimal performance on such a task is achieved by adopting a style of interpretation that favors resolving the ambiguous primes in a manner that yields meanings of this same emotional valence.

The two most common cognitive bias modification tasks used to modify interpretation (CBM-I) differ primarily in terms of whether the initial ambiguous prime information comprises words or sentences. Grey and Mathews (2000) developed a CBM-I variant employing homograph primes. This approach presents an initial homograph, which permits negative or benign interpretation, followed 750 milliseconds (ms) later by a word fragment that can be completed only to yield an associate of one of these two meanings. Participants are instructed to solve the word fragments using the initial word as a clue. In one condition, designed to encourage negative resolutions of ambiguous information (interpret negative condition), target word fragments can be completed only to yield words associ-

ated with the negative meanings of the preceding homographs. In another condition, designed to encourage benign interpretation of ambiguity, the fragments can yield only words associated with non-negative meanings of the ambiguous primes (interpret benign condition). For example: The initial homograph *choke* is presented. In the interpret negative CBM-I condition this homograph would be followed by the target fragment *t-ro-t (throat)*, whereas in the interpret benign CBM-I condition it would instead be followed by the target fragment *eng-n- (engine)*. Participants usually complete between 120 and 240 of these training trials in a CBM-I session. The impact of the CBM-I procedure on interpretive bias then can be determined using an interpretive bias assessment task. This assessment task might be similar to the CBM-I task, but with the training contingency removed to restore it to a bias assessment procedure. Alternatively, quite different task variants can be employed to measure interpretive selectivity following exposure to the CBM-I procedure. Across a series of studies, Grey and Mathews consistently observed that groups of participants exposed to a single session of this CBM-I task in each of these two training conditions came to differ in the patterns of interpretive selectivity they displayed on the subsequent interpretive bias assessment task. Specifically, as intended, participants given the interpret benign CBM-I condition came to exhibit a significantly lesser tendency to impose negative interpretations on ambiguous stimuli than was the case for participants given the interpret negative CBM-I condition.

Mathews and Mackintosh (2000) extended this CBM-I approach by employing as primes ambiguous scenarios that each could be interpreted in either a negative or benign manner. On each trial of this task, participants read a textual description of such an ambiguous scenario, which concludes with an incomplete word fragment. They are then required to rapidly solve this word fragment to provide a meaningful ending to the scenario. In the interpret negative CBM-I condition the fragments yield words that provide such a meaningful ending only if the ambiguous scenario has been interpreted negatively. In the interpret benign

CBM-I condition the fragments yield words that provide meaningful completions to scenarios only if they have been interpreted in a non-negative manner. Across five studies, Mathews and Mackintosh (2000) confirmed that participants consistently exhibited the pattern of selective interpretation these experimental contingencies were designed to encourage. This seminal work has formed the foundation upon which subsequent CBM-I research has been built.

Emotionally Linked Attentional Bias and Its Modification

The development of cognitive bias modification techniques that target attentional bias (CBM-A) has followed a similar trajectory. Attentional bias toward negative information is strongly characteristic of clinically anxious patients and of nonclinical individuals with elevated levels of trait anxiety (cf. Bar-Haim, Lamy, Pergamin, Bakermans-Kranenburg, & van IJzendoorn, 2007). This attentional bias has also been observed in clinically depressed patients and in nonclinical individuals who exhibit elevated levels of trait depression (Baert, De Raedt, Schacht, & Koster, 2010). The tasks employed to measure such attentional bias commonly involve the simultaneous presentation of information that differs in emotional valence, and they seek to assess the distribution of attention between these competing alternatives. Such attentional bias assessment tasks include interference paradigms such as the emotional Stroop (e.g., Rutherford, MacLeod, & Campbell, 2004). Selective attentional bias is revealed on interference paradigms by presenting negative and non-negative stimuli as task-irrelevant distracters and assessing the degree to which each valence of distracter impairs performance on the primary task. This bias can also be assessed using dichotic listening procedures to examine the distribution of attention between the two ears, when one ear is presented with negative and the other with non-negative information (e.g., Wenzel, 2006). Yet another method of assessing attentional bias involves having participants search for target information within arrays of stimuli, with the relative latency to detect targets of differing emotional valence being taken as an indication of the degree to which these targets selectively recruit attention (e.g., Rinck, Becker, Kellermann, & Roth, 2003).

Perhaps the most frequently used method of assessing biased attention has been the visual probe task (MacLeod, Mathews, & Tata, 1986). This task involves the simultaneous brief presentation of negative and non-negative stimuli to different areas of a visual display, before a small visual probe appears in the location vacated by one of the two stimuli. Relative speeding to discriminate the identity of probes appearing in the location of negative versus non-negative stimuli provides an indication of the degree to which attention is selectively drawn to negative information. Using this task, it has been demonstrated repeatedly that individuals with elevated emotional vulnerability and those suffering from emotional pathology display disproportionate speeding to discriminate probes appearing in the same location, as compared to the opposite location, as the negative stimuli, indicating an attentional bias that favors negative information (cf. Bar-Haim et al., 2007).

The development of CBM-A methodologies has involved the introduction of contingencies into these tasks, such that performance will be enhanced by consistently directing attention either toward, or away from, negative stimuli. By far the most frequently used CBM-A approach has been a training variant of the attentional probe task. In the assessment version of this task, probes are presented in the same and opposite location to the negative stimuli with equal frequency. However, the CBM-A variant introduces a contingency between the stimulus position and the probe position, such that probes always appear only in the location of neutral stimuli in the condition designed to encourage attentional avoidance of negative stimuli (avoid negative condition), or else appear only in the locus of negative stimuli in the condition designed to encourage attentional preference for negative stimuli (attend negative condition). In two separate studies MacLeod, Rutherford, Campbell, Ebsworthy, and Holker (2002) exposed participants to 576 attentional probe training trials delivered in either of these two training conditions, using word stimuli. Subsequent attentional bias assessment, using the original format of the attentional probe task, revealed that these participants came to display a pattern of induced attentional selectivity in line with the assigned training contingency. Those exposed to the attend negative CBM-A condition became faster at discriminating probes appearing in the location of negative words rather than neutral words, indicating an attentional bias toward negative information. Those exposed to the avoid negative CBM-A condition instead became faster at discriminating probes appearing in the location of the neutral words rather than the negative words, indicating an attentional bias away from negative information. Subsequent research has also demonstrated that versions of this probe CBM-A task, using negative and non-negative pictorial stimuli, can similarly serve to modify attentional bias (e.g., Eldar, Ricon, & Bar-Haim, 2008).

A great many attention training studies employing this probe CBM-A approach have verified its capacity to modify attentional bias (cf. Hakamata et al., 2010). Recent research also has demonstrated successful modification of attention using a visual search CBM-A methodology. Dandeneau and Baldwin (2004) developed such a task, designed to encourage attentional avoidance of negative stimuli and attentional preference for positive stimuli. This task requires participants to identify a single smiling face within arrays of angry faces. When compared to a control condition involving only nonemotional stimuli, this task has been shown to be effective in encouraging attentional avoidance of negative information, as subsequently assessed using the emotional Stroop task (Dandeneau & Baldwin, 2004; Dandeneau, Baldwin, Baccus, Sakellaropoulo, & Pruessner, 2007) or the attentional probe task (Dandeneau & Baldwin, 2009).

Using these types of CBM-I and CBM-A methodologies, researchers not only have been able to induce systematic change in patterns of interpretive and attentional selectivity, but have gone on to evaluate the impact of such bias change on measures of emotion. In the following sections we describe how such CBM studies have lent support to the hypothesis that these types of selective information processing make a causal contribution to emotional vulnerability and dysfunction.

The Impact of Cognitive Bias Modification on Normal and Abnormal Emotional Experience

Many CBM studies have sought to determine whether interpretive or attentional bias contributes to normal variance in emotional vulnerability, using participants unselected with respect to emotional dysfunction. Other CBM studies, either seeking to address the theoretical hypothesis that such types of processing bias also contribute to emotional pathology, and/or motivated by the possibility that CBM may contribute therapeutically to the treatment of such conditions, instead have been carried out on participants exhibiting subclinical or clinical manifestations of emotional dysfunction. In the following subsections we separately review CBM research conducted on these different populations, in each case covering first those studies that have investigated the impact of interpretive bias modification, before going on to consider those that have examined the impact of attentional bias modification.

Impact of CBM-I on Normal Emotional Experience

Using the fragment-completion CBM-I task with a sample of unselected student participants, Mathews and Mackintosh (2000) demonstrated that those who completed the interpret benign condition came to report significantly lower state anxiety than did those who instead completed the interpret negative condition. Although this finding suggests that the modification of interpretive bias may impact on emotional state, it does not warrant the conclusion that interpretive bias causally contributes to emotional vulnerability. Support for this premise has been strengthened, however, by the demonstration that participants exposed to a single session of these differing CBM-I conditions subsequently report differing levels of trait anxiety, in line with the training contingency, on a questionnaire measure of this emotional disposition (Salemink, van den Hout, & Kindt, 2007, 2009).

Although the finding that CBM-I can induce change in questionnaire measures of trait anxiety is consistent with the hypothesis that interpretive bias makes a causal contribution to anxiety vulnerability, an alternative possibility is that CBM-I training contingencies may simply affect judgments made when responding on such questionnaire measures. Specifically, the modification of selective interpretation may influence individuals' perceptions of the frequency with which anxiety has been experienced in the past, rather than producing genuine change in current susceptibility to anxious mood. More compelling evidence that interpretive bias causally contributes to emotional vulnerability comes from studies that have assessed the impact of CBM-I on emotional reactions to a subsequently administered stressor task. For example, Wilson, MacLeod, Mathews, and Rutherford (2006) delivered 160 trials of Grey and Mathews' (2000) CBM-I task to participants with midrange trait anxiety. Following exposure to either the interpret benign or interpret negative training conditions, these participants viewed four brief video clips depicting emergency situations in which a victim is injured but ultimately rescued. Consistent with the hypothesis that interpretive bias causally underpins emotional vulnerability, participants exposed to the interpret benign and interpret negative CBM-I conditions came to exhibit differentially intense emotional responses to the subsequent stressor. Wilson and colleagues found that immediately following completion of the alternative CBM-I conditions, but prior to exposure to the video stressor, participants who had received the alternative CBM-I conditions did not differ in mood state. However, following the video stressor, those who had undergone the interpret negative CBM-I showed significant elevations on measures of state anxiety and depression, whereas those who had undergone the interpret benign CBM-I did not evidence significant elevations of either anxiety or depression in response to this stressor. Interpretive bias does, therefore, appear to causally contribute to emotional vulnerability, as revealed by emotional reactivity to current stressful events.

Several researchers have used CBM-I to modify patterns of interpretive selectivity in unselected samples of children. Muris, Huijding, Mayer, and Hameetman (2008) developed a CBM-I variant employing ambiguous scenarios designed to engage children's interest. These researchers had children ages 8–13 complete a single session of interpret benign or interpret negative CBM-I before rating how threatening they found new scenarios of a potentially stressful nature. Children who had received the interpret benign CBM-I were found to rate these new situations as significantly less threatening than those who had been given the interpret negative CBM-I. In subsequent research using a modified version of Mathews and Mackintosh's (2000) CBM-I procedure with a group of 13- to 17-year-olds, Lothmann, Holmes, Chan, and Lau (2011) obtained further evidence that interpretive bias modification exerts an emotional impact on young participants. Participants exposed to a single session of interpret benign CBM-I, compared to those given a session of interpret negative CBM-I, not only evidenced more positive interpretations of new scenarios but also displayed a reduction in negative affect.

Impact of CBM-A on Normal Emotional Experience

MacLeod and colleagues (2002) gave the probe CBM-A task to participants with midrange trait anxiety in a study designed to determine whether attentional bias causally contributes to emotional vulnerability. They observed that the attend threat and avoid threat versions of this CBM-A procedure induced differential attentional responses to negative stimuli, as intended. Moreover, although mood state assessed immediately following the CBM-A procedure did not differ between participants given these two CBM-A conditions, the degree to which a subsequent anagram stress task served to elevate anxiety and depression was attenuated for participants who had completed the avoid negative CBM-A, compared to those who had completed the attend negative CBM-A. These findings suggest that selective attentional response to negative information causally influences emotional reactivity to stressful events.

Variants of the attentional probe paradigm using pictorial rather than verbal stimuli have produced similar findings in children. Eldar and colleagues (2008) delivered attend negative or avoid negative CBM-A to unselected 7- to 12-year-olds. Participants given the attend negative CBM-A exhibited significantly more attention to negative pictures than did those given the avoid negative CBM-A. Furthermore, subsequent exposure to a stressful puzzle task served to significantly elevate anxiety only in participants who had been given the attend negative condition, and did not induce a negative emotional response in those who had been given the avoid negative CBM-A. Eldar and colleagues also had independent raters blind to the experimental condition assess the children's behavioral signs of anxiety during the puzzle completion stress task. These raters reported that participants given the avoid negative CBM-A displayed lower levels of anxiety-related behavior than participants given the attend negative CBM-A. Such behavioral data provide verification that the CBM-A manipulation genuinely influenced anxiety reactivity, rather than only affecting self-report. Eldar and colleagues' findings therefore demonstrate that attentional bias functionally contributes to emotional vulnerability in children as well as adults.

Although most CBM-A research has been conducted using variants of the attentional probe paradigm, inducing differential attentional bias by using the visual search variant of CBM-A, described earlier, has also been found to influence emotional vulnerability. For example, Dandeneau and Baldwin (2009) had unselected participants from an adult education center complete 112 trials of this CBM-A task, either in the avoid negative condition or in a control condition containing no training contingency. Exposure to the avoid negative CBM-A, compared to the control condition, induced attentional avoidance of negative images and also served to reduce feelings of rejection subsequently experienced in response to a simulated social interaction. This observation— that the visual search CBM-A condition that reduced selective attention to negative information also ameliorated dysphoric response to a stressor—again supports the hypothesis that attentional bias causally contributes to emotional vulnerability.

Some studies that have examined the capacity of CBM-A to attenuate dysphoric emotional experience in participants unselected with respect to emotional vulnerability have investigated whether such attentional bias modification can attenuate emotional response to stressful life events. For example, Dandeneau and colleagues

(2007) examined the influence of the visual search task CBM-A on emotional response to the high-stress environment of telemarketing workers. They delivered this CBM-A in either the avoid negative condition or in a no-training control condition, each day for 1 week, to telemarketers. Only those who received the avoid negative CBM-A subsequently reported significant reductions in perceived stress and significant increases in self-esteem. Independent assessment of stress reactivity was provided by cortisol measures and by supervisor ratings. Again, only those in the avoid negative CBM-A condition showed reduced cortisol release and were rated by supervisors as becoming more self-confident with clients. These participants also showed a significant increase in their telemarketing sales.

See, MacLeod, and Bridle (2009) also examined the impact of CBM-A on emotional reactivity to a natural stressor in participants unselected with regard to their emotional vulnerability. Students emigrating from their home countries to commence tertiary studies abroad often experience heightened anxiety (Babiker, Cox, & Miller, 1980), and See and colleagues examined whether avoid negative CBM-A could attenuate the emotional impact of such a stressor in participants about to experience this event. In the 2 weeks prior to leaving their home country, participants completed the probe CBM-A procedure online, either in the avoid negative condition or a no-training control condition, on a daily basis. Assessment of attentional bias 1 day prior to departure confirmed that those who had been exposed to avoid negative CBM-A, but not those in the control condition, had come to show attentional avoidance of negative stimuli. When assessed following subsequent transition to the new country, both state anxiety and trait anxiety were found to be significantly attenuated in participants who had completed the avoid negative CBM-A procedure. Furthermore, this effect of avoid negative CBM-A on state and trait anxiety was mediated by its effect on attentional bias.

Such CBM studies, conducted on unselected samples, have provided convincing evidence that attentional and interpretive biases can causally contribute to variations in emotional vulnerability. However, this does not mean that these cognitive biases necessarily contribute to the elevated levels of emotional vulnerability associated with subclinical emotional dysfunction or with emotional pathology. To determine whether this is the case, it becomes necessary to examine whether CBM, designed to modify such processing selectivity, can attenuate this emotional vulnerability in these populations. In the following subsections we review studies that have taken this approach by evaluating the impact of CBM-I and CBM-A on the emotional symptomatology observed in participants selected on the basis of displaying subclinical levels of emotional dysfunction.

Impact of CBM-I on Subclinical Emotional Dysfunction

Using an auditory version of Mathews and Mackintosh's (2000) CBM-I task, Murphy, Hirsch, Mathews, Smith, and Clark (2007) delivered either interpret benign CBM-I or a control condition to participants selected because of their atypically high levels of social anxiety. Participants given the interpret benign CBM-I displayed a reduced tendency to impose negative interpretations on ambiguity, generating significantly more benign interpretations of new ambiguous social situations than did those who had been given the no-training control condition. The participants exposed to the interpret benign CBM-I also subsequently predicted that they would experience less anxiety in response to a future social situation than was the case for those who had received the control condition, suggesting that negative interpretive bias causally contributes to the type of anticipatory anxiety commonly experienced by socially anxious individuals.

Steinman and Teachman (2010) also selected participants on the basis of elevated anxiety vulnerability, specifically recruiting those who reported abnormally high scores on the Anxiety Sensitivity Index (ASI; Reiss, Peterson, Gursky, & McNally, 1986). These participants completed a variant of Mathews and Mackintosh's (2000) CBM-I task. Compared to participants who were exposed to a nontraining control version of the task, those exposed to interpret benign CBM-I made more positive interpretations of ambiguity and also evidenced a reduction

in ASI scores. These individuals also showed a marginally significant attenuation of fear symptoms in response to a subsequent interoceptive exposure task.

Additional evidence that interpretive bias causally contributes to dysfunctional emotional experience comes from CBM-I research using highly worry-prone individuals. Hirsch, Hayes, and Mathews (2009) recruited participants who showed elevated scores on the Penn State Worry Questionnaire (PSWQ; Meyer, Miller, Metzger, & Borkovec, 1990) and had them complete a single session of CBM-I in the interpret benign condition or in a no-training control version of the task. The former group of participants reported fewer negative thought intrusions and reduced levels of state anxiety during the completion of a subsequent breathing focus task than did those in the control condition. Given that worry and intrusive thinking are key features of generalized anxiety disorder (GAD), the finding that CBM-I can attenuate such dysfunctional symptoms suggests not only that interpretive bias may functionally contribute to the symptomatology of GAD, but also that interpret benign CBM-I may be of therapeutic value to GAD patients.

Research utilizing single-session administration of CBM-I has confirmed that selective interpretation contributes to variation in emotional reactions to contrived lab-based stressors. In order to determine whether interpretive bias contributes to elevated emotional vulnerability in real-world settings, it becomes necessary to induce more enduring change in interpretive bias by delivering multiple CBM-I sessions across more extended time periods. A number of studies have now adopted this approach, using participants selected on the basis of heightened emotional vulnerability. Mathews, Ridgeway, Cook, and Yiend (2007) delivered four sessions of interpret benign CBM-I over a 2-week period to individuals selected on the basis of their high-trait anxiety scores. Compared to participants in a test–retest control condition, those who completed the interpret benign CBM-I sessions subsequently demonstrated fewer negative interpretations of novel ambiguous scenarios. Critically, measures taken a full week after this CBM-I program revealed that these individuals also now displayed lower trait anxiety scores than did participants who received the control condition.

Salemink and colleagues (2009) have corroborated these findings using a similar research design. These investigators gave high-trait anxious individuals eight daily sessions of interpret benign CBM-I, or a nontraining control condition, delivered via the Internet. Following completion of the program, those who received the interpret benign CBM-I, compared to those in the control condition, demonstrated more benign interpretations of ambiguous scenarios and reported lower levels of both state and trait anxiety. They also evidenced less general psychopathology according to scores on the Symptom Checklist–90 (SCL-90; Arrindell & Ettema, 1986). Together, these studies suggest that negative interpretive bias does causally contribute to elevated anxiety vulnerability within the real-world setting, and they highlight the potential therapeutic value of CBM-I techniques in attenuating such heighted anxiety vulnerability.

In addition to influencing general anxiety vulnerability, CBM-I has also proven capable of reducing the symptoms of elevated social anxiety. Beard and Amir (2008) delivered eight sessions of interpret benign CBM-I or a nontraining control condition across a 4-week period to individuals selected on the basis of scoring above the 75th percentile on the Social Phobia Scale (SPS; Turner, Beidel, Dancu, & Stanley, 1989). Assessment conducted at the end of this period confirmed that the interpret benign CBM-I was successful in reducing negative interpretive bias, and scores on the SPS revealed that these individuals also showed reduced social anxiety symptoms compared to participants who received the control condition. Of particular interest, the magnitude of the reduction in negative interpretive bias induced by the CBM-I procedure directly accounted for the degree of improvement in social anxiety symptoms.

This finding has since been replicated in children exhibiting heightened social anxiety symptoms. Vassilopoulos, Banerjee, and Prantzalou (2009) recruited 10- and 11-year-old children scoring in the top 25% of the Social Anxiety Scale for Children— Revised (SASC-R; la Greca & Stone, 1993). These participants completed three sessions of CBM-I over 7 days, with posttraining measures gathered 3 to 4 days following the final CBM-I session. Consistent with expectations, participants completing the interpret benign CBM-I procedure evidenced a significant reduction in negative interpretations of ambiguity, whereas those in a control condition revealed no change. Social anxiety symptoms also decreased in the former group, as measured by the SASC-R. Consistent with the findings of Beard and Amir (2008), the magnitude of the CBM-I-induced reduction in the tendency to impose negative interpretations significantly predicted the reduction in SASC-R scores. The results from these CBM-I studies strongly suggest that interpretive bias does make a causal contribution to subclinical levels of emotional dysfunction, and they indicate that CBM-I may yield benefits for nonclinical individuals experiencing elevated levels of emotional vulnerability.

Impact of CBM-A on Subclinical Emotional Dysfunction

Many researchers have sought to determine whether CBM-A also can serve to reduce emotional symptomatology in individuals displaying heightened emotional vulnerability. Amir, Weber, Beard, Bomyea, and Taylor (2008) examined the effects of CBM-A on anxiety responses to a public speaking challenge in participants recruited because of their high levels of social anxiety. Using a pictorial version of the attentional probe task, Amir and colleagues successfully reduced attention to negative information using an avoid negative CBM-A. Participants who received this CBM-A condition also reported significantly lower levels of anxiety in response to a subsequent public speaking challenge than were reported by participants who completed a control condition that contained no attentional training contingency. The impact of the avoid negative CBM-A was corroborated by independent raters, blind to the experimental condition, who assessed the quality of participants' speeches. The speeches presented by individuals who had been exposed to the avoid negative CBM-A were judged to be of a higher quality that those given by participants in the control condition. Furthermore, the degree of reduction in anxiety and the impact of the avoid negative CBM-A on speech performance were statistically mediated by the degree to which they avoid negative CBM-A served to reduce selective attention to social threat stimuli. Li, Tan, Qian, and Liu (2008) delivered a more extended probe CBM-A to undergraduates recruited on the basis of elevated social anxiety symptoms. These participants received either avoid negative CBM-A or a control condition without any training contingency, across 7 consecutive days. Only those exposed to the former condition evidenced reduced selective attention to negative information at the end of this period, and these participants also displayed a significant reduction in scores on the Social Interaction Anxiety Scale.

CBM-A has also been shown to reduce the incidence of negative thought intrusions in individuals predisposed to experience high levels of worry. Hayes, Hirsch, and Mathews (2010) delivered a single session of 480 probe CBM-A trials, in addition to a novel dichotic listening CBM-A variant, to participants selected on the basis of their elevated worry symptoms. The avoid negative CBM-A condition successfully induced attentional avoidance of negative information, compared to a control condition that contained no attentional training contingency. Completion of this avoid negative CBM-A condition also resulted in fewer negative thought intrusions during a subsequent breathing focus task, compared to the control condition. Hazen, Vasey, and Schmidt (2009) also examined the influence of CBM-A on a sample of undergraduates identified as extreme worriers according to the PSWQ (Meyer et al., 1990). Five sessions, each comprising 216 trials of the probe CBM-A procedure, were given to participants across an average of 34 days. When delivered in the avoid negative condition, this series of training sessions was observed to successfully induce attentional avoidance of negative stimuli, an effect that remained evident 7 days after the final attentional training session had been completed. Hazen and colleagues also found that participants exposed to this avoid negative CBM-A also exhibited a significant decrease in a composite index of anxiety, worry, and depression scores, as compared to those who completed the no-training control version of the task.

Najmi and Amir (2010) have reported beneficial effects of CBM-A in a rather different sample of participants exhibiting subclinical symptoms of emotional pathology. They recruited undergraduates reporting high levels of contamination fear, and had them complete a variant of the probe CBM-A task either configured to encourage attentional avoidance of contamination-related stimuli or in a control condition containing no training contingency. The results confirmed that the former condition alone served to reduce attention to contamination related information. During completion of a subsequent exposure-based stress task, it was observed that participants who had received this CBM-A condition were able to approach feared objects more closely than was the case for participants in the control condition. The proximity to which participants were able to approach the feared contaminants was statistically mediated by the degree to which this CBM-A induced attentional avoidance of contamination-related information.

In a follow-up to Eldar and colleagues' (2008) earlier study examining emotional reactivity in unselected children, Bar-Haim, Morag, and Glickman (2011) used a similar design to assess whether inducing attentional avoidance of negative information can also reduce emotional reactions to stressful events in children with heightened anxiety vulnerability. They selected children who showed elevated scores on the Screen for Child Anxiety Related Emotional Disorders (SCARED; Birmaher et al., 1999) and were able to replicate Eldar and colleagues' findings with this sample. Avoid negative CBM-A did serve to induce attentional avoidance of negative information in the anxious children and also attenuated the intensity of their anxiety reactions to a subsequent puzzle stressor task.

Most CBM-A work carried out on emotionally vulnerable participants has examined the capacity of attentional bias modification procedures to reduce elevated levels of anxiety. However, Wells and Beevers (2010) investigated whether CBM-A could reduce depression levels in undergraduate students reporting mild to moderate depression. These individuals were exposed to the probe CBM-A procedure in either the avoid negative or a no-training control condition in four sessions spread across 2 weeks. The avoid negative CBM-A procedure produced a decline in attentional bias to negative information and a significant reduction in depression scores on the Beck Depression Inventory (Beck & Steer, 1993), which was not evident for participants receiving the control condition. Further support for the premise that attentional bias contributes to elevated depression comes from the observation that this reduction in depressive symptoms was mediated by the degree to which the CBM-A induced attentional avoidance of negative information.

Taken together, these CBM studies, carried out on participants selected on the basis of their elevated emotional vulnerability, provide good evidence that interpretive and attentional bias contribute not just to normal variability in emotional disposition, but also to problematic levels of emotional vulnerability. The findings also suggest the possibility that CBM techniques may have potential therapeutic utility in the treatment of emotional pathology. In the following sections, we review more direct evidence that the modification of selective information processing can indeed reduce the symptoms experienced by patients with diagnosed emotional disorders.

Impact of CBM-I on Symptoms of Emotional Pathology

Few studies have yet examined the influence of prolonged CBM-I on clinical psychopathology. However, in an extension of their study on high-worry-prone individuals (Hirsch et al., 2009), Hayes, Hirsch, Krebs, and Mathews (2010) examined the effect of a single CBM-I session on individuals diagnosed with GAD. These clinically anxious participants were exposed to the same CBM-I procedure employed by Hirsch and colleagues (2009), and this was followed by an assessment of negative thought intrusions when performing a breathing focus task both before and after a 5-minute period of instructed worry. It was revealed that the CBM-I condition significantly impacted on the frequency of negative thought intrusions during the breathing focus task, particularly following instructed worry. The patients with GAD who had received the interpret benign CBM-I experienced fewer negative thought intrusions during the breathing task

than did those who received the no-training control condition.

In a small series of A-B design single case studies, Blackwell and Holmes (2010) investigated the impact of interpret benign CBM-I on the symptoms of clinical depression. Seven individuals meeting diagnostic criteria for a major depressive episode had their interpretive bias and their mood state assessed daily for 15 days. Across each of the final 7 days they received 64 trials of CBM-I in the interpret benign condition. Comparison of these baseline and intervention phases led to four of the seven participants being classified as responders, and three of these individuals displayed clinically significant improvement in depression symptomatology across the intervention phase of the study. As the authors acknowledge, there are limitations to the conclusions that can be drawn from this pilot investigation. However, we concur that these findings justify more rigorous testing, within a controlled trial, of the potential contribution CBM-I may make to symptom reduction in clinical depression.

The limited number of CBM-I research studies using clinical samples highlights the need for further research of this nature. Although these early findings certainly are encouraging, they will need further corroboration before it will be possible to confidently conclude that negative interpretive bias causally contributes to emotional pathology, and that CBM-I can make a meaningful therapeutic contribution to the treatment of such pathology.

Impact of CBM-A on Symptoms of Emotional Pathology

There is more compelling evidence that attentional bias causally contributes to emotional pathology, and that CBM-A can exert a therapeutic influence on such clinical dysfunction. Amir, Beard, Burns, and Bomyea (2009) delivered eight, 160-trial sessions of probe CBM-A across a 4-week period to patients diagnosed with GAD. Whereas patients who received a no-training control condition did not evidence improvement in clinical symptoms, those who received avoid negative CBM-A showed a substantial reduction in worry, state anxiety, trait anxiety, social anxiety, and depression.

Indeed, diagnostic interviews revealed that only 50% of those who received avoid negative CBM-A continued to meet diagnostic criteria for GAD at the end of the 4-week intervention, as compared to 87% of those who received the control condition. These findings provide direct evidence that negative attentional bias causally contributes to GAD symptomatology, and they indicate that avoid negative CBM-A may be of value in the treatment of this disorder.

The effectiveness of CBM-A in reducing anxiety pathology is not limited to patients with GAD. Several studies have demonstrated the capacity of avoid negative CBM-A to alleviate the symptoms of social anxiety disorder (SAD). Using a pictorial version of the probe CBM-A procedure, Schmidt, Richey, Buckner, and Timpano (2009) delivered multiple sessions of CBM-A to patients diagnosed with SAD. Across 4 weeks, these patients completed eight sessions of 160 trials in either an avoid negative CBM-A condition or a control condition with no training contingency. Those given the avoid negative CBM-A demonstrated significantly greater reductions in self-reported social anxiety and trait anxiety than did those given the control condition. Furthermore, clinical interviews conducted at completion revealed that 72% of patients given this active CBM-A condition no longer met diagnostic criteria for SAD, compared to only 11% of those given the control condition. Follow-up assessment indicated that these treatment gains were maintained 4 months later.

Schmidt and colleagues (2009) did not assess change in attentional bias. However, measures of attentional selectivity were included in a similar study carried out by Amir, Beard, Taylor, and colleagues (2009), which also delivered eight sessions of either avoid negative CBM-A or a no-training control condition across 4 weeks to patients diagnosed with SAD. Attentional bias assessed posttreatment revealed that patients given the avoid negative CBM-A attended less to negative stimuli than did those who received the control condition. Fifty percent of the former group no longer met diagnostic criteria for SAD postintervention, compared to only 14% of those in the control group. Again, a 4-month follow-up confirmed maintenance of these gains.

More recent research suggests that CBM-A procedures may also be capable of attenuating emotional symptomatology in youth suffering anxiety-related mental health problems. Rozenman, Weersing, and Amir (2011) delivered three avoid negative CBM-A sessions per week, for 4 weeks, to children ages 10–17 with a diagnosis of clinical anxiety (separation anxiety disorder, social phobia, or GAD). Only 25% of the children continued to meet diagnostic criteria at the conclusion of the 4-week CBM-A intervention. These participants also reported a consistent reduction in symptoms of depression, highlighting the potential that depressive symptoms may be responsive to attentional bias modification. As no studies have, to date, examined the impact of CBM-A on the symptoms of patients suffering from clinical depression, this remains an interesting avenue for future research.

Current Issues and Future Directions in CBM Research

The work reviewed in the preceding sections demonstrates that the CBM approach holds considerable promise, both as an investigative methodology capable of illuminating the functional contribution of selective information processing to emotional symptoms of interest, and as a therapeutic technique that may contribute to the alleviation of emotional vulnerability and pathology. The full realization of this promise will depend on investigators now working successfully (1) to broaden the focus of CBM research; (2) to increase understanding of the mechanisms that govern bias modification; and (3) to better exploit the capacity of CBM to yield therapeutic benefits in real-world clinical settings. In this section we consider how work is progressing with respect to each of these three important objectives.

Broadening the Focus of CBM Research

Most CBM studies have sought to modify only selective attention or selective interpretation in participants with heightened emotional vulnerability or dysfunction. However, the types of processing selectivity associated with psychopathology extend beyond attention and interpretation. Hence, it would be appropriate to now broaden the focus of CBM studies by developing tasks capable of modifying other facets of selectivity. Already, as we review in the following sections, such steps are being taken, with encouraging results.

Modification of Other Processing Biases

The range of available CBM techniques is beginning to expand as investigators seek ways of modifying more diverse forms of processing selectivity. Although much of this work is still in its infancy, we briefly consider some of these newer CBM approaches to illustrate their diversity and to communicate the likely flavor of things to come.

CBM Targeting Memory. Given the importance theorists have placed on memory bias in the etiology of psychopathology, value could be gained from CBM procedures capable of directly modifying selective memory retrieval. Joormann and her colleagues have worked to develop a method of training depressed participants to forget negative information. Their approach is based on Anderson and Green's (2001) work, showing that when participants repeatedly encounter cues previously associated with a target memory item, while following the instruction not to think of this target, the representation of the target information thereafter remains suppressed below baseline. Joormann, Hertel, Brozovich, and Gotlib (2005) have employed this approach to induce selective forgetting of negative information in clinically depressed participants. They also have shown that trained forgetting of negative memories is rendered more effective if clinically depressed individuals focus on distracting information during exposure to the cues (Joormann, Hertel, LeMoult, & Gotlib, 2009). It will require further research to determine whether the application of this memory modification procedure will prove effective in attenuating clinically depressed individuals' preferential recollection of negative memories and in reducing their dysphoric emotional symptoms.

CBM Targeting Imagery. The observation that negative mental imagery is a common characteristic of psychological dysfunction (cf. Hackmann & Holmes, 2004) has led Holmes and Mathews (2005) to contend that such imagery makes a particularly strong contribution to emotional vulnerability. If negative imagery exerts an especially potent impact on emotion, then CBM-I designed to modify the degree to which such selective imagery is evoked by ambiguous scenarios should be particularly effective in altering emotion. Holmes, Mathews, Dalgleish, and Mackintosh (2006) have found support for this prediction, using a single-session auditory CBM-I procedure. This procedure was designed to increase benign resolutions of ambiguous scenarios, but in one condition participants were instructed to form mental images of these scenarios during the CBM-I procedure, whereas in the other they were told to process the scenarios in a verbal form. Benign interpretive bias was most strongly induced by the imagery condition, and this imagery version of the CBM-I procedure proved most effective in attenuating negative emotion. This finding has since been replicated by Holmes, Lang, and Shah (2009), who also demonstrated that the imagery version of the CBM-I procedure was more effective than the verbal version in attenuating dysphoric responses to a subsequent mood induction procedure. Hence, it seems likely that the therapeutic benefits of CBM procedures may be augmented when they are designed to alter emotional imagery.

CBM Targeting Appraisal. A central premise underpinning cognitive accounts of psychopathology is that dysfunctional psychological symptoms can reflect the tendency to appraise events in a maladaptive manner (cf. Power & Dalgleish, 2008). Hence researchers are now beginning to investigate whether the use of CBM procedures to modify appraisal style can attenuate such symptoms. In some task variants, participants have been directly instructed to practice appraising scenarios in a particular way. For example, to address the hypothesis that abstract and overgeneral thinking contributes to rumination and dysphoria, Watkins, Baeyens, and Read (2009) presented participants, who had scored high on a measure of depression, with short auditory scenarios and instructed them to practice processing these in a concrete and specific manner.

Across seven daily sessions, these participants reported greater decreases in depressive symptoms than were shown by participants in a no-practice control condition. In a more recent follow-up study, Watkins and colleagues (2012) employed a randomized controlled design to investigate whether the efficacy of a guided self-help intervention for people with a current diagnosis of major depression could be enhanced by the inclusion of this concreteness training. They found that this form of CBM significantly improved symptoms posttreatment and at 3- and 6-month follow-ups. Taking a similar instructional approach, Schartau, Dalgeish, and Dunn (2009) exposed unselected volunteers to potentially distressing film clips and directed them to practice employing a positive appraisal style. This procedure led to a reduction in the distress evoked by the clips, as revealed by self-report and skin conductance measures.

In other cases, researchers have adapted previously used CBM-I methodologies, but have refined their focus to target particular types of negative appraisal. This was the approach taken by Lang, Moulds, and Holmes (2009) in a study designed to test the hypothesis that maladaptive appraisal of negative intrusive memories increases the frequency of such intrusions. On each trial of this CBM procedure, participants were exposed to text describing appraisal of a negative intrusive memory, in which one word was an incomplete fragment and the nature of the communicated appraisal depended on the identity of this word. Participants were instructed to quickly complete the word fragment. In the appraise negative CBM condition, the only words capable of completing the fragments communicated negative appraisal of memory intrusions, whereas in the appraise benign condition these words communicated nonnegative appraisal of such intrusions. Following exposure to this CBM procedure in either condition, participants were shown a distressing film designed to elicit negative memory intrusions. This film evoked less negative memory intrusions across the next 7 days in the participants previously exposed to the appraise benign CBM procedure, compared to those given the appraise negative CBM procedure. In view of recent evidence that the attenuation of intrusive memories can alleviate the symptoms of clinical depression (Kandris & Moulds, 2008), this CBM approach may have practical value in clinical settings.

CBM Targeting Attributional Style. The hopelessness theory of depression proposes that a key causal factor underpinning depressive vulnerability is the tendency to attribute negative events to stable internal causes, whereas resilience to depression results from the tendency to instead attribute them to external transient causes (Abramson, Metalsky, & Alloy, 1989). Peters, Constans, and Mathews (2011) recently developed a CBM task variant specifically designed to modify such attributional style. Each trial in this CBM procedure first described a positive or negative event, with the subsequent completion serving to resolve the initially uncertain cause of this event. In one condition, designed to induce depressogenic attributional style, the resolutions consistently implicated internal stable factors as the causes of negative events and external transient factors as the causes of positive events. In the other condition, designed to induce resilient attributional style, these contingencies were reversed. Following a single CBM session comprising 120 trials of this task, a questionnaire measure confirmed that the groups exposed to these different CBM conditions differed in attributional style, as intended. Furthermore, subsequent exposure to a failure experience served to elevate dysphoria to a significantly lesser extent in those participants who had received the CBM procedure that induced resilient attributional style, compared to those who had received the procedure that induced depressogenic attributional style. These findings provide empirical support for the causal role of attributional style in the moderation of emotional vulnerability, and they suggest that CBM designed to directly alter this attributional style may yield therapeutic benefits.

Illuminating the Mechanisms That Underpin CBM

If we are to optimize the capacity of future CBM interventions to modify cognitive bias, then we must develop a good understanding of the mechanisms through which CBM procedures change such patterns of processing selectivity. Of course, we must be confident that the changes in both the processing bias and symptomatology are genuine and do not represent only a demand effect, reflecting participants' compliance with what they perceive to be the experimenter's expectation. MacLeod and Mathews (2012) offer the following six reasons to doubt the plausibility of demand-effect explanations for CBM-induced change: (1) the patterns of altered task performance that serve to confirm occurrence of the intended cognitive change commonly are not readily evident to participants; (2) simulating this pattern of task performance often would be exceptionally difficult; (3) neurocognitive measures have provided concurrent evidence of CBM-induced cognitive change (e.g., Browning, Holmes, Murphy, Goodwin, & Harmer, 2010; Eldar & Bar-Haim, 2010); (4) CBM-induced symptom change commonly is more highly specific than would be expected if it resulted from demand; (5) such symptom change has also been observed on psychophysiological measures that are not amenable to voluntary control; and (6) direct assessment of participant expectancies has shown that these cannot account for the observed effects of CBM. Hence, it appears that CBM does produce genuine change in processing selectivity.

But through what mechanism is this change produced? It could be argued that CBM-induced change in processing bias might be mediated by mood, given that CBM procedures commonly expose participants to emotional information that could potentially serve to directly influence their mood state. However, the weight of evidence is against this account. The induction of differential mood state does not elicit the cognitive changes produced by CBM (Standage, Ashwin, & Fox, 2010), and these cognitive changes are produced by CBM even when the bias modification procedure itself has no effect on mood (Hoppitt, Mathews, Yiend, & Mackintosh, 2010; Wilson et al., 2006). When CBM does exert an impact on mood, this effect does not statistically account for its impact on cognitive bias (Amir et al., 2008; Hirsch, Mathews, & Clark, 2007), and CBM-induced cognitive changes remain evident for periods of time that far exceed the

duration of any such transient mood effects (Hazen et al., 2009; Mackintosh, Mathews, Yiend, Ridgeway, & Cook, 2006). Neither does the evidence support the idea that CBM may bring about observed changes in cognitive task performance through general affective priming, whereby increased exposure to information of one particular emotional valence during training generally facilitates the processing of subsequent information that shares this same emotional tone. Observed training effects are often more specific than would be predicted by such a semantic priming account, and these effects endure across time periods that greatly exceed the temporal scope of semantic priming (MacLeod & Mathews, 2012).

The most plausible account of CBM-induced cognitive change, articulated in some detail by Hertel and Mathews (2011), is that this change results from transfer of training (Blaxton, 1989). According to this account, after participants have been required to continuously "practice" a specific pattern of selectivity while engaging in the particular cognitive process invoked by the CBM training procedure, this pattern of selectivity then transfers to other tasks that require participants to again employ this same cognitive process. If this is so, then the most effective CBM tasks should be those that generate the most pronounced transfer-of-training effects. Thus, ensuring that CBM-induced change in information processing generalizes beyond the constraints of the CBM training procedure is of paramount importance. One widely adopted method of verifying that CBM training effects generalize beyond the specific stimulus sets used in training involves the inclusion within assessment tasks of new stimulus materials, not previously exposed during the preceding training procedures. To maximize transfer of training to new stimulus materials, it may be prudent to vary the stimuli used across different CBM sessions, such that participants acquire an altered cognitive response to a broad class of stimuli, as opposed to a single subset of stimuli (See et al., 2009).

In addition to the transfer of CBM training across stimuli, it is also desirable that such training transfers across different tasks designed to assess bias in the cognitive process targeted by the CBM procedure. Hence it is appropriate to measure this cognitive process, post CBM, using assessment tasks that differ substantially from those employed to deliver the bias modification. Again, the likelihood that training will transfer across a wide variety of tasks designed to assess the target cognitive process may be maximized by using a broad range of different CBM procedures to induce the desired cognitive change. Thus, for example, rather than restricting CBM-I to a single interpretive training task delivered repeatedly, a battery of interpretive training tasks that share the inclusion of a contingency designed to encourage the same pattern of interpretive selectivity, but that differ in terms of other task parameters and procedures, may produce better generalization of training effects across a wider variety of subsequent bias assessment tasks.

Another issue related to transfer of training concerns the transfer of the CBM-induced change in a targeted cognitive process to other types of information operations. There has been growing experimental interest in evaluating the degree to which the cognitive training effects produced by alternative CBM procedures transfer across different cognitive processes. Recent findings suggest that effective CBM procedures may operate to change processing selectivity at a fundamental level within the cognitive system that spans attentional, interpretive, and memorial processing. Thus, for example, it has been shown that the probe CBM-A training task affects not only selective attention but also exerts an impact on selective interpretation (White, Suway, Pine, Bar-Haim, & Fox, 2011), and that Mathews and Mackintosh's (2000) CBM-I training task influences attentional bias (Amir, Bomyea, & Beard, 2010) and memory bias (Tran, Hertel, & Joormann, 2011) in addition to interpretive bias. As noted by MacLeod and Mathews (2012), the systematic investigation of such CBM transfer-of-training effects should assist future researchers to categorize and fractionate the cognitive mechanisms that underpin the spectrum of psychological disorders. Moreover, it should enable them to identify the CBM variants that exert the most pervasive influence on selective information processing, and so promise to yield the most widespread therapeutic benefits.

Exploiting the Applied Benefits of CBM in Real-World Settings

Our capacity to extract maximum real-world clinical benefits from CBM-based research will be further enhanced by two developments. First, it will be necessary to refine CBM technologies in ways that bolster the magnitude and stability of the changes they induce in their target cognitive biases. Second, these CBM interventions must be packaged in a manner that not only is therapeutically beneficial to patients, but that patients find acceptable within the clinical setting. We conclude by briefly considering how such goals might be pursued and by reviewing recent progress toward these objectives.

For CBM to be a maximally effective therapeutic tool, it is necessary to optimize the emotional impact of CBM-induced change in information processing. In some ways it might be considered paradoxical that CBM procedures designed to induce avoidance of negative information have been shown to be emotionally beneficial, given the evidence that intentional efforts to avoid information and situations that elicit anxiety may be implicated in the development and maintenance of emotional pathology, particularly anxiety-related problems (cf. Barlow, 2002). The resolution to this apparent paradox may lie in the difference between the type of avoidance encouraged by CBM and the type of avoidance that instead characterizes (and possibly contributes to) emotional dysfunction. In the latter case, individuals commonly adopt the explicit goal of intentionally avoiding processing threatening information in an active effort to suppress anxiogenic thoughts. As is well documented from the extensive work of Wegner and colleagues, effortful attempts at suppression frequently evoke the "ironic" effect of increasing the very patterns of thinking they are intended to attenuate (Wegner, Schneider, Carter, & White, 1987). Hence, deliberate efforts to avoid processing negative information might contribute to emotional dysfunction simply because this avoidance intention does not effectively translate into the successful cognitive avoidance of such information, but instead ironically elicits the pattern of cognitive vigilance for negative information typically evidenced by people suffering from such conditions. In contrast, CBM is designed to induce cognitive avoidance of negative information in a manner that does not involve effort or intention at all. Rather, this pattern of cognitive selectivity is encouraged by exposure to a task contingency that generally is not communicated explicitly to participants, but instead is intended to implicitly evoke the desired change in selective information processing. Assessment tasks confirm that CBM is effective in successfully inducing cognitive avoidance of negative information, which contrasts with the widely reported finding that attempts to avoid negative processing through effortful and intentional suppression commonly fail (Wenzlaff & Wegner, 2000). It is plausible, therefore, that the successful cognitive avoidance of negative information, as is induced by CBM, yields emotional benefits, whereas the counterproductive emotional consequences of more effortful attempts to avoid negative information reflect the fact that such efforts can paradoxically induce vigilance for such information.

Although necessarily speculative at the this stage, the above discussion bears upon a potentially important methodological issue concerning whether or not the efficacy of CBM would be impaired or enhanced by making participants explicitly aware of the training contingency and encouraging effortful practice in the desired pattern of processing selectivity. Very few researchers have yet sought to systematically examine whether the adoption of more explicit learning instructions in CBM procedures would serve to impair or to enhance their emotional impact, and early findings are mixed. MacLeod, Mackintosh, and Vujic (2009) have reported that the introduction of explicit learning instructions to their CBM-A procedure increased the magnitude of the attentional training effect on the training task itself, but eliminated transfer of this training to a different measure of attentional selectivity. It also eliminated the impact of the CBM-A procedure on emotional reactivity to a subsequent stressor. In contrast, however, Krebs, Hirsch, and Mathews (2010) found that their CBM-A manipulation had a more powerful impact on worry symptomatology when participants were given explicit learning instructions. Thus, further research is clearly needed to estab-

lish whether it is preferable to design CBM procedures in ways that maximize the contributions of implicit or explicit learning to the underlying cognitive change process.

Not uncommonly, it has been observed that the degree to which a CBM intervention attenuates the dysfunctional symptoms of interest is a direct function of the degree to which it changes the target cognitive bias. Hence the use of CBM approaches that induce cognitive changes of greater magnitude might reasonably be expected to result in more pronounced therapeutic benefits than those that exert a lesser impact on cognitive bias. Few studies have systematically compared alternative variants of CBM approaches to determine which produce the greatest cognitive change, but the field is now at the stage where meta-analysis can serve to usefully inform investigators about such matters (Hakamata et al., 2010; Hallion & Ruscio, 2012). Some of the findings from recent meta-analyses are perhaps unsurprising, such as the observation that the use of more CBM training sessions results in greater cognitive change. However, other factors found to affect the magnitude of cognitive bias modification effects are less self-evident. For example, from their meta-analysis, Hakamata and colleagues (2010) were able to show that probe CBM-A tasks that have separated the valenced stimuli vertically rather than horizontally, and those that have employed verbal rather than pictorial stimuli, produce the most pronounced change in attentional bias. The reasons for this are presently not clear, but candidate explanations, such as the possibility that verbal stimuli may permit participants to generate more personalized mental imagery than do pictorial stimuli, are amendable to future experimental investigation. We anticipate that the refinement of CBM methodologies to maximize cognitive change will be a cyclic process in which meta-analyses play a major role. Meta-analyses can identify which CBM task parameters have been associated with the magnitude of induced cognitive change in previous studies, leading to research designed to illuminate the mechanisms that underpin the enhanced efficacy of particular CBM variations, resulting in a range of more powerful CBM variants, the relative efficacy of which can be contrasted in subsequent meta-analyses.

Even a large change in cognitive bias will have limited therapeutic value if it does not endure across time. Reassuringly, the evidence suggests that a single CBM session can produce surprisingly robust cognitive bias change, particularly in the case of CBM-I. For example, it has been shown that one session of Mathews and Mackintosh's (2000) CBM-I procedure exerts an impact on selective interpretation that endures for at least 24 hours (Yiend, Mackintosh, & Mathews, 2005) and continues to influence emotional vulnerability even after such a delay (Mackintosh et al., 2006). Nevertheless, most researchers concur that the use of multiple CBM sessions will be required to produce truly lasting change in processing selectivity, raising the question of how best to schedule such sessions to yield the most enduring effect. See and colleagues (2009) note that previous work contrasting the persistence of learning acquired through either massed or spaced practice (Cepeda, Pashler, Vul, Wixted, & Rohrer, 2006) suggests that increasing the temporal separation of CBM sessions should increase the stability of the resulting bias change. It also has been proposed that the use of occasional booster CBM sessions, following completion of an initially intensive program of CBM, may contribute to the maintenance of such cognitive change (MacLeod, Koster, & Fox, 2009). Future studies designed to directly test such ideas may serve to enhance the longevity of CBM induced change in cognitive bias.

The continuing accrual of positive findings from small-scale randomized control trials provides good grounds for optimism that CBM will prove to be of value in the clinical context (Beard, Weisberg, & Amir, 2011; Brosan, Hoppitt, Shelfer, Sillence, & Mackintosh, 2011). Indeed, in their meta-analysis Hakamata and colleagues (2010) report that, when delivered to clinically anxious participants, CBM-A yields treatment effect sizes similar to those associated with CBT or selective serotonin reuptake inhibitors (SSRIs). Furthermore, client acceptability studies have confirmed that patients with emotional dysfunction express subjective satisfaction with multisession CBM-A and CBM-I delivered as part of their regular treatment (Beard, Weisberg, Perry, Schofield, & Amir, 2010). There is agreement among most researchers that the time is now ripe for large-scale trials, designed to comply fully with the Consolidated Standards of Reporting Trials guidelines (CONSORT), in order to demonstrate the capacity of CBM to yield meaningful therapeutic benefits for clinical patients in real-world settings (Beard, 2011; MacLeod, 2012).

Closing Comments

As we noted at the outset of this chapter, this is a young field of research. The range of presently available CBM techniques is limited, and almost certainly these do not yet represent the most effective possible means of inducing enduring change in the patterns of processing selectivity they target. In the fullness of time, we can expect to see CBM approaches broaden in terms of methodology, diversify in terms of the biases they target, and strengthen in terms of their capacity to modify these biases in an enduring manner. Nevertheless, on the basis of the seminal work reviewed in this chapter, we can already conclude that the advent of CBM has brought us to an exciting new juncture in our efforts to understand the cognitive basis of psychopathology and to exploit this understanding for therapeutic gain. Researchers seeking to determine whether particular forms of selective attention or selective interpretation contribute to symptoms of interest now can do so by drawing upon newly established techniques with a proven capacity to directly modify such aspects of information processing. When such causal influence is demonstrated, clinical investigators now can incorporate these same bias modification procedures into intervention approaches designed to attenuate such symptoms. The CBM studies reviewed in this chapter provide compelling evidence that attentional bias to negative information, and interpretive bias favoring negative resolutions of ambiguity, do both causally contribute to emotional vulnerability and pathology. Furthermore, CBM interventions designed to alleviate clinical symptoms by directly training target patterns of attentional and interpretive selectivity now have passed the proof of concept stage. These finding amply justify the larger-scale clinical trials that we can expect to see appear in the near future, and we look forward with excitement, anticipation, and no small measure of optimism to this next stage of the CBM journey.

References

Abramson, L. Y., Metalsky, G. I., & Alloy, L. B. (1989). Hopelessness depression: A theory-based subtype of depression. *Psychological Review, 96*(2), 358–372.

Amir, N., Beard, C., Burns, M., & Bomyea, J. (2009). Attention modification program in individuals with generalized anxiety disorder. *Journal of Abnormal Psychology, 118*(1), 28–33.

Amir, N., Beard, C., Taylor, C. T., Klumpp, H., Elias, J., Burns, M., et al. (2009). Attention training in individuals with generalized social phobia: A randomized controlled trial. *Journal of Consulting and Clinical Psychology, 77*(5), 961–973.

Amir, N., Bomyea, J., & Beard, C. (2010). The effect of single-session interpretation modification on attention bias in socially anxious individuals. *Journal of Anxiety Disorders, 24*(2), 178–182.

Amir, N., Weber, G., Beard, C., Bomyea, J., & Taylor, C. T. (2008). The effect of a single-session attention modification program on response to a public-speaking challenge in socially anxious individuals. *Journal of Abnormal Psychology, 117*(4), 860–868.

Anderson, M. C., & Green, C. (2001). Suppressing unwanted memories by executive control. *Nature, 410*(6826), 366–369.

Arrindell, W. A., & Ettema, J. H. M. (1986). *SCL-90: Handleiding bij een multidimensionele psychopathologie-indicator [SCL-90: Manual for a Multidimensional Indicator of Psychopathology]*. Lisse, The Netherlands: Swets & Zeitlinger.

Babiker, I. E., Cox, J. L., & Miller, P. M. C. (1980). The measurement of culture distance and its relationship to medical consultation, symptomatology, and examination performance of overseas students at Edinburgh University. *Social Psychiatry, 15*, 109–116.

Baert, S., De Raedt, R., Schacht, R., & Koster, E. H. (2010). Attentional bias training in depression: Therapeutic effects depend on depression severity. *Journal of Behavior Therapy and Experimental Psychiatry, 41*(3), 265–274.

Bar-Haim, Y. (2010). Research review: Attention bias modification (ADM)—a novel treatment for anxiety disorders. *Journal of Child Psychology and Psychiatry, 51*(8), 859–870.

Bar-Haim, Y., Lamy, D., Pergamin, L., Bakermans-Kranenburg, M. J., & van IJzendoorn, M. H. (2007). Threat-related attentional bias in anxious and nonanxious individuals: A meta-analytic study. *Psychological Bulletin, 133*(1), 1–24.

Bar-Haim, Y., Morag, I., & Glickman, S. (2011). Training anxious children to disengage attention from threat: A randomized controlled trial. *Journal of Child Psychology and Psychiatry, 52*(8), 861–869.

Barlow, D. H. (2002). *Anxiety and its disorders: The nature and treatment of anxiety and panic* (2nd ed.). New York: Guilford Press.

Beard, C. (2011). Cognitive bias modification for anxiety: Current evidence and future directions. *Expert Review of Neurotherapeutics, 11*(2), 299–311.

Beard, C., & Amir, N. (2008). A multi-session interpretation modification program: Changes in interpretation and social anxiety symptoms. *Behaviour Research and Therapy, 46*(10), 1135–1141.

Beard, C., Weisberg, R. B., & Amir, N. (2011). Combined cognitive bias modification treatment for social anxiety disorder: A pilot trial. *Depression and Anxiety, 28*, 981–988.

Beard, C., Weisberg, R. B., Perry, A., Schofield, C., & Amir, N. (2010, June). Feasibility and acceptability of CBM in primary care settings. In C. Beard (Chair), *Cognitive bias modification in anxiety: Targeting multiple disorders, biases, and settings* Symposium presented at the World Congress of Behavioral and Cognitive Therapy, Boston, MA.

Beck, A. T., & Clark, D. A. (1997). An information processing model of anxiety: Automatic and strategic processes. *Behaviour Research and Therapy, 35*(1), 49–58.

Beck, A. T., & Steer, R. A. (1993). *Beck Depression Inventory: Manual*. San Antonio, TX: Psychological Corporation.

Birmaher, B., Brent, D. A., Chiappetta, L., Bridge, J., Monga, S., & Baugher, M. (1999). Psychometric properties of the Screen for Child Anxiety Related Emotional Disorders (SCARED): A replication study. *Journal of the American Academy of Child and Adolescent Psychiatry, 38*(10), 1230–1236.

Blackwell, S. E., & Holmes, E. A. (2010). Modifying interpretation and imagination in clinical depression: A single case series using cognitive bias modification. *Applied Cognitive Psychology, 24*(3), 338–350.

Blaxton, T. A. (1989). Investigating dissociations among memory measures: Support for a transfer-appropriate processing framework. *Journal of Experimental Psychology: Learning, Memory, and Cognition, 15*(4), 657–668.

Brosan, L., Hoppitt, L., Shelfer, L., Sillence, A., & Mackintosh, B. (2011). Cognitive bias modification for attention and interpretation reduces trait and state anxiety in anxious patients referred to an out-patient service: Results from a pilot study. *Journal of Behavior Therapy and Experimental Psychiatry, 42*(3), 258–264.

Browning, M., Holmes, E. A., Murphy, S. E., Goodwin, G. M., & Harmer, C. J. (2010). Lateral prefrontal cortex mediates cognitive modification of attentional bias. *Biological Psychiatry, 67*(10), 919–925.

Cepeda, N. J., Pashler, H., Vul, E., Wixted, J. T., & Rohrer, D. (2006). Distributed practice in verbal recall tasks: A review and quantitative synthesis. *Psychological Bulletin, 132*(3), 354–380.

Dandeneau, S. D., & Baldwin, M. W. (2004). The inhibition of socially rejecting information among people with high versus low self-esteem: The role of attentional bias and the effects of bias reduction training. *Journal of Social and Clinical Psychology, 23*(4), 584–602.

Dandeneau, S. D., & Baldwin, M. W. (2009). The buffering effects of rejection-inhibiting attentional training on social and performance threat among adult students. *Contemporary Educational Psychology, 34*(1), 42–50.

Dandeneau, S. D., Baldwin, M. W., Baccus, J. R., Sakellaropoulo, M., & Pruessner, J. C. (2007). Cutting stress off at the pass: Reducing vigilance and responsiveness to social threat by manipulating attention. *Journal of Personality and Social Psychology, 93*(4), 651–666.

Eldar, S., & Bar-Haim, Y. (2010). Neural plasticity in response to attention training in anxiety. *Psychological Medicine, 40*(4), 667–677.

Eldar, S., Ricon, T., & Bar-Haim, Y. (2008). Plasticity in attention: Implications for stress response in children. *Behaviour Research and Therapy, 46*(4), 450–461.

Eysenck, M. W., Derakshan, N., Santos, R., & Calvo, M. G. (2007). Anxiety and cognitive performance: Attentional control theory. *Emotion, 7*(2), 336–353.

Grey, S., & Mathews, A. (2000). Effects of training on interpretation of emotional ambiguity. *Quarterly Journal of Experimental Psychology A: Human Experimental Psychology, 53A*(4), 1143–1162.

Hackmann, A., & Holmes, E. A. (2004). Reflecting on imagery: A clinical perspective and overview of the special issue of memory on mental imagery and memory in psychopathology. *Memory, 12*(4), 389–402.

Hakamata, Y., Lissek, S., Bar-Haim, Y., Britton, J. C., Fox, N. A., Leibenluft, E., et al. (2010). Attention bias modification treatment: A meta-analysis toward the establishment of novel treatment for anxiety. *Biological Psychiatry, 68*(11), 982–990.

Hallion, L. S., & Ruscio, A. M. (2012). A meta-analysis of the effect of cognitive bias modification on anxiety and depression. *Psychological Bulletin, 137*(6), 940–958.

Hayes, S., Hirsch, C. R., Krebs, G., & Mathews, A. (2010). The effects of modifying interpretation bias on worry in generalized anxiety disorder. *Behaviour Research and Therapy, 48*(3), 171–178.

Hayes, S., Hirsch, C. R., & Mathews, A. (2010). Facilitating a benign attentional bias reduces negative thought intrusions. *Journal of Abnormal Psychology, 119*(1), 235–240.

Hazen, R. A., Vasey, M. W., & Schmidt, N. B. (2009). Attentional retraining: A randomized clinical trial for pathological worry. *Journal of Psychiatric Research, 43*(6), 627–633.

Hertel, P. T., & Mathews, A. (2011). Cognitive bias modification: Past perspectives, current findings, and future applications. *Perspectives on Psychological Science, 6*(6), 521–536.

Hirsch, C. R., Hayes, S., & Mathews, A. (2009). Looking on the bright side: Accessing benign meanings reduces worry. *Journal of Abnormal Psychology, 118*(1), 44–54.

Hirsch, C. R., & Mathews, A. (1997). Interpretive inferences when reading about emotional events. *Behaviour Research and Therapy, 35*(12), 1123–1132.

Hirsch, C. R., Mathews, A., & Clark, D. M. (2007). Inducing an interpretation bias changes self-imagery: A preliminary investigation. *Behaviour Research and Therapy, 45*(9), 2173–2181.

Holmes, E. A., Lang, T. J., & Shah, D. M. (2009). Developing interpretation bias modification as a "cognitive vaccine" for depressed mood: Imagining positive events makes you feel better than thinking about them verbally. *Journal of Abnormal Psychology, 118*(1), 76–88.

Holmes, E. A., & Mathews, A. (2005). Mental imagery and emotion: A special relationship? *Emotion, 5*(4), 489–497.

Holmes, E. A., Mathews, A., Dalgleish, T., & Mackintosh, B. (2006). Positive interpretation training: Effects of mental imagery versus verbal training on positive mood. *Behavior Therapy, 37*(3), 237–247.

Hoppitt, L., Mathews, A., Yiend, J., & Mackintosh, B. (2010). Cognitive mechanisms underlying the emotional effects of bias modification. *Applied Cognitive Psychology, 24*(3), 312–325.

Joormann, J., Hertel, P. T., Brozovich, F., & Gotlib, I. H. (2005). Remembering the good, forgetting the bad: Intentional forgetting of emotional material in depression. *Journal of Abnormal Psychology, 114*(4), 640–648.

Joormann, J., Hertel, P. T., LeMoult, J., & Gotlib, I. H. (2009). Training forgetting of negative material in depression. *Journal of Abnormal Psychology, 118*(1), 34–43.

Kandris, E., & Moulds, M. L. (2008). Can imaginal exposure reduce intrusive memories in depression?: A case study. *Cognitive Behaviour Therapy, 37*(4), 216–220.

Koster, E. H. W., Fox, E., & MacLeod, C. (2009). Introduction to the special section on cognitive bias modification in emotional disorders. *Journal of Abnormal Psychology, 118*(1), 1–4.

Krebs, G., Hirsch, C. R., & Mathews, A. (2010). The effect of attention modification with explicit vs. minimal instructions on worry. *Behaviour Research and Therapy, 48*(3), 251–256.

la Greca, A. M., & Stone, W. L. (1993). Social Anxiety Scale for Children—Revised: Factor structure and concurrent validity. *Journal of Clinical Child Psychology, 22*(1), 17–27.

Lang, T. J., Moulds, M. L., & Holmes, E. A. (2009). Reducing depressive intrusions via a computerized cognitive bias modification of appraisals task: Developing a cognitive vaccine. *Behaviour Research and Therapy, 47*(2), 139–145.

Li, S., Tan, J., Qian, M., & Liu, X. (2008). Continual training of attentional bias in social anxiety. *Behaviour Research and Therapy, 46*(8), 905–912.

Lothmann, C., Holmes, E. A., Chan, S. W., & Lau, J. Y. (2011). Cognitive bias modification training in adolescents: Effects on interpretation biases and mood. *Journal of Child Psychology and Psychiatry, 52*(1), 24–32.

Mackintosh, B., Mathews, A., Yiend, J., Ridgeway, V., & Cook, E. (2006). Induced biases in emotional interpretation influence stress vulnerability and endure despite changes in context. *Behavior Therapy, 37*(3), 209–222.

MacLeod, C. (2012). Cognitive bias modification (CBM) procedures in the management of mental disorders. *Current Opinion in Psychiatry, 25*(2), 114–120.

MacLeod, C., Koster, E. H., & Fox, E. (2009). Whither cognitive bias modification research?: Commentary on the special section articles. *Journal of Abnormal Psychology, 118*(1), 89–99.

MacLeod, C., Mackintosh, B., & Vujic, T. (2009, May). *Does explicit communication of the training contingency enhance the efficacy of CBM.* Expert Meeting on Cognitive Bias Modification Techniques, Ghent, Belgium.

MacLeod, C., & Mathews, A. (2012). Cognitive bias modification approaches to anxiety. *Annual Review of Clinical Psychology, 8*, 189–217.

MacLeod, C., Mathews, A., & Tata, P. (1986). Attentional bias in emotional disorders. *Journal of Abnormal Psychology, 95*(1), 15–20.

MacLeod, C., Rutherford, E., Campbell, L., Ebsworthy, G., & Holker, L. (2002). Selective attention and emotional vulnerability: Assessing the causal basis of their association through the experimental manipulation of attentional bias. *Journal of Abnormal Psychology, 111*(1), 107–123.

Mathews, A. (2012). Effects of modifying the interpretation of emotional ambiguity. *Journal of Cognitive Psychology, 24*(1), 92–105.

Mathews, A., & Mackintosh, B. (2000). Induced emotional interpretation bias and anxiety. *Journal of Abnormal Psychology, 109*(4), 602–615.

Mathews, A., Ridgeway, V., Cook, E., & Yiend, J. (2007). Inducing a benign interpretational bias reduces trait anxiety. *Journal of Behavior Therapy and Experimental Psychiatry, 38*(2), 225–236.

Meyer, T., Miller, M., Metzger, R., & Borkovec, T. D. (1990). Development and validation of the Penn State Worry Questionnaire. *Behaviour Research and Therapy, 28*(6), 487–495.

Muris, P., Huijding, J., Mayer, B., & Hameetman, M. (2008). A space odyssey: Experimental manipulation of threat perception and anxiety-related interpretation bias in children. *Child Psychiatry and Human Development, 39*(4), 469–480.

Murphy, R., Hirsch, C. R., Mathews, A., Smith, K., & Clark, D. M. (2007). Facilitating a benign interpretation bias in a high socially anxious population. *Behaviour Research and Therapy, 45*(7), 1517–1529.

Najmi, S., & Amir, N. (2010). The effect of attention training on a behavioral test of contamination fears in individuals with subclinical obsessive–compulsive symptoms. *Journal of Abnormal Psychology, 119*(1), 136–142.

Peters, K. D., Constans, J. I., & Mathews, A. (2011). Experimental modification of attribution processes. *Journal of Abnormal Psychology, 120*(1), 168–173.

Power, M., & Dalgleish, T. (2008). *Cognition and emotion: From order to disorder* (2nd ed.). New York: Psychology Press.

Reiss, S., Peterson, R. A., Gursky, D. M., & McNally, R. J. (1986). Anxiety sensitivity, anxiety frequency and the predictions of fearfulness. *Behaviour Research and Therapy, 24*(1), 1–8.

Richards, A., & French, C. C. (1992). An anxiety-related bias in semantic activation when processing threat/neutral homographs. *Quarterly Journal of Experimental Psychology A, 45A*(3), 503–525.

Rinck, M., Becker, E. S., Kellermann, J., & Roth, W. T. (2003). Selective attention in anxiety: Distraction and enhancement in visual search. *Depression and Anxiety, 18*(1), 18–28.

Rozenman, M., Weersing, V., & Amir, N. (2011). A case series of attention modification in clinically anxious youths. *Behaviour Research and Therapy, 49*(5), 324–330.

Rutherford, E. M., MacLeod, C., & Campbell, L. W. (2004). Negative selectivity effects and emotional selectivity effects in anxiety: Differential attentional correlates of state and trait variables. *Cognition and Emotion, 18*(5), 711–720.

Salemink, E., van den Hout, M., & Kindt, M. (2007). Trained interpretive bias and anxiety. *Behaviour Research and Therapy, 45*(2), 329–340.

Salemink, E., van den Hout, M., & Kindt, M. (2009). Effects of positive interpretive bias modification in highly anxious individuals. *Journal of Anxiety Disorders, 23*(5), 676–683.

Schartau, P. E., Dalgleish, T., & Dunn, B. D. (2009). Seeing the bigger picture: Training in perspective broadening reduces self-reported affect and psychophysiological response to distressing films and autobiographical memories. *Journal of Abnormal Psychology, 118*(1), 15–27.

Schmidt, N. B., Richey, J., Buckner, J. D., & Timpano, K. R. (2009). Attention training for generalized social anxiety disorder. *Journal of Abnormal Psychology, 118*(1), 5–14.

See, J., MacLeod, C., & Bridle, R. (2009). The reduction of anxiety vulnerability through the modification of attentional bias: A real-world study using a home-based cognitive bias modification procedure. *Journal of Abnormal Psychology, 118*(1), 65–75.

Standage, H., Ashwin, C., & Fox, E. (2010). Is manipulation of mood a critical component of cognitive bias modification procedures? *Behaviour Research and Therapy, 48*(1), 4–10.

Steinman, S. A., & Teachman, B. A. (2010). Modifying interpretations among individuals high in anxiety sensitivity. *Journal of Anxiety Disorders, 24*(1), 71–78.

Tran, T. B., Hertel, P. T., & Joormann, J. (2011). Cognitive bias modification: Induced interpretive biases affect memory. *Emotion, 11*(1), 145–152.

Turner, S. M., Beidel, D. C., Dancu, C. V., & Stanley, M. A. (1989). An empirically derived inventory to measure social fears and anxiety: The Social Phobia and Anxiety Inventory. *Psychological Assessment, 1*, 35–40.

Vassilopoulos, S. P., Banerjee, R., & Prantzalou, C. (2009). Experimental modification of interpretation bias in socially anxious children: Changes in interpretation, anticipated interpersonal anxiety, and social anxiety symptoms. *Behaviour Research and Therapy, 47*(12), 1085–1089.

Watkins, E. R., Baeyens, C. B., & Read, R. (2009). Concreteness training reduces dysphoria: Proof-of-principle for repeated cognitive bias modification in depression. *Journal of Abnormal Psychology, 118*(1), 55–64.

Watkins, E. R., Taylor, R. S., Byng, R., Baeyens, C., Read, R., Pearson, K., et al. (2012). Guided self-help concreteness training as an intervention for major depression in primary care: A Phase II randomized controlled trial. *Psychological Medicine, 42*(7), 1359–1371.

Wegner, D. M., Schneider, D. J., Carter, S. R., & White, T. L. (1987). Paradoxical effects of thought suppression. *Journal of Personality and Social Psychology, 53*(1), 5–13.

Wells, T. T., & Beevers, C. G. (2010). Biased attention and dysphoria: Manipulating selective attention reduces subsequent depressive symptoms. *Cognition and Emotion, 24*(4), 719–728.

Wenzel, A. (2006). Attentional disruption in the presence of negative automatic thoughts. *Behavioral and Cognitive Psychotherapy, 34*(4), 385–395.

Wenzlaff, R. M., & Wegner, D. M. (2000). Thought suppression. *Annual Review of Psychology, 51*, 59–91.

White, L. K., Suway, J. G., Pine, D. S., Bar-Haim, Y., & Fox, N. A. (2011). Cascading effects: The influence of attention bias to threat on the interpretation of ambiguous information. *Behaviour Research and Therapy, 49*(4), 244–251.

Williams, J. M. G., Watts, F. N., MacLeod, C., & Mathews, A. (Eds.). (1997). *Cognitive psychology and emotional disorders* (2nd ed.). Chichester, UK: Wiley.

Wilson, E. J., MacLeod, C., Mathews, A., & Rutherford, E. M. (2006). The causal role of interpretive bias in anxiety reactivity. *Journal of Abnormal Psychology, 115*(1), 103–111.

Yiend, J., Mackintosh, B., & Mathews, A. (2005). Enduring consequences of experimentally induced biases in interpretation. *Behaviour Research and Therapy, 43*(6), 779–797.

Author Index

Subject Index

Page numbers followed by *f* indicate figure; *t* indicate table